Myocardial Preservation

Dennis V. Cokkinos
Editor

Myocardial Preservation

Translational Research and Clinical Application

Springer

Editor
Dennis V. Cokkinos
Heart and Vessel Department
Biomedical Research Foundation
of the Academy of Athens - Gregory Skalkeas
Athens
Greece

ISBN 978-3-319-98185-7 ISBN 978-3-319-98186-4 (eBook)
https://doi.org/10.1007/978-3-319-98186-4

Library of Congress Control Number: 2018965610

This Springer imprint is published by the registered company Springer Nature Switzerland AG
The registered company address is: Gewerbestrasse 11, 6330 Cham, Switzerland

Dedicated to the Memory of
Professor-Academician
Gregory D. Skalkeas
Man of Unequalled Vision
and Unsurpassed Achievement

Foreword

The idea for this book came from the realization, over many years, that the main and determining factor of cardiovascular morbidity and mortality is loss of myocardium. The cardiac muscle, the prime engine of our body, is at a constant danger: before and just after birth from genetically transmitted disease and cardiac defects and at childhood and adolescence from rheumatic fever in developing countries; nonfamilial cardiomyopathy can manifest itself at any time; myocarditis may fell its victim at any age.

Hypertension and valve disease nowadays are not left to progress to myocardial loss; however, at the onset of middle age, coronary heart disease begins to take its toll. An initial or recurrent myocardial ischemic insult or infarct sets the stage for cardiac remodeling and its sequelae, heart failure, and death. In old age together with experience and arguable wisdom comes "presbycardia." Thus, the toil toward cardiac protection is constant and persists throughout a person's lifetime. "Myocardial preservation" is an all-inclusive term, since it encompasses all forms of conditioning, pharmacological therapy, revascularization, both interventional and surgical, and device therapy. Moreover, it entails efforts at preserving cardiac structure and function after initial protective mechanisms have been overwhelmed and cardiac integrity has been compromised. Another important feature to be appreciated is that cardiomyocyte loss from any initial cause eventually follows common pathways and that cardiorestorative efforts are based on similar and parallel mechanisms.

Having complemented my clinical duties with efforts at research with cardiopreservation as its main goal, I felt tempted to write a book with a common unifying thread and concept.

Mr. Grant Weston, who helped me with my previous Springer book *Introduction to Cardiovascular Translational Research*, encouraged me from the start.

It proved a heavy responsibility. Soon I realized that in some subjects I had to enlist the aid of two expert colleagues: Professor Dimitris Tousoulis and Doctor Konstantinos Malliaras and their co-workers. Their efforts have produced excellent fruits. I am deeply indebted to their friendship and help.

The completion of this book on the very tight limits set to me would have been impossible without the expert, extremely efficacious, and friendly secretarial aid of Ms. Athinais Danou.

During the last 52 years, my every effort has been supported through the tolerance afforded to me by my wife Vana who provides me the inspiration for all my undertakings. As an eminent physician herself, she has lent me her criticism and suggestions.

The book was conceived and completed in the friendly and warm academic environment of the Biomedical Research Foundation of the Academy of Athens.

Constant interchange of ideas with my peers, colleagues and young collaborators, has been an invigorating breath of fresh ideas. A continuing collaboration with my former hospital, the Onassis Cardiac Surgery Center, has been fortunate and complementary and has helped advance the collaboration between these two outstanding institutions.

The man who conceived, created, and directed the Biomedical Research Foundation of the Academy of Athens, a giant of our times, a man of unlimited vision and inspired leadership, was Professor-Academician Gregory D. Skalkeas. He encouraged me wholeheartedly to undertake this endeavor. He had been my mentor for more than half a century. I dedicate this book to his memory with respect, admiration, and deep gratitude.

Athens, Greece Dennis V. Cokkinos

Contents

1 **Introduction** 1
Dennis V. Cokkinos

2 **Research: Clinical, Basic, and Translational** 9
Dennis V. Cokkinos

3 **Clinical Research and Evidence-Based Medicine** 37
Dennis V. Cokkinos

4 **The Systems Biology Approach** 53
Dennis V. Cokkinos

5 **Cardiac Hypertrophy** 63
Dennis V. Cokkinos

6 **The Ishemia Reperfusion Injury Challenge** 87
Dennis V. Cokkinos

7 **Cell Death: Many Causes and Many Effects** 105
Dennis V. Cokkinos

8 **Healing of Myocardial Infarction** 151
Nikolaos Papageorgiou and Dimitris Tousoulis

9 **Myocardial Stunning** 171
Dennis V. Cokkinos

10 **Myocardial Hibernation** 185
Dennis V. Cokkinos

11 **The Fetal Phenotype** 203
Dennis V. Cokkinos

12 **Cardiac Remodeling: The Course Toward Heart Failure – I. General Concepts** 215
Dennis V. Cokkinos

13 **Cardiac Remodeling: The Course Towards Heart Failure-II. Diagnostic and Therapeutic Approaches** 247
Dennis V. Cokkinos

14 **Conditioning of the Myocardium** 281
Dennis V. Cokkinos

15 **Fibrosis–Inflammation of the Cardiovascular System** 321
Evangelos Oikonomou and Dimitris Tousoulis

16 **Endogenous Regeneration of the Mammalian Heart** 339
Konstantinos Malliaras

17 **Cell Therapy for Heart Disease: Ready for Prime Time or Lost in Translation?** 355
Konstantinos Malliaras and Dennis V. Cokkinos

18 **Gene Therapy in Cardiac Disease** 377
Styliani Vakrou and Konstantinos Malliaras

Index 393

Chapter 1
Introduction

Dennis V. Cokkinos

The great German poet Johann Wolfgang von Goethe had anatomical knowledge. He discovered the intermaxillary bone or Goethe's Bone in 1784 [1]. In his masterpiece "Faust" he wrote that "Blut ist ein ganz besonderer Saft" which can be translated that "blood is a totally particular humour" or "fluid" in contemporary expression [2].

The author of this book, admitting to being biased as a cardiologist by specialty, can claim that the same holds true for the heart. The heart is one of the single organs of the body, thus it cannot be relieved by a partner at moments of dysfunction, nor can it be removed without the subject's unavoidable immediate demise. It does not rule motionless and supreme, as the brain does, but it must toil incessantly during the 80plus years of the medium life duration of the contemporary human. It is an old pastime to calculate how many times the heart must go into diastole, stasis and systole during a lifetime.

It would be commonplace but true to say that the heart caters to all the organs of the body by sending the "exceptional humour", blood, faithfully to them.

However, this irreplaceable organ is constantly threatened and imperiled during its existence.

A child can be blessed to come to life but burdened by a heart defect which may render its "in utero" or at newborn age correction a necessity.

After birth, rheumatic fever was formerly a world epidemic. I remember as a medical intern honing my skills in auscultation in the Cardiology wards of the "Evangelismos Hospital" in Athens; more than 70% of the patients had mitral or aortic valve disease, a dire legacy of rheumatic fever; the tricuspid at that time, before the advent of echocardiography, was less appreciated. Rheumatic fever may

D. V. Cokkinos (✉)
Heart and Vessel Department, Biomedical Research Foundation,
Academy of Athens - Gregory Skalkeas, Athens, Greece
e-mail: dcokkinos@bioacademy.gr

D. V. Cokkinos (ed.), *Myocardial Preservation*,
https://doi.org/10.1007/978-3-319-98186-4_1

have been eradicated in Western societies, but together with famine various and illnesses threatens young lives all over the developing world countries [3].

Although most of the congenital heart defects can be corrected with little danger and low mortality, cardiomyopathies, the Long QT syndrome and the Brugada syndrome and other rhythm disorders can cut the thread of a young sportive life.

In a recent prospective study, in 5255 middle-school (13 years old) children [4] screened with ECG and cardiac magnetic resonance, the following high-risk conditions were found: Long QT Interval (0.69%, QTc > 0.470 s) anomalous origin of a coronary artery from the opposite sinus (0.44%), dilated cardiomyopathy (0.23%) hypertrophic cardiomyopathy (0.06%), Brugada pattern (0.02%).Apart from dilated cardiomyopathy, in which some forms could be ameliorated as regards their course, if representing the evolution of acute myocarditis, all the others could be protected with early antiarrhythmic prevention.

Although these percentages are low from the statistical viewpoint, they represent a total loss for the young victims' parents.

Some more data in mortality of young people should be given.

In persons 1- 35 years old studied in North Spain, the incidence of sudden unexplained death (SUD) was 0.43/100.000 persons per year, a total of 107. Of these 19 were due to atheromatous coronary disease, 13 to cardiomyopathies, 6 to the abnormalities of the cardiac conduction system; 19 were thought to be due to sudden unexpected death (SUD) [5].

In the 25 year-review of autopsies in 6.3 million military recruits, aged 18-35 years, sudden non traumatic death occurred at a rate of 13.0 per100.000 recruit years [6, 7]. Of these 126 autopsied deaths, over half had an identifiable cardiac abnormality. One-third had an anomalous coronary artery. Importantly, more than one-third of deaths had no explanation.

Here an important diagnostic improvement has occurred. Additionally to the classic autopsy the molecular autopsy is attaining importance in SUD. This technique gives a diagnosis in nearly 30% causes of SUD and 10% in the sudden infant death syndrome. Long QT syndrome, channelopathies and catecholaminergic polymorphic ventricular tachycardia are the most important findings. It can save future lives in family members of victims of SUD [8–13].

However, it does not only concern arrhythmic deaths: It was employed in 17 aortic dissection sudden cardiac death cases [14].

At the young adult life, atherosclerotic cardiovascular disease raises its ugly head.

In autopsy studies in soldiers killed in the Korea war up to 25% [15] and in young male accident victims 20% [16] were found to have severe atherosclerotic heart disease.

Again, the efforts of Public Health experts, nutritionists but also clinicians and lay people with vision have appreciably lowered the incidence of atherosclerotic cardiovascular disease in modern societies. However, with the expected adoption of the "western" type of diet, this epidemic is predicted to replace as a threat malnutrition and infections in the developing world according to the prevalent contemporary statistics. In fact, in China, mortality from ischemic heart disease has risen from

2004 to 2010, mostly in rural males (19.2%/yr) and females (7.0%/yr) and in the age group over 80 years [17].

In a 2010 study of the global burden of disease [3] the following 20-year differences from 1990 where found:

In both 1990 and 2010 ischemic heart disease and stroke were the first two causes of mortality.

Lower respiratory infections and COPD reversed their status as third and fourth respectively.

Lung cancer (5th) and HIV/AIDS (6th) in 2010 replaced diarrhea which now ranks 7th, followed by road injuries (8th), diabetes (9th), and tuberculosis (10th). Interestingly, diabetes ranked only 15th in 1990; with diabetes, cardiovascular disease, especially myocardial infarct prevalence and mortality, heart failure and stroke are affected.

A 2015 update from the same group [18] showed that globally, life expectancy increased from 61.7 years in 1922 to 71.8 years in 2015. However, many geographical differences were seen.

According to the WHO media center fact sheet, updated in January 2017 [18], in 2015, of the 56.4 million deaths worldwide, more than half (54%) of deaths were due to the top 10 causes. Ischemic heart disease and stroke are the world's biggest killers, accounting for a combined 15 million deaths in 2015.

Chronic obstructive pulmonary disease claimed 3.2 million lives in 2015, while lung cancer (along with trachea and bronchus cancers) caused 1.7 million deaths. Diabetes killed 1.6 million people in 2015, up from less than one million in 2000. Deaths due to dementia more than doubled between 2000 and 2015, making it the seventh leading cause of global deaths in 2015.

Lower respiratory infections remained the most deadly communicable disease, causing 3.2 million deaths worldwide in 2015. The death rate from diarrhea diseases almost halved between 2000 and 2015, but still caused 1.4 million deaths in 2015. Similarly, tuberculosis killed fewer people during the same period, but is still among the top 10 causes with a death toll of 1.4 million. HIV/AIDS is no longer among the world's top 10 causes of death, having killed 1.1 million people in 2015 compared to 1.5 million in 2000.

Thus, 10 leading causes of death in 2015 were, in rank order [19].

Ischemic heart disease, stroke, lower respiratory infections, chronic obstructive pulmonary lung disease, trachea, bronchus lung cancers, diabetes mellitus, Alzheimer's disease and other dementias, diarrheal disease, tuberculosis, road injuries.

Heron et al. [20] give a slightly different picture for the 10 leading causes of death in the USA in 2014, as classified by ICD-10.

The 10 leading causes of death in 2014 were, in rank order: Diseases of heart; malignant neoplasms; chronic lower respiratory diseases, accidents (unintentional injuries); cerebrovascular diseases; Alzheimer's disease; diabetes mellitus; influenza and pneumonia; nephritis, nephrotic syndrome and nephrosis; and intentional self-harm (suicide). They accounted for 74% of all deaths occurring in the United States.

Here a word of caution is warranted. In 2015, life expectancy of Americans dipped slightly as compared to the previous year, according to data from the Center for Disease Control and Prevention National Center for Health statistics. For males, life expectancy at birth changed from 76.5 years in 2014 to 76.3 years in 2015, a decrease of 0.2 year, and for females, it decreased 0.1 year from 81.3 years in 2014 to 81.2 in 2015.

Infant mortality did not change [21].

If a person reaches old age with either a completely unblemished or even repaired or convalescing heart, presbycardia is the reward of his or her persistence. Atrial fibrillation, conduction defects, aortic stenosis, beleaguer the strife for survival in the last remaining years.

During the onslaught of all these foes to its integrity, the heart can be maimed or totally destroyed.

Thus, its protection becomes of paramount importance. This protection needs to be constantly applied throughout all these phases, thus it becomes a lifelong effort. It entails and includes prevention against cardiovascular risk factors, protection against myocardial loss during an acute myocardial infarction, protection during cardiac intervention or surgery, in the post-operative period, detection and prevention of a life-threatening arrhythmia, and monitoring of cardiac function during anti-neoplastic therapy which also can damage the heart.

I believe that this incessant strife overreaches the term "cardioprotection" and can be better expressed by the term "myocardial preservation". This term formerly was employed to denote protection of the heart during cardiac surgery. However surgery is declining in favor of interventional techniques, in which "preservation" is not so important due to their short duration and absence of imposed cardiac arrest and restart. However, in the rapidly exploding approach of the TAVR technique, an increase of troponins is routinely found [22, 23] and has prognostic significance. Thus, I believe that the term "myocardial preservation" should rightly attain the wider significance that it deserves, and should render us more aware of its constant importance. I first employed this term in a symposium in Sept. 2009.

In this book I tried to combine basic and clinical knowledge; in fact it is a book with translational approach. This term is overemployed in recent years since its inception in the early 1990's but still remains a sound perception.

The many aspects of myocardial preservation arise in everyday life. Consider a patient with severe coronary artery disease. If he has a chronic decrease of coronary flow reserve he may develop myocardial hibernation with cardiac dysfunction. The discerning clinician will guide him to the appropriate tests and to eventual revascularization.

Our patient may instead develop prodromal angina [24]. Under the right circumstances his myocardium may become preconditioned [25], diminishing the size of an infarction which may occur during the early (1 h) or late phase (24–48 h) protection zone. This protection may diminish the infarct size. Whether this occurs or not, reperfusion will have be carried out in a contemporary medical system. His attending physician and the one performing primary angioplasty is not sure if any drug will be used to it to administer while the patient is "en route" in the ambulance or from "door to needle". Should he benefit from the application of remote preconditioning? After the artery is opened should he undergo local or remote postconditioning? Should he be given cyclosporine in anticipation of more multicenter trials [25–27]? What if he develops ischemia reperfusion injury related no reflow? Will the interventionist trust his level C "expert" experience and give IC Verapamil [28]? If the patient comes to the CCU alive but with a large infarct by ECG and routine echocardiograpy what are the next steps? Shall contrast echocardiography or MRI be used to predict the inexorable road to remodeling? What drugs apart from the "big 4" (beta-blockers, angiotensin converting enzyme inhibitors or angiotensin receptor blockers, aldosterone inhibitors, statins) should be used, from one from more than 20 reported in recent reviews to choose from [29]. Should he receive IC stem cells? Should stem cells be repeated? For how many times if the findings of Bolli's group [30] are verified? Should gene therapy be tried despite the findings of CUPID-2, which showed no benefit with SERCA-2 viral delivery [31]?

If an LBBB is found, should resynchronization be applied? If cardiac dysfunction persists when should LVAD be placed? If it is successful should a donor heart be hoped for or could the heart be expected to be successfully weaned, or should it be left as destination therapy?

One can understand that these are difficult and costly questions. The attending physician cannot rest complacently just offering tender loving care and sympathy but seek and consult all new developments. These are the result of painstaking work by many collaborating centers at sometimes exorbitant cost. This "places the monkey" not only on the shoulder of the clinician but also on that of laboratory researchers.

My hope is that this book will be useful to basic researchers orienting them to the practical/clinical utility of their toil at the bench, and to practicing cardiologists alerting them to the possibility that during the frightful moments of opening an artery in a dying heart they could spare some thought and effort to try a new promising technique of cardiopreservation invented by their "alchemist" peers on the sacrificed laboratory animal or in the "dry lab". Of course, such an intermediating effort may leave both sides dissatisfied, but this is a peril which other authors have faced successfully.

I hope to emulate them.

References

1. Wells GA. Goethe and the inter maxillary bone. Br J Hist Sci. 1967;3:348–61.
2. Johann Wolfgang von Goethe Faust I (Studierzimmer II).
3. Lozano R, Naghavi M, Foreman K, Lim S, Shibuya K, Aboyans V, et al. Global and regional mortality from 235 causes of death for 20 age groups in 1990 and 2010: a systematic analysis for the global burden of disease study 2010. Lancet. 2012;380:2095–128.
4. Angelini P, Uribe C, Masso A, et al. Results of MRI-based screening study of 5130 candidates for sports participation. Am Coll Cardiol. 2017 Scientific Sessions:401–10.

5. Morentin B, Suárez-Mier MP, Aguilera B. Sudden unexplained death among persons 1-35 years old. Forensic Sci Int. 2003;135:213–7.
6. Eckart RE, Scoville SL, Campbell CL, Shry EA, Stajduhar KC, Potter RN, et al. Sudden death in young adults: a 25-year review of autopsies in military. Ann Intern Med. 2004;141:829–34.
7. Balady GJ. Sudden cardiac death in young military recruits: guarding the heart of a soldier. Ann Intern Med. 2004;141:882–4.
8. Tester DJ, Ackerman MJ. The role of molecular autopsy in unexplained sudden cardiac death. Curr Opin Cardiol. 2006;21:166–72.
9. Ackerman MJ. State of postmortem genetic testing known as the cardiac channel molecular autopsy in the forensic evaluation of unexplained sudden cardiac death in the young. Pacing Clin Electrophysiol. 2009;32(Suppl 2):S86–9.
10. Torkamani A, Muse E, Spencer E, Rueda M, Wagner GN, Lucas JR, et al. Molecular autopsy for sudden unexpected death. JAMA. 2016;316:1492–4.
11. Semsarian C, Ingles J. Molecular autopsy in victims of inherited arrhythmias. J Arrhythm. 2016;32:359–65.
12. Hellenthal N, Gaertner-Rommel A, Klauke B, Paluszkiewicz L, Stuhr M, Kerner T et al. Molecular autopsy of sudden unexplained deaths reveals genetic predispositions for cardiac diseases among young forensic cases. ESC 17 Oct 2016.
13. Stattin EL, Westin IM, Cederquist K, et al. Genetic screening in sudden cardiac death in the young can save future lives. Int J Legal Med. 2016;130:59–66.
14. Gago-Díaz M, Ramos-Luis E, Zoppis S, Zorio E, Molina P, Braza-Boïls A, et al. Postmortem genetic testing should be recommended in sudden cardiac death cases due to thoracic aortic dissection. Int J Legal Med. 2017;131:1211–9.
15. Enos WF, Holmes RH, Beyer J. Coronary disease among United States soldiers killed in action in Korea; preliminary report. J Am Med Assoc. 1953;152:1090–3.
16. McGill HC, McMahan CA, Zieske AW, et al. Association of Coronary Heart Disease Risk Factors with microscopic qualities of coronary atherosclerosis in youth. Circulation. 2000;102:374–9.
17. Zhang X, Khan AA, Haq EU, Rahim A, Hu D, Attia J, et al. Increasing mortality from ischaemic heart disease in China from 2004 to 2010: disproportionate rise in rural areas and elderly subjects. 438 million person-years follow-up. Eur Heart J Qual Care Clin Outcomes. 2017;3:47–52.
18. Global, regional, and national life expectancy, all-cause mortality, and cause-specific mortality for 249 causes of death, 1980–2015: a systematic analysis for the global burden of disease study 2015. Lancet. 2016;388:1459–544.
19. The top 10 causes of death. WHO Updated January 2017.
20. Heron M. Deaths: leading causes for 2014. Natl Vital Stat Rep. 2016;65:1–96.
21. National Center for Health Statistics (NCHS). US Life Expectancy Drops for First Time Since 1999. December 08, 2016.
22. Fassa AA, Himbert D, Vahanian A. Mechanisms and management of TAVR-related complications. Nat Rev Cardiol. 2013;10:685–95.
23. Paradis JM, Maniar HS, Lasala JM, Kodali S, Williams M, Lindman BR, et al. Clinical and functional outcomes associated with myocardial injury after transfemoral and transapical transcatheter aortic valve replacement: a subanalysis from the partner trial (placement of aortic transcatheter valves). JACC Cardiovasc Interv. 2015;8:1468–79.
24. Filippo O, Marcello G, Donatella F, Francesco S, Patrizia L, et al. Prodromal angina limits infarct size. A role for Ischemic Preconditioning. Circulation. 1995;91:291–7.
25. Iliodromitis E, Andreadou I, Dagres N, Kremastinos D. Pre- peri- post-conditioning the ischemic myocardium: challenges, confounders and expectations. In: Cokkinos DV, editor. Introduction to translational cardiovascular research. Cham: Springer; 2015. p. 541–52.
26. Cung T-T, Morel O, Cayla G, Rioufol G, Garcia-Dorado D, Angoulvant D, et al. Cyclosporine before PCI in patients with acute myocardial infarction. N Engl J Med. 2015;373:1021–31.

27. Ottani F, Latini R, Staszewsky L, La Vecchia L, Locuratolo N, Sicuro M, et al. Cyclosporine a in reperfused myocardial infarction: the multicenter, controlled, open-label CYCLE trial. J Am Coll Cardiol. 2016;67:365–74.
28. Werner GS, Lang K, Kuehnert H, Figulla HR. Intracoronary verapamil for reversal of no-reflow during coronary angioplasty for acute myocardial infarction. Catheter Cardiovasc Interv. 2002;57:444–51.
29. Cokkinos DV. Le remodelage cardiaque après un infarctus : nouvelles données sur la prévention et le traitement. Bull Acad Natle Med. 2015;199:1383–94.
30. Tokita Y, Tang XL, Li Q, Wysoczynski M, Hong KU, Nakamura S, et al. Repeated administrations of cardiac progenitor cells are markedly more effective than a single administration: a new paradigm in cell therapy. Circ Res. 2016;119:635–51.
31. Greenberg B, Butler J, Felker M, Ponikowski P, Voors A, Desai A, et al. Calcium upregulation by percutaneous administration of gene therapy in patients with cardiac disease (CUPID 2): a randomised, multinational, double-blind, placebo-controlled, phase 2b trial. N Engl J Med. 2016;387:1178–86.

Chapter 2
Research: Clinical, Basic, and Translational

Dennis V. Cokkinos

2.1 Definitions

The explosive increase of knowledge in particular in cardiovascular medicine is considered to be the key to prolongation of life seen in the area of "scientific" medicine; thus, it is recorded that after around 1740 AD, life expectancy increases by 1 year every 5 years [1]. Much of this increase is brought about by improvements in cardiovascular disease management [2] and has been achieved by research. In this setting the term translational research (TR) or translational medicine or science is being increasingly used. As van der Laan and Boenink [3] have pointed out 3 years ago, TR has gained importance because of the awareness that a gap exists between life sciences, which produce great amounts of new data in advanced fields on the molecular level, and clinical medicine, which cannot by definition produce great new knowledge, but is the one expected to gain more from progress in the other side of the gap, i.e., application to patients' diagnosis and therapy; in their Fig. 2.1, they show that from year 2000, the number of medical scientific publications has grown exponentially. This subject was already discussed in 2015 in my book on: "Introduction to Cardiovascular Research" [4, 5].

Before an attempt is made to define TR, one should first try to define research. According to the National Science Foundation [6]:

- Research is planned search or critical investigation aimed at discovery of new knowledge with the hope that such knowledge will be useful in developing a new product or service or a new process or technique or in bringing about a significant improvement to a planned product process.

In the *Oxford English Dictionary*, research is defined more simply as [7]: A search or investigation directed to the discovery of some fact by careful consideration

D. V. Cokkinos (✉)
Heart and Vessel Department, Biomedical Research Foundation,
Academy of Athens - Gregory Skalkeas, Athens, Greece
e-mail: dcokkinos@bioacademy.gr

D. V. Cokkinos (ed.), *Myocardial Preservation*,
https://doi.org/10.1007/978-3-319-98186-4_2

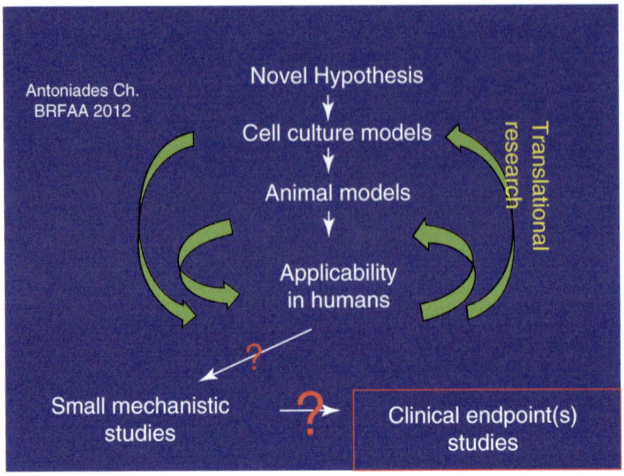

Fig. 2.1 Transferring knowledge from basic science to the clinical area [4]. (Reproduced with permission from Antoniades [4] and Cokkinos [5])

or study of a subject; a course of critical or scientific inquiry. Another definition is given by *Merriam Webster* [8].

Merriam Webster definition of research:

1. Careful or diligent search
2. Studious inquiry or examination; especially: investigation or experimentation aimed at the discovery and interpretation of facts, revision of accepted theories or laws in the light of new facts, or practical application of such new or revised theories or laws
3. The collecting of information about a particular subject

K. Popper in 1972 discussed the philosophy of research. According to him [9], research should follow five steps:

1. Seek a problem
2. Propose a solution
3. Formulate a testable hypothesis from that proposal
4. Attempt to refute the hypothesis by observations and experiments
5. Establish preference between competing theories

Here I would like to propose to young investigators embarking for the long journey of research that it is an intellectual and creative process equal to poetry, literature, music, and the arts. It creates new knowledge.

- Jan Illing [10] proposes the following practical considerations that apply when studying research: the area, the topic, and the general, specific, and data collection questions. She also points out that the important aspects of research are the aim, testing hypothesis, cause and effect, generalizability, adding to existing knowledge, and vigor, viability, and reliability.

Before trying to define TR, which in very plain words is the link between basic and clinical research, one should try to define its two components:

2.1.1 Basic Research

According to the National Science Foundation [6], basic research is performed without practical ends. It results in general knowledge and an understanding of nature and its laws. This general knowledge provides the means of answering a large number of important practical problems, though it may not give a complete specific answer to any one of them.

In other words it is research for the acquisition of knowledge. This would take us to the early Greek philosophers Thales and Empedocles, among others.

However, even those thinkers in the eve of knowledge acquisition must have had a problem in mind, i.e., some potential application toward improving the state of the world they were living in. The function of applied research (to be further defined) is to provide such complete answers [11].

Hecker and Birla [12] gave an excellent review on research only 10 years ago: basic research is the planned systemic approach of new knowledge or understanding toward general application. According to the same authors, applied research is the acquisition of knowledge or understanding to meet a specific recognized need.

Many of the early clinical and recording technique studies, i.e., of the pulse and the ECG, can in some way be considered basic, although undoubtedly Sir Thomas Lewis, Karel Frederik Wenckebach, and Willem Einthoven had therapeutic goals in mind.

Clinical research is much more widely applied. Again one can use the NIH Director's Panel definition [13, 14]. It is tantamount to:

- Patient-oriented research
- Epidemiologic and behavioral studies
- Health services research

According to the NIH National Cancer Institute [15], in clinical research, people, or data or samples of tissue from people, are studied to understand health and disease. Clinical research helps find new and better ways to detect, diagnose, treat, and prevent disease. Types of clinical research include clinical trials, which test new treatments for a disease, and natural history studies, which collect health information to understand how a disease develops and progresses over time.

In a very comprehensive textbook on *Clinical and Translational Science*, Seely and Grinspoon point out [16] that from clinical research are excluded in vitro studies utilizing human tissues that cannot be linked to living individuals. They add that according to the National Institutes of Health (NIH), under patient-oriented research can be included research conducted with human subjects or on material of human origin such as tissues, specimens, and cognitive phenomena for which an investigator (or colleague) directly interacts with human subjects.

Obviously, no definition can be correct or complete in a waterproof manner. Thus, if one investigates or just studies "mechanisms of human disease," without interacting with the patient as an individual, he could well claim to be carrying out basic research.

The US food and drug administration gives a description of different kinds of clinical research [17]:

Treatment, prevention, diagnostic, screening, quality of life, research, genetic studies, epidemiological studies, clinical trials

Clinical research is currently much more widely practiced than the other two types of research described. It is widely divided into retrospective and prospective. Obviously the latter is considered more worthwhile. However, when a clinical question arises, it is easier and faster to look back at already existing data than start acquiring new ones. Of course, only prospective trials can be randomized, and placebo-controlled, thus requiring ethics committee approval and informed consent. Our era has seen the triumph of the multicenter randomized placebo-controlled megatrials. Some concerns about them still exist. Thus Robert M. Califf [18], one of the most experienced clinical trial researchers, points out that less than 15% of major guidance recommendations are evidence-based. It should not be forgotten that since September 2004, it has been announced by the International Committee of Medical Journal Editors that registration of clinical trials is a prerequisite of publication.

Zarin et al. [19] in an update in 2011 reported characteristically that of result records publicly available, 20% reported more than 2 "primary outcomes", and 5% reported more than 5.

2.1.2 Translational Research

The term "translational research" (TR) or science was first used in the 1990 decade and referred to efforts devoted to the discovery of new antitumor genes [20].

It was soon extended to other disciplines and of course to cardiology [14]. Thus, Feldman et al. [21] described examples of drug development programs to provide clues as to potential anticancer drug cardiotoxicity.

Very soon the term "from bench to bedside" was introduced. Other names had been previously employed, i.e., preclinical research, research targeted to the disease [22].

One of the pioneers in the endeavor of establishing the identity of TR, Steven H. Woolf, gives these definitions [23]: Bench-to-bedside enterprise, harnessing basic science to produce new drugs, devices and treatment options for pts.

An Interface between basic science and clinical medicine.

Dische and Saunders [24] mention the definition given by Julie Denekamp: Translational research is the application of scientific method to address a health need.

Barry S. Coller [25] has very simply defined TR as:

- Successful implementation of a laboratory concept into a clinical protocol

He also proposes a revision of the older paradigm of the three-legged stool, in which research is one of the three legs, together with patient care and education, toward the newer paradigm in which research is the cushion that covers a four-legged stool – patient care, education, community service, and global health, being the four legs. He further points out that TR differs from scientific discovery in both its goals and processes. The latter pertain to adding to the store of human knowledge. The former spring from the motivation to improve human health, searching for the identification of discoveries that can fill this need.

Williams and Robertson [26] in the introduction to their excellent book *Clinical and Translational Science* state that TR originally was used to describe the translation of animal studies to humans but that more recently it has applied to a great variety of activities, from cell-based experiment results to whole organs and organisms to epidemiologic data and the delivery of health or health services. The information provided by translating epidemiology data ultimately affects the delivery of health services.

The same authors [27] add the population-based study dimension.

For the academic community, TR signifies the effort to close the gap between knowledge and practice, as well as the transfer of results of research studies to practice [28].

According to the TR Working Group of the National Cancer Institute (NCI), translational research transforms scientific discoveries arising from laboratory, clinical, or population studies into clinical application to reduce cancer incidence, morbidity, and mortality [29].

If one interprets the Institute of Medicine Clinical Research Roundtable [30, 31]:

- T1 (T for translation) is the transfer of new understanding of disease mechanisms gained in the laboratory into the development of new methods for diagnosis and therapy.
- T2 is the translation of results from clinical studies into everyday clinical practice and health decision-making. These authors, and Williams and Robertson, point out [27] that one more subgroup is commonly provided:
- T3 is the dissemination and implementation of research translation into practice/community/large populations.

According to Westfall et al. [32], T1 involves basic research.

T2 includes guideline development, meta-analyses, and systematic reviews, while T3 includes dissemination and implementation research. It is obvious that all these steps are essential if a fruitful transfer of research findings to improved public health is desired.

It is stressed that a continuum exists from basic science to clinical science; in essence, this constitutes the bench-to-bedside process (T1).

Next comes the implementation of findings, from the bedside to practice, i.e., to the general population, health care, and health services (T2 and T3).

Malliaras et al. [33] very opportunely correlate these three stages to phase I, II, and III trials.

Waldman and Terzic [34] maintain that six T steps can be differentiated:

- TO: targets, biomarkers, genes, pathways, mechanisms
- T1: first-in-human phase I–II trials, proof of concept
- T2: phase III trials, clinical efficiency, clinical guidelines
- T3: dissemination, community engagement, health service research,
- comparative effectiveness
- T4: public health, prevention, population health impact, behavioral
- modifications, lifestyle modifications
- T5: social health care, political security, economic opportunity, access to education, access to health care

Of course the problem with definitions and aphorisms is that they can get very pedantic. According to Schteingart [14] and to McGartland Rubio et al. [35], to improve community practice, T2 should cater to the development of new treatments and to the use of new tools to validate diagnosis and treatment. Other aspects to be addressed are comparative effectiveness, the use of bioinformatics to integrate large datasets, and the application of genomics to determine efficacy and safety of drugs. The same authors [35] describe how the members of the ACRT (Association for Clinical Research Training) developed this working definition of TR:

Translational research fosters the multidirectional integration of basic research, patient-oriented research, and population-based research, with the long-term aim of improving the health of the public.

- T1 research expedites the movement between basic research and patient-oriented research that leads to new or improved scientific understanding or standards of care.
- T2 research facilitates the movement between patient-oriented research and population-based research but leads to better patient outcomes, the implementation of best practices, and improved health status in communities.
- T3 research promotes interaction between laboratory-based research and population-based research to stimulate a robust scientific understanding of human health and disease.

They also mention that the NIH has followed another definition in directions about applying for Clinical and Translational Science Awards (CTSA): (http://grants.nih.gov/grants/guide/rfa-files/RFA-RM-07-007.html).

Translational research includes two areas of translation. One is the process of applying discoveries generated during research in the laboratory, and in preclinical studies, to the development of trials and studies in humans. The second area of translation concerns research aimed at enhancing the adoption of best practices in the community. Cost-effectiveness of prevention and treatment strategies is also an important part of translational science.

Again, it is realized according to the NIH Roadmap for Clinical Research that there are three TR models [30]:

- In the unidirectional model, the laboratory findings are applied to the patient and then to the wider public. A good example is the development of a new drug. In the bidirectional model, population findings have to be tested back in the laboratory. The new hypothesis that statins are associated with increased prevalence of type 2 diabetes mellitus, emerging mostly from observational studies, can be studied in the laboratory.

A more realistic model is the multidirectional one in which basic research, patient-oriented research, and population-based research are interconnected [14].

In a pertinent lecture, Walter J. Koch [36] described the following process:

- A clinical observation creates a design for its therapeutic application. Small and large animal models are then studied. The findings from these studies prompt the design of the appropriate clinical trials.
- In another representation, after the "bench" results are applied to the "bedside," the time comes for clinical trials. The knowledge acquired from these is then applied to wide population implementation.

Kieburtz and Olanow propose another approach [37] while describing the experimental translational therapeutic pathway:

- From the in vitro experiments in which mechanisms and candidate interventions are defined, whole animal (in vivo) experiments are carried out to assess efficacy. Safety experiments and drug activity studies follow. Then comes FDA application in the United States and to corresponding organizations elsewhere. After approval, one moves to phase I, II, and III studies. Very important is postmarketing surveillance which further determines both safety and efficacy. As already mentined, Charalambos Antoniades [4] has proposed another roadmap (Fig. 2.1):

Again it must be pointed out that these are definitions given by experienced investigators which are similar among them but differ somewhat according to their creators' backgrounds and research interests.

Hecker and Birla [12] stress that strategy in research consists of two differing directions: the more frequent, especially, I would think, in well-organized departments in the academic setting, is the top-down strategy, in which a vision is set. To ensure successful implementation of this vision, one must set objectives to be attained and research activities to be undertaken.

The same authors describe that in the bottom-up approach, the outcome of experimentation dictates the overall strategic research direction. However, a mixed approach governed by both directions from above, but also readiness to follow ideas from below can be fruitful.

The finding by Murry et al. [38] of ischemic preconditioning is such an example. This latter approach allows for a dynamic environment and promotes creativity. Accordingly, the authors very thoughtfully point out [12] that integration of the two models is quite frequent and can lead to the greatest success.

Of course just establishing definitions for these research patterns does not automatically ensure investigational bliss and clinical success.

Another concept is that TR is very strongly involved in public health. Seals [39] very aptly proposed the term "from molecules to public health." He gives a very nice figure of the continuum (Fig. 2.2).

He advocates translational strategies for presenting vascular endothelial function [40].

The term "translational epidemiology" has also been described to investigate many modalities such as lung and prostate cancer [41] and chronic kidney disease [42].

Translational research has had a great impact on nutrition research [43].

Translational research is very strongly complemented by the emergence of big data analytics which data provide the researchers with quick access to huge amounts of data as will be described later.

Big data provide four Vs, volume, velocity, variety, and veracity (data assurance), and that they can achieve a close integration of routine clinical information systems to allow bidirectional flow between research and practice [44].

According to Iwashyna and Liu [44], the application of big data diminishes inequalities in the provision of health sciences. The same authors also point out that the application of big data can very well integrate data processing toward better care.

Christodoulakis et al. [45] point out that "big data" can be very helpful in assessment of hospitals.

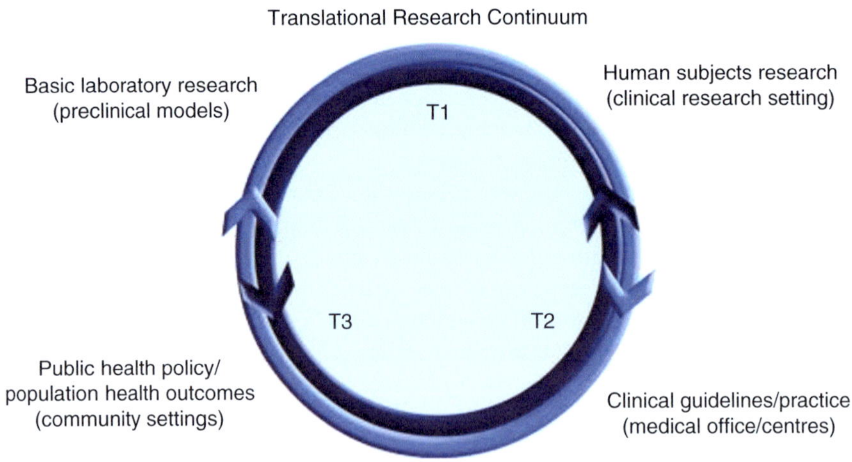

Fig. 2.2 Translational research continuum. Basic science observations are translated initially to the clinical research setting (T1) with subsequent translation for implementation into clinical practice (T2) and public health policy (T3). The process is bidirectional in that observations made initially at higher levels of translation can be studied for underlying mechanisms or other features at the clinical and preclinical levels. (Reproduced with permission from Seals [39])

Of course, this explosive growth of TR creates the need for:

(a) ***Correct Evaluation***

William Trochim [46] addressed this aspect in 2008, evaluating translation of science presentation to the Cornell evaluation network, submitting proposals for the development of culture of evaluation.

(b) ***Appropriate Bioethic Approach***

Hostiuc et al. [47] propose that codes of research ethics require that all biomedical research be carried out under the supervision of a certified physician or other properly qualified health-care professional.

Their proposals for general ethical principles guiding TR are:

- Consequentialist analysis of the TR process
- Translational analysis of the risks associated with the research

2.1.3 Social Justice

In this aspect they address the need for protecting vulnerable populations such as women, children, psychiatry patients, prisoners, and people from developing countries and the need for directions for conducting research in developing countries.

They also point out that vulnerable patients should receive additional benefits.

2.1.4 Data Sharing

This is a very important point. The authors [47] offer two elements of this aspect: the risk of improper dissemination of the information to the media (an example concerns the consequences regarding vaccination practices) and the insurance of reproducibility of results. If the information is not reproducible, according to the authors, the publication could be considered a form of scientific misconduct.

However, this concept is widely advancing and many consortia are devoted to this purpose [48, 49].

2.2 Blocks to Translational Research

Lauer and Scarlatos [31] reiterate the three translational blocks or obstacles identified by the Institute of Medicine Clinical Research Roundtable [24], pertaining to T1, T2, and T3.

Chautard et al. [50] have further defined the first block as this limiting translation of new knowledge into clinical practice and health decision-making towards improved health. As components of the former, they cite lack of willing participants, regulatory burdens, fragmented infrastructures, incompatible databases, and lack of qualified investigators. As components of the latter, they mention career disincentives, practice limitations, high research costs, and lack of funding. A T3 block can be regarded as limitation of dissemination into practice, communities, and large populations.

Here it must be stressed that the NIH itself points out that funding between T1 and T2 is not evenly balanced, to some extent explaining the block between these stages.

Thus, according to some 2007 data, the NIH allots 13 billion dollars to basic research but only 787 million to health services research. The National Cancer Institute stresses another important point, that research dissemination and diffusion are costly by themselves [51].

Hecker and Birla [12] give two interesting additional definitions pertaining to research.

Thus they propose two more entities:

(a) Development is the systematic use of the knowledge or understanding gained from research of practical experience directed toward the production or significant improvement of useful products.
(b) Applied Research is the acquisition of knowledge or understanding to meet a specific recognized need.

According to Vannevar Bush [11], the function of applied research is to give answers which basic research cannot provide.

Another goal of TR which the European Society of Cardiology specifically endorses is innovation, which should be the strong point of discovery.

Deborah Zucker [52] describes that innovation connotes something novel, original, visionary, and hopefully improved. It necessitates the generation of new ideas and hypotheses.

These newer notions signify the quest for the attainment of results and not just the acquisition of new data, which is becoming more pressing with time.

The question then arises, by what measures can TR be carried out and produce favorable results for the improvement of the care of the individual patient and the human populations?

2.3 Organizational Aspects

The evolution toward organizing TR in the United States is interesting and didactic, as presented by Williams and Robertson [26]. They describe how the General Clinical Research Centers (GCRCs) evolved to the Clinical and Translational Science Award (CTSA) program in 2005.

They give a draft of the conceptual framework of the national CTSA consortium.

The CTSA consortium comprises numerous academic health centers (AHCs) in various states.

From their Fig. 2.1, one can readily appreciate the complexity but also the scope of these clinical and translational research institutes.

In 2012, Gordon R. Bernard [53] described the establishment of a new NIH center, the National Center for Advancing Translational Services (NCATS) with a budget of $576.5 million, comprising the Clinical and Translational Science Award (CTSA) program, a consortium of 60 sites.

2.4 The Value of Collaborations: Paradigms

First, the necessity of collaborations must be realized and appreciated. Thus, Lauer and Scarlatos [31] point out in the Progenitor Cell Biology Consortium that collaborations among institutions are essential. They describe the path from discovery (presumably produced through basic research) as producing early (pilot) T1 studies and ancillary studies toward yielding clinical applications.

In the basic research component, this consortium is the main vehicle. A large number of research units are coordinated by the Administrative Coordinating Center, which is the University of Maryland, Baltimore.

As regards clinical applications, the Cardiovascular Cell Therapy Research Network consists of important clinical departments, i.e., Vanderbilt University, the University of Florida, the Cleveland Clinic, and the Texas Heart Institute.

A similar paradigm is offered by the Pediatric Cardiovascular Translational Bench to Bassinet program.

Again one can mark three stages:

- Discovery is managed by the Cardiovascular Development Consortium, managed by four research units (Gladstone, Harvard, Pittsburgh, Utah).
- Early T1 is effected by the Pediatric Cardiac Genomics Consortium, comprising outstanding units (Boston, Columbia, Philadelphia, Mt. Sinai, Yale).
- Finally the clinical application part is implemented by eight clinical sites which constitute the Pediatric Heart Network, a multicenter approach.

Bernard [53] also stresses the importance of collaboration to enable multi-site translational science.

This accent on collaboration brings into focus a consideration by Hecker and Birla [12]. They stress that many investigators or departments have a conception of territorial belonging or ownership of an idea. This narrow outlook is counterproductive and hampers collaboration.

2.5 Training Translational Research Scientists

This brings into focus the question: Can and should TR be taught? The answer to both is yes. Before considering how, let us outline the requirements of becoming a translational researcher.

In the aforementioned excellent and detailed book, *Clinical and Translational Science*, K. E Hartman, E. Heitman, and N. Brown [54] devote a chapter on recommended knowledge bases for T1 and T2 translational research. Not surprisingly the requirements for the former discipline are simpler.

Thus, they describe that for T1, recommended knowledge base includes:

- Human and molecular biology and pathophysiology, animal models, and laboratory techniques.
- The TR translational science components include genomics, proteomics, imaging technology, biomarker development, biomedical informatics, dataset acquisition, and management.

Finally, core competencies additionally include biostatistics, epidemiology, study design, research ethics, writing, and communication.

For a T2 career, health-care epidemiology and other care epidemiology methods are additionally required.

The authors point out that guidelines exist for the education in clinical and translational research of students since 2008 and residents since 2007. They point out that although the mentored/apprentice research prototype still applies, participation into a core didactic curriculum is essential, as well as participation in formal career and leadership development activities. They [54] also describe that some academic medical centers have established training programs in clinical and early translational research, are their majority directed at MDs in post-doctoral training. These curricula vary widely. Moreover, for more advanced training, a few programs offer PhD degrees in clinical and TR per se.

Barry Coller according to David Schteingart [14] proposes that the basic and clinical researchers represent two separate cultures.

Similar specifications are proposed by many authors.

Education programs in TR are being increasingly offered [55, 56].

Thus, according to Williams and Robertson, [57] a TR team should include:

- Laboratory-based investigators
- Clinical investigators
- Statisticians
- Data managers
- Research nurses and coordinators
- Research pharmacists

The same authors propose that the twenty-first-century human research laboratory should have the following picture (Fig. 2.3).

According to Schteingart [14], an appropriate collaborative model should encourage partnerships between researchers, practitioners, and people skilled in translation.

Academician Dimitrios Thanos (personal communication) has given a paradigm how basic and clinical research can be combined in a single center (Fig. 2.4) such as the Biomedical Research Foundation, Academy of Athens.

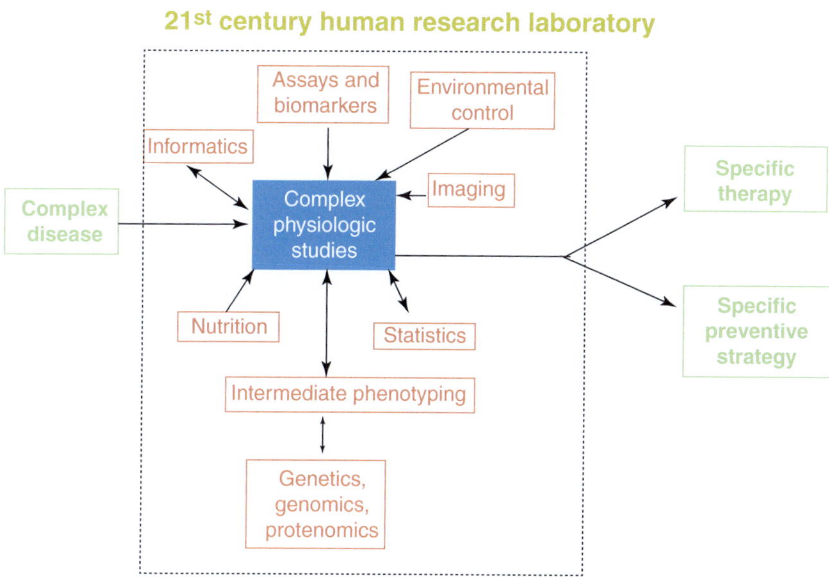

Fig. 2.3 The twenty-first-century human translational investigator's laboratory. (Reproduced with permission from: Williams and Robertson [57])

Fig. 2.4 The Tree of Research. (By permission of Professor-Academician Dimitrios Thanos by Biomedical Research Foundation, Academy of Athens - Gregory Skalkeas)

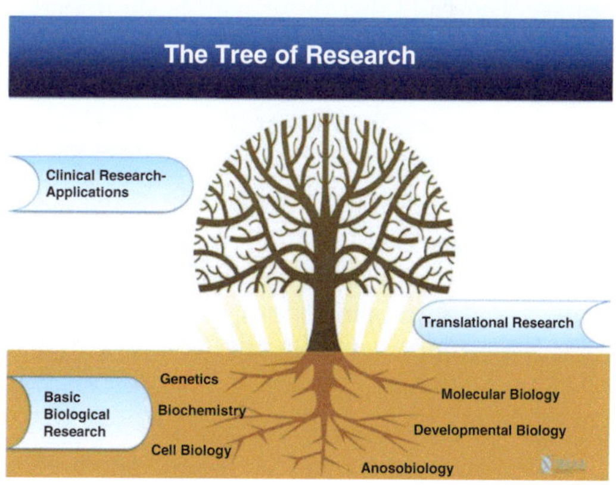

A proposed concept as to who is and who is not a translational investigator is given by Williams and Robertson [57] as adapted from Lee M Nadler, who gives some further thoughts on this subject in 2007 [58].

To produce such results, many medical schools are proposing various teaching courses for producing this type of researchers.

However, it must be realized that there is no formal training to produce a translational researcher. David Schteingart [14] proposes how to train such scientists:

For those coming from a clinical background, he proposes courses and seminars in genetics, molecular biology, computational biology, molecular imaging, epidemiology, and therapeutics.

From those coming from a basic laboratory, he proposes clinical immersion and to learn principles of clinical research. Furthermore, he recommends:

- Translational research training principles
- Multidisciplinary training
- Training customized to an individual's background and skills
- Mentoring by mentoring committees with diverse areas of expertise
- Adaptation to working in multidisciplinary teams

The same author thoroughly accepts that many challenges remain:

- Translational research training challenges
- Career paths uncertain
- Limited number of well-trained mentors
- Competencies still being developed
- Unclear role in the academic research environment
- No specific evaluation criteria

McGartland Rubio et al. [35] discuss the implications for the design of training programs. They stress that since there exists a great diversity of educational background, it may be necessary to design a separate curriculum for every individual trainee. They add that those with basic research background will need to acquire practice in clinical sciences and practice, while clinical background trainees will need additional exposure to basic science. They also stress the importance of mentoring, which will be further discussed. This aspect they consider demanding but highly rewarding.

Bernard [53] stresses the importance of educating and training scientists in clinical and translational research.

Davis et al. [28] stress the importance of both continuing medical education and professional development as promoting knowledge translation primarily in practice centers focusing in evidence-based information.

These activities predispose to change by increasing knowledge or skills and to reinforce this change once it occurs.

At the Biomedical Research Foundation of the Academy of Athens (BRFAA), we have conducted a yearly course, which actually gave the momentum for a previous book *Introduction to Translational Cardiovascular Research*, Springer [5].

2.5.1 *Leadership*

It should be appreciated that, as in all fields of scientific endeavor, correct mentoring of the younger investigators is important and essential. The word "mentor" covers from Homer's Odyssey. The Goddess Athena is disguised as Mentis or Mentor, a friend of Ulysses, who offers to guide his son Telemachus in a journey to gather news about his father (Rhapsodies A and B). What is not appreciated is that Mentor again appears later armed, offering to help Ulysses in his impending fight against the suitors, but again Athena speaks in his person offering first battle and then reconciliation.

A strategy in any department cannot be fruitful unless a sense of leadership is cultivated. Leadership develops leaders at all levels, with as a result exponential growth according to Hecker and Birla [12].

The same authors point out that success in scientific research can be determined by both tangible and, equally important, intangible factors. As tangible factors, one can enumerate publications, impact factor, citations, Hirsch index, invited lectures and articles, positions in committees, grants, patents, and finally return on investment, stock prices, etc.

Intangible rewards are to this and to many authors more important and long-lasting. Hecker and Birla [12] describe them as creating a positive work environment momentum and managing innovation. Additionally, these authors point out that leadership is different from management:

- The latter term is impersonal and concerns resource allocation and accountability, while the former concerns the ability to work and connect with people and to convince them to implement change.

In this sense, in an inspiring article, Verkoeijen and Tabbers point out that good research requires productive theories and guidelines [59].

The PLoS Medicine Editors Tikki Pang and Robert F. Terry stress that in the twenty-first century, it seems astonishing that decisions on health care are still made without solidly grounded research evidence [60].

2.6 The Blocks and Problems

Here, it should be stressed that the effort toward advancing T1 are well delineated and adequately stressed.

However, T2 is also gradually acquiring greater importance, because it is realized that many blocks in its implementation remain.

White et al. [61] and Green et al. [62] point out that the great majority of patients are treated in primary care centers.

Thus, we do not often grasp a real picture of everyday medicine if we only take into account the academic clinical centers, in which an "artificial" atmosphere may be said to exist according to some authors.

To counteract this problem a new concept has emerged: According to Westfall et al. [32]; the NIH Roadmap tries to connect major academic laboratories to physicians and primary physician offices.

The authors further point out that since recommendations and guidelines are created from relatively small centers in selected tertiary centers, their applicability may be limited and not reflect the real-world day-to-day practice.

Martin et al. [63] pointed out 5 years ago that apart from the abovementioned factors, additional patient and trial barriers exist. Patient-specific factors were older age, out-of-state residence, and female gender. Trial-specific barriers that exist were intensive trial-related testing and long anticipation (>6 months).

The first item mentioned, which is essential to the success of clinical trials, is simply the principle of KISS (keep it simple and stupid), since intensive testing militates against adherence.

These considerations become more important currently because of the increasing cost and difficulty of conducting research; a main consideration is how to produce worthwhile results.

However, many researchers, Dirk Brutsaert [64] being a distinguished example, question the future of clinical trials, in this case in chronic heart failure. According to him, most single target-oriented clinical trials are doomed to fail. He advocates that we should incorporate genome-wide association studies (GWAs) and research should be multiscale- and multitarget-based and network medicine-oriented. This is in contrast to the vast majority of multicenter clinical trials. Robert Califf [65] underlines the difficulties facing the planners of clinical trials. He points out the unintended biological targets are common (e.g., intracranial hemorrhage in thrombolysis for acute myocardial infarction) and that interactions among therapies and long-term effects are unpredictable. He points out to the necessity of embedding clinical trials within disease registries.

The Multicenter Research Group [66] realizing the shortcomings and mounting expenses of collaborative clinical trials have advanced many proposals. In accordance with the previous concerns about too much simplicity, they propose the evaluation of the effect of combining different therapies that target diverse pathways or mechanisms in complex medical disorders.

Califf et al. [18] give some further data on clinical trials registered between 2007 and 2010. They remark that during this period, clinical trials registered in clinical trials.gov are dominated by small trials and contain significant heterogeneity in methodological approaches, including data on randomization, blinding, and data monitoring committees.

The observations of Zarin et al. [19] have already been mentioned. They concluded that the usefulness of clinical trials.gov depends on whether responsible investigators and sponsors make urgent efforts to submit complete, timely, accurate, and informative data about their studies.

The large multicenter trials are here to stay. However, because of the problems already described as to their results, the registries' observational studies which according to some investigators better reflect real-life conditions have retained their use and found a new application.

However, as Welke et al. point out [67], data quality assurance mechanisms are very important for the validity of databases.

Sipido et al. [68] propose a clinical trial checklist:

1. Robust number of observations to ensure data care reliability
2. Randomization and blinded observations
3. Correct data processing

In this aspect, Kaul and Diamond [69] point out that research results have many levels of importance. Thus, a finding may be (tough luck) both statistically insignificant and clinically unimportant.

It may be statistically significant but not clinically important; a $p < 0.05$ may not mean anything as it may affect cardiac remodeling after an anterior myocardial infarction as regards end-diastolic volume. The best case scenario would be to have both clinically and statistically important results.

The comparison of the value of observational studies versus RCTs is not new. Benson and Hartz [70] already 17 years ago underline that observational studies show lower cost and greater timelines and concern a broader patient range; however, inherent bias is their main limitation. They mention Chalmers et al. [71] who showed that nonrandomized trials show approximately twice as high favorable treatment effects as compared to blinded randomized, controlled trials.

Although in all classes of the recommendations multiple RCTs and meta-analysis are given a level of evidence A. Tricoci et al. in 2009 [72] examining the scientific evidence underlying the ACC/AHA clinical practice guidelines, remark that they are largely developed from lower levels of evidence or expert opinion. They stress the need to improve the process of writing guidelines and to expand the evidence base from which clinical practice guidelines are derived.

O'Neil et al. [73] studied case examples of systematic reviews in which observational evidence was considered as well as case examples of individual observational studies. They conclude that observational studies may provide moderately to rarely high-strength evidence in systematic reviews. They stress that observational evidence is used when RCTs are infeasible or raise ethical concerns, lack generalizability, or provide insufficient data.

Mentz et al. [74] stress that RCTs have strict enrollment criteria; thus participating pts represent a highly select group of pts not fully representative of real world pts studied in observational studies, selection bias can be reduced by using propensity score analysis. Accordingly the propensity score which calculates the probability that a patient will receive an intervention is calculated using patient population characteristics and is used for analysis adjustment [75]. Propensity score methods give treatment effects estimates closer to the treatment effect than a logistic regression model [76].

Gitt et al. [77] reiterate that RCTs provide the best background for the creation of guideline recommendations. However, they underline that although providing lower evidence level than RCTs, observational studies can provide important evidence when the study outcomes are clinically important and the population studied are representative and provide data from a real-world selection of pts, many of whom would be excluded from RCTs. They provide the key attributes of an effective clinical registry, among which is standardized data collection, in their Table 1.1.

They stress the importance of regression modeling and matching to adjust for imbalances in observed confounders and to control this overt bias. They also point out high-volume, experienced centers in RCTs highly selected pts. They report estimates that less than 1/3 of heart failure pts in clinical practice would qualify for inclusion in RCTs resulting in a lower-risk population [78, 79].

They also cite various instances of disagreement between RCT and registry results, because in the former many pts are excluded as ineligible. An important observation is that large registry populations are ideally placed to assess the incidence of rare adverse events in high-risk groups not identified by RCTs.

A new approach to the problems of both RCTs and Registries maybe the solution of the registry randomized trial.

In an editorial in 2012, James et al. [80] discuss how cardiovascular registries may become novel platform trials. They point out that by including a randomization module in a clinical quality registry, it is possible to combine the best aspects of RCTs and large-scale clinical registries. They designed the TASTE trial on the benefits of thrombus aspiration in primary PCI in acute ST-elevation myocardial infarction.

Lauer and D'Agostino [81] call the randomized registry trial next disruptive technology in clinical research. They underline the fact that many high-quality recently conducted registries exist which have collected huge amounts of data in cardiovascular problems, which, however remain observational studies. They also describe that a registry-based randomized trial was the TASTE trial conducted in Scandinavia. The investigators of this study enrolled patients from a pre-existing high-quality observational registry [82], with a reduction of enrollment time and cost. The authors alert to possible flaws of this type of research, mainly whether the existing electronic health records are of sufficiently high quality, if questions of informed consent can be overcome. The improvement of data keeping by the introduction of "big data" has already been described.

James et al. [83] believe that by "including a randomization module in a large inclusive clinical registry with unselected consecutive enrolment, the advantages of a prospective randomized trial can be combined with the strengths of a large-scale all-comers clinical registry."

One last comment on meta-analyses which constitute I to II level of evidence recommendations. They also must adhere to strict rules. Two types of reporting are proposed, the PRISMA (A) and MOOSE (B), which need no further description. Also consistency or inconsistency in meta-analyses can be measured.

Similarly there exist methods for assessing the quality of report of RCTs. Thus, there is no doubt that evidence-based medicine is here to stay. Also, the RCTs keep multiplying. They form to a large degree the basis for current guidelines always remaining at A level; they also form the basis of meta-analyses, which also constitute class A level.

However, the cost of RCTs can be extremely high. The fact that this cost for the megatrials is to a very large extent covered by industry remains a problem, although admittedly stringent precautions to ensure objectivity are taken. The author still remembers the mute disappointment when the neutral effects of GUSTO-IV and I-PRESERVE had been announced: however, they were faithfully published.

Also, the simultaneous announcement of the results of a megatrial in a large congress and publication in a high-impact journal is always a cause for wonder.

Meta-analyses can be very painstaking to perform but are mark of meticulous researchers. I believe that they actually lend value to the RCTs.

A great improvement in the quality of registries has been marked in recent years. Scandinavian registries are very highly regarded, as well as the registries performed by the European Society of Cardiology. It is a wonder that they still remain level of evidence C. Still their justification maybe the new combination of RCTs and registries, the registry-based RCTs. Finally, is a note from the author: The guidelines are written by avowed exerts. This in a philosophical context they represent a consensus of the opinion of experts, although they firmly adhere to quality criteria.

Some experts of course are proposing different requirements for defining classes and levels of recommendations.

Another reverse way of combining registries and RCTs was reported in 2008 by Olsen et al. in Denmark [84]. An RCT was conducted in 1990 to assess the effect of fish oil on pregnancy duration, maternal prostacyclin and thromboxane production, and essential fatty acid in umbilical blood. After 16 years had passed, information in the offspring of the mothers participating in the study was extracted from the national patient registry using a unique ten-digit personal identification number, to diagnose of fish oil affected allergic asthma the offspring.

2.7 Managing Blocks

Even if RCTs and the registries are successful, implementation of their results is not timely or easy.

This brings again blocks T2 and T3. Balas and Boren [85] point out that it takes an estimated average of 17 years for only 14% of new discoveries to reach clinical practice and patient care.

Contopoulos-Ioannidis et al. [86] examined the life of TR for medical interventions. Even for the most highly published and nonrefuted interventions in first use in human, they found a range of 0–28 years. They propose the following measures to counteract this problem:

- Multidisciplinary collaboration involving both basic and clinical scientists
- Large robust randomized clinical trials to provide proof of effectiveness
- Effort at producing novel agents and new cutting-edge technologies

Antoniades [4] notes that 95% of hypotheses generated by basic science fail in the clinical arena. Translational research is able to filter these observations and is the first priority of funding bodies: ERC/MRC/BHF/BRC. Translational research saves money! Negative findings in translational research are publishable and may be more important than positive.

Many authors have further addressed this question. Morris, Wooding, and Grant [87] commented on the time lag all the 17-year estimated by Balas and Boren [85]. They identified 23 different papers with a mean time lag from 3 to 28 years. They underlined various points considered as limiting the time lag, varying from highly cited publications, guidelines/recommendations, first specific use implementation, and date to market. They cite the finding of Altman and Goodman [88] who found that the time lag for a paper to receive 25 citations is 4–6 years if it described a new technique, but an "expository article" at that time could receive 500 citations.

Young and Borland [89] in 2011 try to identify key barriers to the translation of science into practice and policy. They underline that researchers and practitioners have different "practical ontologies." They stressed the need to consult "generalization gradients" to help practitioners and researchers.

However, while discussing these problems, one should not forget some more encouraging current examples: As the pioneer of the technique, Alain Cribier [90] describes TAVR. For example, the first paper describing TAVR appeared in 2002; by 2006, the technique had been applied as a French experience [91].

Similarly, Farnier [92] describes that since the first report of PCSK9 in 2003 [93], the first studies appeared around 2012 [94].

Additionally, the approach toward reporting the results is changing with the open-access electronic journals which are rapidly multiplying. Also, the practice of presenting results in a large congress and simultaneously publishing them in high-impact journals may change the time lags, especially since many such journals are now publishing more frequently than some years ago.

2.8 A New Concept: The Valley of Death

The difficulties described or blocks T1, T2, and T3 have in the last 5 years been given a new name referring to the Bible or Western films. The Valley of Death concept is the phase between research and successful innovation [95].

Declan Butler [96] describes this valley as an abyss in which neither basic researchers nor physicians busy with patient care are keen to venture. According to this author, lack of communication is the main problem.

2.8.1 Proposed Ways to Cross the Valley of Death

Roberts et al. [97] define the "Valley of Death" as the gap between bench research and clinical application and defined the varied barriers impending the crossing of this valley.

They point out that despite unprecedented US government funding of public research, the dramatic drop of the new drugs and treatments reaching patient use should be of concern. They believe that a major factor is the increasing isolation of basic researchers from clinicians. They believe that clinician-scientists can build bridges across this valley. They point out that up to 2005 more funding goes to PhD than MD scientists.

Coller and Califf [98] again highlight the gap between finding a promising new agent and demonstrating its safety and efficacy. They also point out that basic scientists try to advance from the discovery to the development phase, but their institutions lack systems to support such research.

They propose six categories of questions in an effort to cross the Valley of Death:

1. Is it worth the effort?
2. Is there an adequate potential market?
3. What can be referred from human and animal data about likely safety and efficacy?
4. Can the agent be delivered to its target at an adequate concentration?
5. Is there an industry partner that can develop the agent effectively and efficiently?
6. Can a pivotal trial be designed and completed?

Bodi et al. [99] actually describe three Valleys of Death:

- First: Transition to research in humans
- Second: Preliminary validation in patients
- Third: Use of the model in routine practice

All these studies point out that barriers exist throughout the continuum of TR. Moses et al. [100] already in 2005 pointed out that the study of financial anatomy of biomedical research provides staggering facts. They quantify 10-year funding trends (from 1994 to 2004) in basic, translational, and clinical biomedical research. Funding increased from \$37.1 billion in 1994 to \$94.3 in 2003, doubling when adjusted for inflation. There was an increase from \$4.0 to \$14.2 billion for industry sponsorship of clinical trials, while proportions devoted to basic and applied research were unchanged. These facts underlie the increasing trends for clinical research.

They urge more effective translation of basic research to clinical application, the very essence of TR.

Another interesting aspect is the Matthew effect [101] which signifies that more eminent researchers are given disproportionate credit in instances of collaboration or independent multiple discoveries; this increases their own visibility while reducing the visibility of less well-known researchers.

Merton [101] gave a very pertinent review, considering the reward and communication systems of science.

2.9 New Concepts: The Dry Lab

The spiraling costs of research have highlighted another necessity. According to Quinn and Kohl [102] combining wet and dry research: experience with model development for cardiac mechano-electric structure function studies is important.

The wet lab, i.e., animal experimental work, can be profitably complemented by the "dry" or computational model. In a very far-reaching spotlight review, they point out that this interactive combination of "wet" and "dry" experimentation can be very beneficial, through many processes:

The "wet" investigations (experimental and clinical) help develop experimental and/or clinical theoretical models.

On the other hand, the computational simulation results generate novel hypotheses and predictions. Wet lab studies are used to prove or disprove these model-created hypotheses.

This process is not infallible. More complex models than necessary may be involved; this may necessitate model reduction to appropriate both simplicity and complexity [103].

Newly generated insight is employed to further advance computational models.

Another benefit of this wet/dry integration according to the authors is that computational modeling can help avoid a "fishing expedition." They also very pertinently point out that an eventual mismatch between model prediction and experimental validation can identify directions for subsequent development. This integrative process further promotes translational medicine.

According to the Swedish Academy of Sciences [104] in a report on the occasion of the award of the Nobel Prize in Chemistry for 2013, experiments can be carried out in the laboratory but planned in the computer. The very recent concept of 3D organ printer, which is a transfer of the "dry" lab planning to the "wet" lab (organ production), is a very important paradigm.

Before concluding this chapter, it must still be mentioned that there is hope for the – even near – future. Hudson and Khazragui [105] point out that the "Valley of Death" can be crossed, even with profits. Even though they admit that cooperation between researchers from academia, the pharmaceutical-technical industry, government agencies, and international funding bodies is still far from perfect, many countries are beginning to employ research as a tool for innovation and ultimately for expanding industrial and economic policy. The HORIZON research project is such an example.

Curry [106] offers some thoughts on what is to be expected from translational science over the next 10 years:

- A boost to biomarker research in the universities.
- Transfer of early clinical testing work into academic control.
- Create better opportunities for universities to commercialize their discoveries.
- Promote the regulation of the efficacy and quality of the process and its products.

To give some more concrete ideas of what can be expected from translational cardiovascular research, E. Braunwald [107] describes the following aspects in which hopes exist for the next years from translating research into improved care:

> Research in microRNAs, dilated cardiomyopathy, adaptive immunity in atherogenesis, cardiac hypertrophy and failure, gene therapy, regenerative therapy, sudden cardiac death, myocardial reperfusion injury, and nitrosylation. Actually all of them are addressed in this book.

The deliberations of the Association of Professors of Medicine should be taken into consideration: They specifically refer to the translation of academic discovery into societal benefit which should be the final goal of TR [108].

Finally, in 2017, Douglas L. Mann proposes ways on how Mr. Trump can make TR great again [109].

In conclusion, the author has tried to give an overview on various modalities of research, focusing on translational research.

The obstacles still exist in translation of laboratory findings to patient and population benefits through a multidirectional interactive model.

The need for educating translational research and collaboration of large centers is evident. The integration of wet (animal) and dry (computational) laboratories for greater economy and efficacy is imperative.

References

1. Coller BS. Translating from the rivers of Babylon to the coronary bloodstream. J Clin Invest. 2012;122:4293–9.
2. Fox KA, Steg PG, Eagle KA, Goodman SG, Anderson FA Jr, Granger CB, et al. Decline in rates of death and heart failure in acute coronary syndromes, 1999–2006. JAMA. 2007;297:1892–9.
3. van der Laan AL, Boenink M. Beyond bench and bedside: disentangling the concept of translational research. Health Care Anal. 2015;23:32–49.
4. Antoniades Ch. Bridging the gap between basic science and clinical practice: The role of translational medicine. Lecture presented at the Biomedical Research Foundation Academy of Athens, 31 October 2012.
5. Cokkinos DV. Introduction: what is translational research in: Cokkinos DV, editor. Introduction to translational cardiovascular research. 1st ed. Cham. Springer 2015;p3–16.
6. NSF. Definition of Research. National Science Foundation 2007. http://www.Nsf.gov/statistics/randdef/business.cfm.
7. Oxford English Dictionary (www.oed.com).
8. Merriam Webster, Oxford English Dictionary, Research merriam-webster.com, updated 21 May 2018.
9. Popper KR. Objective knowledge. 2nd ed. Oxford: Clarendon press; 1972. p. 191–205.
10. Jan I. Thinking about research: frameworkers, ethics and scholarships. Edinburgh: Association for the study of Medical Education; 2007. p. 2–37.
11. Bush V (ed.). Science: the endless frontier a report to the president by Vannevar Bush, Director of the Office of Scientific research and Development Washington DC. United states Government Printing office. Jul 1945. Accessed November 13, 2009. Section 3 (The impor-

tance of Basic research), Chapter 3 (Science and the public welfare). http://nsf.gov/about/history/nsf50/vbush1945_content.jsp
12. Hecker L, Birla RV. Intangible factors leading to success in research: strategy, innovation and leadership. J Cardiovasc Trans Res. 2008;1:85–92.
13. Glossary of Themes for Human Subjects Protection and inclusion issues based on the 1997 report of the NIH Director's Panel on clinical research, entry: "clinical research". Accessed November 13 2009. http://grants.nih.gov/grants/peer/tree_glossary.pdf
14. Schteingart DE. Introduction to principles of clinical and translational research. ESCI Core Course on Clinical Research, Athens, 8–10, October 2010.
15. NIH National Cancer Institute NCI Dictionary of Cancer Terms.
16. Seely WE, Grinspoon S. Patient-oriented research: clinical pathophysiology and clinical therapeutics. In: Robertson D, Williams GH, editors. Clinical and translational science. 1st ed. London: Elsevier; 2009. p. 3–12.
17. U.S. Department of Health and Human Services. U.S Food and Drug Administration. What Are the Different Types of Clinical Research?
18. Califf RM, Zarin DA, Kramer JM, Sherman RE, Aberle LH, Tasneem A. Characteristics of clinical trials registered in ClinicalTrials.gov, 2007–2010. JAMA. 2012;307:1838–47.
19. Zarin DA, Tse T, Williams RJ, Califf RM, Ide NC. The ClinicalTrials.gov results database--update and key issues. N Engl J Med. 2011;364:852–60.
20. Karp JE, McCaffrey RP. New avenues of translational research in leukemia and lymphoma: outgrowth of a Leukemia Society of America-National Cancer Institute workshop. J Natl Cancer Inst. 1994;86:1196–201.
21. Feldman AM, Koch WJ, Force TL. Developing strategies to link basic cardiovascular sciences with clinical drug development: another opportunity for translational sciences. Clin Pharmacol Ther. 2007;81:887–92.
22. Littman BH, Di Mario L, Plebani M, Marincola FM. What's next in translational medicine? Clin Sci (Lond). 2007;112:217–27.
23. Woolf SH. The meaning of translational research and why it matters. JAMA. 2008;290:211–3.
24. Dische S, Saunders M. Translational research--a new entity? Acta Oncol. 2001;40:995–9.
25. Coller BS. Translational research: Forging a new cultural identity. Mt Sinai J Med. 2008;75:478–87.
26. Williams GH, Robertson D. Introduction to clinical research. In: Robertson D, Williams GH, editors. Clinical and translational science. 1st ed. London: Elsevier; 2009. p. xvii–xx.
27. Williams GH, Robertson D. Clinical and translational science infrastructure. In: Robertson D, Williams GH, editors. Clinical and translational science. 1st ed. London: Elsevier; 2009. p. 171–81.
28. Davis D, Evans M, Jadad A, Perrier L, Rath D, Ryan D, et al. The case for knowledge translation: shortening the journey from evidence to effect. BMJ. 2003;327(7405):33–5.
29. National Cancer Institute. Translational Research Working Group Definition of Translational Research: http://www.cancer.gov/trwg/TRWG-definition-ND-tr-continuum.
30. Sung NS, Crowley WF Jr, Genel M, Salber P, Sandy L, Sherwood LM, et al. Central challenges facing the national clinical research enterprise. JAMA. 2003;289:1278–87.
31. Lauer M, Scarlatos S. Translational research for cardiovascular diseases at the national heart lung and blood institute. Moving from bench to bedside and from bedside to community. Circulation. 2010;121:929–33.
32. Westfall JM, Mold J, Fagnan L. Practice-based research--"Blue Highways" on the NIH roadmap. JAMA. 2007;297:403–6.
33. Malliaras K, Kreke M, Marbán E. The stuttering progress of cell therapy for heart disease. Clin Pharmacol Ther. 2011;90:532–41.
34. Waldman SA, Terzic A. Clinical and translational science: from bench-bedside to global village. Clin Transl Sci. 2010;5:254–7.
35. McGarland R, Schoenbaum E, Lee S, Schteinggard DE, Marantz PR, Anderson KE, et al. Defining translational research: implications for training. Acad Med. 2010;85:470–5.

36. Koch WJ. Targeting the beta-adrenergic receptor kinase in heart failure. Lecture presented at the 1st International Scientific Conference on Cardiovascular biotechnology: From cell to man, Biomedical Research Foundation of the Academy of Athens. 31 May 2013.
37. Kieburtz K, Olanow CW. Translational experimental therapeutics: the translation of laboratory-based discovery into disease-related therapy. Mt Sinai J Med. 2007;74:7–14.
38. Murry CE, Jennings KA, Reimer KA. Preconditioning with ischemia: a delay of lethal cell injury in ischemic myocardium. Circulation. 1986;74:1124–36.
39. Seals DR. Translational physiology: from molecules to public health. J Physiol. 2013;591:3457–69.
40. Seals DR, Kaplon RE, Gioscia-Ryan RA, TJ LR 2nd. You're only as old as your arteries: translational strategies for preserving vascular endothelial function with aging. Physiology (Bethesda). 2014;29:250–64.
41. Khoury MJ, Gwinn M, Ioannidis JP. The emergence of translational epidemiology: from scientific discovery to population health impact. Am J Epidemiol. 2010;172:517–24.
42. Brück K, Stel VS, Fraser S, De Goeij MC, Caskey F, Abu-Hanna A, et al. Translational research in nephrology: chronic kidney disease prevention and public health. Clin Kidney J. 2015;8:647–55.
43. Kasim-Karakas S, Hyson D, Halsted C, van Loan M, Chedin E, Berglund L. Translational nutrition research at UC Davis--the key role of the Clinical and Translational Science Center. Ann N Y Acad Sci. 2010;1190:179–83.
44. Iwashyna TJ, Liu V. What's so different about big data? A primer for clinicians trained to think epidemiologically. Ann Am Thorac Soc. 2014;11:1130–5.
45. Christodoulakis A, Karanikas H, Billiris A, Thireos E, Pelekis N. "Big data" in health care Assessment of the performance of Greek NHS Hospitals using key performance and clinical workload indicators. Arch Hellenic Med. 2016;33:489–97.
46. Trochim W. Evaluating translational science. Presentation to the Cornell Evaluation Network Presentation to the Cornell Evaluation Network September 29, 2008.
47. Hostiuc S, Moldoveanu A, Dascălu MI, Unnthorsson R6, Jóhannesson ÓI, Marcus I. Translational research-the need of a new bioethics approach. J Transl Med. 2016;14:16. https://doi.org/10.1186/s12967-016-0773-4.
48. Athey BD, Braxenthaler M, Haas M, Guo Y. tranSMART: an open source and community-driven informatics and data sharing platform for clinical and translational research. AMIA J Summits Transl Sci Proc. 2013;2013:6–8.
49. Malin B, Karp D, Scheuermann RH. Technical and policy approaches to balancing patient privacy and data sharing in clinical and translational research. J Investig Med. 2010;58:11–8.
50. Chautard E, Thierry-Mieg N, Ricard-Blum S. Interaction networks: from protein functions to drug discovery. A review. Pathol Biol (Paris). 2009;57:324–33.
51. National Cancer Institute: research dissemination and diffusion. Nov 47, 2007.
52. Zucker DR. What is needed to promote translational research and how do we get it? J Investig Med. 2009;57:468–70.
53. Bernard GR. Preparedness of the CTSA's structural and scientific assets to support the mission of the National Center for Advancing Translational Sciences (NCATS.). Clin Transl Sci. 2012;5:121–9.
54. Hartmann KE, Heitman E, Brown NJ. Training basic, clinical and translational investigators. In: Robertson D, Williams GH, editors. Clinical and translational science. 1st ed. London: Elsevier; 2009. p. 191–9.
55. Pienta KJ. Successfully accelerating translational research at an academic medical center: the University of Michigan-Coulter translational research partnership program. Clin Transl Sci. 2010;3:316–8.
56. Mata HJ, Davis S. Translational health research: perspectives from health education specialists. Clin Transl Med. 2012;1:27.

57. Williams GH, Robertson D. The future of clinical research. In: Robertson D, Williams GH, editors. Clinical and translational science. 1st ed. London: Elsevier; 2009. p. 565–70.
58. Nadler LM, Roberts WC. Lee Marshall Nadler, MD: a conversation with the editor. Proc Bayl Univ Med Cent. 2007;20:381–9.
59. Verkoeijen PPJL, Tabbers HK. Good research requires productive theories and guidelines. Med Educ. 2013;47:858–65.
60. Pang T, Terry RF, The PLoS Medicine Editors WHO/PLoS Collection. No health without research: a call for papers. PLoS Med, 4 e1001008. 2011;8
61. White KL, Williams TF, Greenberg BG. The ecology of medical care. N Engl J Med. 1961;265:885–92.
62. Green LA, Fryer GE Jr, Yawn BP, Lanier D, Dovey SM. The ecology of medical care revisited. N Engl J Med. 2001;344:2021–5.
63. Martin SS, Ou FS, Newby LK, Sutton V, Adams P, Felker GM, Wang TY. Patient- and trial-specific barriers to participation in cardiovascular randomized clinical trials. J Am Coll Cardiol. 2013;61:762–9.
64. Brutsaert D. Heart Failure: Quo Vadis Lecture presented at Cardiovascular Biotechnology: From cell to man Biomedical Research Foundation Academy of Athens, 31 May – 1 June 2013.
65. Califf RM. Clinical trials. In: Robertson D, Williams GH, editors. Clinical and translational science. 1st ed. London: Elsevier; 2009. p. 13–37.
66. Moss AJ, Francis CW, Rayan D. Collaborative clinical trials. N Engl J Med. 2011;364:789791.
67. Welke KF, Ferguson TB Jr, Cooms LP, Dokholygan RS, Murray CJ, Sehrader MI, et al. Validity of the society of thoracic surgeons national adult cardiac surgery database. Ann Thorac Surg. 2004;77:1137–9.
68. Sipido KR, Casadei B, Holvoet P, Janssens S, Luttun A, Sampaolesi M. Bedside to bench: a look at experimental research with a clinical trial checklist. Cardiovasc Res. 2014;101:1–3.
69. Kaul S, Diamond GA. Trial and error. How to avoid commonly encountered limitations of published clinical trials. J Am Coll Cardiol. 2010;55:415–27.
70. Benson K, Hartz AJ. A comparison of observational studies and randomized, controlled trials. N Engl J Med. 2000;342:1878–86.
71. Chalmers TC, Celano P, Sacks HS, Smith H Jr. Bias in treatment assignment in controlled clinical trials. N Engl J Med. 1983;309:1358–61.
72. Tricoci P, Allen JM, Kramer JM, Califf RM, Smith SC Jr. Scientific evidence underlying the ACC/AHA clinical practice guidelines. JAMA. 2009;301:831–41.
73. O'Neil M, Berkman N, Hartling L, Chang S, Anderson J, Motu'apuaka M, et al. Observational evidence and strength of evidence domains: case examples. Syst Rev. 2014;3:35. https://doi.org/10.1186/2046-4053-3-35.
74. Mentz RJ, Kelly JP, von Lueder TG, Voors AA, Lam CS, Cowie MR, et al. Noncardiac comorbidities in heart failure with reduced versus preserved ejection fraction. J Am Coll Cardiol. 2014;64:2281–93.
75. D'Agostino RB. Jr. Propensity scores in cardiovascular research. Circulation. 2007;115:2340–3.
76. Martens EP, Pestman WR, de Boer A, Belitser SV, Klungel OH. Systematic differences in treatment effect estimates between propensity score methods and logistic regression. Int J Epidemiol. 2008;37:1142–7.
77. Gitt AK, Bueno H, Danchin N, Fox K, Hochadel M, Kearney P, et al. The role of cardiac registries in evidence-based medicine. Eur Heart J. 2010;31:525–9.
78. Lenzen MJ, Boersma E, Reimer WJ, Balk AH, Komajda M, Swedberg K, et al. Underutilization of evidence-based drug treatment in patients with heart failure is only partially explained by dissimilarity to patients enrolled in landmark trials: a report from the Euro Heart Survey on Heart Failure. Eur Heart J. 2005;26:2706–13.
79. Masoudi FA, Havranek EP, Wolfe P, Gross CP, Rathore SS, Steiner JF, et al. Most hospitalized older persons do not meet the enrollment criteria for clinical trials in heart failure. Am Heart J. 2003;146:250–7.
80. James S, Fröbert O, Lagerqvist B. Cardiovascular registries: a novel platform for randomised clinical trials. Heart. 2012;98:1329–231.

81. Lauer MS, D'Agostino RB Sr. The randomized registry trial--the next disruptive technology in clinical research? N Engl J Med. 2013;369:1579–81.
82. Fröbert O, Lagerqvist B, Gudnason T, Thuesen L, Svensson R, Olivecrona GK, et al. Thrombus Aspiration in ST-Elevation myocardial infarction in Scandinavia (TASTE trial). A multicenter, prospective, randomized, controlled clinical registry trial based on the Swedish angiography and angioplasty registry (SCAAR) platform. Study design and rationale. Am Heart J. 2010;160:1042–8.
83. James S, Rao SV, Granger CB. Registry-based randomized clinical trials--a new clinical trial paradigm. Nat Rev Cardiol. 2015;12:312–6.
84. Olsen SF, Østerdal ML, Salvig JD, Mortensen LM, Rytter D, Secher NJ, et al. Fish oil intake compared with olive oil intake in late pregnancy and asthma in the offspring: 16 y of registry-based follow-up from a randomized controlled trial. Am J Clin Nutr. 2008;88:167–75.
85. Balas EA, Boren SA. In: Balas EA, editor. Yearbook of medical informatics: managing clinical knowledge for health care improvement. Stuttgart: Shattauer Verlagsgesellschaft mbH; 2000. p. 65–70.
86. Contopoulos-Ioannidis DG, Alexiou GA, Grouvias TC, Ioannidis JPA. Life circle of translational research for medical interventions. Science. 2008;321:1298–9.
87. Morris ZS, Wooding S, Grant J. The answer is 17 years, what is the question: understanding time lags in translational research. J R Soc Med. 2011;104:510–20.
88. Altman DG, Goodman SN. Transfer of technology from statistical journals to the biomedical literature. Past trends and future predictions. JAMA. 1994;272:129–32.
89. Young D, Borland R. Conceptual challenges in the translation of research into practice: it's not just a matter of "communication". Transl Behav Med. 2011;1:256–69.
90. Cribier A. Development of transcatheter aortic valve implantation (TAVI): a 20-year odyssey. Arch Cardiovasc Dis. 2012;105:146–52.
91. Cribier A, Eltchaninoff H, Tron C, Bauer F, Agatiello C, Nercolini D, et al. Treatment of calcific aortic stenosis with the percutaneous heart valve: mid-term follow-up from the initial feasibility studies: the French experience. J Am Coll Cardiol. 2006;47:1214–23.
92. Farnier M. PCSK9: from discovery to therapeutic applications. Arch Cardiovasc Dis. 2014;107:58–66.
93. Seidah NG, Benjannet S, Wickham L, Marcinkiewicz J, Jasmin SB, Stifani S, et al. The secretory proprotein convertase neural apoptosis-regulated convertase 1 (NARC-1): liver regeneration and neuronal differentiation. Proc Natl Acad Sci U S A. 2003;100:928–33.
94. Stein EA, Mellis S, Yancopoulos GD, Stahl N, Logan D, Smith WB, et al. Effect of a monoclonal antibody to PCSK9 on LDL cholesterol. N Engl J Med. 2012;366:1108–18.
95. Hudson J, Khazhragui HF. Into the valley of death; research to innovation. Drug Discov Today. 2012;18:610–3.
96. Butler D. Translational research; crossing the valley of death. Nature. 2008;453:840–2.
97. Roberts SF, Fischhoff MA, Sakowski SA, Feldman EL. Perspective: Transforming science into medicine: how clinician-scientists can build bridges across research's "valley of death". Acad Med. 2012;87:266–70.
98. Coller BS, Califf RM. Traversing the valley of death: a guide to assessing prospects for translational success. Sci Transl Med. 2009;1:10cm9. https://doi.org/10.1126/scitranslmed.3000265.
99. Bodi V, Marrachelli VG, Husser O, Chorro FJ, Viña JR, Monleon D. Metabolomics in the diagnosis of acute myocardial ischemia. J Cardiovasc Trans Res. 2013;6:808–15.
100. Moses H 3rd, Dorsey ER, Matheson DH, Their SO. Financial anatomy of biomedical research. JAMA. 2005;294:1333–42.
101. Merton RK. The Matthew effect in science: the reward and communication systems of science are considered. Science. 1968;159:56–63.
102. Quinn T, Kohl P. Combining wet and dry research: experience with model development for cardiac mechano-electric structure-function studies. Cardiovasc Res. 2013;97:601–11.
103. Garny A, Noble D. Dimensionality in cardiac modelling. Prog Biophys Mol Biol. 2005;87:47–66.

104. The Royal Swedish Academy of Science. Taking permission the experiment to cyberspace. Popular science background. Nobel prize in Chemistry, 2013.
105. Hudson J, Khazragui HF. Into the valley of death: research to innovation. Drug Discov Today. 2013;18:610–3.
106. Curry SH. Translational science: past, present, and future. Bio Techniques. 2008;44:Pii–Pviii.
107. Braunwald E. Cardiovascular science: opportunities for translating research into improved care. J Clin Invest. 2013;123:6–10.
108. Stamler JS, Taber RL, Califf RM. Translation of academic discovery into societal benefit: proposal for a balanced approach--part 1. Am J Med. 2003;115:596–9.
109. Mann DL. Mr. Can. Trump make translational research great again? JACC: Basic to Translational Science. 2017;2:1. https://doi.org/10.1016/j.jacbts.2017.01.001.

Chapter 3
Clinical Research and Evidence-Based Medicine

Dennis V. Cokkinos

3.1 The Emergence of Evidence Based Medicine

It should be stressed that clinical research has led to the emergence of evidence-based medicine (EBM). EBM has been described as conscientious, explicit, and judicious use of the current best evidence in making decisions about the care of individual patients [1].

According to Tenny and Grossman [2], EBM is the use of scientific methods to organize and apply current data and to improve health care decisions. They point out that three parts are included: relevant scientific evidence, clinical judgment, and the patient's values or preferences.

Masic et al. [3] differentiate between EBM, which refers to the individual patient, and evidence-based health care, which refers to evidence primarily at the population level.

Cynthia Farquhar [4], in a recent editorial, attributed the introduction of term to Professor Gordon Guyatt [5], who suggested it in 1992 as an alternative to the use of intuition, nonsystematic clinical experience, and a pathophysiological rationale as sufficient means of clinical decision making [4].

Subsequently, Sackett and Rosenberg [6] described the aforementioned judicious use of evidence in making decisions about the care of the individual patient.

A series in *JAMA* on the subject was published in book form [7].

Cynthia Farquhar also very succinctly describes the Cochrane collaboration, founded in 1993 and named for Archie Cochrane, a Scottish epidemiologist, who led clinical trials on the health of Welsh mining communities and who championed the employment of randomized controlled trials (RCTs).

D. V. Cokkinos (✉)
Heart and Vessel Department, Biomedical Research Foundation,
Academy of Athens - Gregory Skalkeas, Athens, Greece
e-mail: dcokkinos@bioacademy.gr

D. V. Cokkinos (ed.), *Myocardial Preservation*,
https://doi.org/10.1007/978-3-319-98186-4_3

Burns et al. [8] describe very pertinently various levels of evidence and their role in EBM. They mention that various levels of evidence have been described, such as the Canadian Task Force on the Periodic Health Examination's listing of levels of evidence, published in 1979 [9]:

- Level I: Evidence from at least one randomized controlled trial
- Level II-1: Evidence from at least one well-designed cohort study or case–control study, i.e., a controlled trial that is not randomized
- Level II-2: Comparisons between times and places with or without the intervention
- Level III: Opinions of respected authorities, based on clinical experience, descriptive studies, or reports of expert committees

Further levels of evidence were introduced by Sackett in 1989 [10], as follows:

- Level I: Large RCTs with clear-cut results
- Level II: Small RCTs with unclear results
- Level III: Cohort and case–control studies
- Level IV: Historical cohort or case–control studies
- Level V: Case series, studies with no controls

In 1988, the US Preventive Services Task Force further subdivided level II, as follows [11, 12]:

- Level I: Evidence obtained from at least one properly designed randomized controlled trial
- Level II-1: Evidence obtained from well-designed controlled trials without randomization
- Level II-2: Evidence obtained from well-designed cohort or case–control analytical studies, preferably from more than one center or research group
- Level II-3: Evidence obtained from multiple time series designs with or without the intervention; dramatic results in uncontrolled trials might also be regarded as this type of evidence
- Level III: Opinions of respected authorities, based on clinical experience, descriptive studies, or reports of expert committees

Of course, more grading systems have also been described over the years.

In September 2000, the Oxford (UK) levels of evidence were published. They were more complex and addressed not only therapy and prevention but also diagnostic tests, prognostic markers, and the possibility of harm [13]:

- Level 1a: Systematic reviews (with homogeneity) of RCTs
- Level 1b: Individual RCTs (with narrow confidence intervals)
- Level 1c: All-or-none RCTs
- Level 2a: Systematic reviews (with homogeneity) of cohort studies
- Level 2b: Individual cohort studies or low-quality RCTs (e.g., <80% follow-up)
- Level 2c: "Outcomes" research; ecological studies
- Level 3a: Systematic reviews (with homogeneity) of case–control studies
- Level 3b: Individual case–control studies
- Level 4: Case series (and poor-quality cohort and case–control studies)

Table 3.1 Evidence-rating scale for prognostic studies

Level of evidence	Type of evidence
I	High-quality prospective cohort study with adequate power or a systematic review of such studies
II	Lesser-quality prospective cohort, retrospective cohort study, untreated controls from a randomized controlled trial, or a systematic review of such studies
III	Case–control study or a systematic review of such studies
IV	Case series
V	Expert opinion; case report or clinical example; or evidence based on physiology, bench research, or "first principles"

Adapted from the American Society of Plastic Surgeons [14]

- Level 5: Expert opinion without explicit critical appraisal or based on physiology, bench research, or "first principles"

As Burns et al. [8] point out, guidelines have also been published for prognostic studies, such as the rating scale published by the American Society of Plastic Surgeons [14] (Table 3.1).

One should remember the suggestions of David L. Sackett [15], the pioneer in this field, on how the process of EBM creates the need for clinically important information and how we should:

1. Convert these information needs into answerable questions
2. Track down, with maximum efficiency, the best evidence with which to answer them (and make increasing use of secondary sources of the best evidence)
3. Critically appraise that evidence for its validity (closeness to the truth) and usefulness (clinically applicability)
4. Integrate the appraisal with clinical expertise and apply the results in clinical practice
5. Evaluate [our] own performance

Dunning et al. [16], referring to the best evidence topic (BestBET) for cardiothoracic surgery, also proposes five somewhat different levels of evidence.

Finally, the American College of Cardiology/American Heart Association (ACC/AHA) have come up with the following classification of indications (classes I–III) and levels of evidence (A–C). It is interesting that although they use the term "guidelines" in the titles of their publications, in the actual text they use the term "recommendations." In more detail, the ACC/AHA guidelines for coronary angiography give the following indications [17]:

- Class I: Conditions for which there is evidence and/or general agreement that this procedure is useful and effective
- Class II: Conditions for which there is conflicting evidence and/or a divergence of opinion about the usefulness/efficacy of performing the procedure
- Class IIa: The weight of evidence/opinion is in favor of usefulness/efficacy
- Class IIb: Usefulness/efficacy is less well established by evidence/opinion
- Class III: Conditions for which there is evidence and/or general agreement that the procedure is not useful/effective and in some cases may be harmful

The weight of evidence in support of the recommendation for each listed indication is presented as follows:

- Level of Evidence A: The presence of multiple randomized clinical trials
- Level of Evidence B: The presence of a single randomized trial or nonrandomized studies
- Level of Evidence C: Expert consensus

The 2014 AHA/ACC guidelines for the management of patients with non-ST-elevation acute coronary syndromes give somewhat different recommendations [18]. They recommend three levels of evidence, to estimate the certainty (precision) of the treatment effect:

- Level A: Multiple populations evaluated—data derived from multiple randomized clinical trials or meta-analyses
- Level B: Limited populations evaluated—data derived from a single randomized trial or nonrandomized studies
- Level C: Very limited populations evaluated—only consensus opinion of experts, case studies, or standard of care

with four classes of evidence:

- Class I: Benefit > > > risk—the procedure/treatment should be performed/administered
- Class IIa: Benefit > > risk—additional studies with focused objectives are needed
- Class II: Benefit ≥ risk—additional studies with broad objectives are needed; additional registry data would be helpful
- Class III: No benefit, or harm

The 2017 European Society of Cardiology (ESC) guidelines for the management of acute myocardial infarction [19] give slightly different levels of evidence:

- Level of evidence A: Data derived from multiple randomized clinical trials or meta-analyses
- Level of evidence B: Data derived from a single randomized clinical trial or large nonrandomized studies
- Level of evidence C: Consensus of opinion of experts and/or small studies, retrospective studies, registries

but also four classes:

- Class I: Evidence and/or general agreement that a given treatment or procedure is beneficial, useful, and effective
- Class II: Conflicting evidence and/or a divergence of opinion about the usefulness/efficacy of the given treatment or procedure
- Class IIa: Weight of evidence/opinion in favor of usefulness/efficacy
- Class IIb: Usefulness/efficacy less well established by evidence/opinion
- Class III: Evidence or general agreement that the given treatment or procedure is not useful/effective and in some cases may be harmful

As Masic et al. [3] point out, the reason for the great interest in EBM is the awareness that in many cases medical practice cannot keep pace with the available clinical practice.

Obviously, one can find many similar types of evidence. What is important to discuss is what progress has been achieved a quarter century on, as suggested by Djulbegovic and Guyatt [20]. They highlight the role of EBM in the development of standards for clinical research measuring practice.

In this context, Masic et al. [3] stress that EBM is not "cookbook" medicine. It integrates the best external evidence with individual clinical expertise.

Very succinctly, Djulbegovic and Guyatt [20] point out that the first EBM epistemological principle is that not all evidence is created equal, and that medicine should be based on the best available evidence. According to these authors, the second principle endorses the philosophical view that the pursuit of truth is best accomplished by evaluating the totality of evidence and not selecting evidence that favors a particular claim [21]. They note that many investigators have given examples of biased research leading to suboptimal medical research, and that EBM, since its inception, has developed processes for assessing the quality of evidence [22]. They give a very succinct description of the hierarchy of evidence, comparing traditional EBM and the Grading of Recommendations Assessment, Development, and Evaluation (GRADE) classification of the quality of evidence [20] (Fig. 3.1).

They point out that earlier formulations classified systematic reviews at the top, above RCTs, which is misguided. However, they accept that systematic reviews are essential for developing clinical practice guidelines and for forming the design of new research studies. Thus, an international prospective register of "systematic

a

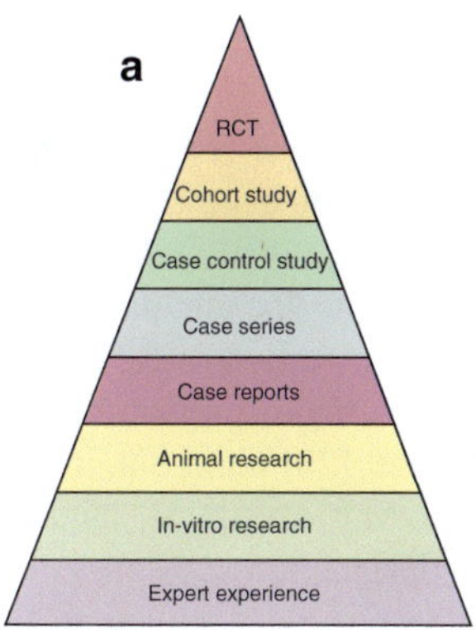

b

Quality of evidence	Study design	Lower quality if*	Higher quality if†
High	Randomised trial	Study limitations -1 serious -2 very serious	Large effect + 1 large + 2 very large
Moderate		Inconsistency -1 serious -2 very serious	Dose response + 1 evidence of a gradient
Low	Observational study	Indirectness -1 serious -2 very serious	All plausible confounders + Would reduce a demonstrated effect or + Would suggest a spurious effect when results show no effect
Very low		Imprecision -1 serious -2 very serious Publication bias -1 likely -2 very likely	

Fig. 3.1 Hierarchy of evidence: comparison of the traditional evidence-based medicine (EBM) hierarchy of evidence (1991–2004) and the Grading of Recommendations Assessment, Development, and Evaluation (GRADE) classification of the quality of evidence (confidence, certainty; 2004 to the present). (**a**) Traditional EBM hierarchy of evidence. (**b**) GRADE classification of the quality of evidence. RCT randomized controlled trial. *Quality of study moves down one or two grades. †Quality of study moves up one or two grades. (Reproduced from Djulbegovic and Guyatt [20], with permission)

reviews" has been created, with increasing sophistication of methods [23]. Also, systematic reviews help in avoiding duplicate research. Djulbegovic and Guyatt [20] describe how the Cochrane collaboration was instrumental for advances in systematic review methodology [24]. They also describe how the recognition of variation in medical practice [25] led the US Institute of Medicine to call for the development and application of clinical practice guidelines [26].

Data from the USA suggest that 30% of health care is inappropriate or wasteful, that only 55% of needed health services are delivered, and that a third of all deaths occur annually as a result of medical errors.

GRADE was first published in 2004 [27, 28] and, according to Djulbegovic and Guyatt [20], it provides a much more sophisticated hierarchy of evidence. It provides guidance for assessing the quality of evidence not only in therapy but also for diagnosis, prognosis, animal studies, and network meta-analysis [25]. According to the same authors [20, 29], the factors that determine decision making are the effect of:

1. The context or framing
2. Situational or contextual factors
3. The individual characteristics of the decision maker [30]

The same authors point out, correctly, that what determines the decision is evidence in the context of values and preferences. Finally, they [20] discuss three major criticisms of EBM.

The first is that the evidence hierarchy pyramid, as shown in Fig. 3.1, is narrow and simplistic [31].

The second is that EBM promotes "cookbook medicine," leading to automatic decision making, and encourages logarithmic approaches [32], leading away from the focus on the individual. However, Djulbegovic and Guyatt [20] and the author of this chapter point out that EBM encourages consideration for the individual patient and provides guides for subgroup analysis [33]. In fact, Masic et al. [3] comment that any guidelines must be integrated with individual clinical expertise. Tenny and Gossman [2] point out that clinicians must use their professional and clinical expertise to extrapolate the scientific evidence as it applies to the specific patient.

A third criticism is that there is no strong evidence that application of EBM has improved patient care. Here the time lag already described, from publication to application is reminded. However, as Djulbegovic and Guyatt [20] point out, it has discouraged many ineffective therapies. In fact, according to Masic et al. [3], another claim is that EBM is inspired by industry interests, and that many RCTs are conducted by industry. I am of the opinion that waiting for the results of the last RCT before guidelines are finalized by an expert group seems to be overreaching.

Masic et al. [3] point out EBM can assist family medicine.

In 2016, Sheridan and Julian [34] discussed the achievements and limitations of EBM, and they noted that EBM has extended its influence over the past two decades, which is a notable achievement. They pointed out that the Cochrane collaboration is the most prominent result of the efforts of EBM. As Djulbegovic and Guyatt [20] comment the Cochrane collaboration has marshaled over 3700 collaborators from more than 130 countries [31] and, apart from reviewing RCTs, it also includes observational studies. As Masic et al. [3] point out, the Cochrane library is a collection of databases in medicine and other health care specialties. The Cochrane library had almost four million downloads in 2010 [16].

Sheridan and Julian [34] also point out that clinical guidelines are intimately connected to EBM, providing the means to disseminate what EBM advocates. EBM also increases awareness of "overdiagnosis" which, although it has very importantly addressed prostate [35] and breast cancer, has also been a feature of other campaigns. Also, they stress that EBM has contributed to efforts to reform medical ethics and professionalism [36]. EBM has also addressed inefficient, inaccurate, and wasteful therapies. Sheridan and Julian [34] also point out that one of the limitations of EBM is that it gives a restricted view of evidence in that it proposes that clinical judgment and mechanistic reasoning are less reliable forms of medicine [37].

Some limitations of clinical trials are described in Chap. 12. They are recapitulated here.

Nonrepresentativeness of trial subjects: It was observed by Lee et al. [38] that although 37% of patients admitted with acute myocardial infarction are older than 75 years of age, they accounted for only 2% of patients with acute coronary syndromes in trials from 1966 to 1990 and only 9% of those from 1991 to 2000; women were also underrepresented.

Long-term therapy: Although many drugs have been used for many years, clinical trial evidence is available for only 5–10 years.

Many patients with morbidities are excluded from clinical trials [39]. Statistical significance, as opposed to clinical significance, must be mentioned. Sheridan and Julian [34] point out that a skilled statistician can, by introducing "corrections," change a p value from 0.051 to 0.049; they mention the Metoprolol in Acute Myocardial Infarction (MIAMI) trial [40] and a low-dose aspirin trial [41].

Misleading results: Sheridan and Julian [34] stress that clinical guidelines depend mainly on meta-analysis, and systematic review bias is well recognized [42]; also, there is a reluctance on the part of journals to publish negative results. They [34] also discuss the contrasting conclusion of two systematic reviews on β-blockers. Maggioni et al. [43] concluded that there was a significant reduction in mortality (in 27,536 patients), while Freemantle et al. [44], in a systematic review of 29,260 patients, showed no significant reduction in mortality.

Some adverse effects of EBM are further mentioned by Sheridan and Julian [34].

Bias of the easily measurable: This refers to omission of elements that are more difficult to quantify, such as quality of care, patients' experience of illness, respect for human dignity, and contribution to the knowledge base. It must be remembered that in many trials, greatly variable results are seen in different countries and different geographical regions.

They [34] also describe differences of views between epidemiologists and clinicians. Tenny and Grossman [2] cite another example: Is a randomized trial needed to prove that parachutes save lives?

Bias in commissioned research: There is a contrast between the view that scientists should lead research [24] and the view advocating that government departments that fund research should commission and oversee the research.

Comparative research versus original science: They [34] describe that EBM tries to determine the best available treatment whereas original science seeks to explore and discover new knowledge.

Also, they poignantly point out the need to avoid overdiagnosis and overtreatment, as in the case of prostatic cancer, which remains a major case of death in males. In my view, too much methodology may stifle the quest for new progress. For example, I have not followed the recommendation from the American Urological Society that patients over 70 years of age should no longer undergo prostate-specific antigen (PSA) testing; nor have I instructed my cardiological patients to forego such testing, with all due respect to statistical research–based guidelines.

Another aspect of the creation of guidelines is that despite I–V and A–D levels and classes, finally a consensus/compromise is reached.

Interestingly, both Djubelgovic and Guyatt [20] and Sheridan and Julian [34] try to foresee the future of EBM. The latter [34] stress that the concept is an explicit element of professionalism. They also remark that EBM should also be applied to health policy and reforms. Also, EBM must be independent in terms of selection of the topics that are addressed, and it must not be subject to the motive of "research commissioners," whether commercial or political. Djubelgovic and Guyatt [20] try to foresee the next 25 years of EBM. They stress that more efficient production and dissemination of both systematic reviews and practice guidelines will be needed [41, 45]. This will require improvement of research teams and writing efficiency [46], and strong electronic platforms. It will have to utilize the evidence generated by big data [47], as discussed elsewhere in this chapter. The development of a continuously learning health care system [48] is considered a necessity.

In conclusion, research has become more complicated, necessitating integrative efforts such as the systems-based approach. Larger databases, acquired much faster, are indispensable.

Finally, if all of this unprecedented wealth of knowledge is to be useful and beneficial for the individual patient or health care systems, it must be evaluated using the evaluation methods provided by EBM.

3.2 Precision Medicine

Precision medicine (Pr Med) is an aspect of personalized medicine. It has already been discussed that EBM does not preclude personalized medicine. A definition has been given by the National Academy of Sciences, as referred to by Giardino et al. [49]:

> Precision medicine refers to the tailoring of medical treatment to the individual characteristics of each patient, encompassing the ability to classify individuals into subpopulations that differ in their susceptibility to a particular disease, in the biology and/or prognosis of those diseases that may develop, or in their response to a specific treatment.

The first definition, used by Collins et al. [50, 51], was "using information about a person's genetic makeup to tailor strategies for the detection, treatment, or prevention of disease."

Actually the term "personalized medicine" was probably first used in 1971 by Gibson [52].

According to a recent special review by Giardino et al. [53], Pr Med takes into account individual viability in genetic and environmental factors. Jameson and Longo [54] point out that in Pr Med, treatments are tailored for genetic, biomarker, phenotypical, or psychosocial characteristics that distinguish individual patients from others with similar clinical features. The same authors also state that the ultimate aim of application of Pr Med is to improve clinical outcomes, and they point out that the terms "precision medicine," "personalized medicine," and "individualized medicine" are often used interchangeably. As Monsieur Jourdain complains in *Le Bourgeois Gentilhomme*, published by Molière in 1670, "I have been speaking prose for more than 40 years without knowing it." Many physicians, especially in previous generations, have believed that they have always practiced personalized medicine, which is certainly true with regard to the patient but actually not to the disease context. Technological advances are obligatory drivers of Pr Med. In their Table 3.1, they [54] give examples in which Pr Med has been used: chronic myeloid leukemia, lung cancer, thrombosis, human immunodeficiency virus/acquired immune deficiency syndrome (HIV/AIDS), coronary artery disease, cystic fibrosis, kidney transplant rejection, hepatitis C, hyperlipidemia, autoimmune encephalitis, alcohol use disorder, smoking cessation, and Leber congenital amaurosis. The diagnosis of these disorders is based on definite biomarkers.

As Giardino et al. [53] stress, the acceptance of Pr Med is boosted by advances in genomics, molecular biology, information technology, and imaging. As reported by the National Human Research Institute, a high-quality "draft" whole-genome sequence costed less than $1500 as of July 2016. In a similar vein, Hayden wrote about a $1000 genome study [55]. Hunt and Jha [56] postulated that Pr Med may reduce overdiagnosis and promote selection of the best therapies for the right patient at the right time [8].

There is a momentum toward making personalized medicine more precise [57].

3.3 Artificial Intelligence

With regard to the application of Pr Med in cardiovascular medicine, Krittanawong et al. [58] describe the role of artificial intelligence (AI) in precision cardiovascular medicine. They state that AI is a field of computer science that aims to mimic human thought processes, learning capacity, and knowledge storage. They offer a very illustrative general estimation on how AI can aid precision cardiovascular medicine. Geoffrey Pitt [59] offers many paradigms of how Pr Med advances will aid cardiology, including heart failure treatment, the CHA_2DS_2-VASc scoring system, and identification of specific genetic loci for long-QT syndrome (LQTS) and genetic polymorphisms affecting clopidogrel efficacy.

As Joyner [60] recently pointed out, Pr Med includes ideas about generating new targets for therapeutic intervention and development of new drug classes. As compared with "personalized medicine," Pr Med implies greater accuracy; it can offer increased accuracy on top of personal treatment that attempts to consider the multifactorial nature of the individual circumstances. Joyner [60] considers application of Pr Med in diseases with a genetic component, diagnostics, preventive medicine, pharmacogenomics, and gene and drug therapy. He believes that the question as to whether this can reduce costs is still open, since economic projections of potential cost savings are challenging and subject to frequent revisions [61, 62].

Antman and Loscalzo [63] underline that new tools will be needed for describing the cardiovascular health status of individuals and populations, including "-omics" data, the exposome, social determinants of health, the microbiome, behaviors and motivations, patient-generated data, and data from electronic medical records.

Claude Lenfant [64], a former director of the National Heart, Lung, and Blood Institute (NHLBI) at the National Institutes of Health (NIH), wrote in 2013 about the prospects of personalized medicine in cardiovascular disease (CVD). He stresses that knowledge of the genetic determinants of traits or diseases contributes to "personalized" medicine. He underlines that knowledge of genetic determinants must be coupled with examination of environmental factors and knowledge of the patients' medical and family history, physical status, and lifestyle. He emphasizes some important points regarding genome-wide association studies (GWAS):

> They are useful to identify large numbers of genetic variants associated with CVD, but they have failed to explain mechanisms of such associations, predict preclinical diagnosis and offer directions of prevention and therapy [65].

Lenfant [64] also points out that pharmacogenetics research has been accelerated by GWAS. He mainly stresses research on statins and clopidogrel. However, he underlines that the use of genotyping is not widely practiced yet. He also describes epigenetics as modifications that modify and regulate gene expression by DNA methylation and microRNA mechanisms. He refers to the conclusion of Guttmacher and Collins [66]:

> that all physicians will need to understand the concept of genetic variability in the context of its interaction with the environment.

Favalli et al. [67] question if personalized medicine and Pr Med represent a dream comes true. They stress that this new concept offers its best results in single gene disease models such as cystic fibrosis or pure restrictive cardiomyopathy. They describe that multifactorial CVDs share a similar pathological background but their causes may differ, and they may represent the end phenotypes of different diseases. Also, Favalli et al. [67] emphasize that the molecular bases of modifiable risk factors are only partially appreciated. Personalized medicine, which cannot be classified as the offspring of Pr Med, can have practical approaches. Thus, Savoia et al. [68] point out that data-driven studies have facilitated the evolution of these new modalities in hypertension. Kashyap et al. [69] point out that characterization of the "microbiome," which includes all of the microbes that reside within and upon the human organism, allows us to develop new preventive and therapeutic strategies by using next-generation sequencing. They conclude that the microbiome represents a potentially modifiable factor amenable to targeting by therapeutics.

The concept of Pr Med is interwoven with other very important new approaches to disease diagnosis and management, such as systems biology, which is discussed in Chap. 4.

DeVries et al. [70] describe that as the genomic field expands and medicine becomes more personalized, identification of methods to protect data content needs to be established. Thus, they expand on the systems-based approach to managing data in research core facilities. They stress that recognition of the need for specialized support for data management has become a critical component of institutional services.

Bland et al. [71] point out that in chronic disease, the current predominant health care approach is inappropriate, ignores the subclinical stage of disease development, and lacks the ability to properly address disease-promoting lifestyles. They propose personalized lifestyle medicine as first-line therapy and discuss the need to harness -omics technologies in personalized lifestyle medicine. For example, they describe that in research on prevention of recurrent colorectal adenomas, [72] prevention of overweight [73], specific single-nucleotide polymorphisms (SNPs) have been found. They mention that in the Data-as-a-Service Platform for Healthy Lifestyle and Preventive Medicine (DAPHNE) project, management of the obesity epidemic will be attempted via personalized lifestyle medicine [74].

Also, the pioneering 100 Person Wellness Project will integrate longitudinal information from whole-genome sequencing, clinical and functional lab testing, gut microbiome analysis, and quantified self-measures [75, 76] to optimize health management and affect disease prevention.

The concepts of data management advanced by DeVries et al. [70] again bring into scope the emerging field already mentioned by Krittanawong et al. [58]. Thus, McCue and McCoy [77] ascribe the increased interest in the application of big data to health care to advances in high-throughput molecular biology and electronic health records. According to those authors, big data promises more personalized medicine and Pr Med, with improved accuracy and earlier diagnosis.

Another concept is that of the contribution of AI to medical practice. Miller and Brown [78] offer a very succinct review. They stress that AI offers diagnostic speed and accuracy exceeding those of the "experts." Machine learning directly from medical data could avert clinical errors due to human cognitive biases. However, Miller and Brown [78] stress that because AI is neither astute nor intuitive, physicians will remain essential to cognitive medical practice, and they mention that combining pathologists and deep learning has been shown to optimize performance and reduce human error by 85% [79].

In this sense, Krittanawong [80]—one of the researchers greatly involved in this subject—discusses the rise of AI and the uncertain future for physicians. He stresses that physicians can analyze big data but this requires much time and supercomputers, which few doctors utilize. He believes that while AI could assist physicians in many ways, it is unlikely to replace physicians in the foreseeable future. Hamet et al. [81] give a simple definition of AI, implying the use of a computer to model intelligent behavior with no or minimal human intervention. They stress that it has two main branches: The *virtual branch* includes informatics approaches, from deep learning information management to control of health management systems, including electronic health records and active guidance of doctors in their therapeutic decisions. In the *physical branch*, robots and nanorobots are listed.

The connection of AI with personalized medicine has been referred to previously by Hamburg and Collins [82]. They underline that the NIH and the US Food and Drug Administration (FDA) have personalized medicine as a main goal. They also stress that moving from concept to clinical use requires basic, translational, and regulatory science. The former two types of science have already been described. The FDA is developing the regulatory science standards and evidence needed for use in drug and genetic information, in drug and device development, and in clinical decision making.

In this chapter I have tried to describe the various aspects of research and how they can affect personal, community, and world health. The problems are getting more complex, but the goals are becoming greater and continuously more important.

In conclusion, in a 2017 review on AI in cardiology, Bonderman [83] describes that in cardiovascular biomedicine, four big data sources are important:

1. Functional phenotypes (demographics, electrocardiography (ECG), echo, imaging)
2. Molecular profiles
3. Medical records
4. Literature knowledge

She stresses that many ethical aspects are associated with the use of AI, including transparency in ethical efforts, threats to privacy, human rights, and even robot rights.

Johnson et al. [84] also stress that AI in cardiovascular medicine can aid in research and development, clinical practice, and population health.

Since big data have been mentioned, it should be noted that Hemingway et al. [85] recently described their importance for electronic health records and the challenges and potential for cardiovascular translational research.

References

1. Sackett DL, Rosenberg WM, Gray JA, Haynes RB, Richardson WS. Evidence based medicine: what it is and what it isn't. BMJ. 1996;312:71–2.
2. Tenny S, Gossman WG. Evidence based medicine (EBM). Treasure Island: StatPearls Publishing, 2018.
3. Masic I, Miokovic M, Muhamedagic B. Evidence based medicine—new approaches and challenges. Acta Inform Med. 2008;16:219–25.
4. Farquhar C. Evidence-based medicine—the promise, the reality. Aust N Z J Obstet Gynaecol. 2018;58:17–21.

5. Guyatt G, Cairns J, Churchill D, et al. Evidence-based medicine: a new approach to teaching the practice of medicine. JAMA. 1992;268:2420–5.
6. Sackett DL, Rosenberg WM. Evidence based medicine: what it is and what it isn't. BMJ. 1996;13:71–2.
7. Guyatt G, Rennie D, editors. Users' guides to the medical literature: a manual for evidence-based clinical practice. Chicago: American Medical Association; 2002.
8. Burns PB, Rohrich RJ, Chung KC. The levels of evidence and their role in evidence-based medicine. Plast Reconstr Surg. 2011;128:305–10.
9. The periodic health examination. Canadian Task Force on the Periodic Health Examination. Can Med Assoc J. 1979;121:1193–254.
10. Sackett DL. Rules of evidence and clinical recommendations on the use of antithrombotic agents. Chest. 1989;95:2S–4S.
11. Robert Lawrence, US Preventive Services Task Force Edition. Guide to clinical preventive services. Darby: Diane; 1989. ISBN 1568062974. Retrieved 9 Dec 2014.
12. US Preventive Services Task Force. Guide to clinical preventive services: report of the US Preventive Services Task Force. Darby: Diane; 1989. p. 24. ISBN 978-1-56806-297-6. Appendix A.
13. Centre for Evidence-Based Medicine. Oxford Centre for Evidence-Based Medicine—levels of evidence (March 2009). https://www.cebm.net/2009/06/oxford-centre-evidence-based-medicine-levels-evidence-march-2009/. Accessed 25 Mar 2015.
14. Adapted from the American Society of Plastic Surgeons. http://www.plasticsurgery.org/Medical_Professionals/Health_Policy_and_Advocacy/Health_Policy_Resources/Evidence-based_GuidelinesPractice_Parameters/Description_and_Development_of_Evidence-based_Practice_Guidelines/ASPS_Evidence_Rating_Scales.html.
15. Sackett DL. Evidence-based medicine. Semin Perinatol. 1997;21:3–5.
16. Dunning J, Prendergast B, Mackway-Jones K. Towards evidence-based medicine in cardiothoracic surgery: best BETS. Interact Cardiovasc Thorac Surg. 2003;2:405–9.
17. Scanlon PJ, Faxon DP, Audet AM, Carabello B, Dehmer GJ, Eagle KA, et al. ACC/AHA guidelines for coronary angiography: executive summary and recommendations. A report of the American College of Cardiology/American Heart Association Task Force on Practice Guidelines (Committee on Coronary Angiography) developed in collaboration with the Society for Cardiac Angiography and Interventions. Circulation. 1999;99:2345–57.
18. Amsterdam EA, Wenger NK, Brindis RG, et al. 2014 AHA/ACC guideline for the management of patients with non-ST-elevation acute coronary syndromes: executive summary. A report of the American College of Cardiology/American Heart Association Task Force on Practice Guidelines. Circulation. 2014;130:2354–94.
19. Ibanez B, et al. 2017 ESC guidelines for the management of acute myocardial infarction in patients presenting with ST-segment elevation: the Task Force for the Management of Acute Myocardial Infarction in Patients Presenting with ST-Segment Elevation of the European Society of Cardiology (ESC). Eur Heart J. 2018;39(2):119–77.
20. Djulbegovic B, Guyatt GH. Progress in evidence-based medicine: a quarter century on. Lancet. 2017;390:415–23.
21. Djulbegovic B, Guyatt GH, Ashcroft RE. Epistemologic inquiries in evidence-based medicine. Cancer Control. 2009;16:158–68.
22. Atkins D, Best D, Briss PA, Eccles M, Falck-Ytter Y, Flottorp S, et al. Grading quality of evidence and strength of recommendations. BMJ. 2004;328:1490.
23. PROSPERO. International registry of systematic reviews. http://www.crd.york.ac.uk/prospero. Accessed 21 Apr 2016.
24. Chalmers I. The Cochrane collaboration: preparing, maintaining, and disseminating systematic reviews of the effects of health care. Ann N Y Acad Sci. 1993;703:156–63; discussion 163–5.
25. Wenneberg J. Which rate is right? N Engl J Med. 1986;314:310–1.

26. Institute of Medicine (US) Committee to Advise the Public Health Service on Clinical Practice Guidelines. In: Field MJ, Lohr KN, editors. Clinical practice guidelines: directions for a new agency. Washington, DC: National Academy Press; 1990.
27. Atkins D, Eccles M, Flottorp S, et al. Systems for grading the quality of evidence and the strength of recommendations I: critical appraisal of existing approaches. The GRADE Working Group. BMC Health Serv Res. 2004;4:38.
28. GRADE Working Group. List of GRADE Working Group publications and grants. 2016. http://www.gradeworkinggroup.org. Accessed 21 Aug 2016.
29. Djulbegovic B. A framework to bridge the gaps between evidence-based medicine, health outcomes, and improvement and implementation science. J Oncol Pract. 2014;10:200–2.
30. Appelt KC, Milch KF, Handgraaf MJJ, Weber EU. The decision making individual deferences inventory and guidelines for the study of individual deferences in judgment and decision-making research. Judgm Decis Mak. 2011;6:252–62.
31. Montori VM, Guyatt GH. Progress in evidence-based medicine. JAMA. 2008;300:1814–6.
32. Greenhalgh T, Howick J, Maskrey N. Evidence based medicine: a movement in crisis? BMJ. 2014;348:g3725.
33. Sun X, Briel M, Walter SD, Guyatt GH. Is a subgroup effect believable? Updating criteria to evaluate the credibility of subgroup analyses. BMJ. 2010;340:c117.
34. Sheridan DJ, Julian DG. Achievements and limitations of evidence-based medicine. J Am Coll Cardiol. 2016;68:204–13.
35. Dahm P, Kunz R, Schünemann H. Evidence-based clinical practice guidelines for prostate cancer: the need for a unified approach. Curr Opin Urol. 2007;17:200–7.
36. Royal College of Physicians. Doctors in society: medical professionalism in a changing world. Report of a working party of the Royal College of Physicians of London. 2005. https://cdn.shopify.com/s/files/1/0924/4392/files/doctors_in_society_reportweb.pdf?15745311214883953343. Accessed 4 May 2016.
37. Guyatt GH. Evidence-based medicine. ACP J Club. 1991;114:A16.
38. Lee PY, Alexander KP, Hammill BG, Pasquali SK, Peterson ED. Representation of elderly persons and women in published randomized trials of acute coronary syndromes. JAMA. 2001;286:708–13.
39. Jadad AR, To MJ, Emara M, Jones J. Consideration of multiple chronic diseases in randomized controlled trials. JAMA. 2011;306:2670–2.
40. MIAMI Trial Research Group. Long-term prognosis after early intervention with metoprolol in suspected acute myocardial infarction: experiences from the MIAMI Trial. J Intern Med. 1991;230:233–7.
41. Roncaglioni MC, Collaborative Group of the Primary Prevention Project (PPP). Low-dose aspirin and vitamin E in people at cardiovascular risk: a randomised trial in general practice. Lancet. 2001;357:89–95.
42. Reveiz L, Chapman E, Asial S, Munoz S, Bonfill X, Alonso-Coello P. Risk of bias of randomized trials over time. J Clin Epidemiol. 2015;68:1036–45.
43. Maggioni AP, Latini R, Tognoni G, et al. Pain relief, general management and other adjunctive treatments. In: Yusuf S, Cairns JA, Camm AJ, et al., editors. Evidence based cardiology. 2nd ed. London: BMJ; 2003. p. 482.
44. Freemantle N, Cleland J, Young P, et al. B blockade after myocardial infarction: systematic review and meta regression analysis. BMJ. 1999;318:1730–7.
45. Black N. A national strategy for research and development: lessons from England. Annu Rev Public Health. 1997;18:485–505.
46. Schünemann HJ, Moja L. Reviews: rapid! rapid! rapid!…and systematic. Syst Rev. 2015;4:1–3.
47. Sim I. Two ways of knowing: big data and evidence-based medicine. Ann Intern Med. 2016;164:562–3.
48. Eddy DM. Evidence-based medicine: a unified approach. Health Aff (Millwood). 2005;24:9–17.
49. National Research Council. Washington, toward precision medicine: building a knowledge network for biomedical research and a new taxonomy of disease. Washington, DC: National Academies Press, 2011.

50. Collins FS, Varmus H. A new initiative on precision medicine. N Engl J Med. 2015;372:793–5.
51. Collins FS, Green ED, Guttmacher AE, Guyer MS, US National Human Genome Research Institute. A vision for the future of genomics research. Nature. 2003;422:835–47.
52. Gibson WM. Can personalized medicine survive? Can Fam Physician. 1971;17:29–88.
53. Giardino A, Gupta S, Olson E, Sepulveda K, Lenchik L, Ivanidze J, et al. Role of imaging in the era of precision medicine. Acad Radiol. 2017;24:639–49.
54. Jameson JL, Longo DL. Precision medicine—personalized, problematic, and promising. N Engl J Med. 2015;372:2229–34.
55. Hayden EC. Technology: the $1,000 genome. Nature. 2014;507(7492):294–5.
56. Hunt S, Jha S. Can precision medicine reduce overdiagnosis? Acad Radiol. 2015;22:1040–1.
57. Katsnelson A. Momentum grows to make 'personalized' medicine more 'precise'. Nature Med. 2013;19:249.
58. Krittanawong C, Zhang H, Wang Z, Aydar M, Kitai T. Artificial intelligence in precision cardiovascular medicine. J Am Coll Cardiol. 2017;69:2657–64.
59. Pitt GS. Cardiovascular precision medicine: hope or hype? Eur Heart J. 2015;36:1842–23.
60. Joyner MJ. Precision medicine, cardiovascular disease and hunting elephants. Prog Cardiovasc Dis. 2016;58:651–60.
61. Lord J, Willis S, Eatock J, Tappenden P, Trapero-Bertran M, Miners A, et al. Economic modelling of diagnostic and treatment pathways in National Institute for Health and Care Excellence clinical guidelines: the Modelling Algorithm Pathways in Guidelines (MAPGuide) project. Health Technol Assess. 2013;17(58):v–vi, 1–192.
62. Burgers LT, Redekop WK, Severens JL. Challenges in modelling the cost effectiveness of various interventions for cardiovascular disease. Pharmacoeconomics. 2014;32:627–37.
63. Antman EM, Loscalzo J. Precision medicine in cardiology. Nat Rev Cardiol. 2016;13:591–602.
64. Lenfant C. Prospects of personalized medicine in cardiovascular diseases. Metabolism. 2013;62(Suppl 1):S6–10.
65. O'Donnell CJ, Nabel EG. Genomics of cardiovascular disease. N Engl J Med. 2011;365: 2098–109.
66. Guttmacher AE, Collins FS. Genomic medicine—a primer. N Engl J Med. 2002;347:1512–20.
67. Favalli V, Serio A, Giuliani LP, Arbustini E. 'Precision and personalized medicine,' a dream that comes true? J Cardiovasc Med (Hagerstown). 2017;18(Suppl 1):e1–6.
68. Savoia C, Volpe M, Grassi G, Borghi C, Agabiti Rosei E, Touyz RM. Personalized medicine—a modern approach for the diagnosis and management of hypertension. Clin Sci (Lond). 2017;131:2671–85.
69. Kashyap PC, Chia N, Nelson H, Segal E, Elinav E. Microbiome at the frontier of personalized medicine. Mayo Clin Proc. 2017;92:1855–64.
70. DeVries M, Fenchel M, Fogarty RE, Kim BD, Timmons D, White AN. Name it! Store it! Protect it! A systems approach to managing data in research core facilities. J Biomol Tech. 2017;28:137–41.
71. Bland JS, Minich DM, Eck BM. A systems medicine approach: translating emerging science into individualized wellness. Adv Med. 2017;2017:1718957.
72. Barry EL, Peacock JL, Rees JR, Bostick RM, Robertson DJ, Bresalier RS, et al. Vitamin D receptor genotype, vitamin D3 supplementation, and risk of colorectal adenomas: a randomized clinical trial. JAMA Oncol. 2017;3:628–35.
73. Huang T, Qi Q, Li Y, Hu FB, Bray GA, Sacks FM, et al. FTO genotype, dietary protein, and change in appetite: the Preventing Overweight Using Novel Dietary Strategies trial. Am J Clin Nutr. 2014;99:1126–30.
74. Gibbons C, Bailador Del Pozo G, Andrés J, Lobstein T, Manco M, Lewy H, et al. Data-as-a-service platform for delivering healthy lifestyle and preventive medicine: concept and structure of the DAPHNE project. JMIR Res Protoc. 2016;5:e222.
75. Hood L, Lovejoy JC, Price ND. Integrating big data and actionable health coaching to optimize wellness. BMC Med. 2015;13:4.
76. Price ND, Magis AT, Earls JC, Glusman G, Levy R, Lausted C, et al. A wellness study of 108 individuals using personal, dense, dynamic data clouds. Nat Biotechnol. 2017;35:747–56.

77. McCue ME, McCoy AM. The scope of big data in one medicine: unprecedented opportunities and challenges. Front Vet Sci. 2017;4:194.
78. Miller DD, Brown EW. Artificial intelligence in medical practice: the question to the answer? Am J Med. 2018;131:129–33.
79. Wang D, Khosa A, Gargeya R, Irshad H, Beck AH. Deep learning for identifying breast cancer. Proceedings of the International Society on Biomedical Imaging. 2016.
80. Krittanawong C. The rise of artificial intelligence and the uncertain future for physicians. Eur J Intern Med. 2018;48:e13–4.
81. Hamet P, Tremblay J. Artificial intelligence in medicine. Metabolism. 2017;69S:S36–40.
82. Hamburg MA, Collins FS. The path to personalized medicine. N Engl J Med. 2010;363:301–4.
83. Bonderman D. Artificial intelligence in cardiology. Wien Klin Wochenschr. 2017;129:866–8.
84. Johnson KW, Torres Soto J, Glicksberg BS, Shameer K, Miotto R, Ali M, et al. Artificial intelligence in cardiology. J Am Coll Cardiol. 2018;71:2668–79.
85. Hemingway H, Asselbergs FW, Danesh J, Dobson R, Maniadakis N, Maggioni A, et al. Big data from electronic health records for early and late translational cardiovascular research: challenges and potential. Eur Heart J. 2018;39:1481–95.

Chapter 4
The Systems Biology Approach

Dennis V. Cokkinos

4.1 General Knowledge

Albert Einstein (1879–1955) wrote among others that: Things should be as simple as possible but not simpler.

Actually, "things" have become much more complicated in cardiovascular research.

As Lusis and Weiss [1] pointed out already 8 years ago, traditional biological and biochemical studies involve relatively few components. However, the addition of new data has increased explosively. To explain and integrate all of them, we need a more global analysis and integrative quantitative mathematical models. The new branch of biology, "systems biology," introduces this approach [2].

According to the Department of Systems Biology of the Harvard Medical School [3]:

- Systems biology is the study of systems of biological components, which may be molecules, cells, organisms or entire species. Living systems are dynamic and complex, and their behavior may be hard to predict from the properties of individual parts.

Lusis [4] describes that "systems level" means a biologic analysis that looks beyond individual genes or proteins or lipids to the ensemble of multiple elements of the system.

In a perspicacious editorial in 2013, Mayr [5] highlights this process: from data gathering to systems medicine.

He underlines that the "omics" technology, genomics, transcriptomics, proteomics, and metabolomics, creates the necessity to understand this complex interplay [6].

D. V. Cokkinos (✉)
Heart and Vessel Department, Biomedical Research Foundation,
Academy of Athens - Gregory Skalkeas, Athens, Greece
e-mail: dcokkinos@bioacademy.gr

D. V. Cokkinos (ed.), *Myocardial Preservation*,
https://doi.org/10.1007/978-3-319-98186-4_4

Lusis and Weiss [1] define as a central concept of systems biology that networks rather than classical linear pathways characterize biological processes.

These biological networks occur in many different levels, i.e., gene transcripts, proteins, metabolites, organelles, cells, organs, whole organisms, and even social systems.

In fact, every type of complex and interinfluencing process can be described as a network.

According to Chautard et al. [7], this emergent field, called systems biology, is the study of an organism, viewed as an integrated and interacting networking of genes, proteins, and biochemical reactions which give rise to life.

Chuang et al. [8], describing "a decade of systems biology," point out that systems approaches by necessity involve systematic data. It is a framework for using genome-scale experiments to perform predictive, hypothesis-driven science.

According to Albert Laszlo Barabasi, cited by Lusis and Weiss [1], "If there is any area in which a network thinking could trigger a revolution, I believe that biology is it."

As Shreenivasaiah et al. [9] describe, systems biology allows the coordinated study of biological systems by studying the components of cellular networks and interactions. These can be affected through high-throughput omics data and with use of computation methods (Fig. 4.1).

According to Lusis and Weiss [1], system-based definition of the approach involves four steps:

1. Systems to be examined (e.g., a cardiomyocyte)
2. The components of the system
3. How the components interact with each other
4. To determine the dynamics of the networks mathematically (i.e., how they change over time or responds to various perturbations)

These authors [1] give an excellent paradigm of the components of cardiovascular disease, which represents a network of many and varied processes.

They reproduce the phenotypic database network proposed by Hidalgo et al. [10], showing all diseases connected to hypertension and ischemic heart disease.

Dirk Brutsaert [11] has pointed out already that Heart Failure management is aided by Network Medicine. Thus, there exist interactions in the cell-organ system and disease networks.

According to Kalamatianos [12], systems biology is modeling: model-driven analysis is the application of experimental and computational tools, to produce new data.

Ideker et al. [2] stress that implementation of these systems follows a fundamental framework which involves many steps:

1. Definition of all the components
2. Assessment of perturbations and global monitoring of the components
3. Reconciliation of experimentally absent responses to those predicted by the model
4. Design and performance of new perturbation experiments to distinguish between multiple and competing model hypotheses

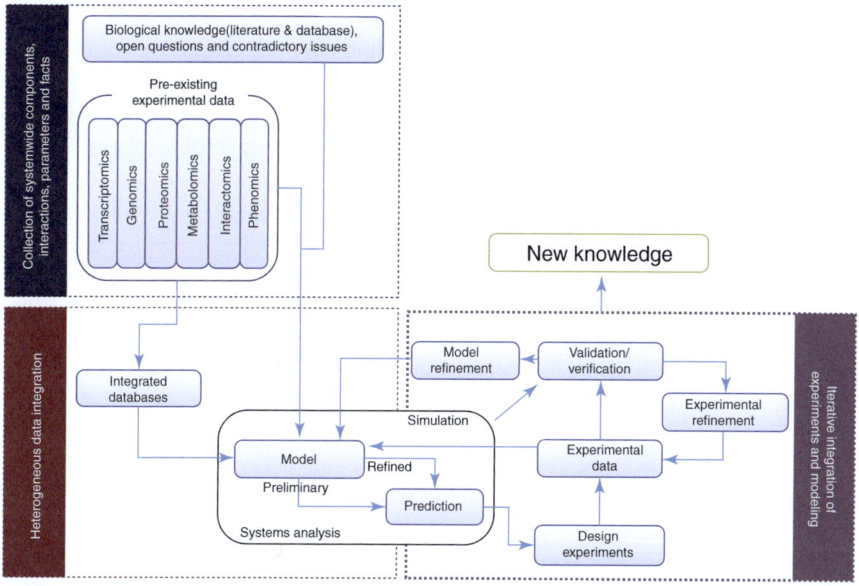

Fig. 4.1 Framework of systems biology: previous experimental and biological knowledge is used to formulate initial components and their relationships and to derive parameters for the selected biological questions. Further all these are systematically exploited to construct initial mathematical models to describe a biological phenomenon. Comparisons between experimental data generated and predicted results from various models can help in screening a valid model which best describes the data. In case of inconsistencies with the previously built model, existing models can be refined with the help of existing data, or one may also design new experiments to derive required parameters. The experimental data thus generated can be used to refine the model by integrating the data into the model. These iterative processes of matching experimental observation against model prediction can continue, until it results in a new knowledge. (Reproduced by permission from Shreenivasaiah et al. [9])

Weiss et al. [13] stress the necessity for all the elements to be studied and that systems biology involves a strategic interplay between discovery and hypothesis-driven science.

One of the concepts of systems biology is that instead of the linear pathways, networks best express biological processes. Components are called nodes, and their interactions are called edges or links. Some nodes have more interconnections and are called hubs. Networks are characterized by robustness, adaptability, and redundancy so that they are more protected than a linear pathway which can be more easily interrupted.

In this context Weiss et al. [12] describe the topology of network, i.e., the relationship between nodes and links and edges.

An elementary description of networks is necessary. According to Lusis and Weiss [1], one of the central concepts in systems biology is that networks, rather than classic linear pathways, underline biological processes: the interaction follows a much shorter way in the network than the linear pathway concept. Moreover, the linear approach may be efficient because it is simpler, but it sacrifices adaptability, because cutting just one link disrupts the chain.

A random network is characterized by a random, not preferential relationship.

An exponential network results after a random network grows over time: Older nodes will have a statistically greater probability to acquire more links.

The author is not an expert in translational research; however, while trying to comprehend this complex field during the last 20 year, hopes that his thoughts may help other interested learners even novices.

Barabasi, one of the fathers of the concept systems biology, and Bonabeau gave an excellent review 15 years ago [14].

A description of this well-simplified article is here attempted. For many of the previous years, systems were modeled by the random network type. This type consists of nodes with randomly placed connections. Most nodes have approximately the same number of links. It is a "democratic" type of network. The links to a node follow the Poisson distribution (bell-shaped), very few nodes having a large number of links [13].

Barabasi and Bonabeau [14] parallel this type of network to the US highway system. In this system if one connection fails, the corresponding node is isolated, and if a critical number of nodes are removed, the system breaks into small, non-communicable areas. The scale-free network resembles the airline system; if one even short and effective connection fails, the same airport can be reached through other although longer and more costly routes.

As Weiss et al. [13] describe when the "random network" begins to grow, the "older" nodes we will have a strategically greater chance to acquire new links, following an exponential instead of a Poisson distribution. This more complex network is characterized by more links. As this more advanced model grows further, new links preferentially are attached to already busy nodes, which become very busy and are now called "hubs." The model now becomes "scale free" [15].

Barabasi and Bonabeau [14] describe that in scale-free networks, as many 80% of the routes can fail and still a compact cluster can be maintained. However, although they are resistant to accidental failure, they are vulnerable to coordinated attacks.

Ravasz et al. [16] point out that living cells are dynamically interconnected especially as regards their metabolism; a fully connected biochemical network is described.

Both Barabasi and Bonabeau [14] and Weiss et al. [13] again stress that scale-free networks are more robust as compared to the random ones because since hubs have many links disruption of one or more links will not completely disconnect the node. Up to 80% of nodes or links can be randomly disrupted without having a major impact on the conductivity of the network.

However, these networks are vulnerable to targeting attacks: they can be disrupted if 5–15% of hubs are simultaneously eliminated [17].

If further growth occurs, more nodes acquire more numerous connections becoming "hubs," and the network becomes scale-free. Besides becoming much more difficult to disrupt, a new situation arises: Thus, the "rich get richer," since busier hubs develop "the lion's share" of connections. Robert K. Merton called this the Matthew effect [18] which may serve to heighten the visibility of contributions to science by scientists of acknowledged standing and to reduce the visibility of contributions by authors who are less well known.

Barabasi and Bonebeau stress [14] that 40 years ago networks were considered completely random, following a Poisson distribution with a bell shape. The scale-free theory was introduced by them in 1998.

4.2 Applications in Cardiovascular Disease

Lusis and Weiss [1] offer approaches as regards cardiovascular disease. Some pertinent examples include inflammation and macrophage activation as implicated in atherogenesis and the network mediated by TLRs, as described by Ramsey et al. [19].

A network of genes mediates the development of advanced atherosclerotic lesions in mice as described by Skogsberg et al. [20].

The genetic perturbation of the inflammatory network is associated with atherosclerosis [21].

The functional network for the cardiovascular system describes traits characterizing exercise and cardiac structure and function [22].

Systems biology also applies to genetics. Common forms of cardiovascular disease are due to both genetic and environmental factors, which both perturb molecular phenotypes, which in turn affect the cellular and physiological state contributing to the disease [23, 24].

Lusis and Weiss [1] created a graph of components (nodes-hubs-traits) and their interactions (connecting lines) in cardiovascular disease. Thus, they link metabolic factors, and atherogenesis factors to heart failure and myocardial infarction, as derived from work by Lusis et al. [20] and Topol et al. [25]. Important nodes are:

- Blood pressure levels, endothelium and smooth muscle, lipids, insulin, inflammation and gender, which lead to vascular instability leading to acute myocardial infarction which also affects platelets, coagulation, reperfusion injury, formation of collateral vessels, leading to functional derangements (arrhythmias)and structural derangements (hypertrophy, remodeling), leading to heart failure.

In a very pertinent review, Loscalzo et al. [26] propose a complex systems approach to human pathology to attain human disease classification in the postgenomic area. They stress that contemporary classification of human disease stems from correlation between pathological analysis and clinical syndromes. However, they believe that this strategy demonstrates both lack of sensitivity in identifying preclinical disease and lack of specificity in unequivocally defining disease. They also try to define disease phenotype. They give a diagram indicating associations among genetic and environmental factors. They also give many examples of network approaches to human disease (Fig. 4.2). They also describe that network analysis has been employed to characterize the spread and control of epidemics [27, 28] and novel targets to influence the metastatic propensity and lethality of prostate carcinoma [29], neurodegenerative disorders causing ataxia [30], and allergic asthma [31].

They also describe network approaching to therapeutics, with the aim of identifying new drug targets, determining appropriate dosage based on metabolomic profiling [32], and determining the causes of resistance or increased toxicity to drugs [33].

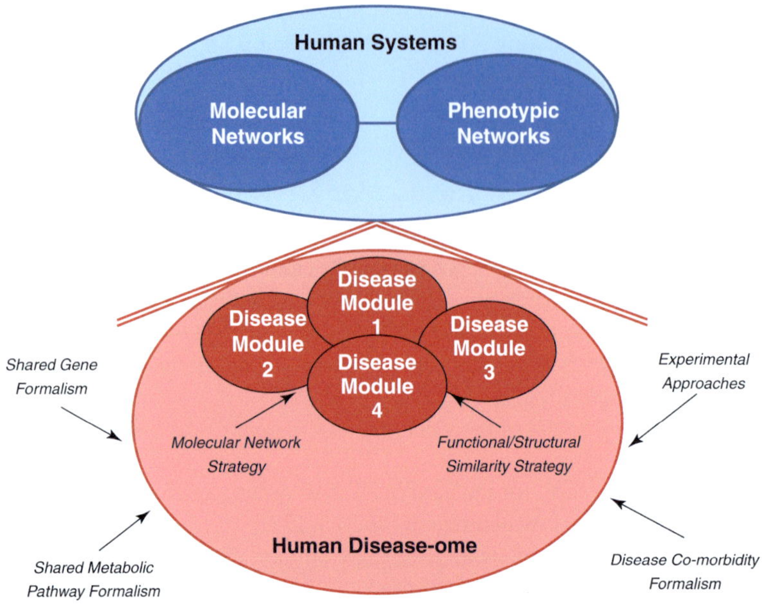

Fig. 4.2 The Human Systems Biology Universe. Human systems comprise molecular and phenotypic networks, which are related to, but distinct from, each other, as indicated by the separate linked ovals. The human diseasome represents a collection of subnetworks, the disease modules, which are identified by one of two strategies, the molecular network-based strategy or the functional and structural similarity-based strategy. The assembly of disease modules into the diseasome can be determined by bioinformatics-based approaches—the shared gene formalism, the shared metabolic pathway formalism, or the disease comorbidity formalism—or by laboratory-based experimentation. (Reproduced with permission from Loscalzo J et al. on Wiley Interdiscip Rev. Syst Biol Med. 2011;3:619–27)

Butcher et al. [34] in 2004 gave a very elegant perspective already in 2004 of how systems biology can aid drugs discovery. Huan et al. [35] used network-driven integrative analysis, using whole blood gene expression profiles from 188 pts with coronary heart disease and 188 controls to identifying related genes and their molecular interactions.

West, Geneston, and Grigolin [36] stress that complex networks include and "overarch" all traditional scientific descriptions. As examples they mention transportation, i.e., networks of planes, highways, and railroads, the economy networks of global finance and stock markets, social networks (governments, business, churches, terrorism), physical networks (global warming, telephones, Internet, earthquakes), and biological networks (gene regulation, human body, clusters of neurons). All these share universal properties, the more as they become more complex.

Our group [37] has proposed the creation of an "obesidome" to describe obesity interactions.

After offering so much, sometimes difficult to assimilate information, a very thoughtful commentary from Marc Kirschner [38] is appropriate. He reminds that in the beginning molecular biology was claimed to hardly differ from biochemistry.

He points out that systems biology offers an opportunity to study how the phenotype is generated from the genotype and with it a glimpse of how evolution has crafted the phenotype.

He underlines the importance of high-throughput biology and attempts a simple definition "that systems biology is the study of the behavior of complex biological constituents."

In conclusion, I would like to bring the reader's attention to a very pertinent article by Dennis Noble in 2005 [39]. In this he points out that real founders of the field were Hodgkin and Huxley [40], who first identified the systems of interactions between cell electrical potential and ion channel activity. They won the Nobel Prize in 1963 for this. In the same article, Noble stresses that he has employed systems biology for 40 years, since 1960 [41].

He remarks that a bottom-up analysis, i.e., starting from genes, making proteins from them, and building an organism, is practically impossible and that nature rather employs a *downward causation* with many feedback loops between levels. He refers to heart cell models and incorporation of cellular models into anatomically detailed models of the whole organ (Fig. 4.3).

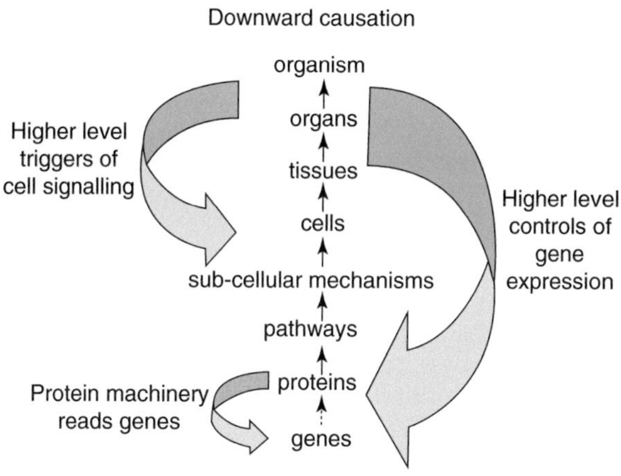

Fig. 4.3 The upward arrows show the sequence envisaged by bottom-up reconstruction of the functioning of biological systems. Genes code for proteins, which form pathways and subcellular machinery, incorporated into cells, tissues, organs, and systems, reaching up to the whole organism. The downward arrows show that there are many feedback loops between the levels. Systems analysis respects these loops in a way that bottom-up approaches would not. (Reproduced with permission from Noble [39])

He concludes by predicting that the computer modeling of biological systems (silico biology) has many possibilities, to exploit the data generated through rapid gene sequencing and proteomic mapping to create the physiome.

The “omics” revolution proved him right.

With the employment of systems biology, a better description of the various models that underline heart disease at all levels can be provided. Of course this new paradigm creates complexity but can immensely aid our understanding of interactions among contributing mechanisms.

References

1. Lusis AJ, Weiss JN. Cardiovascular networks: systems-based approaches to cardiovascular disease. Circulation. 2010;121:157–70.
2. Ideker T, Galitski T, Hood L. A new approach to decoding life: systems biology. Annu Rev Genomics Hum Genet. 2001;2:343–72.
3. Department of Systems Biology Harvard Medical School. https://sysbio.med.Harvard.edu.
4. Lusis AJ. A thematic review series: systems biology approaches to metabolic and cardiovascular disorders. J Lipid Res. 2006;47:1887–90.
5. Mayr M. From data gathering to systems medicine. Cardiovasc Res. 2013;97:599–600.
6. Arrell DK, Terzic A. Systems proteomics for translational network medicine. Circ Cardiovasc Genet. 2012;5:478.
7. Chautard E, Thierry-Mieg N, Ricard-Blum S. Interaction networks: from protein functions to drug discovery. A review. Pathol Biol (Paris). 2009;57:324–33.
8. Chuang HY, Hofree M, Ideker T. A decade of systems biology. Annu Rev Cell Dev Biol. 2010;26:721–44.
9. Shreenivasaiah PK, Rho SH, Kim T, Kim DH. An overview of cardiac systems biology. J Mol Cell Cardiol. 2008;44:460–9.
10. Hidalgo CA, Blumm N, Barabási AL, Christakis NA. A dynamic network approach for the study of human phenotypes. PLoS Comput Biol. 2009;5:e1000353.
11. Brutsaert D. Heart Failure: Quo Vadis Lecture presented at Cardiovascular Biotechnology: From cell to man Biomedical Research Foundation Academy of Athens, 31 May – 1 June 2013.
12. Kalamatianos D. MCQs Systems Biology Approaches and Applications in Cardiovascular Diseases. Introduction to Translational Cardiovascular Research, 25 Jan 2013.
13. Weiss JN, Yang L, Qu Z. Network perspectives of cardiovascular metabolism. J Lipid Res. 2006;47:2355–66.
14. Barabási AL, Bonabeau E. Scale-free networks. Sci Am. 2003;288:60–9.
15. Barabási AL, Oltvai ZN. Network biology: understanding the cell's functional organization. Nat Rev Genet. 2004;5:101–13.
16. Ravasz E, Somera AL, Mongru DA, Oltvai ZN, Barabási AL. Hierarchical organization of modularity in metabolic networks. Science. 2002;297:1551–5.
17. Jeong H, Tombor B, Albert R, Oltvai ZN, Barabási AL. The large-scale organization of metabolic networks. Nature. 2000;407:651–4.
18. Merton RK. The Matthew effect in science: the reward and communication systems of science are considered. Science. 1968;159(3810):56–63.
19. Ramsey SA, Klemm SL, Zak DE, Kennedy KA, Thorsson V, Li B, et al. Uncovering a macrophage transcriptional program by integrating evidence from motif scanning and expression dynamics. PLoS Comput Biol. 2008;4:e1000021.
20. Skogsberg J, Lundström J, Kovacs A, Nilsson R, Noori P, Maleki S, et al. Transcriptional profiling uncovers a network of cholesterol-responsive atherosclerosis target genes. PLoS Genet. 2008;4:e1000036.

21. Gargalovic PS, Imura M, Zhang B, Gharavi NM, Clark MJ, Pagnon J, et al. Identification of inflammatory gene modules based on variations of human endothelial cell responses to oxidized lipids. Proc Natl Acad Sci U S A. 2006;103:12741–6.
22. Nadeau JH, Burrage LC, Restivo J, Pao YH, Churchill G, Hoit BD. Pleiotropy, homeostasis, and functional networks based on assays of cardiovascular traits in genetically randomized populations. Genome Res. 2003;13:2082–91.
23. Machleder D, Ivandic B, Welch C, Castellani L, Reue K, Lusis AJ. Complex genetic control of HDL levels in mice in response to an atherogenic diet. Coordinate regulation of HDL levels and bile acid metabolism. J Clin Invest. 1997;99:1406–19.
24. Lusis AJ, Attie AD, Reue K. Metabolic syndrome: from epidemiology to systems biology. Nat Rev Genet. 2008;9:819–30.
25. Topol E. Textbook of cardiovascular medicine. 3rd ed. Philadelphia, PA: Lippincott Williams and Wilkins; 2007. Mentioned in Ref. [1].
26. Loscalzo J, Kohane I, Barabasi AL. Human disease classification in the postgenomic era: a complex systems approach to human pathobiology. Mol Syst Biol. 2007;3:124.
27. Pastor-Satorras R, Vespignani A. Epidemic dynamics and endemic states in complex networks. Phys Rev E Stat Nonlinear Soft Matter Phys. 2001;63:066117.
28. Eubank S, Guclu H, Kumar VS, Marathe MV, Srinivasan A, Toroczkai Z. Modelling disease outbreaks in realistic urban social networks. Nature. 2004;429:180–4.
29. Ergün A, Lawrence CA, Kohanski MA, Brennan TA, Collins JJ. A network biology approach to prostate cancer. Mol Syst Biol. 2007;3:82.
30. Lim J, Hao T, Shaw C, Patel AJ, Szabó G, et al. A protein-protein interaction network for human inherited ataxias and disorders of Purkinje cell degeneration. Cell. 2006;125:801–14.
31. Lu X, Jain VV, Finn PW, Perkins DL. Hubs in biological interaction networks exhibit low changes in expression in experimental asthma. Mol Syst Biol. 2007;3:98.
32. Nicholson JK. Global systems biology, personalized medicine and molecular epidemiology. Mol Syst Biol. 2006;2:52.
33. Kitano H. A robustness-based approach to systems-oriented drug design. Nat Rev Drug Discov. 2007;6:202–10.
34. Butcher EC, Berg EL, Kunkel EJ. Systems biology in drug discovery. Nat Biotechnol. 2004;22:1253–9.
35. Huan T, Zhang B, Wang Z, Joehanes R, Zhu J, Johnson AD, et al. A systems biology framework identifies molecular underpinnings of coronary heart disease. Arterioscler Thromb Vasc Biol. 2013;33:1427–34.
36. West BJ, Geneston EL, Grigolini P. Maximizing information exchange between complex networks. Phys Rep. 2008;468:1–99.
37. Geronikolou S, Pavlopoulou A, Albanopoulos K, Cokkinos D, Chrousos G. Kisspeptin and Stress induced obesidome. P052 IFSO 2018 eBook of Abstracts Springer 2018 p104. 8th Congress of the Int Fed for the surgery of obesity and metabolic disorders-eur chapter, Athens, May 17–19th 2018.
38. Kirschner MC. The meaning of systems biology. Cell. 2005;121:503–4.
39. Noble D. Systems biology and the heart. Biosystems. 2006;83:75–80.
40. Hodgkin AL, Huxley AF. A quantitative description of membrane current and its application to conducting and excitation in nerve. J Physiol. 1952;117:500–44.
41. Noble D. Cardiac action and pacemaker potentials based on the Hodgkin Huxley equations. Nature. 1960;188:495–7.

Chapter 5
Cardiac Hypertrophy

Dennis V. Cokkinos

The definition of cardiac hypertrophy (HYP) is an increase in heart mass. Normally, as the organism grows, in parallel with the functional work load [1], the cardiac mass increases.

This normal growth is termed by some authors "eutrophy" [2].

Heart growth above this level can be called "hypertrophy." A lot of work has been devoted to differentiate physiological or adaptive hypertrophy vs pathological or maladaptive hypertrophy. Some important reviews from experts in the field will be discussed.

Frey and Olson [3] point out that the hypertrophic response eventually normalizes the increase in wall tension, if it is produced by an initial stimulus, as will be discussed [4].

Dorn et al. [2] underline that the terms "compensated" versus "decompensated" are based on left ventricular contractility and pump performance and the prospect of a course toward an inexorable deterioration [5].

Dorn [6] points out that both compensated or decompensated hypertrophy are followed by alterations in cardiac size and shape and function. He gives three examples of physiological HYP:

(a) An exotic and rare but physiologically relevant paradigm is the postprandial hypertrophic response of the Burmese python [7].

The python feeds only periodically but when happening on a large meal can increase its metabolic rate 40-fold and oxygen consumption 7-fold. These increases are followed by a 40% increase in ventricular mass and stroke volume with an increase in protein content per cardiomyocyte [8].

D. V. Cokkinos (✉)
Heart and Vessel Department, Biomedical Research Foundation,
Academy of Athens - Gregory Skalkeas, Athens, Greece
e-mail: dcokkinos@bioacademy.gr

D. V. Cokkinos (ed.), *Myocardial Preservation*,
https://doi.org/10.1007/978-3-319-98186-4_5

Ventricular mass returns to normal within 28 days after the meal. As Dorn [6] points out, postprandial cardiac hypertrophy has not been attested in humans. However, increases in cardiac workload have been found during digestion [9, 10].

Another universal paradigm, affecting approximately half the humans sometime in their lives, is the physiological hypertrophy of pregnancy. During the second and third trimester of pregnancy, cardiac output increases; thus volume overload is seen corresponding to increased placental flow.

A moderate eccentric hypertrophy is seen [11]. Classically, these alterations are completely reversible after delivery; also in the mouse, fetal gene expression is not seen during pregnancy [12].

Thus, pregnancy hypertrophy can be considered physiological. However, two points must be mentioned.

(a) During pregnancy, QT prolongation is seen, and an overexpression of Kv4.3 is seen [13].

(b) Also, an overexpression of src tyrosine, which is a pathological gene it noted [14]. This may justify considering the heart in pregnancy “less than completely physiological” according to Dorn [6]. It cannot be said if the recently intensively studied peripartum cardiomyopathy can be considered an extension of possibly not physiological changes during pregnancy.

5.1 The Heart and Exercise

The benefits of chronic exercise have been extensively studied, especially those of endurance exercise.

The hypertrophy which it produces corresponds to eccentric hypertrophy and volume overload, especially with chronic endurance training.

In the experimental animal, exercise mitigates pathological HYP [15]. It also reduces cardiac remodeling in the experimental animal [16] and in the human [17].

Our group has actually shown that even in pts. with an LVAD placement, exercise improves the molecular profile of the tissue hypothyroidism [18].

5.2 The Athlete’s Heart

This concept appeared in the late nineteenth century, with the question if prolonged exercise could cause excessive hypertrophy and cardiomegaly which can be noxious [19].

As regards strength exercise, there have been reports that it causes concentric hypertrophy and increased peripheral vascular resistance.

Concerning athlete’s heart thickness, a seminal article by Peliccia et al. [20] showed that elite rowers and cyclists and cross-country skiers predominate, although a left ventricular wall thickness of 1.3 cm is the upper limit [20].

Peliccia et al. [21] have found that athletes can develop ventricular remodeling which in 20% does not reverse even after 5 years of deconditioning [21].

Apart from the abnormalities of the LV, structural abnormalities of the left atrium have been described [22].

In the experimental animal, prolonged and severe exercise can induce pathological genes [23]. In rats, very intense exercise for 16 weeks can cause ventricular remodeling, fibrosis and arrhythmias [24]. The findings in spontaneously hypertensive rats are very interesting: Moderate exercise improves their cardiac function [25]. However, prolonged exercise in the same model produces a decrease in LVEF, LV dilation, and fibrosis [26].

Dorn's laboratory [27] has described already in 2001 that physiological hypertrophy was represented in the mouse by protein kinase Cε [28], while pathological hypertrophy by expression of Gq and calcineurin [30].

Iemitsu et al. [23] differentiated between cardiac hypertrophy produced by swimming in rats and that seen in spontaneously hypertensive rats, which is by definition pathological.

They described genes upregulated in pathological hypertrophy, such as brain natriuretic peptide, angiotensin-converting enzyme, endothelin receptor, and β-adrenergic receptor kinase [31].

However, as already mentioned, they found that β-adrenergic receptor mRNA was increased in both physiological and pathological hypertrophy.

Kong et al. [32] carried out similar experiments. They compared genes regulated with daily exercise and Dahl salt-sensitive rats on high-salt diet, which progressed to heart failure. Of ~ 3000 known genes that they studied, 159 were regulated in both physiological and pathological hypertrophy. In figure 3 Dorn [6] gives a Venn diagram showing this overlap. Strøm et al. [33] performed a similar study with treadmill exercise in rats. They did not find upregulation of fetal cardiac genes, such as atrial natriuretic factor, α skeletal actin, and β-myosin heavy chain [33], or collagen (fibrosis) gene expression. Genes that were upregulated in both paradigms of hypertrophy were those for extracellular matrix and cytoskeletal proteins, ribosomal proteins, and genes required for cardiomyocyte protein synthesis and structural growth. However, the gene for G-protein receptor kinase-2 which is increased in pathological hypertrophy [34] was downregulated by exercise.

Hill and Olson [35], in a seminal review with the title "cardiac plasticity," specifically stress the role of neurohumoral activation but also of myocardial injury.

Thyroid hormone receptors [36] and α versus β-myosin heavy chain isoforms [37] are regulated in opposite directions in exercise versus pressure overload Kinugawa et al [36] propose that in pathological HYP, a relative hypothyroidism is seen.

Also, collagen is not increased in physiological HYP as stressed by Dorn [6].

Strøm et al. [33] have also described that some genes involved in fatty acid metabolism are upregulated in physiological hypertrophy; importantly, they are downregulated in pathological hypertrophy and remodeling [38, 39]. Here I must stress that many elements of pathological cardiac hypertrophy are discussed in the chapters on myocardial remodeling and the fetal phenotype.

The uncoupling protein UCP2 which induces mitochondrial heat generation instead of ATP production [40] is upregulated in pathological hypertrophy but downregulated by treadmill exercise [38].

Dorn [6] points out that UCP2 is normalized by β-adrenergic receptor blockade [41] and ACE inhibition [42].

The question of ACE therapy brings to mind observations by many authors who found that in athletes [43] the presence of the D allele is associated with a greater ventricular mass index.

Dorn [6] describes the signaling pathways in physiological hypertrophy, especially this caused by exercise: It involves PI3k/Akt pathway and the IGF and growth hormone. These two are main determinants for both physiological hypertrophy and normal growth [44, 45].

However, as already pointed out in the chapter on myocardial remodeling, although the PI3K/Akt pathway induces physiological/adaptive hypertrophy [46], it can also induce hypertrophy with pathological features and fibrosis [47].

Dorn [6] also in figure 4 of his review depicts many pathways in which physiological and pathological hypertrophy cross-regulate each other. He stresses that membrane phosphatidylinositol biphosphate is a substrate for physiological HYP through PI3K phosphorylation and pathological HYP through hydrolysis by phospholipase C. Also, he describes that an alternate form of PI3K is activated through the Gq pathways [49].

He stresses that an important paradigm of signal cross talk between the two types of HYP occurs at the level of GSK: thus, GSK-3β, a negative growth activator inhibits both normal heart growth and isoproterenol [50] and pressure overload hypertrophy [51].

Thyroid hormones, a subject close to my heart, typically induce physiological HYP [52].

However, we have shown that excess T3 can produce excessive cardiac remodeling through Akt overexpression [54].

Another modulator of Akt signaling is the family of sirtuins. Some of these (SIRT3 and 6) are involved in regulating the aging process in mammals and SIRT3 attenuates cardiac hypertrophy.

Interestingly, the behavior of SIRT follows a pattern similar to that of Akt: Excessive upregulation of SIRT1 induces pathological cardiac hypertrophy and dysfunction, while less marked induction attenuates age-related hypertrophy [55].

5.3 Pathological Hypertrophy

Unfortunately this form of HYP is the more frequent. Frey and Olson [3] and Kontaridis et al. [56] describe the pathways seen in Fig 5.1.

5.4 Calcineurin/NFAT

Calcineurin is a serine-threonine phosphatase. In T-cells it is an activator or immune response through IL-2 [56] (Fig. 5.1).

It appears to be involved in most if not all etiologies of pathological HYP [57]. It is calcium and calmodulin dependent. Its activity is inhibited by the immunosuppressive drugs cyclosporine A and FK506 [58]. In this context, questions have been raised whether its inhibition by cyclosporine A is beneficial, as Hill et al. [59] have found, or noxious [60, 61].

5.5 G-Protein-Coupled Receptors

They are the largest class of cell surface receptors. They regulate adaptation to changes in a hemodynamic burden [62].

They include adrenergic and muscarinic receptors. Their classification is difficult and complicated for the nonexperts. Thus I will only describe some of their associations:

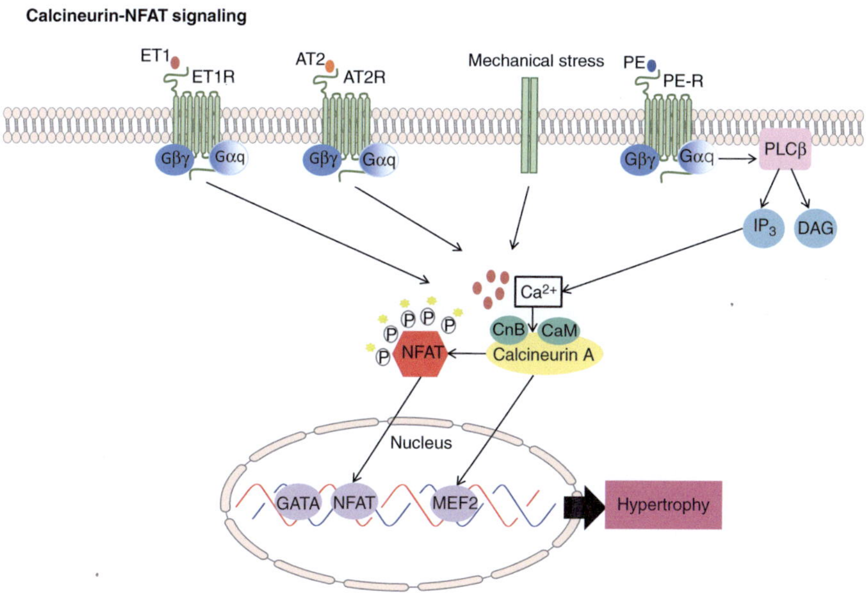

Fig. 5.1 The calcineurin pathway to myocardial hypertrophy. Calcineurin/NFAT signaling. Upon stimulation of Gαq-coupled receptors (i.e., ET1R, AT2R, or PE) or mechanical stress, the levels of intracellular calcium increase. Calcium then binds to calmodulin, thereby activating calcineurin through sustained elevations in intracellular calcium. This leads to nuclear localization of NFAT transcription factors as well as direct activation of nuclear MEF2 factors. Subsequent cardiac muscle hypertrophy follows. (Reproduced with permission from Kontaridis et al. [56])

Beta receptors: the most abundant, as already described in cardiac remodeling, is β1 which activates adenylate cyclase. Its overexpression initially increases contractility and chronotropy but can lead to hypertrophy, fibrosis, and dysfunction [63, 64].

β2 overexpression is only deleterious at very high levels (>100-fold), while moderate levels improve basal contractility [64].

On the contrary, β3 receptors are simulated at high catecholamine, doses and levels are cardioprotective in pressure overload hypertrophy and heart failure. Niu et al. [65] found that the β3 agonist, BRL37344 reduced hypertrophy produced by transverse aortic constriction; neural NOS was upregulated twofold and superoxide generation was suppressed.

In heart failure there occurs a decrease of receptor numbers together with functional uncoupling [66], which is affected by beta-adrenoceptor kinase 1 [67].

With β-blocker therapy, with its well-known beneficial effects, a downregulation of hypertrophic genes and upregulation of SERCA 2α and a-MHC has been found [68].

Angiotensins I and II and endothelin receptors [69, 70], serotonin receptors, and α-adrenergic receptors also belong to this class.

As Kontaridis et al [56] remark, these receptors, apart from sharing their function to control hypertrophy in response to stress, have additional important properties. Thus, they point out that α1 adrenergic receptors modulate Na + -H+ exchange transporter regulators, while angiotensin receptors control Ca2+ signaling and collagen synthesis/deposition, and endothelin-1 mediates cardiac rhythm and collagen expression [71]. These receptors also participate in the embryonic phenotype reactivation described in the corresponding chapter and over time lead to maladaptive hypertrophy and failure [72].

According to Kontaridis et al. [56], a good translational paradigm is the benefit of ACE inhibition which targets GPO signaling [73]. They also describe that the cells have mechanisms to turn off GPCR signaling. These are:

(a) Vesicular translocation in which the receptor is engulfed by a clathrin-coated vesicle, removed and disassembled from its agonist, and then recycled or degraded. (b) The other mechanism is desensitization by β-arrestin.

According to Kontaridis et al. [56], the most recently studied class of heterotrimeric G-proteins is the Rho family of small G-proteins, members of when activate JNK-MAP in response to two typical stimuli of pathological hypertrophy, phenylephrine [74], and the Rho family of small G-proteins consist of Rho, Rac, and Cdc42 subfamilies, which regulate the cytoskeleton organization of non-cardiomyocytes but also cardiomyocytes [76].

5.6 MAPK Pathways

They are divided into three subfamilies:

ERK 1/2. It has been discussed if its overexpression results into physiological [77] or pathological HYP.

Thus, in transgenic mice, overexpression of MEK 1, which activates ERK1/2 but not JNKs or p38 MAPKs, as will be described later, results into hypertrophy with supernormal systolic function, constituting a mode of physiological HYP [78].

5.6.1 *JNK*

According to Bernardo et al. [79], It may be a necessary regulator of pathological HYP, activated by stretching [80], endothelin I [81], phenylephrine [82], or angiotensin II [83].

p38 – MAPK; it is a component of stress response pathways. It leads to the expression of the fetal gene program. It seems to cause fibrosis, dysfunction, and the development of a form of dilated cardiomyopathy. Still, many questions as to its cardioprotective versus deleterious roles exist [84].

PI3K (p110γ) signaling. This isoform is coupled to the already mentioned GPCRs, which are considered as including Ang-II, adrenergic, and endothelin receptors. Although it has a protective role [85], it on the whole may reduce cardiac contractility [86].

Protein kinases: Pressure overload activates PKIC and D; they trigger hypertrophic responses [87].

PKC includes at least 12 isoforms of which α, β, δ, and ε are involved in cardiac hypertrophy. Interestingly, in transgenic mice overexpressing PKCε, it had a protective role in response to ischemia-induced damage, while PKCδ exacerbated this response [88].

5.7 Insulin/Insulin Receptor/Akt Signaling

Shimizu and Minamino [89] stress that although the insulin pathway promotes physiological hypertrophy, its activation can disturb homeostasis and induce pathological hypertrophy through Ang-II signaling [90]. Maintained cardiac insulin activation can cause myocardial hypoxia and dysfunction when pressure overload is applied [91].

5.8 Inflammation

Shamak et al. [92] point out that this process is prominent in HYP [93]:

> Pathological HYP is characterized by interstitial inflammatory cell infiltration such as macrophages and T-lymphocytes. Also cytokines such as interleukin IL-6, IL-1β, IL-1RA, and TNFα and activation of NF-kβ are prominent [94].

Another interesting cytokine is cardiotrophin-1 which activates many hypertrophic characteristics; it activates gr 130 and LIFR tyrosine.

As regards inflammatory cells, Shamak et al. [92] dedicate a paragraph to macrophages MΦ which are mononuclear phagocytes, divided into pro-inflammatory M1 and anti-inflammatory M2 [96, 97].

M1 liberate cytokines and induce apoptosis;while M2 stimulate cardiac reparation and angiogenesis [98].

Xu and Brink [99] describe the inflammatory signaling of cardiomyocyte in response to stress.

They describe that the mammalian target of rapamycin (mTOR) regulates NF-kβ activity; it may produce fibrosis; pressure overload induces expression of TNFα and its receptors [100], which activate NF-kB.

In this context, rapamycin diminishes HYP caused by pressure overload [101] and reverses

SERCA-2α decreases, as well as αMHC decreases [102] and diminishes fibrosis [103].

5.8.1 *The Role of TLRs*

Even completely mechanical stresses such as hypertension and aortic constriction stimulate inflammatory signaling.

In this context, the comparatively recently described role of Toll-like receptors (TLRs) in myocardial HYP is interesting. TLRs are pattern recognition receptors which are very important for innate immunity by recognition of endogenous pattern-associated molecular patterns [104].

They activate NF-kB [105]. Ha et al. [106] performed aortic banding in TLR-4-deficient and wild-type mice. The former developed significantly less hypertrophy, with less NF-kB binding capacity. Ehrentrant et al. [108] reported similar findings [107]. Higashikuni et al. [108] found the same in TLR-2-deficient mice; they also found that HSP70 can activate TLR2 signaling; actually, administration of anti-HSP70 antibodies impaired HYP in wild-type mice.

Tollip (Toll- interacting protein) is an endogenous negative modulator of TLR signaling [109].

Liu et al. [110] found that Tollip limited angiotensin II induced HYP. Transgenic mice overexpressing Tollip developed less hypertrophy, fibrosis, and dysfunction after aortic banding.

In fact, Abrahao and Carneiro-Ramos [111] found cross talk between TLRs and the RAS system in a HYP model.

In accordance to their findings that TLR-4 deficiency protects against cardiac pressure overload-induced hyperinflammation [107], Ehrentraut et al. [112] found that the TLR-4 antagonist eritoran reduced cardiac hypertrophy in mice subjected the transverse aortic constriction and inhibited natriuretic peptide mRNA elevation, together with inhibition of the increase of IL-10 and IL-6 mRNA and protein elevation [112].

Eritoran also increased the cardioprotective IL-1β, and interestingly in placebo animals, MMP activity was increased. Of course as has been discussed in the chapter in cardiac remodeling, MMPs increase after an experimental myocardial infarction [113], and volume overload [114], but MMP inhibition also had a beneficial impact on pressure overload [115].

Frey and Olson [3] describe that the cardiac helicase is activated by MEF2 protein (CHAMP): its overexpression abrogates cardiomyocyte growth and ANF expression caused by phenylephrine treatment [116].

The Na+/H+ exchanger (NHE) activity is induced in pressure overload [117]. Its upregulation increases intracellular calcium via the Na+/Ca2+ exchanger, with the already described results [118].

5.8.2 Redox Signaling

Oxidative stress has been associated with HYP; ROS activate a great number of the aforementioned hypertrophic signaling pathways. Also, they mediate the hypertrophic effects of angiotensin II [119] and norepinephrine [120].

Moreover, antioxidant treatment abolishes TNF-α induced hypertrophy [121]. Also, ROS contribute to apoptosis which will be further described [122].

Seddon et al. [123] describe the effects of ROS on the development of HYP: They point out that ROS are involved in the response to HYP induced by angiotensin II, endothelin 1, norepinephrine, TNFα, or pulsatile mechanical stretch. They also remind that NADPH oxidases are the key sources of ROS. Thus, in pressure overload, increased NADPH oxidase parallels MAPK activation [124].

They also reiterate the already mentioned findings that ROS contribute to contractile dysfunction and also to diastolic dysfunction through the inactivation of endothelial-derived NO [125]. Also, they describe the contribution of ROS to fibrosis, which is inhibited by the NADPH oxidase inhibitor apocynin [126].

Two more mechanisms involved in HYP: a. Energy metabolism changes.

As already discussed in the chapter 12 in cardiac remodeling a shift in energy production occurs in HYP, in the sense that fatty acid oxidation is suppressed and glucose utilization increased; these result in a decrease of O2 consumption per mole of ATP generation. Moreover, this impaired fatty acid utilization results to their accumulation in the heart [127]. The genes involved in fatty acid oxidation are regulated by the peroxisome proliferator-activated receptor (PPAR) family of transcription factors. Three PPAR isoforms have been described, α, β/δ, and γ. PRARα is the predominant isoform in the heart and is involved in hypertrophic signaling: It is downregulated during pressure overload HYP; this may be an adaptive response, leading to contractile dysfunction [128].

b. With the discussion of the noxious effects of ROS, we come to the description of various forms of cell death in HYP. Of course, much greater detail is given in the corresponding chapter 7.

Balakumar and Singh [129] describe that in maladaptive cardiac HYP, apoptosis is seen through over-activation of caspase 3.

The same authors found an upregulation of caspase 3 in pathological pressure overload-induced HYP, but not in swimming-induced physiological HYP.

Interestingly, autophagy which on the whole is a protective process can be maladaptive and associated with cardiac dysfunction in the pressure overload model [130].

Moreover, autophagy protein 5, encoded by Atrogin 5 (Atg) deletion, induces cardiac hypertrophy, systolic dysfunction, and cardiac dilation [131].

However, whole body deletion of atrogin-1 together with suppression of the autophagic response leads to cardiac HYP and fibrosis [132].

Li et al. [133] discuss in a review the role of autophagy in cardiac HYP. They remind that its role in

HYP remains controversial. They describe the following processes:

TAC-induced HYP promotes autophagy in the heart, through upregulation of Atg 5, Atg 16, LC3-II, and beclin-1.

They underline various conflicting findings:

Mitigation of autophagy could improve right ventricular function after pulmonary artery constriction [134].

Decreased autophagy causes a deterioration of cardiac hypertrophy, while high levels of autophagy ameliorate cardiac hypertrophy. They concluded that while basal autophagy is essential for maintenance of cellular homeostasis, excess or frustrated autophagic activity can cause deterioration of HYP and predispose to heart failure [135].

Angiogenesis: according to Shimizu and Minamino [136], a symmetrical and coordinated myocardial growth, differenciates physiological HYP from the pathological. In the former the number of the capillaries is maintained or even increases, while in the latter capillary rarefaction is seen [136].

VEGF is initially upregulated in the adaptive phase of HYP, while disruption of the symmetrical advance of ventricular mass and angiogenesis leads to the transition to heart failure [137].

Akt, which in the majority of instances promotes physiological HYP, is a significant regulator of angiogenesis by production of NO [136]. Angiogenesis increase can induce HYP via NO-dependent or independent mechanisms [136].

Oka et al. [139] also describe the importance of angiogenesis in cardiac hypertrophy toward maintaining normal cardiac function. They reiterate that in adaptive hypertrophy capillary microvasculature and myocytes grow in proportion to the heart mass increase [140].

They also remarked that myocardial angiogenesis induces HYP. They advance the hypothesis of increased delivery of nutrients and oxygen, and endothelium-derived enhanced NO production, since an NO synthase inhibitor and NG-nitro-L-arginine methyl ester could prevent HYP [141].

Moreover, they describe that myocardial angiogenesis is regulated by VEGF, angiopoietin-1 and angiopoietin-2, fibroblast growth factors, and transforming growth and platelet growth factors, and refer again to the study by Shiojima et al. [137] which suggests that cardiomyocytes produce angiogenic growth factors. The role of short or long action of Akt on the myocardium has already been described.

Phung et al. [142] describe that in endothelial cells, prolonged Akt activation resulted in unorganized blood cell formation similar to tumor vasculature.

Oka et al. [139] address special attention to the role of VEGF: transverse aortic constriction in VGEF-deficient mice induces HYP accompanied by capillary rarefaction and cardiac decompensation [143], while its administration in the failing heart maintained cardiac contractility [144]: antiapoptotic GATA4 is essential for both HYP [145] and angiogenesis [146]. Its cardiomyocyte specific overexpression in the adult heart increased capillary density [146] and induced VGEF secretion.

Oka et al. [139] again stressed the fact that capillary rarefaction characterizes transition from compensated HYP to decompensated heart failure, in the pressure-overloaded heart. Sano et al. [147] describe that eventually the myocardium becomes ischemic and the hypoxia-inducible factor (HIF-1) is downregulated together with VEGF [147], a very important mechanism. In the hypertrophic myocardium, p53 is overexpressed in response to hypoxic stress [148]; it has also been found to be overexpressed post-MI [148]. HIF-1 is required for hypoxia-induced p53 overexpression [149]. Oka et al. [139] also describe the two major roles of p53 in the heart:

Cell cycle arrest [150], and inhibition of new vessel formation [151]; p53 has another noxious effect in that it inhibits HIF-1 and promotes progression to maladaptive heart failure [147]. p53 is also pro-apoptotic under specific circumstances [147, 152]. Oka et al. [139] in their figure 3 suggest that in the hypertrophied heart VEGF is increased by HIF-1, while in the failing heart HIF-1 is inhibited by p53 accumulation in the myocardium.

When addressing angiogenesis, it is useful to remember that from the structural aspect, HYP is classified in two types:

Concentric hypertrophy (Fig. 5.2) is the result of pressure overload characterized by the addition of sarcomeres in parallel and increased relative wall thickness with no appreciable change in cavity size.

According to Dorn et al. [2], in eccentric HYP cavity volume is increased and sarcomeres are added in series with longitudinal cell growth (Fig. 5.2).

Profound cardiomyocyte HYP [153] is found in dilated cardiomyopathy [153]. Dorn et al. [154] report that in concentric HYP in the compensated state, overall cardiac performance is maintained, but cardiomyocyte contractility is depressed. It should also be reminded that in both forms of HYP, wall thickness is actually increased. There has been much discussion about which type of hypertrophy is more benign for the myocardium.

You et al. recently [155] compared models of experimental transverse aortic constriction (TAC) and aortic regurgitation (AR) in mice. TAC was associated with more significant fibrosis and apoptosis, and AR with more significant angiogenesis; MAPK family, β-arrestin-2, Akt, and Ca2+ signaling pathways were activated to a much greater degree in TAC.

This object has already been addressed in Chap. 12 on cardiac remodeling. My view is that the degree of fibrosis, which usually is more pronounced in pressure overload HYP, determines prognosis. From the clinical standpoint, it must be

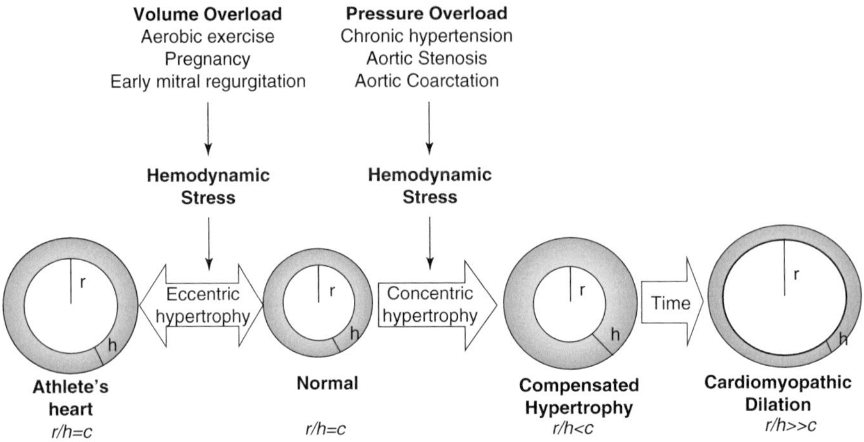

Fig. 5.2 Stimulus-specific hypertrophic responses of the heart and how they affect wall stress (c), which, at equal pressures, is proportional to the ratio of internal ventricular radius at end-diastole (r) and ventricular wall thickness (h). (Reproduced with permission from Dorn [6])

remembered that aortic stenosis is nowadays reaching operative mortality of about zero; it is not commonly allowed to deteriorate to left ventricular dilation.

This brings into focus the clinical standpoint: Can echocardiography help toward differentiation physiological from pathological HYP?

Derumeaux et al. [156] assigned Wistar rats to sedentary state, swimming, and abdominal aortic banding. After 2 months, they did not find differences in conventional left ventricular fractional shortening and dP/dt max. However, the myocardial velocity gradient was lower in the rats with banding as compared to the other two groups; this normalized after debanding. The authors postulate that tissue Doppler imaging is more sensitive than conventional echocardiography for assessing early myocardial dysfunction in pressure overload HYP. From the clinical standpoint, Galanti et al. [157] found that diastolic TDI parameters could easily differentiate between elite athletes and mild hypertensive subjects.

Afonso et al. [158] studied with two-dimensional strain or speckle tracking pts with hypertrophic cardiomyopathy (HCM), hypertensive HYP, professional athletes, and normal controls. HCM pts. had significantly lower regional and average global peak longitudinal systolic strain compared to controls and other forms of LV HYP. Olah et al. [159] used both echocardiographic and hemodynamic measurements (LV pressure volume analysis) to differentiate between physiological HYP induced by swimming and pathological HYP produced by abdominal aortic banding.

Their observations were supported by histological and molecular examination. The degree of myocardial HYP was similar by echocardiography in the two groups.

Physiological HYP was characterized by increased stroke volume: Active relaxation was ameliorated by exercise but impaired in the pathological form. Fractional shortening was higher in exercise. By P-V loops, many sensitive contractility parameters, including dP/dt max-EVD, were increased in both HYP models with no differences between them. Also, mechanical efficiency and ventricular-arterial coupling were improved in physiological HYP but unchanged in the pathological form.

5.8.3 Arrhythmic Consequences

Schiattarella and Hill [160] also describe arrhythmic remodeling in HYP, characterized by an increase of the action potential duration and from a clinical aspect showing increased susceptibility to malignant arrhythmias.

5.9 Gender Differences

Another aspect which has clinical undertones is the gender difference. Thus, in the experimental protocol, Douglas et al. [161] subjected 16 male and 18 female weanling rats to ascending aortic banding or sham surgery. At 6 weeks, hypertrophy and function were similar in the 2 genders, but at 20 weeks only male rats showed an early transition to heart failure and importantly loss of concentric remodeling. Weinberg et al. [162] from the same group found that at 6 weeks after ascending aortic banding, contractile reserve was depressed only in the male animals. Moreover, the male hearts expressed higher β-MHC and ANF mRNA and lower SERCA 2α.

These findings have a clinical counterpart; women with aortic stenosis tend to develop less wall tension than males [163].

Lee et al. [164] found greater left ventricular mass and the LV remodeling index in aortic stenosis in men. Using CMR Threibel et al. [165] found more normal geometry in women as well as concentric remodeling, while concentric and eccentric hypertrophy was more prevalent in men, who also had more clinical decompensation, lower ejection fraction, higher NT-proBNP, and fibrosis.

These data suggest that aortic stenosis maybe better tolerated in women than in men. They also bring into focus another aspect of clinical importance:

Is cardiac HYP a therapeutic target?

A very distinguished group on this subject addressed this question in 2004 [166].

These authors, gathering evidence from clinical trials comparing blood pressure-lowering drugs, point out that ACE inhibition and AT1 receptor blockade maybe the more desirable interventions. Similarly, in aortic stenosis, HYP has been found to confer a worse prognosis [167].

In this sense the group of Verdecchia [168] found that left ventricular hypertrophy regression predicted a more favorable course [168].

Schiattarella and Hill [160] (Fig. 5.3) also consider inhibition of hypertrophy as a good therapeutic strategy in ventricular pressure overload.

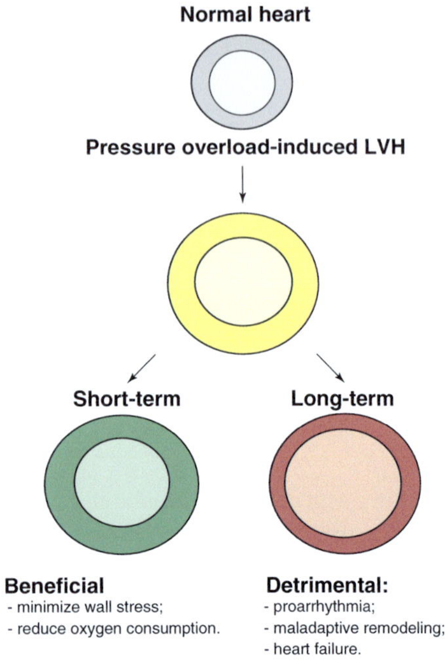

Fig. 5.3 Canonical 3-stage model of hypertrophic transformation of the heart. This model posits short-term hypertrophy as a beneficial event and long-term hypertrophy as detrimental. LVH indicates left ventricular hypertrophy. (Reproduced with permission from Schiattarella and Hill [160])

Apart from the drugs already being used, and which are also described in chapter 13 on Cardiac Remodeling, a recent concept for treating HYP is small molecular therapies [169], which targets intracellular targets.

Reid et al. [174] give a recent review.

They suggest that some drugs used for other purposes such as bromocriptine (used currently for peripartum cardiomyopathy) [175], imipramine, escitalopram, dipyridamole, imatinib, and many others have promise.

However, when discussing therapies addressed to the cardiomyocyte, it should not be forgotten that as Kontaridis et al. point out [56], other cells are also involved in HYP, i. e.,

Cardiac fibroblasts, which together with their activated form as myofibroblasts, are the most numerous cells the myocardium. They produce extracellular matrix proteins; they also regulate HYP response to pressure overload by producing cytokines and growth factors such as PDGF and IGF-1 [176].

TGF-β levels are correlated with fibrosis; it also acts downstream of angiotensin II to promote cardiomyocyte growth [177].

Endothelial cells interact directly with adjacent cardiomyocytes. They release NO, endothelin 1, angiotensin II, and prostaglandin I2 [174].

Vascular smooth muscle cells also express various growth factors, especially when injured, such as fibroblast growth factor, platelet-derived, and epidermal growth factor [175].

5.10 MicroRNAs and HYP

These ubiquitous small (18–25 nucleotides) noncoding RNAs are also involved in cardiac HYP. Wang and Yang [176] give a pertinent review. They state that miRs are closely involved in HYP. They mention many paradigms.

miRs regulated by thyroid hormones

The role of these hormones inducing HYP has already been described. A family of pro-hypertrophic miRs (miR-208α, miR-208b, and miR-499) is regulated by thyroid hormones.

miRs regulated by IGF-1 signaling
miR-1 and miR-133 are pro-hypertrophic
miRs regulated by TGF-β signaling; this factor protects the heart from HYP and fibrosis. It inhibits the expression of miR-23α/miR-27α/miR-24-2 and miR-23b/miR-27b/miR-24-1 clusters at the transcriptional level [177].
miR-27b is pro-hypertrophic and causes cardiac dysfunction [178].
miR-24 is upregulated in HYP by aortic constriction or expression of activated calcineurin; it also induces HYP in cardiomyocytes in vitro [179].
miRs regulated by calcineurin signaling
miR-23α is upregulated by NFATc3. An upregulation is also caused by isoproterenol and aldosterone [180].

On the other hand miR-133 loss of function leads to increased NFAT expression and HYP [181].

Da Costa Martins and De Windt [182] also describe the control of miRs in cardiac HYP. They list the following anti-hypertrophic miRs: miR-1, miR-133, miR-26, miR-9, miR-98, and miR-29; the following miRs are pro-hypertrophic: miR-143, miR-199α, miR-208, miR-23α, miR-499, and miR-21.

Sadiq et al. [183] recently also described the role of miRs in the hypertrophic heart: They mention the following miRs involved in pathological HYP: miR-19α/b, miR-22, miR-23α, miR-34α, miR-133, miR-155, miR-208,miR-214, miR-328, miR-350, miR-378, and miR-489.

Finally, Xu et al. [184] used bioinformatics analysis to find miRs regulating biological pathways is exercise induced physiological HYP: The collected 23 miRs from 8 published studies; 12 where upregulated, 14 were downregulated while 3 miRs showed different results in different reports.

In all the reviews mentioned above the possible therapeutic roles of miRs are also discussed.

In conclusion, the very recent review of Nakamura and Sadoshima [185] should be mentioned. They stress some still unresolved issues: First, the growing list of the identified molecular factors contributing to HYP. Integration bioinformatics analysis might allow identification of the most crucial mechanisms and determine their therapeutic priorities.

Second, a better understanding of the role of hypertrophy and the role of cardiac adaptation could be very useful.

Thus cardiac HYP is a master factor determining structure and function of the myocardium. It may be beneficial and noxious, adaptive or maladaptive. It is evident that, as seen in many biological processes concerning the myocardium, it should be moderate short acting and reversible to be defined as beneficial. Maladaptive HYP is by definition associated with a compromised prognosis.

References

1. Zak R. Development and proliferative capacity of cardiac muscle cells. Circ Res. 1974;35(suppl II):17–26.
2. Dorn GW 2nd, Robbins J, Sugden PH. Phenotyping hypertrophy: eschew obfuscation. Circ Res. 2003;92:1171–5.
3. Frey N, Olson EN. Cardiac hypertrophy: the good, the bad, and the ugly. Annu Rev Physiol. 2003;65:45–79.
4. Grossman W, Jones D, McLaurin LP. Wall stress and patterns of hypertrophy in the human left ventricle. J Clin Invest. 1975;56:56–64.
5. Meerson FZ. On the mechanism of compensatory hyperfunction and insufficiency of the heart. Cor Vasa. 1961;3:161–77.
6. Dorn GW 2nd. The fuzzy logic of physiological cardiac hypertrophy. Hypertension. 2007;49:962–70.
7. Andersen JB, Rourke BC, Caiozzo VJ, Bennett AF, Hicks JW. Physiology: postprandial cardiac hypertrophy in pythons. Nature. 2005;434:37–8.
8. Secor SM, Hicks JW, Bennett AF. Ventilatory and cardiovascular responses of a python (Python molurus) to exercise and digestion. J Exp Biol. 2000;203:2447–54.
9. Baliga RR, Rosen SD, Camici PG, Kooner JS. Regional myocardial blood flow redistribution as a cause of postprandial angina pectoris. Circulation. 1998;97:1144–9.
10. Berlinerblau R, Shani J. Postprandial angina pectoris: clinical and angiographic correlations. J Am Coll Cardiol. 1994;23:627–79.
11. Schannwell CM, Zimmermann T, Schneppenheim M, Plehn G, Marx R, Strauer BE. Left ventricular hypertrophy and diastolic dysfunction in healthy pregnant women. Cardiology. 2002;97:73–8.
12. Eghbali M, Deva R, Alioua A, Minosyan TY, Ruan H, Wang Y, et al. Molecular and functional signature of heart hypertrophy during pregnancy. Circ Res. 2005;96:1208–16.
13. Lechmanová M, Kittnar O, Mlcek M, Slavícek J, Dohnalová A, Havránek S, et al. QT dispersion and T-loop morphology in late pregnancy and after delivery. Physiol Res. 2002;51:121–9.
14. Takeishi Y, Huang Q, Abe J, Glassman M, Che W, Lee JD, et al. Src and multiple MAP kinase activation in cardiac hypertrophy and congestive heart failure under chronic pressure-overload: comparison with acute mechanical stretch. J Mol Cell Cardiol. 2001;33:1637–48.
15. Wisløff U, Loennechen JP, Currie S, Smith GL, Ellingsen Ø. Aerobic exercise reduces cardiomyocyte hypertrophy and increases contractility, Ca2+ sensitivity and SERCA-2 in rat after myocardial infarction. Cardiovasc Res. 2002;54:162–74.
16. Chicco AJ, McCune SA, Emter CA, Sparagna GC, Rees ML, Bolden DA, et al. Low-intensity exercise training delays heart failure and improves survival in female hypertensive heart failure rats. Hypertension. 2008;51:1096–102.
17. Giannuzzi P, Temporelli PL, Corrà U, Tavazzi L, ELVD-CHF Study Group. Antiremodeling effect of long-term exercise training in patients with stable chronic heart failure: results of the Exercise in Left Ventricular Dysfunction and Chronic Heart Failure (ELVD-CHF) Trial. Circulation. 2003;108:554–9.

18. Adamopoulos S, Gouziouta A, Mantzouratou P, Laoutaris ID, Dritsas A, Cokkinos DV, et al. Thyroid hormone signalling is altered in response to physical training in patients with end-stage heart failure and mechanical assist devices: potential physiological consequences? Interact Cardiovasc Thorac Surg. 2013;17:664–8.
19. Thompson PD. D. Bruce Dill Historical lecture. Historical concepts of the athlete's heart. Med Sci Sports Exerc. 2004;36:363–70.
20. Pelliccia A, Maron BJ, Spataro A, Proschan MA, Spirito P. The upper limit of physiologic cardiac hypertrophy in highly trained elite athletes. N Engl J Med. 1991;324:295–301.
21. Pelliccia A, Maron BJ, De Luca R, Di Paolo FM, Spataro A, Culasso F. Remodeling of left ventricular hypertrophy in elite athletes after long-term deconditioning. Circulation. 2002;105:944–9.
22. Toutouzas K, Trikas A, Pitsavos C, Barbetseas J, Androulakis A, Stefanadis C, et al. Echocardiographic features of left atrium in elite male athletes. Am J Cardiol. 1996;78:1314–7.
23. Iemitsu M, Miyauchi T, Maeda S, Yuki K, Kobayashi T, Kumagai Y, et al. Intense exercise causes decrease in expression of both endothelial NO synthase and tissue NOx level in hearts. Am J Physiol Regul Integr Comp Physiol. 2000;279:R951–9.
24. Benito B, Gay-Jordi G, Serrano-Mollar A, Guasch E, Shi Y, Tardif JC, Brugada J, et al. Cardiac arrhythmogenic remodeling in a rat model of long-term intensive exercise training. Circulation. 2011;123:13–22.
25. Emter CA, McCune SA, Sparagna GC, Radin MJ, Moore RL. Low-intensity exercise training delays onset of decompensated heart failure in spontaneously hypertensive heart failure rats. Am J Physiol Heart Circ Physiol. 2005;289:H2030–8.
26. Schultz RL, Swallow JG, Waters RP, Kuzman JA, Redetzke RA, Said S, et al. Effects of excessive long-term exercise on cardiac function and myocyte remodeling in hypertensive heart failure rats. Hypertension. 2007;50:410–6.
27. Aronow BJ, Toyokawa T, Canning A, Haghighi K, Delling U, Kranias E, et al. Divergent transcriptional responses to independent genetic causes of cardiac hypertrophy. Physiol Genomics. 2001;6:19–28.
28. Aronow BJ, Toyokawa T, Canning A, Haghighi K, Delling U, Kranias E, et al. Divergent transcriptional responses to independent genetic causes of cardiac hypertrophy. Physiol Genomics. 2001;6:19–28.
29. D'Angelo DD, Sakata Y, Lorenz JN, Boivin GP, Walsh RA, Liggett SB, et al. Transgenic Galphaq overexpression induces cardiac contractile failure in mice. Proc Natl Acad Sci U S A. 1997;94:8121–6.
30. Molkentin JD, Lu JR, Antos CL, Markham B, Richardson J, Robbins J, et al. A calcineurin-dependent transcriptional pathway for cardiac hypertrophy. Cell. 1998;93:215–28.
31. Dorn GW 2nd, Force T. Protein kinase cascades in the regulation of cardiac hypertrophy. J Clin Invest. 2005;115:527–37.
32. Kong SW, Bodyak N, Yue P, Liu Z, Brown J, Izumo S, et al. Genetic expression profiles during physiological and pathological cardiac hypertrophy and heart failure in rats. Physiol Genomics. 2005;21:34–42.
33. Strøm CC, Aplin M, Ploug T, Christoffersen TE, Langfort J, Viese M, et al. Expression profiling reveals differences in metabolic gene expression between exercise-induced cardiac effects and maladaptive cardiac hypertrophy. FEBS J. 2005;272:2684–95.
34. Choi DJ, Koch WJ, Hunter JJ, Rockman HA. Mechanism of beta-adrenergic receptor desensitization in cardiac hypertrophy is increased beta-adrenergic receptor kinase. J Biol Chem. 1997;272:17223–9.
35. Hill JA, Olson EN. Cardiac plasticity. N Engl J Med. 2008;358:1370–80.
36. Kinugawa K, Yonekura K, Ribeiro RC, Eto Y, Aoyagi T, Baxter JD, et al. Regulation of thyroid hormone receptor isoforms in physiological and pathological cardiac hypertrophy. Circ Res. 2001;89:591–8.
37. Scheuer J, Malhotra A, Hirsch C, Capasso J, Schaible TF. Physiologic cardiac hypertrophy corrects contractile protein abnormalities associated with pathologic hypertrophy in rats. J Clin Invest. 1982;70:1300–5.

38. Stanton LW, Garrard LJ, Damm D, Garrick BL, Lam A, Kapoun AM, et al. Altered patterns of gene expression in response to myocardial infarction. Circ Res. 2000;86:939–45.
39. Tan FL, Moravec CS, Li J, Apperson-Hansen C, McCarthy PM, Young JB, et al. The gene expression fingerprint of human heart failure. Proc Natl Acad Sci U S A. 2002;99:11387–92.
40. Nicholls DG, Locke RM. Thermogenic mechanisms in brown fat. Physiol Rev. 1984;64:1–64.
41. Gaussin V, Tomlinson JE, Depre C, Engelhardt S, Antos CL, Takagi G, et al. Common genomic response in different mouse models of beta-adrenergic-induced cardiomyopathy. Circulation. 2003;108:2926–33.
42. Murakami K, Mizushige K, Noma T, Tsuji T, Kimura S, Kohno M. Perindopril effect on uncoupling protein and energy metabolism in failing rat hearts. Hypertension. 2002;40:251–5.
43. Rizzo M, Gensini F, Fatini C, Manetti P, Pucci N, Capalbo A, et al. ACE I/D polymorphism and cardiac adaptations in adolescent athletes. Med Sci Sports Exerc. 2003;35:1986–90.
44. Duerr RL, Huang S, Miraliakbar HR, Clark R, Chien KR, Ross J Jr. Insulin-like growth factor-1 enhances ventricular hypertrophy and function during the onset of experimental cardiac failure. J Clin Invest. 1995;95:619–27.
45. Lupu F, Terwilliger JD, Lee K, Segre GV, Efstratiadis A. Roles of growth hormone and insulin-like growth factor 1 in mouse postnatal growth. Dev Biol. 2001;229:141–62.
46. Kemi OJ, Ceci M, Wisloff U, Grimaldi S, Gallo P, Smith GL, et al. Activation or inactivation of cardiac Akt/mTOR signaling diverges physiological from pathological hypertrophy. J Cell Physiol. 2008;214:316–21.
47. Matsui T, Li L, Wu JC, Cook SA, Nagoshi T, Picard MH, et al. Phenotypic spectrum caused by transgenic overexpression of activated Akt in the heart. J Biol Chem. 2002;277:22896–901.
48. O'Neill BT, Abel ED. Akt1 in the cardiovascular system: friend or foe? J Clin Invest. 2005;115:2059–64.
49. Dorn GW 2nd, Force T. Protein kinase cascades in the regulation of cardiac hypertrophy. J Clin Invest. 2005;115:527–37.
50. TA ACLMK, Frey N, Kutschke W, McAnally J, Shelton JM, et al. Activated glycogen synthase-3 beta suppresses cardiac hypertrophy in vivo. Proc Natl Acad Sci U S A. 2002;99:907–12.
51. Michael A, Haq S, Chen X, Hsich E, Cui L, Walters B, et al. Glycogen synthase kinase-3beta regulates growth, calcium homeostasis, and diastolic function in the heart. J Biol Chem. 2004;279:21383–93.
52. Dillmann W. Cardiac hypertrophy and thyroid hormone signaling. Heart Fail Rev. 2010;15:125–3.
53. Cokkinos D, Pantos C. Les hormones thyroïdiennes. Activation sur le myocardie. Bull Acad Med. 2009;193:327–38.
54. Mourouzis I, Mantzouratou P, Galanopoulos G, Kostakou E, Roukounakis N, Kokkinos AD, et al. Dose-dependent effects of thyroid hormone on post-ischemic cardiac performance: potential involvement of Akt and ERK signalings. Mol Cell Biochem. 2012;363:235–43.
55. Alcendor RR, Gao S, Zhai P, Zablocki D, Holle E, Yu X, et al. Sirt1 regulates aging and resistance to oxidative stress in the heart. Circ Res. 2007;100:1512–21.
56. Kontaridis MI, Geladari EV, Geladari CV. Pathways to myocardial hypertrophy. In: Cokkinos DV, editor. Introduction to translational cardiovascular research. London: Springer; 2015. p. 167–86.
57. Crabtree GR, Olson EN. NFAT signaling: choreographing the social lives of cells. Cell. 2002;109(Suppl):S67–579.
58. Wilkins BJ, Dai YS, Bueno OF, Parsons SA, Xu J, Plank DM, et al. Calcineurin/NFAT coupling participates in pathological, but not physiological, cardiac hypertrophy. Circ Res. 2004;94:110–8.
59. Hill JA, Karimi M, Kutschke W, Davisson RL, Zimmerman K, Wang Z, et al. Cardiac hypertrophy is not a required compensatory response to short-term pressure overload. Circulation. 2000;101:2863–9.
60. Oie E, Bjørnerheim R, Clausen OP, Attramadal H. Cyclosporin A inhibits cardiac hypertrophy and enhances cardiac dysfunction during postinfarction failure in rats. Am J Physiol Heart Circ Physiol. 2000;278:H2115–23.

61. Meguro T, Hong C, Asai K, Takagi G, McKinsey TA, Olson EN, et al. Cyclosporine attenuates pressure-overload hypertrophy in mice while enhancing susceptibility to decompensation and heart failure. Circ Res. 1999;84:735–40.
62. Rockman HA, Koch WJ, Lefkowitz RJ. Seven-transmembrane-spanning receptors and heart function. Nature. 2002;415:206–12.
63. Bisognano JD, Weinberger HD, Bohlmeyer TJ, Pende A, Raynolds MV, Sastravaha A, et al. Myocardial-directed overexpression of the human beta(1)-adrenergic receptor in transgenic mice. J Mol Cell Cardiol. 2000;32:817–30.
64. Dorn GW 2nd, Tepe NM, Lorenz JN, Koch WJ, Liggett SB. Low- and high-level transgenic expression of beta2-adrenergic receptors differentially affect cardiac hypertrophy and function in Galphaq-overexpressing mice. Proc Natl Acad Sci U S A. 1999;96: 6400–5.
65. Niu X, Watts VL, Cingolani OH, Sivakumaran V, Leyton-Mange JS, Ellis CL, et al. Cardioprotective effect of beta-3 adrenergic receptor agonism: role of neuronal nitric oxide synthase. J Am Coll Cardiol. 2012;59:1979–87.
66. Bristow MR, Ginsburg R, Minobe W, Cubicciotti RS, Sageman WS, Lurie K, et al. Decreased catecholamine sensitivity and beta-adrenergic-receptor density in failing human hearts. N Engl J Med. 1982;307:205–11.
67. Rockman HA, Chien KR, Choi DJ, Iaccarino G, Hunter JJ, Ross J Jr, et al. Expression of a beta-adrenergic receptor kinase 1 inhibitor prevents the development of myocardial failure in gene-targeted mice. Proc Natl Acad Sci U S A. 1998;95:7000–5.
68. Lowes BD, Gilbert EM, Abraham WT, Minobe WA, Larrabee P, Ferguson D, et al. Myocardial gene expression in dilated cardiomyopathy treated with beta-blocking agents. N Engl J Med. 2002;346:1357–65.
69. Yoshida H, Kakuchi J, Yoshikawa N, Saruta T, Inagami T, Phillips JA 3rd, et al. Angiotensin II type 1 receptor gene abnormality in a patient with Bartter's syndrome. Kidney Int. 1994;46:1505–9.
70. Sadoshima J, Xu Y, Slayter HS, Izumo S. Autocrine release of angiotensin II mediates stretch-induced hypertrophy of cardiac myocytes in vitro. Cell. 1993;75:977–84.
71. Feuerstein GZ, Rozanski D. G proteins and heart failure: is Galphaq a novel target for heart failure? Circ Res. 2000;87:1085–6.
72. Mishra S, Ling H, Grimm M, Zhang T, Bers DM, Brown JH. Cardiac hypertrophy and heart failure development through Gq and CaM kinase II signaling. J Cardiovasc Pharmacol. 2010;56:598–603.
73. Chrysant SG. Current status of dual Renin Angiotensin aldosterone system blockade for the treatment of cardiovascular diseases. Am J Cardiol. 2010;105:849–52.
74. Maruyama Y, Nishida M, Sugimoto Y, Tanabe S, Turner JH, Kozasa T, et al. Galpha (12/13) mediates alpha(1)-adrenergic receptor-induced cardiac hypertrophy. Circ Res. 2002;91:961–9. endothelin 1 (75)
75. Arai K, Maruyama Y, Nishida M, Tanabe S, Takagahara S, Kozasa T, et al. Differential requirement of G alpha12, G alpha13, G alphaq, and G beta gamma for endothelin-1-induced c-Jun NH2-terminal kinase and extracellular signal-regulated kinase activation. Mol Pharmacol. 2003;63:478–88.
76. Hoshijima M, Sah VP, Wang Y, Chien KR, Brown JH. The low molecular weight GTPase Rho regulates myofibril formation and organization in neonatal rat ventricular myocytes. Involvement of Rho kinase. J Biol Chem. 1998;273:7725–230.
77. van Berlo JH, Maillet M, Molkentin JD. Signaling effectors underlying pathologic growth and remodeling of the heart. J Clin Invest. 2013;123:37–45.
78. Bueno OF, De Windt LJ, Tymitz KM, Witt SA, Kimball TR, Klevitsky R, et al. The MEK1-ERK1/2 signaling pathway promotes compensated cardiac hypertrophy in transgenic mice. EMBO J. 2000;19:6341–50.
79. Bernardo BC, Weeks KL, Pretorius L, McMullen JR. Molecular distinction between physiological and pathological cardiac hypertrophy: experimental findings and therapeutic strategies. Pharmacol Ther. 2010;128:191–227.

80. Komuro I, Kudo S, Yamazaki T, Zou Y, Shiojima I, Yazaki Y. Mechanical stretch activates the stress-activated protein kinases in cardiac myocytes. FASEB J. 1996;10:631–6.
81. Choukroun G, Hajjar R, Kyriakis JM, Bonventre JV, Rosenzweig A, Force T. Role of the stress-activated protein kinases in endothelin-induced cardiomyocyte hypertrophy. J Clin Invest. 1998;102:1311–20.
82. Ramirez MT, Zhao XL, Schulman H, Brown JH. The nuclear deltaB isoform of Ca2+/calmodulin-dependent protein kinase II regulates atrial natriuretic factor gene expression in ventricular myocytes. J Biol Chem. 1997;272:31203–8.
83. Yano M, Kim S, Izumi Y, Yamanaka S, Iwao H. Differential activation of cardiac c-jun amino-terminal kinase and extracellular signal-regulated kinase in angiotensin II-mediated hypertension. Circ Res. 1998;83:752–60.
84. Wang Y, Huang S, Sah VP, Ross J Jr, Brown JH, Han J, et al. Cardiac muscle cell hypertrophy and apoptosis induced by distinct members of the p38 mitogen-activated protein kinase family. J Biol Chem. 1998;273:2161–8.
85. Oudit GY, Sun H, Kerfant BG, Crackower MA, Penninger JM, Backx PH. The role of phosphoinositide-3 kinase and PTEN in cardiovascular physiology and disease. J Mol Cell Cardiol. 2004;37:449–71.
86. Kerfant BG, Zhao D, Lorenzen-Schmidt I, Wilson LS, Cai S, Chen SR, et al. PI3Kgamma is required for PDE4, not PDE3, activity in subcellular microdomains containing the sarcoplasmic reticular calcium ATPase in cardiomyocytes. Circ Res. 2007;101:400–8.
87. Dorn GW 2nd, Force T. Protein kinase cascades in the regulation of cardiac hypertrophy. J Clin Invest. 2005;115:527–37.
88. Chen L, Hahn H, Wu G, Chen CH, Liron T, Schechtman D, et al. Opposing cardioprotective actions and parallel hypertrophic effects of delta PKC and epsilon PKC. Proc Natl Acad Sci U S A. 2001;98:11114–9.
89. Shimizu I, Minamino T. Physiological and pathological cardiac hypertrophy. J Mol Cell Cardiol. 2016;97:245–62.
90. Samuelsson AM, Bollano E, Mobini R, Larsson BM, Omerovic E, Fu M, et al. Hyperinsulinemia: effect on cardiac mass/function, angiotensin II receptor expression, and insulin signaling pathways. Am J Physiol Heart Circ Physiol. 2006;291:H787–96.
91. Shimizu I, Minamino T, Toko H, Okada S, Ikeda H, Yasuda N, et al. Excessive cardiac insulin signaling exacerbates systolic dysfunction induced by pressure overload in rodents. J Clin Invest. 2010;120:1506–14.
92. Shamak M, Fatullayev J, Sabashnikov A, Zeriouh M, Schmack B, Farag M, et al. Cardiac hypertrophy: an introduction to molecular and cellular basis. Med Sci Monit Basic Res. 2016;22:75–9.
93. Yang F, Dong A, Mueller P, Caicedo J, Sutton AM, Odetunde J, et al. Coronary artery remodeling in a model of left ventricular pressure overload is influenced by platelets and inflammatory cells. PLoS One. 2012;7:e40196.
94. Kuusisto J, Kärjä V, Sipola P, Kholová I, Peuhkurinen K, Jääskeläinen P, et al. Low-grade inflammation and the phenotypic expression of myocardial fibrosis in hypertrophic cardiomyopathy. Heart. 2012;98:1007–13.
95. Wollert KC, Chien KR. Cardiotrophin-1 and the role of gp130-dependent signaling pathways in cardiac growth and development. J Mol Med (Berl). 1997;75:492–501.
96. Takeda N, Manabe I. Cellular interplay between cardiomyocytes and nonmyocytes in cardiac remodeling. Int J Inflam. 2011;2011:535241.
97. Mosser DM, Edwards JP. Exploring the full spectrum of macrophage activation. Nat Rev Immunol. 2008;8:958–69.
98. van den Akker F, de Jager SC, Sluijter JP. Mesenchymal stem cell therapy for cardiac inflammation: immunomodulatory properties and the influence of toll-like receptors. Mediat Inflamm. 2013;2013:181020.
99. Xu L, Brink M. mTOR, cardiomyocytes and inflammation in cardiac hypertrophy. Biochim Biophys Acta. 1863;2016:1894–903.
100. Mann DL. Innate immunity and the failing heart: the cytokine hypothesis revisited. Circ Res. 2015;116:1254–68.

101. Shioi T, McMullen JR, Tarnavski O, Converso K, Sherwood MC, Manning WJ, et al. Rapamycin attenuates load-induced cardiac hypertrophy in mice. Circulation. 2003;107:1664–70.
102. McMullen JR, Sherwood MC, Tarnavski O, Zhang L, Dorfman AL, Shioi T, et al. Inhibition of mTOR signaling with rapamycin regresses established cardiac hypertrophy induced by pressure overload. Circulation. 2004;109:3050–5.
103. Gao XM, Wong G, Wang B, Kiriazis H, Moore XL, Su YD, et al. Inhibition of mTOR reduces chronic pressure-overload cardiac hypertrophy and fibrosis. J Hypertens. 2006;24:1663–70.
104. Medzhitov R, Preston-Hurlburt P, Janeway CA Jr. A human homologue of the Drosophila Toll protein signals activation of adaptive immunity. Nature. 1997;388:394–7.
105. Baeuerle PA, Baltimore D. NF-kappa B: ten years after. Cell. 1996;87:13–20.
106. Ha T, Li Y, Hua F, Ma J, Gao X, Kelley J, et al. Reduced cardiac hypertrophy in toll-like receptor 4-deficient mice following pressure overload. Cardiovasc Res. 2005;68:224–34.
107. Higashikuni Y, Tanaka K, Kato M, Nureki O, Hirata Y, Nagai R, et al. Toll-like receptor-2 mediates adaptive cardiac hypertrophy in response to pressure overload through interleukin-1β upregulation via nuclear factor κB activation. J Am Heart Assoc. 2013;2: e000267.
108. Ehrentraut H, Felix Ehrentraut S, Boehm O, El Aissati S, Foltz F, Goelz L, et al. Tlr4 deficiency protects against cardiac pressure overload induced hyperinflammation. PLoS One. 2015;10:e0142921.
109. Burns K, Clatworthy J, Martin L, Martinon F, Plumpton C, Maschera B, et al. Tollip, a new component of the IL-1RI pathway, links IRAK to the IL-1 receptor. Nat Cell Biol. 2000;2:346–51.
110. Liu Y, Jiang XL, Liu Y, Jiang DS, Zhang Y, Zhang R, et al. Toll-interacting protein (Tollip) negatively regulates pressure overload-induced ventricular hypertrophy in mice. Cardiovasc Res. 2014;101:87–96.
111. Abrahao M, Carneiro-Ramos M. Cross-talk between Toll-like receptors and renin angiotensin system in a cardiac hypertrophy model induced by renal ischemia/reperfusion. FASEB J. 2014;Abstr. Nr.4045
112. Ehrentraut H, Weber C, Ehrentraut S, Schwederski M, Boehm O, Knuefermann P, et al. The toll-like receptor 4-antagonist eritoran reduces murine cardiac hypertrophy. Eur J Heart Fail. 2011;13:602–10.
113. Spinale FG, Coker ML, Heung LJ, Bond BR, Gunasinghe HR, Etoh T, et al. A matrix metalloproteinase induction/activation system exists in the human left ventricular myocardium and is upregulated in heart failure. Circulation. 2000;102:1944–9.
114. Chancey AL, Brower GL, Peterson JT, Janicki JS. Effects of matrix metalloproteinase inhibition on ventricular remodeling due to volume overload. Circulation. 2002;105:1983–8.
115. Asakura M, Kitakaze M, Takashima S, Liao Y, Ishikura F, Yoshinaka T, et al. Cardiac hypertrophy is inhibited by antagonism of ADAM12 processing of HB-EGF: metalloproteinase inhibitors as a new therapy. Nat Med. 2002;8:35–40.
116. Liu ZP, Olson EN. Suppression of proliferation and cardiomyocyte hypertrophy by CHAMP, a cardiac-specific RNA helicase. Proc Natl Acad Sci U S A. 2002;99:2043–8.
117. Takewaki S, Kuro-o M, Hiroi Y, Yamazaki T, Noguchi T, Miyagishi A, et al. Activation of Na(+)-H+ antiporter (NHE-1) gene expression during growth, hypertrophy and proliferation of the rabbit cardiovascular system. J Mol Cell Cardiol. 1995;27:729–42.
118. Cingolani HE. Camilión de Hurtado MC.Na(+)-H(+) exchanger inhibition: a new antihypertrophic tool. Circ Res. 2002;90:751–3.
119. Amin JK, Xiao L, Pimental DR, Pagano PJ, Singh K, Sawyer DB, et al. Reactive oxygen species mediate alpha-adrenergic receptor-stimulated hypertrophy in adult rat ventricular myocytes. J Mol Cell Cardiol. 2001;33:131–9.
120. Kuster GM, Pimentel DR, Adachi T, Ido Y, Brenner DA, Cohen RA, et al. Alpha-adrenergic receptor-stimulated hypertrophy in adult rat ventricular myocytes is mediated via thioredoxin-1-sensitive oxidative modification of thiols on Ras. Circulation. 2005;111:1192–8.
121. Higuchi Y, Otsu K, Nishida K, Hirotani S, Nakayama H, Yamaguchi O, et al. Involvement of reactive oxygen species-mediated NF-kappa B activation in TNF-alpha-induced cardiomyocyte hypertrophy. J Mol Cell Cardiol. 2002;34:233–40.

122. Kwon SH, Pimentel DR, Remondino A, Sawyer DB, Colucci WS. H(2)O(2) regulates cardiac myocyte phenotype via concentration-dependent activation of distinct kinase pathways. J Mol Cell Cardiol. 2003;35:615–21.
123. Seddon M, Looi YH, Shah AM. Oxidative stress and redox signalling in cardiac hypertrophy and heart failure. Heart. 2007;93:903–7.
124. Li JM, Gall NP, Grieve DJ, Chen M, Shah AM. Activation of NADPH oxidase during progression of cardiac hypertrophy to failure. Hypertension. 2002;40:477–84.
125. MacCarthy PA, Grieve DJ, Li JM, Dunster C, Kelly FJ, Shah AM. Impaired endothelial regulation of ventricular relaxation in cardiac hypertrophy: role of reactive oxygen species and NADPH oxidase. Circulation. 2001;104:2967–74.
126. Park YM, Park MY, Suh YL, Park JB. NAD(P)H oxidase inhibitor prevents blood pressure elevation and cardiovascular hypertrophy in aldosterone-infused rats. Biochem Biophys Res Commun. 2004;313:812–7.
127. Barger PM, Kelly DP. PPAR signaling in the control of cardiac energy metabolism. Trends Cardiovasc Med. 2000;10:238–45.
128. Lehman JJ, Barger PM, Kovacs A, Saffitz JE, Medeiros DM, Kelly DP. Peroxisome proliferator-activated receptor gamma coactivator-1 promotes cardiac mitochondrial biogenesis. Clin Invest. 2000;106:847–56.
129. Balakumar P, Singh M. The possible role of caspase-3 in pathological and physiological cardiac hypertrophy in rats. Basic Clin Pharmacol Toxicol. 2006;99:418–24.
130. Rothermel BA, Hill JA. Autophagy in load-induced heart disease. Circ Res. 2008:103–1363.
131. Nakai A, Yamaguchi O, Takeda T, Higuchi Y, Hikoso S, Taniike M, et al. The role of autophagy in cardiomyocytes in the basal state and in response to hemodynamic stress. Nat Med. 2007;13:619–24.
132. Zaglia T, Milan G, Ruhs A, Franzoso M, Bertaggia E, Pianca N, et al. Atrogin-1 deficiency promotes cardiomyopathy and premature death via impaired autophagy. J Clin Invest. 2014;124:2410–24.
133. Li L, Xu J, He L, Peng L, Zhong Q, Chen L, et al. The role of autophagy in cardiac hypertrophy. Acta Biochim Biophys Sin Shanghai. 2016;48:491–500.
134. Qipshidze N, Tyagi N, Metreveli N, Lominadze D, Tyagi SC. Autophagy mechanism of right ventricular remodeling in murine model of pulmonary artery constriction. Am J Physiol Heart Circ Physiol. 2012;302:H688–96.
135. Rifki OF, Hill JA. Cardiac autophagy: good with the bad. J Cardiovasc Pharmacol. 2012;60:248–52.
136. Shimizu I, Minamino T. Physiological and pathological cardiac hypertrophy. J Mol Cell Cardiol. 2016;97:245–62.
137. Shiojima I, Sato K, Izumiya Y, Schiekofer S, Ito M, Liao R, et al. Disruption of coordinated cardiac hypertrophy and angiogenesis contributes to the transition to heart failure. J Clin Invest. 2005;115:2108–18.
138. Dimmeler S, Fleming I, Fisslthaler B, Hermann C, Busse R, Zeiher AM. Activation of nitric oxide synthase in endothelial cells by Akt-dependent phosphorylation. Nature. 1999;399:601–5.
139. Oka T, Akazawa H, Naito AT, Komuro I. Angiogenesis and cardiac hypertrophy: maintenance of cardiac function and causative roles in heart failure. Circ Res. 2014;114:565–71.
140. Anversa P, Levicky V, Beghi C, McDonald SL, Kikkawa Y. Morphometry of exercise-induced right ventricular hypertrophy in the rat. Circ Res. 1983;52:57–64.
141. Jaba IM, Zhuang ZW, Li N, Jiang Y, Martin KA, Sinusas AJ, et al. NO triggers RGS4 degradation to coordinate angiogenesis and cardiomyocyte growth. J Clin Invest. 2013;123:1718–31.
142. Phung TL, Ziv K, Dabydeen D, Eyiah-Mensah G, Riveros M, Perruzzi C, et al. Pathological angiogenesis is induced by sustained Akt signaling and inhibited by rapamycin. Cancer Cell. 2006;10:159–70.
143. Izumiya Y, Shiojima I, Sato K, Sawyer DB, Colucci WS, Walsh K. Vascular endothelial growth factor blockade promotes the transition from compensatory cardiac hypertrophy to failure in response to pressure overload. Hypertension. 2006;47:887–93.

144. Friehs I, Barillas R, Vasilyev NV, Roy N, McGowan FX, del Nido PJ. Vascular endothelial growth factor prevents apoptosis and preserves contractile function in hypertrophied infant heart. Circulation. 2006;114:I290–5.
145. Oka T, Maillet M, Watt AJ, Schwartz RJ, Aronow BJ, Duncan SA, et al. Cardiac-specific deletion of Gata4 reveals its requirement for hypertrophy, compensation, and myocyte viability. Circ Res. 2006;98:837–45.
146. Heineke J, Auger-Messier M, Xu J, Oka T, Sargent MA, York A, et al. Cardiomyocyte GATA4 functions as a stress-responsive regulator of angiogenesis in the murine heart. J Clin Invest. 2007;117:3198–210.
147. Sano M, Minamino T, Toko H, Miyauchi H, Orimo M, Qin Y, et al. p53-induced inhibition of Hif-1 causes cardiac dysfunction during pressure overload. Nature. 2007;446:444–8.
148. Naito AT, Okada S, Minamino T, Iwanaga K, Liu ML, Sumida T, Nomura S, et al. Promotion of CHIP-mediated p53 degradation protects the heart from ischemic injury. Circ Res. 2010 Jun 11;106:1692–702.
149. An WG, Kanekal M, Simon MC, Maltepe E, Blagosklonny MV, Neckers LM. Stabilization of wild-type p53 by hypoxia-inducible factor 1alpha. Nature. 1998;392:405–8.
150. Carr AM. Cell cycle. Piecing together the p53 puzzle. Science. 2000;287:1765–6.
151. Muller PA, Vousden KH. p53 mutations in cancer. Nat Cell Biol. 2013;15:2–8.
152. Shizukuda Y, Matoba S, Mian OY, Nguyen T, Hwang PM. Targeted disruption of p53 attenuates doxorubicin-induced cardiac toxicity in mice. Mol Cell Biochem. 2005;273:25–32.
153. Gerdes AM. Cardiac myocyte remodeling in hypertrophy and progression to failure. J Card Fail. 2002;8:S264–8.
154. Dorn GW 2nd, Robbins J, Ball N, Walsh RA. Myosin heavy chain regulation and myocyte contractile depression after LV hypertrophy in aortic-banded mice. Am J Phys. 1994;267:H400–5.
155. You J, Wu J, Zhang Q, Ye Y, Wang S, Huang J, et al. Differential cardiac hypertrophy and signaling pathways in pressure versus volume overload. Am J Physiol Heart Circ Physiol. 2018;314:H552–62.
156. Derumeaux G, Mulder P, Richard V, Chagraoui A, Nafeh C, Bauer F, et al. Tissue Doppler imaging differentiates physiological from pathological pressure-overload left ventricular hypertrophy in rats. Circulation. 2002;105:1602–8.
157. Galanti G, Toncelli L, Del Furia F, Stefani L, Cappelli B, De Luca A, et al. Tissue doppler imaging can be useful to distinguish pathological from physiological left ventricular hypertrophy: a study in master athletes and mild hypertensive subjects. Cardiovasc Ultrasound. 2009;7:48.
158. Afonso L, Kondur A, Simegn M, Niraj A, Hari P, Kaur R, et al. Two-dimensional strain profiles in patients with physiological and pathological hypertrophy and preserved left ventricular systolic function: a comparative analyses. BMJ Open. 2012;2:e001390.
159. Oláh A, Németh BT, Mátyás C, Hidi L, Lux Á, Ruppert M, et al. Physiological and pathological left ventricular hypertrophy of comparable degree is associated with characteristic differences of in vivo hemodynamics. Am J Physiol Heart Circ Physiol. 2016;310: H587–97.
160. Schiattarella GG, Hill JA. Inhibition of hypertrophy is a good therapeutic strategy in ventricular pressure overload. Circulation. 2015;131:1435–47.
161. Douglas PS, Katz SE, Weinberg EO, Chen MH, Bishop SP, Lorell BH. Hypertrophic remodeling: gender differences in the early response to left ventricular pressure overload. J Am Coll Cardiol. 1998;32:1118–25.
162. Weinberg EO, Thienelt CD, Katz SE, Bartunek J, Tajima M, Rohrbach S, et al. Gender differences in molecular remodeling in pressure overload hypertrophy. J Am Coll Cardiol. 1999;34:264–73.
163. Bech-Hanssen O, Wallentin I, Houltz E, Beckman Suurküla M, Larsson S, Caidahl K. Gender differences in patients with severe aortic stenosis: impact on preoperative left ventricular geometry and function, as well as early postoperative morbidity and mortality. Eur J Cardiothorac Surg. 1999;15:24–30.

164. Lee JM, Park SJ, Lee SP, Park E, Chang SA, Kim HK, et al. Gender difference in ventricular response to aortic stenosis: insight from cardiovascular magnetic resonance. PLoS One. 2015;10:e0121684.
165. Treibel TA, Kozor R, Fontana M, Torlasco C, Reant P, Badiani S, et al. Sex dimorphism in the myocardial response to aortic stenosis. JACC Cardiovasc Imaging. 2017;pii:S1936-878X(17)30907-5. https://doi.org/10.1016/j.jcmg.2017.08.025.
166. Frey N, Katus HA, Olson EN, Hill JA. Hypertrophy of the heart: a new therapeutic target? Circulation. 2004;109:1580–9.
167. Cioffi G, Faggiano P, Vizzardi E, Tarantini L, Cramariuc D, Gerdts E, et al. Prognostic effect of inappropriately high left ventricular mass in asymptomatic severe aortic stenosis. Heart. 2011;97:301–7.
168. Verdecchia P, Angeli F, Gattobigio R, Sardone M, Pede S, Reboldi GP. Regression of left ventricular hypertrophy and prevention of stroke in hypertensive subjects. Am J Hypertens. 2006;19:493–9.
169. McKinsey TA, Kass DA. Small-molecule therapies for cardiac hypertrophy: moving beneath the cell surface. Nat Rev Drug Discov. 2007;6:617–35.
170. Reid BG, Stratton MS, Bowers S, Cavasin MA, Demos-Davies KM, Susano I, et al. Discovery of novel small molecule inhibitors of cardiac hypertrophy using high throughput, high content imaging. J Mol Cell Cardiol. 2016;97:106–13.
171. Hilfiker-Kleiner D, Haghikia A, Berliner D, Vogel-Claussen J, Schwab J, Franke A, et al. Bromocriptine for the treatment of peripartum cardiomyopathy: a multicentre randomized study. Eur Heart J. 2017;38:2671–9.
172. Vivar R, Humeres C, Varela M, Ayala P, Guzmán N, Olmedo I, et al. Cardiac fibroblast death by ischemia/reperfusion is partially inhibited by IGF-1 through both PI3K/Akt and MEK-ERK pathways. Exp Mol Pathol. 2012;93:1–7.
173. Dobaczewski M, Chen W, Frangogiannis NG. Transforming growth factor (TGF)-β signaling in cardiac remodeling. J Mol Cell Cardiol. 2011;51:600–6.
174. Brutsaert DL. Cardiac endothelial-myocardial signaling: its role in cardiac growth, contractile performance, and rhythmicity. Physiol Rev. 2003;83:59–115.
175. Crowley ST, Ray CJ, Nawaz D, Majack RA, Horwitz LD. Multiple growth factors are released from mechanically injured vascular smooth muscle cells. Am J Phys. 1995;269:H1641–17.
176. Wang J, Yang X. The function of miRNA in cardiac hypertrophy. Cell Mol Life Sci. 2012;69:3561–70.
177. Sun Q, Zhang Y, Yang G, Chen X, Zhang Y, Cao G, et al. Transforming growth factor-beta-regulated miR-24 promotes skeletal muscle differentiation. Nucleic Acids Res. 2008;36:2690–9.
178. Wang J, Song Y, Zhang Y, Xiao H, Sun Q, Hou N, et al. Cardiomyocyte overexpression of miR-27b induces cardiac hypertrophy and dysfunction in mice. Cell Res. 2012;22:516–27.
179. van Rooij E, Sutherland LB, Liu N, Williams AH, McAnally J, et al. A signature pattern of stress-responsive microRNAs that can evoke cardiac hypertrophy and heart failure. Proc Natl Acad Sci U S A. 2006;103:18255–60.
180. Lin Z, Murtaza I, Wang K, Jiao J, Gao J, Li PF. miR-23a functions downstream of NFATc3 to regulate cardiac hypertrophy. Proc Natl Acad Sci U S A. 2009;106:12103–8.
181. Dong DL, Chen C, Huo R, Wang N, Li Z, Tu YJ, et al. Reciprocal repression between microRNA-133 and calcineurin regulates cardiac hypertrophy: a novel mechanism for progressive cardiac hypertrophy. Hypertension. 2010;55:946–52.
182. Da Costa Martins PA, De Windt LJ. MicroRNAs in control of cardiac hypertrophy. Cardiovasc Res. 2012;93:563–72.
183. Sadiq S, Crowley TM, Charchar FJ, Sanigorski A, Lewandowski PA. MicroRNAs in a hypertrophic heart: from foetal life to adulthood. Biol Rev Camb Philos Soc. 2017;92:1314–31.
184. Xu J, Liu Y, Xie Y, Zhao C, Wang H. Bioinformatics analysis reveals MicroRNAs regulating biological pathways in exercise-induced cardiac physiological hypertrophy. Biomed Res Int. 2017;2017:2850659.
185. Nakamura M, Sadoshima J. Mechanisms of physiological and pathological cardiac hypertrophy. Nat Rev Cardiol. 2018;15:387–407.

Chapter 6
The Ishemia Reperfusion Injury Challenge

Dennis V. Cokkinos

The advent of thrombolysis in acute myocardial infarction (AMI) gave the first possibility of establishing reperfusion of an occluded coronary artery [1, 2].

Early at that time, apart from resolution of ST-T segment elevation, which together with the course of enzymes in the serum was a means of assessing the success of recanalization, a concern timidly raised its head. This was the emergence of reperfusion arrhythmias [3], which actually were considered as a sign of reperfusion. These had already been noted in animal experiments by Tennant and Wiggers in 1935 [4].

In the clinical arena, ventricular fibrillation was more common in primary angioplasty than in thrombolysis [5].

Already in 1985, two leading figures on the subject, Braunwald and Kloner [6] had expressed concerns, proposing myocardial reperfusion as a "double-edged sword".

In 1995, Grech et al. [7] also expressed concerns that reperfusion may have clinically important adverse effects [7].

Braunwald and Kloner [6] discuss the much older but pertinent findings of Jennings et al. [8], who had postulated that reperfusion may actually hasten the necrotic process of irreversibly injured cardiomyocytes. Since then the problem has been reviewed by many experts. A main contribution has been that of Yellon and Hausenloy [9].

They describe four types of cardiac complications caused by the myocardial reperfusion injury. The first discribed by Braunwald and Kloner in 1982 [10] is myocardial stunning, which will be further discussed in the respective chapter.

The second is the no-reflow phenomenon, which apart from its basic research considerations, has a negative influence on prognosis after PCI in AMI [11].

D. V. Cokkinos (✉)
Heart and Vessel Department, Biomedical Research Foundation,
Academy of Athens - Gregory Skalkeas, Athens, Greece
e-mail: dcokkinos@bioacademy.gr

D. V. Cokkinos (ed.), *Myocardial Preservation*,
https://doi.org/10.1007/978-3-319-98186-4_6

The no-reflow phenomenon remains a major problem for which no practical treatment exists currently [12]; according to a very pertinent review of Hausenloy and Yellon [13] the major determinants of this phenomenon are many and varied.

Capillary damage, is a main factor. The coronary vascular endothelium undergoes damage similar to that of the myocardium together with impaired vasodilatation, compression of the capillaries by swelling of the cardiomyocytes apart from the swelling of the endothelial cells themselves. The debris released from the atherosclerotic plaque, platelet microhrombi, and the release of various factors which have vasoactive and thrombogenic actions, as well as plugging by neutrophils play an additive role. Also, within the endothelium, ischemia further promotes proinflammatory gene production and bioactive substances such as endothelin and thromboxane [14].

This complication is demonstrated by routine angiography in around 25% or pts. [15]. It can be assessed by scintigraphy [15] and is a major cause of cardiac remodeling [16] as already mentioned, and as Hausenloy and Yellon [13] point out, it can be missed clinically but detected by myocardial contrast echocardiography, myocardial perfusion scanning [17] or contrast enhanced MRI [18].

Bulluck and Hausenloy [19] characterize microvascular obstruction as "the bane" of myocardial reperfusion. They reiterated –in 2015-that currently there was no effective therapy available for this complication.

According to van Kranenburg [18] in a meta-analysis including more than 1000 pts., it was found by MRI in 54.9% in pts. with angiographic normal coronary flow.

In 2017, the very prominent group of Kloner [20] discuss the management of this phenomenon in the laboratory which they describe as occurring in 5–60% of published data, especially in degenerating vein grafts. In addition to the already discussed mechanisms they mention microvascular spasm. They mention that the efficacy of intracoronary adenosine, calcium channel blockers and nitroprusside is yet to be established.

As regards thrombus aspiration, they refer to the neutral meta-analysis over 14 trials by Mongeon et al. [21]. However, in the more recent meta-analysis by Mancini [22] a lower incidence of no-reflow was seen, but without long-term clinical benefit.

According to Rezkalla et al. [20] routine aspiration should be avoided and only tried in the presence of angiographically visible thrombus.

The third type concerns the emergence cardiac arrhythmias, which do not currently represent a main threat.

Cell death is the forth expression of IRI. As regards the "cost" of reperfusion the following estimation is given by Hausenloy and Yellon [9–13]. As they point out the following percentages: as regards infarct size:

- If myocardial ischemia only exists in the absence of reperfusion, the infarct size can be estimated at 70%; if reperfusion is applied, the infarct size decreases to 40%, which is a great Improvement but still is a substantial loss of myocardium.
- If appropriate preventive measures prove successful, they infarct size can be reduced by a further 25% which is substantial. Garcia-Dorado et al. [23] believe

that necrosis is the main cause of cell death in IRI. They discuss however that apoptosis can be important especially in larger animals and that the time window to salvage the myocardium appears to be wider in patients than animals.

More details are given in the chapter on cardiomyocyte death.

The following factors are considered to be operative in lethal reperfusion injury [9, 12, 13].

Oxidative stress, otherwise termed oxygen paradox, as described by Hearse et al. [24].

6.1 Oxidative Stress

Thus, reoxygenation can increase the injury produced by ischemia [24]. However, antioxidant therapy has not fulfilled its promise [25].

The "energy paradox": this postulates that replenishing mitochondrial ATP increases cellular damage [26], either by causing breaking of membranes or by new damage to energy production. Here older studies must be reiterated, from the seminal work of Jennings and Reimer [27].

They mention that very early (15–20 s) after an arterial occlusion anaerobic glucosis emerges as the sole source of high energy phosphate. This can meet only the most basic energy demands; within 60–90 min the ischemic area develops contracture-rigor. At reperfusion although mitochondrial oxidative phosphorylation is restored, contractility returns less promptly to normal. This constitutes myocardial stunning which is described in the corresponding chapter.

During reperfusion an overshoot in fatty acid oxidation is seen which inhibits glucose oxidation, resulting into an imbalance between glycolysis and glucose oxidation. This "uncoupling" is a source of net H+ production.

Thus, one could also invoke the "acidosis paradox": during ischemia. H+ accumulates in the intracellular space, as a result of anaerobic glycolysis. After flow is restored and reperfusion occurs it returns to the extracellular space, with a resultant increase of intracellular Na + Ca2+ exchanger with the calcium paradox occurring.

Piper and Garcia-Dorado [28] also describe cardiomyocyte death during IRI. Frank et al. [29], as well as Hausenloy and Yellon [13] have already stressed [15] describe the "metabolic modulation", which consists of overshoot of fatty acid oxidation, impaired pyruvate oxidation and accelerated anaerobic glycolysis; the already described increase of fatty acid oxidation inhibits glucose oxidation, resulting in imbalance between glycolysis and glucose oxidation, accompanied by further inhibition of pyruvate oxidation, with as a result an increased H+ and Ca2+ as well as the disruption of the mitochondrial membrane potential leading to the production of ROS. As will be further described a therapeutic effort is the shift from fatty acid towards glucose metabolism [30].

They already described [9, 13] oxidative stress-induced membrane damage and the sarcoplasmic reticulum dysfunction lead to an abrupt increase of intercellular

Ca2+. According to the acidosis paradox, restoration of pH at reperfusion is noxious to the cell by permitting mPTP opening [31]. Thus, if at reperfusion an acidic buffer is used, infarct size can be reduced [32].

6.2 Calcium Paradox

Calcium overload leads to hypercontracture and mPTP opening [26]. Attenuation of this overload can decrease infarct size up to 50%. This can be effected either by the mitochondrial Ca2+ uniporter or the Na + H+ exchanger [33, 34].

Also, through the already described mechanisms, the accumulation of hydrogen, sodium and calcium in the cell causes hyperosmolality which leads to entry of water in the cytoplasm and cell swelling [35].

In the context of the aforementioned ROS overproduction, Neri et al. [36] mention the detrimental role which nitric oxide can play in IRI. They remind that at high concentrations it can be cytotoxic, pro- apoptotic and cause senescence [37–39].

Wu et al. [35] describe that all types of NOS (neuronal, endothelial and inducible) produce NO, which in up to moderate concentrations has antioxidative and anti-inflammatory functions.

However, in a hypoxic state NOS is converted to NOS uncoupling and produces ROS.

Schulz et al. [40] already in 2004 pointed out that data as regards NO involvement in IRI were inconsistent. This could be ascribed to the following confounding factors:

1. Lack of characterization of the degree of the involvement of the three NOS isoforms in various animal species.
2. The lack of direct measurements of myocardial concentration and/or NOS activity and the lack of the production of nonenzymatic NO production as a potential source of NO.
3. The absence of plasma measurements or blood components.

Neri et al. [36] postulate that during IRI, an increase in NO release can occur [41] causing injury either through direct toxicity or due to the formation of toxic peroxynitrite (ONOO2) [42, 43].

These data correspond to a nitrosative not just oxidative stress.

Neri et al. [36] also stress the role of calpains in the induction of cardiomyocyte death. They also describe that IRI, oxidative stress and nitrosative stress, involving ONOO- activate metalloproteinases (MMPs) and inactivate TIMP. MMP-2 apart from degrading collagen has additional deleterious efforts such as a proapoptotic role through β-AR simulation and can cause mitochondrial dysfunction [44, 45].

It can also cause platelet aggregation [46] and vasoconstriction through endothelin 1 [47] and the calcitonin gene-related peptide [48].

Another interesting action of MMP-2 may explain the confusion occasionally emerging in acute coronary syndromes: It may result in partial proteolysis of the thin filament regulatory troponin I thus characterizing stunned but not necrotic myocardium [49–52].

Another metalloproteinase, MMP-9, is involved in inappropriate ECM degradation, activation of inflammatory mediators, and an increase of capillary permeability [53, 54] It has been associated with an increase of infarct size [55] and expansion [56].

MMP-9 also activates cytokines such as IL-1β and chemokines [57].

All families the four TIMP family members have biological properties independent of MMPs [58].

6.3 Other Factors of IRI

6.3.1 Inflammation (INFL)

It is still being debated whether infl is the cause of IRI or a result/reaction to myocardial injury [59, 60].

Here it must be re-iterated that INFL by itself is one more double- edged sword, since it is basically a host defense against invading pathogens, and is also vital to tissue repair, since macrophages remove cellular debris.

IRI produces a "sterile INFL" in the setting of an AMI as neutrophils infiltrate the myocardium.

According to Wang and Frangogiannis [61] activated neutrophils produce ROS, release hydrolytic enzymes, and secrete pore-forming molecules. The stimulus to neutrophil infiltration is tissue necrosis, which by releasing cell contents into the extracellular tissue elicits the INFL response. Additionally, perivascular cells become activated. Through their activation they release many mediators, i.e. TNFα and other cytokines.

6.3.2 Innate Immunity

Innate immunity activation has been widely studied during the last years. Many groups have worked extensively on this subject.

A main consideration of the induction of innate immunity is that it begets a wide inflammatory response which triggers widespread atherosclerosis activation [62]. Indeed, it has recently been stated that myocardial infarction begets myocardial infarction [63, 64].

Mediators released by IRI are listed as damage associated molecular patterns (DAMPs). When cells undergo necrosis; DAMPs are released into the extracellular space and elicit the inflammatory response, by binding to TLRs. According to Wang and Frangogiannis [61] of the 13 known (11 human) mammalian TLRs, TLRs −2,-3 and-4 have been found to play roles in inflammation of the infarcted heart [65–67].

6.4 Monocytes and Macrophages

They are sequentially recruited in the infarct area, through the chemokine receptor CCR2 with phagocytic properties [68], complement, TGF- β, free radicals, and other chemokines. The recruited monocytes undergo many changes finally becoming mature macrophages through the macrophage colony-stimulating factor (M-CSF) and the granulocyte macrophage colony stimulating Factor (GM-CSF) [69].

- 3. Neutrophils. They are recruited to the reperfusion- injured tissues. They adhere to the microvascular endothelium. As already mentioned they secrete ROS, cytokines (mainly TNFα) and chemokines such as the interleukin family (IL-1, interleukin 6, interleukin 12) IFNγ and the monocyte chemotactic factor – 1 elastin and collagenase.
- 4. Lymphocytes. The role of the T and B cells has been well discussed.
- T helper (Tn) lymphocytes are mainly represented by $CD4^+$ cells; they accumulate in the injured tissue [70].
- They also secrete cytokines either pro-inflammatory, by the Th1 cells (IL-2, IL-12, IF Nα, TnFa) or anti-inflammatory, by the Th 2 cells. $CD4^+$ T cells further promote neutrophil recruitment and adhesion.
- B-cells have also been found to participate in IRI.
- Suppression or regulatory T cells (Treg) also participate in IRI being protective through secretion of anti-inflammatory IL-10.
- Mast cells are multifunctional cells which when activated can release cytokines, growth factors, tryptase, chymase, histamine, serotonin, TnFa which promote fluid leakage and edema, with recruitment of leucocytes, monocytes, macrophages, Kupffer cells. The last mentioned family of cells can both promote and limit inflammation [71]. Further details are beyond the scope of this description.

6.4.1 Microparticles

These have acquired recognition and importance during the last few years. They are actually membrane vesicles of 0.1-1 min diameter. They are released from many types of cells such as platelet, erythrocytes, leukocytes, and endothelial cells; these cells are activated by inflammatory stimuli or thrombin activation. They are procoagulant on their own and bind various tissue factors. Apart from this activity, the microparticles transport signaling agents intercellularly, such as arachidonic acid, bioactive lipids, chemokines, [72–74] cytokines, gluten factors, proteases, such as calpain, integrins, caspases and various DNA.

6.4.2 Endothelial Cells

Endothelial cells strongly influence polymorphonuclear leukocyte infiltration into tissues, by allowing passage through the endothelial barrier.

The endothelium also actively controls vasomotor tone; when it is injured in IRI vasodilation is decreased and constriction increased [75].

The underling mechanism of this phenomenon is the already described decrease of NO production and availability.

It should be remembered that the endothelium normally exhibits an anticoagulant action. On the contrary, at IRI this protective action becomes prothrombotic and increases platelet aggregation through expression of endothelial tissue factor, which induces micro thrombus activation. This may be one of the factors, inducing the already described no-reflow phenomenon [76].

6.4.3 Therapeutic Approaches

Many thoughtful reviews have been offered.

Monassier [77] points out that the main efforts have been towards early reperfusion. There is no doubt that primary PCI decreases infarct size and subsequent cardiac remodeling and heart failure.

The very pertinent approach of “conditioning” is described extensively in the corresponding Chapter.

It must be mentioned that a very large number of pharmaceutical substances has been proven effective in the experimental setting [13]. A main consideration, which has practical consequences, is if a drug can be effective when given before or after reperfusion has begun. Of course, practically, while a patient is being prepared for primary PCI the drug can be administered both before and after the artery is open to achieve higher tissue concentrations.

Fröhlich et al. [78] use a characteristic title: Looking beyond primary PCI.

As regards pharmaceutical and general interventions, a very expert group in 2013 concluded that: Currently no effective therapy against IRI exists. They recorded 17 neutral, 14 positive and 15 promising therapies [79].

The same group in 2017 [80] described new 13 new neutral studies,

However, some drugs must be mentioned:

- Results of Adenosine trials AMISTAD I [81] AMISTAD II [82] and ATTACC [83] were on the whole neutral. The exact dose is still discussed. It is not widely used in clinical practice.

In a meta-analysis of randomized clinical trial Bulluck et al. [84] postulate that it has a beneficial long-term effect as regards less subsequent heart failure.

Nicorandil, it is a combination of nitrate and an ATP- sensitive K+ channel activator, with excellent experimental results [85]. However, it is not given routinely during primary PCI or thrombolysis.

Campo et al. [86] analyzing the results of randomized clinical trials for Nicorandil did not find a benefit from the use of this drug.

They report the same for Cyclosporine: This drug raised great hopes in the initial trial when given before primary PCI [87]. Unfortunately the much larger CIRCUS [88] trial and the CYCLE trial [89] were ineffective, yielding a severe blow to the hopes engendered by the initial favorable results.

It is difficult to expect that a new big trial with this drug will come soon.

Gerd Heusch in 2017 [90] mentions many other drugs such as TRO403 03 and interventions such as hypothermia which have not achieved significant acceptance.

He stresses that timing and dosage are important, as in the case of metoprolol, which was protective in higher doses [91] but ineffective in lower doses [92].

6.4.4 Combination of Drugs

Hausenloy and Yellon [93] in a recent editorial raise once more the importance of cardioprotective drug combination. They refer to a very recent study by Pasupathy et al. [94] who propose one more combination therapy in AMI, in this case of N-acetylcysteine with nitrate, two already widely used drugs.

Collard and Gelman [95] mention three other approaches which have being more or less widely tried:

6.4.5 Antioxidant Therapy

They mention superoxide dismutase, catalase, mannitol, allopurinol, vitamin E, N-acetylcysteine, iron chelation, ACE, calcium channel antagonists. No definite positive results to prompt widespread use have emerged.

6.4.6 Anticomplement Therapy

The C3 convertase inhibitor soluble complement receptor one has been shown effective in the rat model [96]. Anti-C5 antibody is also being tried; together these data suggest that this therapy may have promise [97].

6.4.7 Antileukocyte Therapy

In on-pump surgery, leukocyte trapping is widely used with favorable results mentioned. An excellent review is given by Boodram and Evans [98].

Pharmaceutical approaches against leukocytes include lipoxins which are triggered by aspirin [99]. They attenuate neutrophil mediated changes in vascular permeability. Efforts are also directed against leukocyte molecule synthesis and cytokine expression and leukocyte endothelial adhesion.

6.5 The Deliberations of Expert Groups

At the 30th anniversary of IPC leading pioneers in the field discussed the state of the art on this field in a meeting in Barcelona in May 2016 [100]. As regards IRI some observations to be noted are:

Platelet deposition is an important factor. Endothelial cells are more tolerant to ischemia than cardiomyocytes, since they are independent of mitochondrial respiration.

Importantly, this expert group comment that APO plays little role in IRI cell death. IRI is associated with additional Ca2+ influx and ROS generation High Ca2+ for the opening of the mPTP. They point out that cyclosporine A prevents this opening.

They underline the fact that the RISK pathway may not equally apply to rodents and large animal models; the SAFE pathway is confirmed in both large and small animals.

Also, they postulate that pharmacological conditioning mimetic agents may limit IRI through the SAFE pathway activation. In humans the STAT- 5 isoform maybe the main pathway. They make a plea towards combination therapy, trying to influence both the RISK and SAFE pathways and combining non-pharmacologic and also pharmacologic conditioning approaches.

Another Expert Group meeting in 2016 in Mexico [101] with the aim of protecting the cardiovascular system from ischemia included the following major topics:

New targets in cardioprotection, inflammatory mechanisms, microRNAs, and biodirectional exchange between bench and bedside as discussed in other chapters of this book.

Another meeting of experts was held in the same year in Singapore [102].

They point out that during tissue hypoxia, nuclear proteins (histones, HSPs, amphoterin) as well as nuclear, mitochondrial and ribosomal DNA and microRNAs are liberated. The innate immune system tries to neutralize danger signals by activating inflammatory pathways.

They introduced the theranostics, a term which includes many interventions including pluripotent stem cells and conditioning, which is discussed in the corresponding chapter (Fig. 6.1).

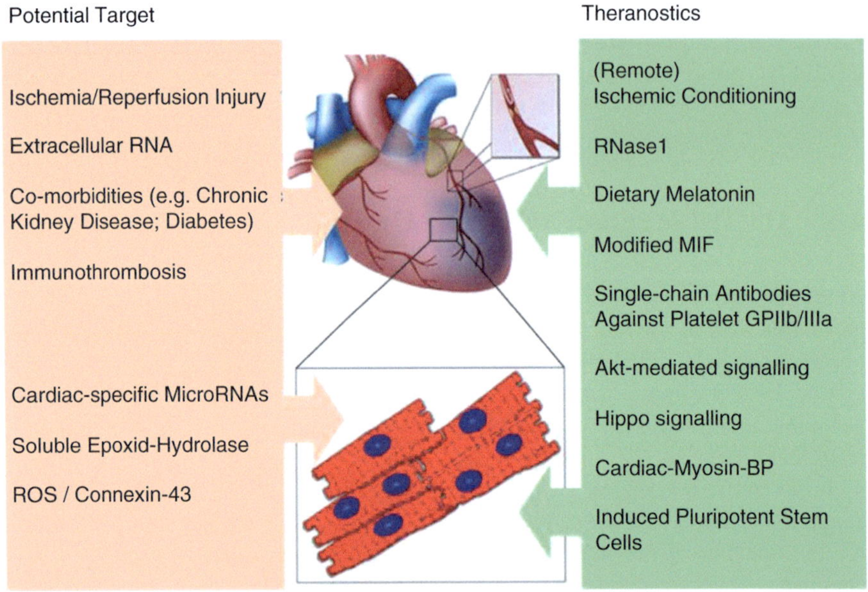

Fig. 6.1 Potential new targets and theranostics in cardio-protection. The basic mechanisms, preclinical models and some clinical applications of several cardio-destructive pathologies and cardiovascular diseases (red box) are discussed in the text. Existing and novel antagonistic procedures as well as the related theranostics (green box), both in vitro and in experimental models, were found to promote cardio-protection on different molecular levels, particularly improving the functional status of cardiomyocytes (ROS reactive oxygen species, MIF macrophage migration inhibition factor, GP glycoprotein, BP binding protein). (Reproduced with permission from Cabrera-Fuentes et al. [102]. https://doi.org/10.1007/s00395-016-0586-x. Copyright © 2016, The Authors)

6.6 Approaches for Myocardial Protection in Heart Surgery

Mentzer et al. [103] mention the following drugs used in Phase II trials: adenosine (+), GIK-2 (+), nicorandil (1+, 1 neutral), isoflurane and sevoflurane (both+), pyridoxal - 5 - phosphate (+). They also mention the following phase III trials: Cariporide (2 trials+), pexelizumab (neutral), Acadesine (2 neutral), pyridoxal - 5 -phosphate (neutral).

6.7 A Natural Paradigm

As a clinical counterpart of abrogation of the ischemia reperfusion injury, cases of "aborted myocardial infarction" have been reported, defined as a ≥ 50% ST elevation resolution, noted initially with thrombolysis and subsequently with primary PCI.

Dianati Maleki et al. [104] in 2014 analyzing the results of the STREAM trial note that early fibrinolysis more often "aborts" MI than PCI; the total ischemic time in "aborted infarcts" was shorter, and prognosis better. Pyda et al. [105] in 119 consecutive pts. treated with primary PCI note 16pts with "aborted" MI(13.4%) They had half the time to treatment (101 vs 220 min) and lower IL-6 and MCP-1 serum levels, and a higher EF at 6 months without mortality, vs 13/103 deaths in non-aborted infarcts. Another mechanism of this difference could be more gradual or "gentle" reperfusion, which may lessen IRI [106, 107].

6.8 The Role of the microRNAs

Sluijter et al. [108] in a detailed review discuss the aspect of epigenetics as expressed by microRNAs. Thus, miR-1 and miR-133α were down-regulated in the infarct areas of deceased post MI pts while miR-208 was upregulated [109]; miR – 92 was upregulated in the infarct area [110], as was miR 34α [111].

The therapeutic aspect of microRNAs manipulation is currently being intensively investigated.

6.9 Clinical Perspectives

Acute myocardial infarction is still a major source for cardiac morbidity, (leading to cardiac failure in surviving patients) and mortality: currently, despite the explosive increase in the employment of primary angioplasty mortality in acute myocardial infarction was reported in an excellent clinical trial as 4.4–4.6% [112]. Post-infarction remodeling in anterior infarcts still occurring in up to 30% is as mentioned in the Chapter on Cardiac Remodeling.

Obviously, we need to improve these numbers. Similarly, during cardiac bypass surgery myocardial preservation may be of great importance in patients with already compromised cardiac function. Obviously, no perfect approach exists. The following steps should be considered. As early application of primary PCI as possible; while preparing for PCI, RPC can be tried; metoprolol may be given as soon as possible. Thrombus aspiration can be tried in heavily thrombosed occluded lesions. Once the artery is opened, IC adenosine or nicorandil may be administered.

In conclusion these are only postulations which have to be proven by further experimentation and still larger trials. We still need a long way to go to diminish both acute mortality and long-term morbidity, which actually is determined at the time of the acute attack.

References

1. Chazov EI, Matveeva LS, Mazaev AV, Sargin KE, Sadovskaia GV, Ruda MI. Intracoronary administration of fibrinolysin in acute myocardial infarct. Ter Arkh. 1976;48:8–192. Reatrop
2. Rentrop P, Blanke H, Karsch KR, Kaiser H, Köstering H, Leitz K. Selective intracoronary thrombolysis in acute myocardial infarction and unstable angina pectoris. Circulation. 1981;63:307–17.
3. Goldberg S, Greenspon AJ, Urban PL, Muza B, Berger B, Walinsky P, et al. Reperfusion arrhythmia: a marker of restoration of antegrade flow during intracoronary thrombolysis for acute myocardial infarction. Am Heart J. 1983;105:26–32.
4. Tennant R, Wiggers CJ. The effect of coronary occlu- sion on myocardial contraction. Am J Phys. 1935;12:351–61.
5. Grines CL, Browne KF, Marco J, Rothbaum D, Stone GW, O'Keefe J, et al. A comparison of immediate angioplasty with thrombolytic therapy for acute myocardial infarction. The Primary Angioplasty in Myocardial Infarction Study Group. N Engl J Med. 1993;328:673–9.
6. Braunwald E, Kloner RA. Myocardial reperfusion: a double-edged sword? J Clin Invest. 1985;76:1713–9.
7. Grech ED, Jackson MJ, Ramsdale DR. Reperfusion injury after acute myocardial infarction. BMJ. 1995;310:477–8.
8. Jennings RB, Sommers HM, Smyth GA, Flack HA, Linn H. Myocardial necrosis induced by temporary occlusion of a coronary artery in the dog. Arch Pathol. 1960;70:68–78.
9. Yellon DM, Hausenloy DJ. Myocardial reperfusion injury. N Engl J Med. 2007;357:1121–35.
10. Braunwald E, Kloner RA. The stunned myocardium: prolonged, postischemic ventricular dysfunction. Circulation. 1982;66:1146–9.
11. Ito H. No-reflow phenomenon and prognosis in patients with acute myocardial infarction. Nat Clin Pract Cardiovasc Med. 2006;3:499–506.
12. Monassier JP. Reperfusion injury in acute myocardial infarction: from bench to cath lab. Part I: Clinical issues and therapeutic options. Arch Cardiovasc Dis. 2008;101:565–75.
13. Hausenloy DJ, Yellon DM. Myocardial ischemia-reperfusion injury: a neglected therapeutic target. J Clin Invest. 2013;123:92–100.
14. Vishwakarma VK, Upadhyay PK, Gupta PK, Yadav HN. Pathophysiologic role of ischemia reperfusion injury: a review. JICC. 2017;7(3):97–104. j.jicc.2017.06.017
15. Morishima I, Sone T, Okumura K, Tsuboi H, Kondo J, Mukawa H, et al. Angiographic no-reflow phenomenon as a predictor of adverse long-term outcome in patients treated with percutaneous transluminal coronary angioplasty for first acute myocardial infarction. J Am Coll Cardiol. 2000;36:1202–9.
16. Ito H, Tomooka T, Sakai N, Yu H, Higashino Y, Fujii K, et al. Lack of myocardial perfusion immediately after successful thrombolysis. A predictor of poor recovery of left ventricular function in anterior myocardial infarction. Circulation. 1992;85:1699–705.
17. Schofer J, Montz R, Mathey DG. Scintigraphic evidence of the "no reflow" phenomenon in human beings after coronary thrombolysis. J Am Coll Cardiol. 1985;5:593–8.
18. van Kranenburg M, Magro M, Thiele H, de Waha S, Eitel I, Cochet A. Prognostic value of microvascular obstruction and infarct size, as measured by CMR in STEMI patients. JACC Cardiovasc Imaging. 2014;7:930–9.
19. Bulluck H, Hausenloy DJ. Microvascular obstruction: the bane of myocardial reperfusion. Rev Esp Cardiol. 2015;68:28–34.
20. Rezkalla SH, Stankowski RV, Hanna J, Kloner RA. Management of no-reflow phenomenon in the catheterization laboratory. JACC Cardiovasc Interv. 2017;10:215–23. Esp Cardiol (Engl Ed). 2015;68:919–20
21. Mongeon FP, Bélisle P, Joseph L, Eisenberg MJ, Rinfret S. Adjunctive thrombectomy for acute myocardial infarction: a bayesian meta-analysis. Circ Cardiovasc Interv. 2010;3:6–16.

22. Mancini JG, Filion KB, Windle SB, Habib B, Eisenberg MJ. Meta-analysis of the long-term effect of routine aspiration thrombectomy in patients undergoing primary percutaneous coronary intervention. Am J Cardiol. 2016;118:23–31.
23. Garcia-Dorado D, Ruiz-Meana M, Piper HM. Lethal reperfusion injury in acute myocardial infarction: facts and unresolved issues. Cardiovasc Res. 2009;83:165–8.
24. Hearse DJ, Humphrey SM, Bullock GR. The oxygen paradox and the calcium paradox: two facets of the same problem? J Mol Cell Cardiol. 1978;10:641–68.
25. Downey JM. Free radicals and their involvement during long-term myocardial ischemia and reperfusion. Annu Rev Physiol. 1990;52:487–504.
26. Piper HM, García-Dorado D, Ovize M. A fresh look at reperfusion injury. Cardiovasc Res. 1998;38:291–300.
27. Jennings RB, Reimer KA. The cell biology of acute myocardial ischemia. Annu Rev Med. 1991;42:225–46.
28. Piper HM, García-Dorado D. Prime causes of rapid cardiomyocyte death during reperfusion. Ann Thorac Surg. 1999;68:1913–9.
29. Frank A, Bonney M, Bonney S, Weitzel L, Koeppen M, Eckle T. Myocardial ischemia reperfusion injury: from basic science to clinical bedside. Semin Cardiothorac Vasc Anesth. 2012;16:123–13230. Horowitz JD, Chirkov YY, Kennedy JA, Sverdlov AL. Modulation of myocardial metabolism: an emerging therapeutic principle. Curr Opin Cardiol. 2010;25:329–334.
30. Horowitz JD, Chirkov YY, Kennedy JA, Sverdlov AL. Modulation of myocardial metabolism: an emerging therapeutic principle. Curr Opin Cardiol. 2010;25:329–34.
31. Lemasters JJ, Bond JM, Chacon E, Harper IS, Kaplan SH, Ohata H, et al. The pH paradox in ischemia-reperfusion injury to cardiac myocytes. EXS. 1996;76:99–114.
32. Qian T, Nieminen AL, Herman B, Lemasters JJ. Mitochondrial permeability transition in pH-dependent reperfusion injury to rat hepatocytes. Am J Phys. 1997;273(6 Pt 1):C1783–92.
33. Klein HH, Pich S, Lindert S, Nebendahl K, Warneke G, Kreuzer H. Treatment of reperfusion injury with intracoronary calcium channel antagonists and reduced coronary free calcium concentration in regionally ischemic, reperfused porcine hearts. J Am Coll Cardiol. 1989;13:1395–401.
34. Murphy E, Steenbergen C. Mechanisms underlying acute protection from cardiac ischemia-reperfusion injury. Physiol Rev. 2008;88:581–609.
35. Wu MY, Yiang GT, Liao WT, Tsai AP, Cheng YL, Cheng PW, et al. Current mechanistic concepts in ischemia and reperfusion injury. Cell Physiol Biochem. 2018;46:1650–67.
36. Neri M, Riezzo I, Pascale N, Pomara C, Turillazzi E. Ischemia/reperfusion injury following acute myocardial infarction: a critical issue for clinicians and forensic pathologists. Mediat Inflamm. 2017;2017:7018393.
37. Thomas DD, Ridnour LA, Isenberg JS, Flores-Santana W, Switzer CH, Donzelli S, et al. The chemical biology of nitric oxide: implications in cellular signaling. Free Radic Biol Med. 2008;45:18–31.
38. Förstermann U, Sessa WC. Nitric oxide synthases: regulation and function. Eur Heart J. 2012;33:829–37, 837a–837d.
39. Phillips L, Toledo AH, Lopez-Neblina F, Anaya-Prado R, Toledo-Pereyra LH. Nitric oxide mechanism of protection in ischemia and reperfusion injury. J Investig Surg. 2009;22:46–55.
40. Schulz R, Kelm M, Heusch G. Nitric oxide in myocardial ischemia/reperfusion injury. Cardiovasc Res. 2004;61:402–13.
41. Zweier JL, Fertmann J, Wei G. Nitric oxide and peroxynitrite in postischemic myocardium. Antioxid Redox Signal. 2001;3:11–22.
42. Radi R, Beckman JS, Bush KM, Freeman BA. Peroxynitrite-induced membrane lipid peroxidation: the cytotoxic potential of superoxide and nitric oxide. Arch Biochem Biophys. 1991;288:481–7.

43. van der Vliet A, O'Neill CA, Halliwell B, Cross CE, Kaur H. Aromatic hydroxylation and nitration of phenylalanine and tyrosine by peroxynitrite. Evidence for hydroxyl radical production from peroxynitrite. FEBS Lett. 1994;339:89–92.
44. Menon B, Singh M, Singh K. Matrix metalloproteinases mediate beta-adrenergic receptor-stimulated apoptosis in adult rat ventricular myocytes. Am J Physiol Cell Physiol. 2005;289:C168–76.
45. Zhou HZ, Ma X, Gray MO, Zhu BQ, Nguyen AP, Baker AJ, Simonis U, et al. Transgenic MMP-2 expression induces latent cardiac mitochondrial dysfunction. Biochem Biophys Res Commun. 2007;358:189–95.
46. Sawicki G, Salas E, Murat J, Miszta-Lane H, Radomski MW. Release of gelatinase A during platelet activation mediates aggregation. Nature. 1997;386:616–9.
47. Fernandez-Patron C, Radomski MW, Davidge ST. Vascular matrix metalloproteinase-2 cleaves big endothelin-1 yielding a novel vasoconstrictor. Circ Res. 1999;85:906–11.
48. Fernandez-Patron C, Stewart KG, Zhang Y, Koivunen E, Radomski MW, Davidge ST. Vascular matrix metalloproteinase-2-dependent cleavage of calcitonin gene-related peptide promotes vasoconstriction. Circ Res. 2000;87:670–6.
49. Cheung PY, Sawicki G, Wozniak M, Wang W, Radomski MW, Schulz R. Matrix metalloproteinase-2 contributes to ischemia-reperfusion injury in the heart. Circulation. 2000;101:1833–9.
50. Gao WD, Atar D, Liu Y, Perez NG, Murphy AM, Marban E. Role of troponin I proteolysis in the pathogenesis of stunned myocardium. Circ Res. 1997;80:393–9.
51. Wang W, Schulze CJ, Suarez-Pinzon WL, Dyck JR, Sawicki G, Schulz R. Intracellular action of matrix metalloproteinase-2 accounts for acute myocardial ischemia and reperfusion injury. Circulation. 2002;106:1543–9.
52. Pipikos T, Kapelouzou A, Tsilimigras DI, Fostinis Y, Pipikou M, Theodorakos A, et al. Stronger correlation with myocardial ischemia of high-sensitivity troponin T than other biomarkers. J Nucl Cardiol. 2018; https://doi.org/10.1007/s12350-018-1199-6.
53. Lindsey M, Wedin K, Brown MD, Keller C, Evans AJ, Smolen J, et al. Matrix-dependent mechanism of neutrophil-mediated release and activation of matrix metalloproteinase 9 in myocardial ischemia/reperfusion. Circulation. 2001;103:2181–7.
54. McMillan WD, Tamarina NA, Cipollone M, Johnson DA, Parker MA, Pearce WH. Size matters: the relationship between MMP-9 expression and aortic diameter. Circulation. 1997;96: 2228–32.
55. Heymans S, Luttun A, Nuyens D, Theilmeier G, Creemers E, Moons L, et al. Inhibition of plasminogen activators or matrix metalloproteinases prevents cardiac rupture but impairs therapeutic angiogenesis and causes cardiac failure. Nat Med. 1999;5:1135–42.
56. Rohde LE, Ducharme A, Arroyo LH, Aikawa M, Sukhova GH, Lopez-Anaya A, et al. Matrix metalloproteinase inhibition attenuates early left ventricular enlargement after experimental myocardial infarction in mice. Circulation. 1999;99:3063–70.
57. Ducharme A, Frantz S, Aikawa M, Rabkin E, Lindsey M, Rohde LE, et al. Targeted deletion of matrix metalloproteinase-9 attenuates left ventricular enlargement and collagen accumulation after experimental myocardial infarction. J Clin Invest. 2000;106:55–62.
58. Vanhoutte D, Heymans S. TIMPs and cardiac remodeling: 'Embracing the MMP-independent-side of the family'. J Mol Cell Cardiol. 2010;48:445–53.
59. Vinten-Johansen J. Involvement of neutrophils in the pathogenesis of lethal myocardial reperfusion injury. Cardiovasc Res. 2004;61:481–97.
60. Kalogeris T, Baines CP, Krenz M, Korthuis RJ. Cell biology of ischemia/reperfusion injury. Int Rev Cell Mol Biol. 2012;298:229–317.
61. Wang J, Frangogiannis NG Repair of the infarcted myocardium. Introduction to translational cardiovascular research. Cham: Springer 2015, p 279–97.
62. Dutta P, Nahrendorf M. Monocytes in myocardial infarction. Arterioscler Thromb Vasc Biol. 2015;35:1066–70.
63. Joshi NV, Toor I, Shah AS, Carruthers K, Vesey AT, Alam SR, et al. Systemic atherosclerotic inflammation following acute myocardial infarction: myocardial infarction begets myocardial infarction. J Am Heart Assoc. 2015;4:e001956.

64. Nahrendorf M, Swirski FK. Innate immune cells in ischaemic heart disease: does myocardial infarction beget myocardial infarction? Eur Heart J. 2016;37:868–72.
65. Shishido T, Nozaki N, Yamaguchi S, Shibata Y, Nitobe J, Miyamoto T, et al. Toll-like receptor-2 modulates ventricular remodeling after myocardial infarction. Circulation. 2003;108:2905–10.
66. Timmers L, Sluijter JP, van Keulen JK, Hoefer IE, Nederhoff MG, Goumans MJ, et al. Toll-like receptor 4 mediates maladaptive left ventricular remodeling and impairs cardiac function after myocardial infarction. Circ Res. 2008;102:257–64.
67. Lu C, Ren D, Wang X, Ha T, Liu L, Lee EJ, et al. Toll-like receptor 3 plays a role in myocardial infarction and ischemia/reperfusion injury. Biochim Biophys Acta. 1842;2014:22–31.
68. Dewald O, Zymek P, Winkelmann K, Koerting A, Ren G, Abou-Khamis T, et al. CCL2/Monocyte Chemoattractant Protein-1 regulates inflammatory responses critical to healing myocardial infarcts. Circ Res. 2005;96:881–9.
69. Frangogiannis NG, Mendoza LH, Ren G, Akrivakis S, Jackson PL, Michael LH, et al. MCSF expression is induced in healing myocardial infarcts and may regulate monocyte and endothelial cell phenotype. Am J Physiol Heart Circ Physiol. 2003;285:H483–92.
70. Hofmann U, Frantz S. Role of T-cells in myocardial infarction. Eur Heart J. 2016;37:873–9.
71. Somasundaram P, Ren G, Nagar H, Kraemer D, Mendoza L, Michael LH, et al. Mast cell tryptase may modulate endothelial cell phenotype in healing myocardial infarcts. J Pathol. 2005;205:102–11.
72. Bernal-Mizrachi L, Jy W, Jimenez JJ, Pastor J, Mauro LM, Horstman LL, et al. High levels of circulating endothelial microparticles in patients with acute coronary syndromes. Am Heart J. 2003;145:962–70.
73. Boulanger CM, Scoazec A, Ebrahimian T, Henry P, Mathieu E, Tedgui A, et al. Circulating microparticles from patients with myocardial infarction cause endothelial dysfunction. Circulation. 2001;104:2649–52.
74. Ozaki M, Kawashima S, Hirase T, Yamashita T, Namiki M, Inoue N, et al. Overexpression of endothelial nitric oxide synthase in endothelial cells is protective against ischemia-reperfusion injury in mouse skeletal muscle. Am J Pathol. 2002;160:1335–44.
75. Loscalzo J. Endothelial injury, vasoconstriction, and its prevention. Tex Heart Inst J. 1995;22:180–4.
76. Nieswandt B, Pleines I, Bender M. Platelet adhesion and activation mechanisms in arterial thrombosis and ischaemic stroke. J Thromb Haemost. 2011;9(Suppl 1):92–104.
77. Monassier JP. Reperfusion injury in acute myocardial infarction: from bench to cath lab. Part II: Clinical issues and therapeutic options. Arch Cardiovasc Dis. 2008;101:565–75.
78. Fröhlich GM, Meier P, White SK, Yellon DM, Hausenloy DJ. Myocardial reperfusion injury: looking beyond primary PCI. Eur Heart J. 2014;34:1714–22.
79. Hausenloy DJ, Erik Bøtker H, Condorelli G, Ferdinandy P, Garcia-Dorado D, Heusch G, et al. Translating cardioprotection for patient benefit: position paper from the Working Group of Cellular Biology of the Heart of the European Society of Cardiology. Cardiovasc Res. 2013;98:7–27.
80. Hausenloy DJ, Garcia-Dorado D, Bøtker HE, Davidson SM, Downey J, Engel FB, et al. Novel targets and future strategies for acute cardioprotection: Position Paper of the European Society of Cardiology Working Group on Cellular Biology of the Heart. Cardiovasc Res. 2017;113:564–85.
81. Mahaffey KW, Puma JA, Barbagelata NA, DiCarli MF, Leesar MA, Browne KF, et al. Adenosine as an adjunct to thrombolytic therapy for acute myocardial infarction: results of a multicenter, randomized, placebo-controlled trial: the Acute Myocardial Infarction STudy of ADenosine (AMISTAD) trial. J Am Coll Cardiol. 1999;34:1711–20.
82. Ross AM, Gibbons RJ, Stone GW, Kloner RA, Alexander RW, AMISTAD-II Investigators. A randomized, double-blinded, placebo-controlled multicenter trial of adenosine as an adjunct to reperfusion in the treatment of acute myocardial infarction (AMISTAD-II). J Am Coll Cardiol. 2005;45:1775–80.
83. Quintana M, Hjemdahl P, Sollevi A, Kahan T, Edner M, Rehnqvist N, et al. Left ventricular function and cardiovascular events following adjuvant therapy with adenosine in acute

myocardial infarction treated with thrombolysis, results of the ATTenuation by Adenosine of Cardiac Complications (ATTACC) study. Eur J Clin Pharmacol. 2003;59:1–9.
84. Bulluck H, Sirker A, Loke YK, Garcia-Dorado D, Hausenloy DJ. Clinical benefit of adenosine as an adjunct to reperfusion in ST-elevation myocardial infarction patients: an updated meta-analysis of randomized controlled trials. Int J Cardiol. 2016;202:228–37.
85. Wu H, Ye M, Yang J, Ding J, Yang J, Dong W, et al. Nicorandil protects the heart from ischemia/reperfusion injury by attenuating endoplasmic reticulum response-induced apoptosis through PI3K/Akt signaling pathway. Cell Physiol Biochem. 2015;35:2320–32.
86. Campo G, Pavasini R, Morciano G, Lincoff MA, C Gibson M, Kitakaze M, et al. Data on administration of cyclosporine, nicorandil, metoprolol on reperfusion related outcomes in ST-segment Elevation Myocardial Infarction treated with percutaneous coronary intervention. Data Brief. 2017;14:197–205.
87. Mewton N, Croisille P, Gahide G, Rioufol G, Bonnefoy E, Sanchez I, et al. Effect of cyclosporine on left ventricular remodeling after reperfused myocardial infarction. J Am Coll Cardiol. 2010;55:1200–5.
88. Cung TT, Morel O, Cayla G, Rioufol G, Garcia-Dorado D, Angoulvant D, et al. Cyclosporine before PCI in Patients with Acute Myocardial infarction. N Engl J Med. 2015;373:1021–31.
89. Ottani F, Latini R, Staszewsky L, La Vecchia L, Locuratolo N, Sicuro M, et al. Cyclosporine A in reperfused myocardial infarction: the multicenter, controlled, open-label CYCLE trial. J Am Coll Cardiol. 2016;67:365–74.
90. Heusch G. Critical issues for the translation of cardioprotection. Circ Res. 2017;120:1477–86.
91. Ibanez B, Macaya C, Sánchez-Brunete V, Pizarro G, Fernández-Friera L, Mateos A, et al. Effect of early metoprolol on infarct size in ST-segment-elevation myocardial infarction patients undergoing primary percutaneous coronary intervention: the Effect of Metoprolol in Cardioprotection During an Acute Myocardial Infarction (METOCARD-CNIC) trial. Circulation. 2013;128:1495–503.
92. Roolvink V, Ibáñez B, Ottervanger JP, Pizarro G, van Royen N, Mateos A, et al. Early intravenous beta-blockers in patients with ST-segment elevation myocardial infarction before primary percutaneous coronary intervention. J Am Coll Cardiol 2016;67:2705–2715.
93. Hausenloy DJ, Yellon DM. Combination therapy to target reperfusion injury after ST-segment-elevation myocardial infarction: a more effective approach to cardioprotection. Circulation. 2017;136:904–6.
94. Pasupathy S, Tavella R, Grover S, Raman B, NEK P, Du YT, et al. Early use of N-acetylcysteine with nitrate therapy in patients undergoing primary percutaneous coronary intervention for ST-segment-elevation myocardial infarction reduces myocardial infarct size (the NACIAM trial [N-acetylcysteine in acute myocardial infarction]). Circulation. 2017;136:894–903.
95. Collard CD, Gelman S. Pathophysiology, clinical manifestations, and prevention of ischemia-reperfusion injury. Anesthesiology. 2001;94:1133–8.
96. Weisman HF, Bartow T, Leppo MK, Marsh HC Jr, Carson GR, Concino MF, et al. Soluble human complement receptor type 1: in vivo inhibitor of complement suppressing post-ischemic myocardial inflammation and necrosis. Science. 1990;249:146–51.
97. Vakeva AP, Agah A, Rollins SA, Matis LA, Li L, Stahl GL. Myocardial infarction and apoptosis after myocardial ischemia and reperfusion: role of the terminal complement components and inhibition by anti-C5 therapy. Circulation. 1998;97:2259–67.
98. Boodram S, Evans E. Use of leukocyte-depleting filters during cardiac surgery with cardiopulmonary bypass: a review. J Extra Corpor Technol. 2008;40:27–42.
99. Chiang N, Gronert K, Clish CB, O'Brien JA, Freeman MW, Serhan CN. Leukotriene B4 receptor transgenic mice reveal novel protective roles for lipoxins and aspirin-triggered lipoxins in reperfusion. J Clin Invest. 1999;104:309–16.
100. Hausenloy DJ, Barrabes JA, Bøtker HE, Davidson SM, Di Lisa F, Downey J, et al. Ischaemic conditioning and targeting reperfusion injury: a 30 year voyage of discovery. Basic Res Cardiol. 2016;111:70.

101. Cabrera-Fuentes HA, Alba-Alba C, Aragones J, Bernhagen J, Boisvert WA, Bøtker HE, et al. Meeting report from the 2nd International Symposium on New Frontiers in Cardiovascular Research. Protecting the cardiovascular system from ischemia: between bench and bedside. Basic Res Cardiol. 2016;111:7.
102. Cabrera-Fuentes HA, Aragones J, Bernhagen J, Boening A, Boisvert WA, Bøtker HE, et al. From basic mechanisms to clinical applications in heart protection, new players in cardiovascular diseases and cardiac theranostics: meeting report from the third international symposium on "New frontiers in cardiovascular research". Basic Res Cardiol. 2016;111:69.
103. Mentzer RM Jr. Myocardial protection in heart surgery. J Cardiovasc Pharmacol Ther. 2011;16:290–7.
104. Dianati Maleki N, Van de Werf F, Goldstein P, Adgey JA, Lambert Y, Sulimov V, et al. Aborted myocardial infarction in ST-elevation myocardial infarction: insights from the STrategic Reperfusion Early After Myocardial infarction trial. Heart. 2014;100:1543–9.
105. Musiolik J, van Caster P, Skyschally A, Boengler K, Gres P, Schulz R, Heusch G. Reduction of infarct size by gentle reperfusion without activation of reperfusion injury salvage kinases in pigs. Cardiovasc Res. 2010;85:110–7.
106. Beyersdorf F. The use of controlled reperfusion strategies in cardiac surgery to minimize ischaemia/reperfusion damage. Cardiovasc Res. 2009;83:262–8.
107. Pyda M, Grajek S, Oleśkowska-Florek F, Lesiak M, Siniawski S, Gwizdała A, et al. Aborted myocardial infarction in patients undergoing primary percutaneous coronary intervention. J Med Science. 2015;84:27–32.
108. Sluijter JP, Condorelli G, Davidson SM, Engel FB, Ferdinandy P, Hausenloy DJ, et al. Novel therapeutic strategies for cardioprotection. Pharmacol Ther. 2014;144:60–70.
109. Bostjancic E, Zidar N, Stajer D, Glavac D. MicroRNAs miR-1, miR-133a, miR-133b and miR-208 are dysregulated in human myocardial infarction. Cardiology. 2010;115:163–9.
110. Bonauer A, Carmona G, Iwasaki M, Mione M, Koyanagi M, Fischer A, et al. MicroRNA-92a controls angiogenesis and functional recovery of ischemic tissues in mice. Science. 2009;324:1710–3.
111. Boon RA, Iekushi K, Lechner S, Seeger T, Fischer A, Heydt S, et al. MicroRNA-34a regulates cardiac ageing and function. Nature. 2013;495:107–10.
112. Armstrong PW, Gershlick AH, Goldstein P, Wilcox R, Danays T, Lambert Y, et al. Fibrinolysis or primary PCI in ST-segment elevation myocardial infarction. N Engl J Med. 2013;368:1379–87.

Chapter 7
Cell Death: Many Causes and Many Effects

Dennis V. Cokkinos

7.1 Definitions

Cell death (CD) can be seen in all aspects of heart disease. In the myocardium, its various forms lead to cardiomyocyte loss, which, especially when replaced by fibrotic tissue, leads to cardiac remodeling (REM), congestive heart failure (CHF), and death.

Marin-Garcia [1] describes the three major cell death modalities (apoptosis, necrosis, and autophagy).

However, it must also be realized that during organ and specifically cardiac development, many cells and cellular formations disappear or are transformed through various processes.

Galluzzi et al. [2] describe that in human health and disease conditions, CD plays a very prominent role; thus myocardial infarction (MI), stroke, inflammation, atherosclerosis, immunologic factors, and AIDS are involved in the cardiovascular field. In the chapter of oncology, interplay is vastly more complex. It seems that cell death in cancer cells and cardiomyocytes do not necessarily follow the same steps.

Before trying to describe the various modalities, the difficulty in their definition should be underlined. The Nomenclature Committee on Cell Death in 2005 and in more detailed reports in 2009 and 2018 [3, 4], in order to circumvent these difficulties, which any reader who is not an expert in this field will duly appreciate, actually decided to use purely morphological criteria (Table 7.1), although as Galluzzi et al. [2] point out that, CD can also be classified apart from morphologic appearance according to enzymological criteria and functional aspects, as programmed or accidental, physiological, pathological, or immunological characteristics. The Nomenclature

D. V. Cokkinos (✉)
Heart and Vessel Department, Biomedical Research Foundation,
Academy of Athens - Gregory Skalkeas, Athens, Greece
e-mail: dcokkinos@bioacademy.gr

D. V. Cokkinos (ed.), *Myocardial Preservation*,
https://doi.org/10.1007/978-3-319-98186-4_7

Table 7.1 Distinct modalities of cell death

Cell death mode	Morphological features	Notes
Apoptosis	Rounding-up of the cell Retraction of pseudopodes Reduction of cellular and nuclear volume (pyknosis) Nuclear fragmentation (karyorrhexis) Minor modification of cytoplasmic organelles Plasma membrane blebbing Engulfment by resident phagocytes in vivo	"Apoptosis" is the original term introduced by Kerr et al. [14] to define a type of cell death with specific morphological features. Apoptosis is *not* a synonym of programmed cell death or caspase activation
Autophagy	Lack of chromatin condensation Massive vacuolization of the cytoplasm Accumulation of (double-membraned) autophagic vacuoles Little or no uptake by phagocytic cells: in vivo	"Autophagic cell death" defines cell death occurring with autophagy, though it may misleadingly suggest a form of death occurring by autophagy as this process often promotes cell survival [15, 16]
Cornification	Elimination of cytosolic organelles Modifications of plasma membrane Accumulation of lipids in F and L granules Extrusion of lipids in the extracellular space Desquamation (loss of corneocytes) by protease activation	"Cornified envelope" formation or "keratinization" is specific of the skin to create a barrier function. Although apoptosis can be induced by injury in the basal epidermal layer (e.g., UV irradiation), cornification is exclusive of the upper layers (granular layer and stratum corneum) [17, 18]
Necrosis	Cytoplasmic swelling (oncosis) Rupture of plasma membrane Swelling of cytoplasmic organelles Moderate chromatin condensation	"Necrosis" identifies, in a negative fashion, cell death lacking the features of apoptosis or autophagy. Note that necrosis can occur in a regulated fashion, involving a precise sequence of signals

Reproduced with permission from Kroemer et al. [3]

Committee itself [4] expresses the wish that morphological aspects should be replaced by biochemical and functional criteria.

Also, in their more recent report, they express the confidence that correct use of regulated cell death-related terms [4] will help toward finding more effective therapies in the future.

The term CD includes the three main modalities already mentioned.

Some atypical forms will be described at the end of this chapter.

According to Galluzi et al. [4] in the latest recommendations of the Nomenclature Committee on Cell Death 2018, the preferred term is regulated cell death (RCD) which relies on a dedicated molecular machinery, in the sense that it can be modulated by pharmacological or genetic interventions.

RCD differs importantly from accidental cell death (ACD) which is an instantaneous and catastrophic death in cells exposed to severe insults.

The overlap found between these two modalities will be further discussed.

RCD is involved according to Galluzzi et al. [2, 4] in two different situations:

(a) Without the influence of any exogenous perturbation, occurring as a physiological process of tissue turnover. This is characterized as programmed cell death and occurs in animal development [5].
(b) RCD is caused by perturbations of intra- or extracellular microenvironment [6].

The authors also delineate the classification of cell death into three different forms which will be further discussed.

1. Type I cell death or apoptosis
2. Type II cell death or autophagy
3. Type III cell death or necrosis (N), in which there is no phagocytic or lysosomal involvement [2]

7.1.1 Apoptosis

Here it must be reminded, as Whelan et al. [7] and other authors point out, that apoptotic programmed CD in the nematode *Caenorhabditis elegans* has been conserved over 600 million years during the development of this organism.

Moreover, since it involves the mitochondria (MITO), it gives a significant insight into the function of these important organelles, as will be further described.

Its name derives from the Greek, meaning falling (ptosis)-off (apo). While necrosis (N) is characterized by cell swelling due to plasma membrane rupture, this membrane in apoptosis (APO) remains intact (not to be confused with the rupture of the outer mitochondrial membrane), while the cell shrinks, together with the nucleus. Morphologic characteristics of the nucleus in APO are chromatin condensation and nuclear fragmentation. In a further stage, the nucleus breakup is also called karyorrhexis (rhexis = rupture).

The cells emit processes or pseudopodia (budding) which contain pyknotic nuclear fragments, as described 20 years ago by Majno and Joris [8] who mention that the first microscopic description of APO probably appeared in 1886. These “buds” are phagocytosed by local resident cells, usually without causing an inflammatory response.

Kroemer et al. [3] as well as Kostin [9] describe plasma membrane “blebs” as typical of APO.

Apoptotic bodies contain fragments of both cytoplasm and nucleus.

Whelan et al. [7] describe the two pathways which mediate cell death in APO and which are intimately entwined:

(a) *The intrinsic pathway* or canonical or mitochondrial pathway. It also involves the endoplasmic reticulum (ER). This combines extracellular and intracellular stresses of any type; however in the former, deficiency of nutrients, radiation, drugs, and physical stress predominate, while in the latter, the main factors are oxidative stress (ROS), DNA damage, and protein misfolding. Both types of signals are transmitted to the MITO by the BH3-only proteins which will be further described. These stimulate the release of cytochrome c and other apoptogens as described by Baines [10].

(b) *Extrinsic pathway* or death receptor (DR) pathway [10]. This is effected by the binding of death ligands, Fas and TNF-α being prime examples. Fas binds to the cell surface receptors, binding to the adaptor protein FADD (Fas-associated via death domain). FADD recruits procaspase-8 and procaspase-10 through the DISC (multiprotein death-inducing complex) which activates procaspase-3 and Bid (BH3 interacting-domain death agonist) which activates procaspase-3.

- Kostin [9] has also given a concise description of the two pathways. The death receptor activation is affected, apart from Fas and TNFα, by AT II and β1 adrenergic receptors, which are further discussed.
- The critical step is irreversible and widespread mitochondrial outer membrane permeabilization (MOMP).

Apoptotic stimuli are ultimately mediated through the proapoptotic Bcl-2 protein family. This family is differentiated as follows:

1. *The antiapoptotic members*, of which Bcl-2 (B cell leukemia/lymphoma 2) and Bcl-XL (long isoform) are the representatives.
2. *The proapoptotic members*, which include many proteins:

- Main players are Bax (Bcl-2-associated X protein), Bak (Bcl-2- homologous antagonist killer), and BH3-only (Bcl-2 homology domain 3-only) proapoptotic proteins: Bid (BH3 interacting-domain death agonist); Bad (Bcl-2-antagonist of cell death); Bim (Bcl-2-interacting mediator of cell death); Bmf (Bcl-2 modifying factor); Noxa and Smac/DIABLO which will be discussed further on; Puma (p 53 upregulated modulator of APO), which is essential for DNA damage-induced APO; and Bcl-2/adenovirus E1B 19 kDa protein-interacting protein 3 (BNIP3). Either Bax or Bak is necessary for this process; they are translocated to the mitochondrial outer membrane (MOM). They stimulate the release of cytochrome c and other apoptogenic mitochondrial proteins into the cytosol. Bax activation may be mediated through calpain; as this protein will also be mentioned as an effector of N, its participation in both processes may represent another link in the cross talk of the two processes. Bax and Bak, which are located at the ER as well as the MITO, increase ER Ca^{2+} stores, while Bcl-2 decreases them. The increased ER Ca^{2+} increases the release of Ca^{2+} in the cytoplasm, causing APO [8].

Cytochrome c and other apoptogens (importantly procaspase-9) are gathered in the apoptosome, activating pro-caspase-9, which activates caspase-3, the main mediator of apoptotic CD. Many other effectors are involved in this process, as described by Whelan et al. [7].

According to the same author, the main inhibitors of APO in the intrinsic pathway are the Bcl-2 proteins. However, the IAP proteins (inhibitor of APO protein family) are also important, since they inhibit activated caspase-3 and -7.

Other APO inhibitors are FLIP (FLICE-like Fas-associated death domain protein-like interleukin-1-converting enzyme like inhibitory protein) and ARC (apoptosis repressor with a CARD).

Apart from their role in APO, several BH3-only members also regulate cell cycle, DNA repair, and metabolism but are also involved in the crosstalk of APO with the third cell death process to be discussed next, autophagy (AUTO), by liberating Beclin-1 from its binding within the Bcl-2/Bcl-XL complexes.

Crompton [12] underlines the multifaceted actions of the Bcl-2 family proteins, with the Bcl-2/Bax ratio determining resistance to APO. This ratio is very widely used in remodeling myocardium studies.

The JNKs (superfamily of MAP kinases) are instrumental in both cell proliferation and APO; the balance can be tilted by many factors.

Dhanasekaran and Reddy [13] point out that JNK signals APO by various mechanisms: It increases expression of TNF-α, Fas, and Bak. It also phosphorylates the p53 family of proteins. It is also critical for the release of cytochrome c and induces cleavage of Bid; it promotes the release of Smac/DIABLO, which antagonizes cytosolic inhibitor of apoptosis proteins (IAPs), from the intermembrane space to the cytosol, stimulating caspase activation.

The mitochondria occurrence of APO is to a large extent mediated by the MITO. A description of their structure and function is considered helpful:

They are located into the intermyofibrillar spaces, underneath the sarcolemma. Their location permits more efficient ATP supply to the myofibrils.

The MITO drive two different CD mechanisms (APO and N) through the mitochondrial permeability transition pore (MPTP). They are surrounded by two membranes [9, 11, 12, 14], with a narrow intermembrane space between them.

7.2 The Outer Membrane (MOM or OMM), Which Drives APO

It has many pores based on protein, which allow passage of ions and molecules.

This is the action site of the already mentioned pro-death members of the Bcl-2 family. Under the response to noxious stimuli, Bax, which normally resides in the cytosol, is translocated to MOM and the endoplasmic reticulum (ER).

Thus it causes MOM permeabilization and the release of proapoptotic proteins from the intermembrane space into the cytosol, such as cytochromes, Smac/DIABLO, and endonuclease G (endoG). Cytochrome c binds to the cytosolic protein apaf 1 and thus causes the formation of the "apoptosome" which activates the caspase-9 and -3 system [9].

7.3 The Inner Membrane (MIM or IMM)

This has more restricted permeability, much like the cell plasma membrane. It is involved in electron transport and ATP synthesis and is spanned by the mitochondrial permeability transition pore (MPTP) which drives necrosis.

This pore is inhibited by low pH <7.0; thus it is closed during ischemia, which corresponds clinically to persistent artery occlusion. When reperfusion occurs, there is restitution of pH and acceleration of cytosolic Ca^{2+} increase (which is slow during ischemia). The cell deals with this explosive Ca^{2+} increase by taking it up into the mitochondria via the MITO Ca^{2+} uniporter, a protein that uses the negative $\Delta\Psi m$ to drive Ca^{+2} into the matrix [15].

There exist many MPTP activators, such as Ca^{2+}, ROS, and Pi (inorganic phosphate), which emerge after adenine nucleotides are depleted after the onset of ischemia and a reduction of the ATP/ADP ratio. From the pharmacological agents, cyclosporine A is a typical inhibitor; its beneficial effects on I/R injury [12] will be discussed later.

The MPTP is very well described by Baines [10], Crompton [12], Lemasters et al. [14], and Weiss et al. [16]: They state that the MITO use electron transport to develop an electrochemical gradient across the MIM (membrane space and matrix). This is formed by the MIM membrane potential ($\Delta\Psi m$ or $\Delta Cm \approx -200$ mV) and a proton gradient (ΔpH) according to Weis et al. [16]. The electrochemical gradient is employed by ATP synthase to phosphorylate ADP to ATP. When MPTP opens, $\Delta\Psi m$ depolarizes, and the synthase actually starts consuming ATP in an attempt which however is ineffective to restore the proton gradient, solutes up to 15 kDa pass the MIM, and cause MITO swelling. As MITO swell, the MIM stretches, but actually it is the MOM which ruptures: The surface of MIM is enhanced by the cristae, parallel invaginating membrane structures. The MOM rupture effects the release of proapoptotic proteins from the intermembrane space, notably cytochrome c, Smac/DIABLO, and endonuclease G (endoG). Cytochrome c binds to the cytosolic protein apaf1, creating the "apoptosome" which activates the caspase-9 and -3 protease system, while EndoG translocates to the nucleus, mediating DNA fragmentation, as described by Baines [10] who also points out that the Bcl-2 proteins permeabilize the MOM, while ROS and Ca^{2+} the MIM. The role of ROS production is complex. MITO ROS can trigger MPTP opening, with further ROS release creating a cascading process known as ROS-induced ROS release mechanism.

Some further molecular characteristics of the MPTP should be given:

(a) The voltage-dependent anion channel (VDAC) resides in the MOM. This protein facilitates efficient transport of ATP/ADP across the MOM. According to Baines [10], this protein, although very abundant, is not an essential component of the MPTP.

(b) The adenine nucleotide translocase (ANT) family resides in the MIM and facilitates the exchange of ATP and ADP across it. It is considered an essential factor, although recently some doubts have emerged about its central role. Crompton [12] points out that VDAC and ANT can interact strongly in junctional sites between the two membranes. They form a complex which can recruit additional proteins. One of these is:

7.4 Cyclophilin D (CyPD)

This protein resides in the MITO matrix. Its activation opens the MPTP, while its inhibition (by cyclosporine A (CsA) or sanglifehrin A is cardioprotective [15]. Interestingly according to Lemasters et al. [10], CsA prevents both N and APO.

The MITO phosphate carrier (PiC) is a CypD-interacting protein which regulates ATP synthesis. Its overexpression induces APO.

Apart from the MPTP, another death channel has been described, the mitochondrial apoptosis channel, which is regulated by the Bcl-2 protein family [15]:

The mitochondrial calcium uniporter (MCU); by its action Ca^{2+} normally enters the MITO. As Pan et al. [17] describe, under normal conditions, entry of Ca^{2+} in the MITO augments their ATP production to match its demand up to 10–20-fold. However, larger increases can induce CD. Normally, most unstimulated cells maintain Ca^{2+} in the range of 100–200 nM in the cytosol and the MITO through the function of pumps in the plasma membrane and the ER.

The MCU blockade can prevent abnormal increase Ca^{2+} (and Fe^{2+}) entry.

Thus it is suggested that MCU is required to cope with increased Ca^{2+} cycling.

During ischemia, the closed state of the MPTP, affected by a decrease in pH, activation of Pi, and only a mild increase of Ca^{2+} and ROS, results in limited damage. At reperfusion, the opening of the MPTP is characterized by an increase of the pH, the Pi, and the Ca^{2+} and an explosive increase of ROS resulting in irreversible damage.

Lemasters et al. [14] recapitulate that the MPTP is involved in both APO and N.

Another question which has been advanced is whether APO can be induced without the all-important caspase-3 activation [5, 15].

Studies in mice and *C. elegans* provide evidence for caspase-independent CD. The apoptosis-inducing factor (AIF) is such a candidate.

Susin et al. [18] have shown that AIF can cause a picture of mitochondrial-effected APO which cannot be prevented by a wide-ranging caspase inhibitor. It does not need Apaf-1 or procaspase-9 for its action. However, AIF is required for cell death mediated by poly-ADP ribose polymerase (PARP), which is a main component of N, as will be further described. It also triggers the release of cytochrome c and caspase-9. They suggest that it has a direct effort on isolated nuclei, effecting chromatin condensation and fragmentation which can be caspase-independent. They also postulate that BH3-domain-only protein may act independently of Apaf-1 and caspases.

7.5 Other Pathways Involved in APO

7.5.1 *The Tumor Suppressor p53*

It exerts its proapoptotic action through activation of multiple proapoptotic genes, i.e., Bax, Bid, Puma, Apaf-1, caspase-6, and Fas.

The endoplasmic (or sarcoplasmic in muscle cells) reticulum (ER) pathway regulates the kinetics of intracellular Ca^{2+}; its stores are increased by Bax and Bak which – apart from the outer mitochondrial membrane – are also located in the ER, together with the antiapoptotic Bcl-2 which has an opposing effect.

The HSP-70 which is a well-known cardioprotective chaperone reduces ER stress. It also reduces the apoptosome formation and AIF activation.

Galluzzi et al. [4] describe some additional forms of apoptosis:

- *Ferroptosis,* which is initiated by lipid peroxidation through ROS generation and iron availability [19, 20].

It is interesting from a clinical standpoint that ferroptosis can be prevented by some well-known antioxidants such as vitamin E, coenzyme Q10, and iron chelators [21].

7.5.2 *Pyroptosis*

It is related to innate immunity. It has some different features from apoptosis, i.e., a peculiar form of chromatin condensation and cellular swelling resulting in plasma membrane permeability [22].

According to Cookson and Brennan [23], this form of regulated cell death is dependent on caspase-1.

Subsequent studies have shown that caspase-3 can also drive this form of death [24].

Caspases 4, 5, and 11 have also been implicated. It is frequently associated with IL-1β and IL-18 secretion [25, 26] and is triggered by LPS [27].

Parthanatos is involved in the action of HSPs [15, 22]. This form of apoptosis occurs through prolonged alkylating DNA damage but also oxidative stress, hypoxia, hypoglycemia, or inflammation [28, 29].

7.5.3 *Entotic Cell Death*

According to Overholtzer et al. [30], it is a nonapoptotic cell death but is described here. It is seen in neoplasms, demonstrating an oncosuppressor effect [30, 31]. It is executed by lysosomes [31].

Neutrophil extracellular traps (NETs) are produced as a response to microbial and sterile actions or upon stimulation of various receptors including [32] TLRs. According to Galluzzi et al. [4], this is a ROS-dependent modality of regulated cell death depending on components of the necroptotic apparatus.

7.6 Necrosis

Necrosis (N) to the non-researcher has been considered as the prevalent form of CD. It is derived from the Greek word νεκρός, which means corpse or dead person. It is usually considered to be non-programmed, in contrast to the two forms of programmed cell death (PCD), apoptosis and autophagy.

However it will be subsequently shown that this distinction is not absolute.

Thus, some authors are bringing back the originally employed term *oncosis,* which is a predominantly morphologic term [6, 15]. The morphologic differences of the two modalities are well presented by Feuerstein et al. [33] (Fig. 7.1).

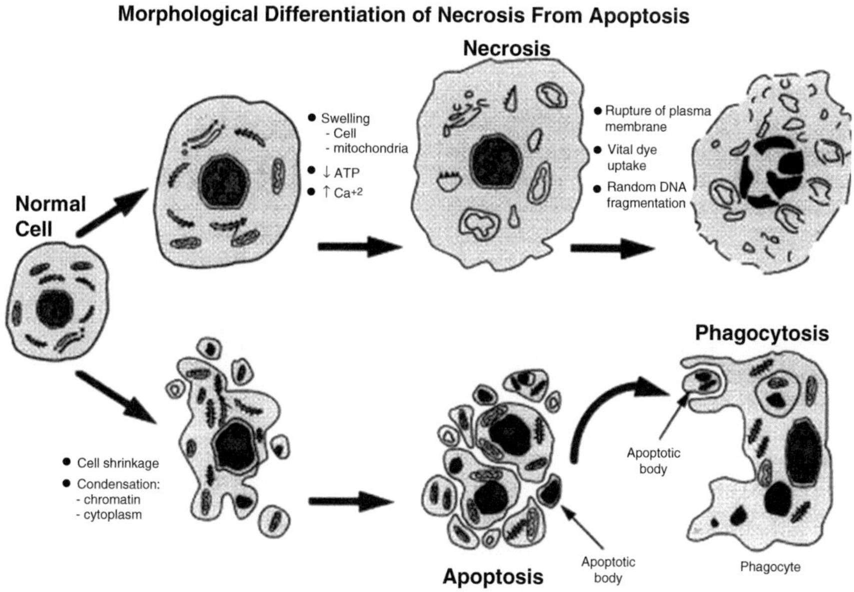

Fig. 7.1 Morphological differentiation of necrosis from apoptosis. The figure illustrates cardinal features of the histological appearances of cell death by either necrosis or apoptosis. The integrity of the plasma membrane and cell swelling are marked in necrosis, whereas cell shrinkage and fragmentation are most common in apoptosis. Most notable is the discrete process of phagocytosis of the "apoptotic bodies" by resident cells eliminating apoptosis, whereas cell eruption and content leakage (events triggering inflammation) are the final outcome of necrosis. (Reproduced by permission from Feuerstein et al. [33])

The main causes of N are:

- The impact of a stress or insult beyond the protective capacity of the cell causes rupture of the plasma membrane and swelling of the MITO and endoplasmic reticulum (this is why the term oncosis has also been used). It is accompanied by nuclear pyknosis. However, the nuclear chromatin condensation is not as intense as seen in APO.

The increased membrane permeability and rupture have two results: cellular and extracellular.

1. Cellular

   The cell and its organelles swell, as already described.

2. Extracellular

   Necrotic cells release their intracellular content; thus they induce inflammatory reactions, both of adjacent cells but also systemically. This causes activation of innate immunity, as will be further described.

N occurs because ATP cellular supply is exhausted. In what sequence this is associated with membrane rupture is difficult to ascertain, as will be further discussed. The decline in function of the ATP-dependent ion pumps in the membrane leads to the opening of the "death channel" which results in colloid osmotic forces and entry of cations inside the membrane.

The "death channel" is selectively permeable to cations and inhibitable by glycine [34].

Hotchkiss et al. [15] very pertinently point out that acute and profound decreases in ATP induce N, while modest yet chronic decreases of ATP induce APO.

Various types of insults have been described: Loss of blood flow is what mostly concerns the cardiologist, but physical trauma, heat, and radiation are also significant factors.

In what instances is N seen in the heart?

In the cardiovascular context, it is mainly caused by the abrupt interruption of blood flow, especially during coronary occlusion in the course of an acute myocardial infarction (AMI). The emergence of APO was widely identified when reperfusion was introduced in the therapy of AMI.

Baines [10] reviews work showing that the MPTP is inhibited by low pH, and that it is quiescent during ischemia (occlusion).

However N is also seen as a result of a combination of ischemic and reperfusion injury.

Early on it must be stressed that the limits between N and APO are becoming less distinct. Thus, very experienced workers refer to cell death as occurring through "necrosis or apoptosis" in I/R [35].

A main component of cell N is calcium overload during reperfusion [5, 6].

Also, Baines [10] points out that if a stress is severe and/or prolonged, ATP (which is required for APO) will be significantly depleted and N will occur.

It is proposed that the hypercontraction caused by I/R in early experiments is a characteristic component of contraction band necrosis [5].

It is postulated that Ca^{2+} overload at higher magnitudes can cause N and at lower APO. Garcia-Dorado et al. [36] believe that APO is not a main component of CD induced by Ca^{2+} overload. Due to the increase of membrane permeability, the necrotic cells swell, while they characteristically shrink in APO. The mitochondria also swell. As already stated, cellular contents during N spill into the extracellular space and can be detected in the periphery (plasma). They induce an inflammatory response [17]. This is mostly ascribed to molecules such as high-mobility group protein B1 (HMGB 1).

Zong and Thompson [37] point out that N may enter the fate cycle of a cell and that the inflammation that it elicits may be a warning response. Thus, according to Whelan et al. [5], some authors have used the term necroptosis, which will be discussed later on.

Galluzzi et al. [2, 4], Whelan et al. [7], and Hotchkiss et al. [15] stress an intriguing point: that N may be less accidental and more regulated than originally thought.

Thus Galluzzi et al. [2] postulate that there exists a stereotyped cascade of events in the various models of N. Another aspect which they refer to is that N can occur during mammalian development, i.e., the death of chondrocytes during bone growth, or in the adult the loss of intestinal epithelial cells.

Luke et al. [38] have described that the intracellular serpin-6 which "regulates" N exhibits a prosurvival function by blocking N, protecting against hypotonic shock, heat shock, oxidative stress, and cation channel hypertrophy, thus casting doubt on its completely accidental nature.

7.6.1 Necrotic Pathways

According to Whelan et al. [7], N can be signaled by two pathways:

1. The first involves death receptors, such as tumor necrosis factor-α receptor 1 (TNFR1). This receptor can promote survival, APO, or N. Laster et al. [39] stress the complex nature of the cytotoxic response that it can induce: In the rat fibroblast F17 cell line, it induced typical APO, while in the L-M line, it caused N. Further details are beyond the scope of this review. However, one interesting aspect must be mentioned, the role of procaspase-8, which when activated can induce APO, but when inhibited, the result is N, through an increase of ROS production.
2. The second necrotic mechanism is affected by the mitochondrial permeability transition pore (MPTP) which as already stated is situated in the inner mitochondrial membrane, actually on the leaf facing the intermembrane space.

This process is regulated by cyclophilin D. MPTP can be opened by increases in oxidative stress, increased phosphate concentration, adenine nucleotide depletion, and importantly an increase of the matrix Ca^{2+}.

Its opening causes the breakdown of intracellular ATP.

Cyclophilin D regulates MPTP pore opening and swelling of the mitochondria, hallmark of N, and cell death.

Cytoplasmic Ca^{2+} through MPTP opening can lead to N, in the worm and in the mammal through the proteases calpains, which are activated by Ca^{2+}, and cathepsins which are released from the lysosomes during stress.

According to Zong and Thompson [37], calpain activation leads to N through cleavage of the Na^+/Ca^{2+} exchanger in the plasma membrane and a sustained secondary intracellular Ca^{2+} overload.

However, according to Whelan et al. [7], calpain can also induce APO, through Bax and Bid, and autophagy, through cleavage of Atg5 (autophagy-related 5 homologue) which will be described later. According to the same authors, the lysosomal cathepsins leak out explosively from the lysosomes, digest molecules, and lead to N. Under less abrupt conditions, partial lysosomal rupture leads to APO. They point out that N, APO, and AUTO can be initiated by the lysosomes, whose integrity is preserved by HSP70.

Syntichaki et al. [40] point out that they are the result of perturbation of intercellular Ca^{2+}.

Hotchkiss et al. [15] delineate the following mediators of N: ROS and Ca^{2+}-activated non-lysosomal proteases calpains and cathepsins. These proteases are activated by oxidative stress and Ca^{2+} overload. Prolonged elevation of catecholamines, Ang II, and other vasoactive hormones may well be involved.

Whelan et al. [3] describe how ischemia-induced hypoxia increases intracellular acidosis, which extrudes H^+ from the cell by Na^+/H^+ exchange leading to an increase of intracellular Na^+, which through the Na^+/Ca^{2+} exchanger leads to an intercellular Ca^{2+} increase, with the cell swelling, effects which have already been described.

At reperfusion, Ca^{2+}-induced Ca^{2+} release is effected through the ER (SR), or sarcoplasmic reticulum, and MPTP opening is induced in some forms of N, such as DNA damage from alkylating agents mainly through ATP depletion. They also describe that HMGB1, which as already stated is released as an inflammatory elicitor during N, can provide a switch from APO to N.

Opening of the MPTP pore is a major component of necrotic cell death. At R, APO cell death occurs at a lower incidence than N, but for a more extended time: APO occurs as early as 30 min and as late as 3 days after R initiation [41].

According to Whelan et al. [7], Poly-ADP-ribose-polymerase (PARP) is a main player in N occurring through DNA damage from alkylating agents.

7.7 Autophagy

This term derived from the Greek (auto = self and phagy = eat) delineates a process of death triggered by a sublethal stress involving nutrient deprivation. This causes the cell to recycle its own nonessential redundant or damaged organelles. Kroemer et al. [3] point out that probably one should define CD not occurring through, but with AUTO. The same authors point out that cells with the characteristics of autophagic CD can still recover when the noxious stimulus is withdrawn.

According to Clarke [42], AUTO occurs regularly during the development of an organism, as in the amphibian tail during metamorphosis.

Three forms have been described: *Macroautophagy* will be the one further discussed. *Chaperone-mediated AUTO* refers to a process mediated through chaperone proteins, such as HSC70 and heat shock protein (HSP) 70; these bind selectively to the substrate and deliver it to the lysosomes for degradation.

Interestingly, Pedrozo et al. [43] have shown that this form of cell death is responsible for ryanodine receptor 2 degradation.

In microautophagy, the material to be phagocytized is surrounded by invagination of the lysosomal membrane [44]. From this point on, *macroautophagy* will be described, in which the material to be phagocytized is sequestered within the characteristic body, the "autophagosome" contained by a double-membrane vesicle.

Lavandero et al. [44] point out that autophagy is seen in cardiac fibroblast and the cardiomyocytes.

They remind that autophagy is important for normal cardiac development.

This autophagosome can be well seen with electron microscopy. Its formation is governed by autophagy-regulating (ATG) proteins, one of which is Beclin-1(ATG 6) [45]. Characteristically Beclin-1 is a BH3-only protein already described to be active in APO. Moreover, the antiapoptotic proteins Bcl-2 and Bcl-XL can also inhibit starvation-induced AUTO.

Thus Bcl-2 plays a dual role: It can be pre-survival in the MITO, by blocking APO, and detrimental in the ER, by inhibiting AUTO.

Additional factors are the phosphatidylinositol-3-kinase (PI-3 K) and the mammalian target of rapamycin (mTOR) which inhibits autophagosome formation.

Whelan et al. [7] point out that under energy availability (fed condition), mTOR inhibits AUTO by phosphorylating and activating ATG proteins.

However, under starvation, reduced PI3K-Akt signaling decreases mTOR activity and activates AUTO.

After inclusion in the autophagosome, its components are lysed by the action of the lysosomes, providing the cell with the aminoacids, free fatty acids, and energy.

Nucleus pyknosis can be seen, but is not so prominent as in APO. Autophagosomes fuse with the lysosomes, the enclosed cytoplasmic material is degraded by acid hydrolysis, and the nutrients are released to the cytosol for recycling.

Wang et al. [46] describe the multiple ways in which AUTO participates in metabolic remodeling: It provides aminoacids, nucleotides, sugars, and lipids. The former enter the tricarboxylic (TCA) acid cycle. Nucleotides can be recycled into new nucleic acids or enter the pentose phosphate pathway (PPP). Sugars can participate into new glucose synthesis and glycolysis, while lipids undergo β-oxidation. Together with energy production, the above processes contribute to new membrane generation biosynthesis. Starvation nutrient deprivation, hypoxia, ROS, damaged organelles, and protein aggregates can induce AUTO, in an mTOR-dependent process.

According to Dhesi et al. [47], the process of AUTO involves five steps:

1. Formation of the isolation membrane or phagophore.
2. Expansion of the phagophore.
3. Formation of the double membrane.
4. Fusion of the autophagosome with a lysosome to form the autolysosome.
5. Digestion of the content together with the inner membrane layer by the lysosome hydrolases.

However, there is some discussion if these processes can actually cause CD, converting AUTO from a survival to a death process, if overexpressed. The increased number of autophagosomes in dying cells might signify that they are associated with CD, but it can well be a sign of failure of the cell to survive despite sacrificing its vital components, according to Hotchkiss et al. [15].

Thus, Dhesi et al. [47] believe that it is a beneficial process under most conditions. They also describe ER-phagy, or reticulophagy which selectively targets the ER, which actually forms the dual membranes described.

Gottlieb and Mentzer [48] also point out that it is a beneficial process under most conditions. Notably they enumerate many cardioprotective agents which induce AUTO (diazoxide, ranolazine, rapamycin, statins). They describe an additional term, mitophagy, which is a specialized form which causes elimination of the MITO, which have been reported to be contained within the autophagosomes. Thus, they could be protected from “a mitochondrial stampede” causing widespread cell death by the “ROS begetting ROS production” process already described. They further stress that this may be the more important mechanism, since the amount of energy production may not be critical. They further enlarge upon the adaptive versus maladaptive instances, some of which will be further described. They conclude that the bulk of available evidence supports the protective role of AUTO.

Another question has arisen whether AUTO can be an adaptive response in desmin-related cardiomyopathy which is characterized by overexpression of mutated αβ-crystallin (cry ABR120G). It is being discussed by two investigative groups:

Tannous et al. [49] believe that AUTO is upregulated by twofold in order to cope with the increase of misfolded protein aggregates seen in this disorder. Blunting AUTO dramatically hastened progression to heart failure.

Maloyan et al. [50] remark that mice with this cardiomyopathy show progressive MITO abnormalities and activation of CD through APO. By preventing APO through crossing these mice with transgenic strains with cardiac-specific Bcl-2 overexpression, they found decreased MITO abnormalities, attenuation of APO, reduction of protein aggregation, restitution of cardiac function, prevention of cardiac hypertrophy, and a prolongation of survival by 20%. However, the animals still died prematurely; thus inhibition of APO resulted in AUTO upregulation and increased N according to the authors, as detected by an increase of Evans blue dye cells, a technique which detects necrotic CD-related abnormalities. It is not clear from their work if CD is overall reduced or not.

Zhu et al. [51] have a different opinion as regards hemodynamic stress and AUTO: They consider that AUTO increases after transverse aortic constriction representing a maladaptive process. These questions will be further addressed when the three forms of death are assessed in the principal cardiological conditions.

Ferdous et al. [52] provide a very comprehensive review. They differentiate among three forms of AUTO activity:

Basal, which is adaptive, includes homeostatic protein control, ROS detoxification, and removal of defective MITO. *Maladaptive* consists of excessive catabolism, MITO elimination, and adverse REM and reduced cell survival, and *adaptive*.

These authors point out the role of FoxO (Forehand box-containing protein, O subfamily) in governing AUTO.

Cao et al. [53] describe the role of this protein, which is activated by mechanical unloading and acts through the AUTO-lysosomal and ubiquitination-proteasome pathways to produce cardiac atrophy. Interestingly, it triggers BNIP-3 (Bcl-2 and 19 kDa-interacting protein 3) which is also involved in APO Zhang and Ney [54] describe the role of BNIP3 and NIX in autophagy and mitophagy. BNIP has homology to Bcl-2 in the BH3 domain.

BNIP3 has a proapoptotic action through a mitochondrial "pathway" but also regulates autophagy in response to hypoxia.

NIX also has proapoptotic activity but can induce autophagy, which according to the authors can be protective but also can induce cell death. In the same vein, Feng et al. [55] show that hypoxia suppresses the survival pathway of the myocardium through HIF-1A-IGFBD-3 signaling. They showed that BNIP3 activation by prolonged hypoxia could induce autophagy and mitochondria department apoptosis in cardiomyocyte.

Another factor involved in inducing autophagy is REDD1, a protein ubiquitously involved in various human tissues [56]. It has been found to attenuate hypertrophy in primary neonatal ventricular cardiomyocytes exposed to phenylephrine. Its sustained overexpression leads to lung cancer cell survival through Akt activation [57].

Another important aspect of cell death is lysosome-dependent cell death.

According to Galluzzi et al. [4], this is a subroutine of RCD initiated by perturbation of intracellular homeostasis, and it is characterized by permeabilization of lysosomal membranes. According to Aits and Jäättelä [58], after lysosome membrane permeabilization (LMP), leakage of the lysosomal content, which includes proteolytic enzymes of the cathepsin family into the cytosol, leads to this form of cell death.

According to some observations, LMP is an epiphenomenon of intrinsic apoptosis [59]. Additionally, Bax recruitment causes LMP. ROS play an important role [60].

Other processes involved in LMP are calpain proteases. Interestingly, HSP70, which is a lysosome stabilizer, is a target of calpain [61].

Activation of apoptotic caspases, especially caspase-9, caspase-8, and caspase-2 [58] is another cause.

Lipids and their metabolites play an important role: Excess of either sphingomyelin or sphingosine has a destabilizing effect, while sphingosine-1-phosphate (S1P) processes lysosomal function. LMP can also be caused by phospholipase A2 (PLA2) [62].

The apoptotic factor p53 can also trigger LMP [63].

Finally, proapoptotic Bcl-2 family members might contribute to LMP in some cases. All in all, lysosome-dependent cell death shares many pathways with apoptosis.

The Role of the Ubiquitin Proteasome System (UPS)

It is often mentioned, but its actual role has not been adequately defined. Schuler and Green [64] provide a recent inclusive review. They describe that this system, in parallel with the various mechanisms involved in CD, has definite roles in cell-cycle control, protein turnover and quality control, cell signaling, and APO.

According to the authors, the system is closely involved in myocardial ischemia. Its four components include the proteasome, the ubiquitin (UB), the ubiquitination machinery, and the deubiquitinases. It is an energy-requiring (ATP) process.

The proteasome can be involved in the removal and clearing of oxidized and damaged proteins. It can also form a hybrid, the "immunoproteasome," since the ubiquitin system is also involved in immune response and antigen presentation.

Ubiquitin (Ub) is involved in protein degradation.

The UPS and specifically the proteasome become dysfunctional in ischemia, both myocardial and cerebral. Its ATP-dependent activity is mainly affected, decreasing proteasome activity.

The UPS becomes dysfunctional during ischemia, while its function is preserved by ischemic preconditioning.

The UPS exerts a parallel function to AUTO, which also prevents proteotoxic stress, but targets mostly macromolecular structures and organelles. Moreover, AUTO is upregulated while the UPS becomes dysfunctional at ischemia. Actually, it is suggested that there is an inverse relationship between UPS and autophagic flux.

7.8 Efforts at CD Modality Clarification

It must be pointed out that the efforts to further clarify the various modalities of CD continue.

Thus the Nomenclature Committee on Cell Death has issued recommendations in 2005 and 2009 [3]. They state that it is important to discriminate between *dying* as a process and *death* as an end point.

They also suggest that exact description of various characteristics should replace the mention of the modality itself, i.e., TUNEL-positive cells % instead of APO %. Similarly they recommend that "double-membraned microvesicles" should be described instead of AUTO.

Galluzzi et al. [2], as many other authors have pointed out, describe that N is a negative definition, i.e., cell death with no signs of APO or AUTO. Moreover they suggest limiting the use of the term oncosis. However, Kostin [9] extensively uses this term.

The Committee authors [3] also describe the term:

- *Mitotic catastrophe,* which occurs after a dysregulation of failed mitosis and is morphologically accompanied by micro- and multinucleosis.

Also in Table 7.1, they describe "cornification," which affects epidermal keratinocytes.

They also comment on the validity of the term "programmed cell death."

They point out that "genetic programming" characterizes APO during development and aging. They recommend that the terms developmental, etoposide, osmotic shock-induced cell death, etc. should be used.

Moreover, they give a useful suggestion as to when a cell can be considered dead:

1. When it has lost the integrity of its plasma membrane.
2. When, including the nucleolus, it has undergone complete fragmentation into discrete bodies.
3. Its corpse or its fragments has been engulfed by an adjacent cells in vivo.

In Table 7.1 they give morphologic characteristics of APO, AUTO, and N.

7.9 Crosstalk Among Processes

Before finishing this description of the various forms of CD, the common pathways of the crosstalk among the three processes, which has already been referred to and addressed by most expert groups [1–4, 7], must be further discussed.

Kung et al. [65] described experiments both in *C. elegans* and mammalian cells.

They stress that the process of N is as old as APO and that Virchow first described the "unregulated" or "accidental" form of N. They describe that in APO the main mechanism is permeabilization of the MOM, while in N the opening of the MPTP, which spans the MIM. They also point out that the same death ligands that can activate APO (TNFα, Fas ligand, TRAIL – TNF-related APO-inducing ligand) can also stimulate N and that TNFα can induce survival, APO, or N. They also remind how, when caspase-8 is deleted or inhibited, APO cannot be initiated and programmed N emerges through TNFR1 ligation. They also remind that apart from Ca^{2+} overload, Fe^{2+}cystolic increase can lead to TNFα-induced N, and that APO and N are connected at the death receptor and MITO pathways, and that the MOM and MIM are separated by only microns, promoting these crosstalks.

A number of expert researchers have been discussing to what extent N death can be considered to be programmed.

Konstantinidis et al. [66] from the Richard N. Kitsis group also stress that the MITO and the ER are central to both APO and N signaling; the Bcl-2 family proteins can be implicated both in APO and N. Also, they stress that the ER can mediate both APO and N and that the proapoptotic proteins Bax and Bak have been shown to also regulate N.

Proskuryakov et al. [67] underline that various stimuli (cytokines, ischemia, heat, irradiation, pathogens) can cause both APO and N. Also, protective mechanisms (Bcl-2/Bcl-XL, HSPs) are equally effective against both forms of CD. Finally, they stress that a main difference between the two forms of CD is the inflammatory response caused by N. This will be further discussed.

The question whether and how much N can be programmed – thus merging toward APO – is being posed with increasing frequency.

Kung et al. [65] and Konstantinidis et al. [66] point out a significant difference: In APO the central mitochondrial event is permeabilization of the MOM, while in N it is the opening of the MIM and the MPTP, which is regulated by cyclophilin D.

The same authors describe that programmed N can be activated by the same ligands as APO (TNFa, FasL, TRAIL) and that the intrinsic mitochondrial death pathway is the more ancient, conserved in *C. elegans*.

They also stress that regulated – or programmed – N is an important factor of CD in acute myocardial infarction or congestive heart failure, as will be further discussed.

Linkermann and Green [68] use another term for programmed cell death – *necroptosis* – which is dependent on the activity of the receptor-interacting protein 3 (RIP3) which through various death processes binds to the TNF and FADD. This kinase is necessary for programmed N. In contrast, necrostatin (Nec)-1 is a small-molecule inhibitor of programmed N, which inhibits the kinase activity of the RIP kinase 3 (RIPK3).

Necroptosis was initially recognized as a defensive mechanism against viral infection. However, according to the authors, it is operative also in I/R injury, myocardial infarction, and atherosclerosis, among others. It is characterized by the necrosome. It is caspase-independent and can actually be triggered by TNF in the presence of caspase-8 inhibition. It is inhibited by necrostatin-1 which is an inhibitor of RIPK1 (receptor increasing protein kinase 1) which after a series of interactions promotes CD. The authors point out that necroptosis and APO may occur in the same organ.

Finally, it should be realized that N death is predominant in the ubiquitous cardiovascular involvement of atherosclerosis, but APO also contributes.

The great majority of dying cells in human atherosclerotic plaques undergo N. Oxidative stress, depletion of ATP, and increased Ca^{2+} together with decreased clearance of APO cells promote this process, which in turn, through the release of various substances, further promotes inflammation.

On this subject some more pertinent points should be stressed.

Karch and Molketin [69] in 2015 described regulated necrotic cell death in which they state that mitochondria are important mediators of both apoptosis and necrosis. They clarify that opening of the outside mitochondrial membrane is specific for apoptosis, where inner membrane opening produces necrosis. Otherwise stated, mitochondrial dysfunction occurs during necrosis because of prolonged opening of the MPTP. However if a small proportion of mitochondria undergo MPTP opening, the remaining may still provide enough high-energy phosphates for apoptotic cell death to occur.

Nikoletopoulou et al. [70] postulate that there exists a crosstalk between the three forms, which were previously thought to represent mutually exclusive cellular states.

They describe the following indications of cross talk between necrosis and apoptosis. They reiterate the term necroptosis, which describes the cases where necrosis represents a regulated and programed and not accidental form of cell death. They stress that this picture may emerge when apoptosis has been blocked (by caspase inhibitors) or under low levels of ATP, as will be described further.

It can also be initiated by activation of the innate immunity mechanisms which recognize the pathogen-associated molecular patterns (PAMPs). They also describe that TNFα can induce APO and necrosis by distinct signaling pathways [70] and that apoptosis occurs when the action of caspase-8 is by anyway impeded.

They stress that Akt can have variable actions, since it can prevent APO but also facilitate necroptosis. The authors describe the role of ATP: If its levels remain high, APO is formed; low levels favor necrosis.

It is of interest, however, that complete ATP deletion promotes a different picture, which Skulachev [71] has described as "mitochondrial suicide."

They further postulate that TNF intrinsic APO is the one determining cardiomyocyte fate in heart failure. Sustained TNF signaling activated the intrinsic cell death pathway, while overexpression of Bcl-2 blunted this process.

Micheau and Tschopp [72] report that TNF-induced apoptosis is induced by TNFR1.

Nikoletopoulou et al. [70] also extensively describe the role of p53 in APO; and p53, is a central agent influenced by many noxious stimuli, such as DNA, oxidative stress, and ischemia. It can also induce permeabilization of the mitochondrial outer membrane (MOMK) which promotes APO through the Bcl-2 family. They also describe a setting similar to cardiac APO and ischemic brain infarction. In this setting, an apoptotic "border zone" termed in the neurological terminology as "penumbra" surrounds a necrotic center.

The authors advance the view that p53 can promote not only APO but also necrosis through various transcriptional mechanisms.

Xia et al. [73] point out that the distinction of the three commonly reported types of cell death goes far back. They point out that the Nomenclature Committee on Cell Death has recommended that the various types of CD should be defined according to their distinct biochemical characteristics [3, 74]. According to these, APO is defined as a caspase-dependent, genetically controlled form of death that can be modulated by genetic or pharmacologic interventions.

According to the same authors, autophagic cell death is associated with lipidation of microtubule-associated protein light chain 3 (CL3) and degradation of the sequestome 1, also known as p62 [75].

Necroptosis is dependent on receptor-interacting protein kinases 1 and 3 (RIPK1/R1PK3) [76].

Xia et al. [73] differentiate that the intrinsic apoptosis (mitochondrial) pathway, which is caused by intracellular stress such as oxidative stress, calcium overload, and DNA damage, leads to Bax-/Bak-induced MITO outer membrane permeabilization and release of cytochrome c from the MITO into the cytosol, which together with the apoptotic protease-activating factor1 (Apaf1) form the apoptosome, with resultant activation of caspase 9.

Conversely, the extrinsic pathway APO is initiated by extracellular stress signals, i.e., TNF-α, Fas ligand (FasL), and TNF-related APO-inducing ligand (TRAK); these bind to their respective receptors, which recruit Fas-associated death domain (FADD) and procaspase 8 into the death-inducing signaling complex leading to caspase 8 activation and the activation of effector caspases 3, 6, and 9.

The same authors [73] summarize the signaling pathways regulating APO.

7.10 PI3K/Akt Pathway

This pathway is discussed in many chapters. It protects against APO by phosphorylation and inactivation of the BH3-only proapoptotic protein BAD. Here one should reflect that some proteins such as Akt are activated, while others inactivated by phosphorylation.

This pathway is also involved in the protective action of ischemic preconditioning and many other factors. PTEN (dual protein/lipid phosphatase and tensin homologue) inhibits Akt activation. Its overexpression leads to caspase activation [37]. Akt is also inhibited (dephosphorylated) by PH domain leucine-rich repeat protein phosphatase (PHLPP), which significantly is activated by isoproterenol. The same authors point out that the Bcl-2 family, which play a typical APO role can also be involved in necroptosis; overexpression of Bcl-2 can prevent both APO and necrosis in a rat insulin-producing cell line but also other types of cells.

Nikoletopoulou et al. [70] also point out that crosstalk exists between autophagy and APO. They point out that autophagy may be protective in cancer cells but noxious in non-cancer cells. Also mTOR kinase inhibition which typically induces autophagy may have pleiotropic effects on APO depending on the cellular context. Also, they point out that caspases, typical inducers of APO, can also modulate autophagy. Finally, the authors point out that crosstalk exists between autophagy and necrosis. Thus, the typical necrosis-mediator PARP can also promote autophagy.

Apart from the various descriptions of cardiomyocyte death, the original term "necrosis" which around 60 years ago was considered as the only modality of cell death has found a new use. The Society of Toxicologic Pathology in 1999 [77] recommended that this term be used to signify changes after cell death, regardless of the pathway leading to death.

In addition to the mixed term necroptosis, Takemura et al. [78] have proposed the term "autophagic necrosis" to describe a combination of the morphological features of both autophagy and necrosis as an end result of failure of the autophagic process.

The behavior of the MPTP can tilt the modality of cell death toward apoptosis, necrosis, or necroptosis.

Kostin [79] has also estimated that in a human heart with ischemic heart disease and chronic hibernation, dilated cardiomyopathy, or even aortic stenosis, a total annual loss of 20% of cardiomyocytes is predicted. This should be a factor in timing of revascularization, possibly resynchronization and aortic valve replacement or TAVR, respectively. Vigliano et al. [80] recently postulated that autophagy may also be a noxious and not just compensatory process.

Piek et al. [81] point out another not well-appreciated aspect of cardiomyocyte death: that fibrosis by itself begets cell death. Fibrosis as already described in the respective chapter is characteristic of REM.

Fibrosis (F) can be divided according to these authors into:

- Interstitial, replacement, and perivascular fibrosis.
- It is defined as expansion of the ECM without cardiomyocyte loss.
- Replacement F is a response to tissue death.

Perivascular F collagen accumulates in the adventitia of coronary arteries. This fibrotic response limits myocardial blood flow and reserve and promotes myocardial ischemia especially in conditions of increased myocardial metabolic needs. Perivascular fibrosis is a cause of decreased capillary density. It may thus cause further cell death.

A common aspect of F is the activation in differentiation of fibroblasts into myofibroblasts, which are not present in healthy cardiac tissue but only in heart valves. Transforming growth factor (TGF) is the most potent activator of this transition. Alpha smooth muscle actin (aSMA) is a marker of myofibroblasts, but it is also expressed in SMCs. However, fibroblasts are also derived from endothelial cells [82].

It is interesting that myofibroblasts produce many factors which induce pathological cardiomyocyte hypertrophy including TGFβ, TNFα, GF1, and ET-1 and may culminate in cell death. It is interesting that TGFβ prevents myofibroblast apoptosis via the prosurvival PI3K/Akt pathway. Also, a feedback seems to occur, since cardiomyocytes at overload conditions induce the fibrotic response of myofibroblasts.

Xia et al. [73] review that many signaling pathways can be involved in cardiomyocyte apoptosis. They describe the following main pathways:

The PI3k/Akt pathway which has an antiapoptotic action. It is strongly activated by insulin and IGF-1. Here the work by our group and others mentioned in the chapter on cardiac REM has suggested that prolonged overexpression of Akt-1 can be deleterious, causing fibrosis and exacerbation of IRI. Chaanine et al. [83] point out that in pressure overload produced by aortic clamping, Akt is activated but JNK is increased to a greater degree.

Akt is activated by many cardioprotective agents such as conditioning, estrogens, leukemia inhibitory factor, neuregulin, adrenomedullin, kallikrein, isoflurane, urotensin II, and GLP1.

Akt activation is inhibited by PTEN (protein/lipid phosphatase and tensin homologue). Its overexpression leads to caspase activation [84].

It is also inhibited by PHLPP (PH domain leucine-rich repeat protein phosphatase), which significantly is increased with angina and isoproterenol infusion.

GSK-3 (glycogen synthase kinase-3). Its inactivation is cardioprotective. It seems that a delicate balance exists: transient and partial inhibition of GSK-3 is cardioprotective, while complete loss is deleterious. Pim 1 is a serine-threonine kinase upregulated by IGF-1. Its downexpression exacerbates APO, while upregulation reduces infarct size [85]. Its deficiency increased APO after an AMI and reduced autophagy. It also complexes the cardioprotective yes-associated protein (YAP) and is antioxidative. Another member FoxO3α is also antiapoptotic. Knockdown of FoxO1 also exaggerates APO.

The mitogen-activated protein kinase (MAPK) pathway [86].

This include the following:

- Extracellular signal-regulated kinases 1 and 2 (ERK1/2). Activation is cardioprotective and antiapoptotic. However, doxorubicin-induced persistent ERK1/2 activation can contribute to apoptosis [87].

7.11 Stress-Activated Protein Kinases

These include JNK and MAPK p38. They are proapoptotic; they respond to outside stress influences.

JNK has a definite a proapoptotic activity and its inhibition protects against IRI. However, under some circumstances, it may protect against hypoxia/deoxygenation APO. According to Shao et al. [88], this action may occur throughout Akt activation. JNK increases with pressure overload, and it activates the aforementioned apoptotic factor FoxO3α.

The role of MAPK p38 has also been the subject of intense investigation. It leads to cardioprotection and increase of the antiapoptotic Bcl-2 family. Its behavior in ischemic preconditioning suggests that it may be activated by short cycles of simulated ischemia/reoxygenation but that in the preconditioned heart [89], p38 is actually lower. It is also prohypertrophic. The use of the classical inhibitor of this kinase SB203580 attenuates apoptosis [89].

7.11.1 Integrins/FAK

β1 integrin is antiapoptotic. Since integrins do not possess an intracellular domain, to transduce their signals, they depend on cytosolic kinases, one of which is the focal adhesion kinase (FAK) [90]. Its activation protects against APO through Bcl-2 family upregulation. This kinase also protects against doxorubicin-induced APO.

7.11.2 TNFα/NF-kB

This cytokine has already been described. It has a strong proapoptotic activity together with its proinflammatory action. Here it must be stressed that TNFα exerts its action through two receptors: TNFR1 mediates most of the detrimental effect of TNFα, while some of its reported cardioprotection effect is exerted through TNFR2 [91].

NFkB is a central inflammatory agent. It is a main effector of Toll-like receptors TLR2 and 4. Its chronic activation causes APO [92] and a form of inflammatory dilated cardiomyopathy [93]. Again, in connection with the data presented for TNFα, its overstimulation may be cardioprotective.

7.12 G-Protein-Coupled Receptors (GPCRs)

This is a very important family. They include the following important receptors:

β-adrenergic receptors, α1 adrenergic receptors, endothelin, angiotensin, and adenosine receptors.

7.12.1 Adrenergic Receptors

In the myocardium, β1 (≈70%), β2 (≈20%), and α1 (≈10%) predominate [94]. β3 receptors have been relatively recently described. β1 stimulation causes APO, through the activation of many factors: PKA [95], calcineurin Ca^{2+}/calmodulin kinase II, and synthesis of TNF. Stimulation of β2 suppresses APO through P13K/Akt activation. β3 stimulation is cardioprotective.

α1 stimulation with phenylephrine is antiapoptotic in up to moderate doses, while much greater doses can cause APO [96].

Endothelin-1 exerts its action through two receptors: types A and B. The majority of studies suggest that receptor A has a proapoptotic action [97].

Angiotensin-II exerts proapoptotic and pro-fibrotic actions through its type 1 receptor [98].

The *adenosine receptors* are anti-antiapoptotic through the PI3K/Akt and MEK/ERK1/2 pathways [99, 100].

Protein kinase C (PKC). This is a large family; its isoforms have been counted up to 12. PKCα causes hypertrophy and is associated with decreased contractility but also apoptosis. PKCε is anti antiapoptotic, as well as PKCj PCkδ may be pro-apoptotic, as well as PKCβ [101].

Cyclic AMP-dependent protein kinase (PKA). It is pro-apoptotic, mostly through β1 adrenergic activity.

7.13 Calcium Cycling and Cell Survival/Death

Calcium cycling is essential for cardiomyocyte function. However, while being the key factor influencing cardiac contraction and relaxation, it can cause both necrosis and APO. It can also cause pathological hypertrophy, through the calcineurin-NFAT and CaMKII pathways [102, 103].

It is protective against APO in some studies, as against doxorubicin [104]. However, the majority of studies have shown that it is proapoptotic [103, 104].

Zhivotovsky and Orrenius [105] and Hajnóczky et al. [106] mention that apart from necrotic and apoptotic signaling, calcium overload can also cause anoikis and autophagy cell death.

HAX-1. This is an antiapoptotic protein which increases during IRI in both the brain and the myocardium. Interestingly it has been shown to interact with the SERCA2/PLN complex and to promote cell survival through modulation of SERCA2 protein levels and ER Ca^{2+} stores according to Vafiadaki et al. [107]. These authors also found that overexpression of SERCA2 abrogated the protective effects of HAX-1 on cell survival but that HAX-1 overexpression downregulated SERCA2 levels. Further work by this group showed that HAX-1 overexpression reduced SERCA2 pump activity and contractility [108].

7.14 The Induction of Inflammation by Various Modalities of CD

Traditionally, as already described, N has been considered as causing inflammation through the rupture of the cell membrane and the spilling of intracellular contents in the intercellular space.

APO was traditionally considered as not causing inflammation, actually causing "anergy" [15, 109]. Konstantinidis et al. [66] characteristically describe that in APO, when phagocytosis by macrophages or occasionally neighboring cells is efficient, inflammation is avoided.

The inflammatory response after I/R is well known. Again, this process is not solely noxious, because it contributes to healing, as pointed by Timmers et al. [110].

These authors refer to the endogenous alarm signals produced by I/R as danger-associated molecular patterns. These include HSPs, high-mobility group box-1, hyaluronic acid, and fibronectin fragments.

Here it must be pointed out that the activation of Toll-like receptors (TLRs) can also have a beneficial effect, if not prolonged. Otherwise, it exerts a deleterious action.

However, APO has another effect: It contributes to the production and secretion of microparticles which modulate the innate and acquired immune system.

Kostin [9] remarks that an essential part of APO is timely removal of the dying cell before it causes a secondary inflammation.

Here it must be stressed again that the role of CD is not the same for all pathologic conditions. What is bad for the heart may be good for cancer.

As regards AUTO, it was also long regarded a "clean" process. However, Oka et al. [111] showed that mitochondrial DNA escaping from AUTO lead to TLR-9 mediated inflammatory cardiomyocyte responses.

On the other hand, inflammation itself can trigger APO [112].

Kung et al. [65] further describe "silent" vs "noisy" removal. In the former, phagocytosis is predominant. In "noisy" removal, N factors released (protein and nucleic acid) modify the inflammation response. The high-mobility group protein β1(HMG β1) is such a protein [113] which acts through the well-known TLRs and RAGEs (receptor for advanced glycation end products).

Linkermann and Green [68] point out that N triggers inflammation and innate and adaptive immune responses. They further describe that *necroptosis*, as already described, is a main element of ischemia-reperfusion injury and alloimmune injury in organ transplantation. They [68] also note that RIPK3 confers resistance against a viral load. However, absence of these mechanisms prevented various types of inflammatory lesions (intestinal epithelial cells, atherosclerotic lesions through high-fat diets). The authors consider necroptosis as a second-line defense mechanism against viruses which however can result in a maladaptive inflammatory response.

Probably the form of "immunogenic cell death" should be described in this context. It can be initiated by viral infections and some chemotherapeutic agents such as anthracyclines, radiation, and photodynamic therapy. Through their action a series of danger-associated molecular patterns (DAMPs) is released, such as calreticulin [114], ATP [115], the already mentioned high-mobility group box 1 (HMGβ1) [116], type I IFN [117], cancer cell-derived nucleic cells [118], and annexin A1 [119].

7.15 The Role of HSPs

These protective chaperones delay lysosome membrane permeabilization (LMP) and N induced by TNF and oxidative stress. LPM leads to a release of ROS, free cytosolic iron which is important for TNFα-induced N, and release of cathepsins which leads to N.

Kroemer et al. [3] give some more additional definitions of atypical CD.

Pyroptosis is an APO type of death seen in macrophages infected with *Salmonella* Typhimurium, *Yersinia*, *P. aeruginosa*, and other pathogens, mainly through caspase-1 activation. The macrophages involved exhibit morphological features of APO but also some traits of N. It is induced by the inflammasome [120]. *Excitotoxicity* is a death of neurons through glutamate or related aminoacids. It overlaps with APO and N.

7.16 Cell Death in Various Conditions

As already mentioned CD is the cause of myocardial dysfunction in the great majority of cardiac disorders.

7.16.1 Acute Myocardial Infarction (AMI)

Currently, in the vast majority of cases, reperfusion (R) is employed, either by thrombolysis or by primary angioplasty. It is thus very interesting that most descriptions are based on the work of Kajstura et al. [41] which is 22 years old and concerns permanent ligation. They studied AMI post left coronary artery ligation in rats. At that time they studied only APO and N, not AUTO. They found that at 2 h the former was responsible for the death of 2.8 million (M) cells, while the latter for the death of only 90,000. APO was still the major component of cardiomyocyte death at 4.5 h, killing 6.6 M myocytes. Myocytes showing both APO and N were prominent only after 6 h. N peaked at 1 day, involving 1.1 M myocytes, remained elevated up to 2 days, and decreased sharply at 7 days. However, it must be noted that the researchers did not study the border zone, which is an important area between necrotic and remote myocardium.

The most important point concerning this work is that the authors used permanent coronary artery ligation without reopening it, i.e., without employing reperfusion. Few direct comparisons exist, between permanent occlusion and occlusion/reperfusion. Gottlieb et al. [35] performed such a study in the rabbit: They compared animals undergoing 30 min of ischemia (I) and 4 h of reperfusion (R) compared to those undergoing 4.5 h of continuous I only. They also studied other groups of animals which will be discussed further on.

Their main findings can be summarized as follows:

Seven rabbits underwent I/R. They all showed a typical nucleosome ladder on DNA electrophoresis, in the ischemic LV area but not outside it. In this group 50% of cells developed CD in the ischemic area at risk, by TTC (triphenyltetrazolium chloride) staining, which mainly signifies N. In the five rabbits undergoing continuous occlusion, no nucleosome cleavage suggestive of APO was detected. This is in agreement with the suggestions of Baines [10] that APO cannot occur with persistent ischemia, during which he suggests that the MPTP is quiescent.

Gotlieb et al. [35] also studied two more subgroups:

At 5 min of ischemia only, no CD was detected nor was APO detected at only 5 min of ischemia and 4 h R. Additionally, the authors subjected three animals to 30 min I only without R. No DNA nucleosomal fragmentation was found. They did not specifically study N in this subgroup.

The authors also postulate that APO may be converted to N by polymorphonuclear attachment to the ischemic area activation. This brings into focus an aspect of the I/R injury discussed by Whelan et al. [7]: They note that both the extrinsic and intrinsic pathways are involved, with the latter playing a more central role, as evidenced by the effects of various manipulations of Bcl-2 and Bax and their inhibitors. In describing N, the authors point out that cyclophilin D, a factor affecting APO, is also involved in N through explosive MPTP opening.

One aspect that has not been adequately discussed is the contribution of inflammation in the I/R injury. Yellon and Hausenloy [121] gave a very detailed review. They describe the following potential mediators of reperfusion injury.

7.16.2 The Impact of Inflammation

The release of chemoattractant factors attracts neutrophils into the infarct zone. These cells have very important effects: They induce vascular plugging and also release degrading enzymes and ROS.

It has already been described that during N, due to the rupture of the cytoplasmic membrane, cell contents leaking into the intercellular space elicit a systemic reaction. Timmers et al. [110] have termed it an innate immunity activation.

Dutta et al. [122] showed that an index MI accelerates atherosclerosis. They ascribe this finding to activation of sympathetic nervous system and signaling expression of interleukin-6, MMP-9, myeloperoxidase, and LY-6c in atherosclerosis plaques after an acute infarct.

Another protective mechanism which sheds light on I/R injury is the active protein phosphatase-1 inhibitor-1 which attenuates the ER stress response, which, when induced in the ischemic heart, contributes to APO through altered Ca^{2+}homeostasis [123]. Murphy and Steenbergen [124] discuss the relative roles of the CD modalities in I/R. They also stress that this injury can be a mixture of all three and that the MPTP is a major regulator of both APO and N.

Further evidence suggesting that at I/R both APO and N are induced is given by other authors.

Ong and Gustafsson et al. [125] stress that N, APO, and AUTO all contribute to cell death in the reperfused heart. They reiterate that during ischemia N is the main component, due to long-lasting oxygen deprivation and ATP depletion. At reperfusion both APO and N are rapidly activated.

Park and Lucchesi [126] point out, in accordance with the findings of Gottlieb et al. [35], that N occurs only if R is initiated after 20 min of occlusion. They also stress the activation of the complement cascade, which triggers the already mentioned innate immunity, and the neutrophil/endothelium interaction as a major component of the inflammatory response.

Eltzsching and Eckle [127] stress the role of the innate immune responses, which represent a "sterile inflammation."

They further underline that I/R is not seen only during the course of an acute MI. The kidney, intestine, and brain undergo similar processes, while cardiac and vascular surgery creates similar conditions.

Additionally, multi-organ I/R injury may be seen in trauma, resuscitation after cardiac arrest, sickle cell disease, and sleep apnea.

In accordance with this, Whelan et al. [7] state that cyclophilin D, a major factor in APO, according to Crompton [12], is also involved in N. They additionally describe the role of necrostatin-1, which reduces infarct size after I/R through RIP1-RIP3 signaling.

Whelan et al. [5] also suggest that during occlusion AMPK is activated inhibiting the AUTO inhibitor mTOR; thus AUTO is induced. However at reperfusion Beclin-1-induced AUTO as already suggested by Matsui et al. [128] may be detrimental.

Again, the interplay between AUTO and APO in hypoxia has been described by Azad et al. [129] in cancer cells which underwent cell death hypoxia. This was reduced by AUTO but not with caspase inhibitors. This autophagic death was effected through a mechanism involving BNIP3.

Konstantinidis et al. [66] point out that many paradigms of pharmacologic or genetic manipulations of CD exist in the setting of MI. Thus, lack of Fas and Bax and Bak in mice results into smaller infarcts; the same is seen with Bcl-2 overexpression. The lack of cyclophilin D has the same effect. The protective role of cyclophilin D inhibition by cyclosporine A or sanglifehrin A has already been discussed.

7.17 Myocardial Remodeling

The development of post-MI CHF is linked to the emergence of myocardial remodeling (REM).

Mani and Kitsis [130] in an editorial cite animal and human studies in which APO is a main factor.

Sam et al. [131], studying the mouse heart, have very pertinently shown that at 6 months post-MI REM, APO can coexist with increased wall thickness in areas remote from the infarct.

APO is mainly expressed in the border zone surrounding the infarct, in the experimental animal [132], and in the human [133].

However, although the post-MI is the prime paradigm of REM and CHF in which APO is strongly involved, other causes have been noted. Thus, pacing-induced HF involves APO, i.e., caspase-3, AIF, and the nuclear-localized markers p53 and p21, according to Marin-Garcia et al. [134] who stress that:

In rapid atrial fibrillation induced for 3 weeks in the dog, an increase of APO TUNEL and molecular markers caspases-3 and 8, reduced Bcl-2 is seen at the atria.

APO can be seen in volume overload produced by an A-V shunt in rats, especially the males [135].

Pressure overload can also produce APO, in the spontaneous hypertensive rat and after aortic banding [136].

The antineoplastic drug doxorubicin significantly induces APO, characterized by caspase-3 activation [137].

7.18 The Aging Heart

In Fischer 344 rat hearts, Kajstura et al. [138] in the left ventricular free wall at 24 months found 13,600 myocytes undergoing N but only 874 cells undergoing APO. A combination of both processes involved 14,500 cells. Olivetti et al. [139] in 106 human hearts found that in aging men 64 M cells had been lost in both right (19 M) and left (45 M) sides. They did not differentiate between N and APO.

Galluzzi et al. [4] in their very recent reviews describe that cellular senescence cannot be considered as a form of regulated cell death.

Shirakobe et al. [140] describe that autophagy is decreased in the aging heart.

Myocarditis is an uncommon but significant cause of acute heart failure. Its main manifestation is the presence of necrotic myocytes. In the subacute phase, the myocardium is infiltrated by natural killer cells. TNFα and IL-1 B and IL-2 are produced. Cytotoxic T lymphocytes can lyse virus-infected cardiomyocytes [141].

Brunner et al. [142] have shown APO in virus-induced dilated cardiomyopathy in mice.

Apoptosis was also seen in pts with acute myocarditis [143]; interestingly pts with functional recovery had higher apoptosis rates than those without recovery and than normal hearts.

It is interesting that a vicious feedback cycle has been postulated in acute myocarditis, since cardiac myosin, liberated through an initial insult, can promote chronic immunity and chronic inflammation through TLRs [144].

As Whelan et al. [7] point out, autophagosomes are increased in this condition; however it cannot be determined whether this is compensatory or deleterious. This has already been discussed in the context of hemodynamic overload states.

Knaapen et al. [145] in cardiac tissue of pts with terminal CHF due to both ischemic and dilated cardiomyopathy have found autophagic cell death by granular cytoplasmic ubiquitin inclusions but no APO or N indications.

Park et al. [146] addressed the question: are cardiomyocytes the only heart cells involved in cardiac injury?

They point out that, by cell number, 75% of cells in the heart are nonmyocytes. In a primate model of chronic heart failure produced first by experimental MI and subsequently rapid pacing for 2–6 months, they found, as expected, an increase in APO with the emergence of HF. However, the TUNEL-positive nonmyocytes were eightfold higher than cardiomyocytes in the border zone and ninefold higher in the remote area.

7.19 Therapeutic Implications

This is the translational investigator's dream.

Whelan et al. [7] and Hotchkiss et al. [15] dedicate parts in their extensive reviews. The first group of authors [7] concentrates mostly on acute MI, which according to their postulation requires treatment for a limited period of time. They focus on the promise of small-molecule polycaspase inhibitors which reduce infarct size by 21–52% following I/R. In the already cited review by Whelan et al. [7], the following findings can be underlined: Bcl-2 overexpression, Bax ablation, and caspase inhibition reduce I/R injury, through APO reduction.

They also mention that Akt reduces infarct size. However, adenoviral transduction seems difficult to apply. On this subject of acute MI, excellent reviews have been written:

- The Working Group of Cellular Biology of the Heart of the European Society of Cardiology states that "there is currently no effective therapy for protecting the heart against the detrimental effects of acute I/R injury" [147].

The same group in 2017 arrives to similar conclusions [148].

Possibly the drug giving the greatest promise is cyclosporine A, which inhibits N by inhibiting MPTP [149]. This clinical beneficial result is supported by experimental data with cyclosporine A but also by sanglifehrin A, another powerful inhibitor by the MPTP. However, they were clinically disappointing as described in Chap. 6 on IRI. Hydrogen sulfide is a drug which in small doses may protect against I/R injury [150].

Necrostatin-1 which decreases N by inhibiting the activity of RIP1 may prove a promising agent [151].

It is interesting that a modality widely employed in the past therapeutics, glucose-insulin-potassium reduces APO in AMI by soluble Fas and sFas measurements [152].

7.20 Mechanisms of Conditioning and Cell Death

This very important cytoprotective mechanism, a universal phenomenon, decreases CD in all its three forms (N, APO, and AUTO).

A review is given in the Chap. 14 on conditioning and recently by Ovize et al. [153].

The major signaling pathways underlying cardioprotection are noted. The authors point out that "conditioning" (pre-, peri-, and post-) is effected by two endogenous cardioprotective pathways:

- RISK: Reperfusion injury salvage kinase.
- SAFE: Survival activating factor enhancement.

The former is exerted through MEK1/2-ERK1/2 and PI3K-Akt while the latter by the TNFα receptor and STAT3.

Both pathways relay these signals from cell membrane receptors to the MITO and MPTP opening inhibition [154].

7.20.1 Other Cardioprotective Interventions

Hypothermia has been tried against both myocardial and cerebral ischemia. It was found to ameliorate APO in rat hearts undergoing experimental transplantation [155].

In the human it is used to protect the brain during resuscitation after a cardiac arrest [156].

Exercise training can upregulate AUTO [157].

7.20.2 Pharmaceutic Interventions

Minocycline protects against hypoxia-ischemia reperfusion-induced APO: It inhibits MITO Ca^{2+} uptake [158].

Chen et al. [159] have shown that T3 treatment for 3 days in experimental MI in rats decreased border area APO through phosphorylation of Akt.

We have shown the same results with thyroid hormones but at 2 weeks after AMI in the rat [160].

Ferreyra et al. have shown the same in acute tubular necrosis induced by I/R in the rat kidney [161].

This approach is now being used in a multicenter European trial in post-infarct patients as described in the chapter on cardiac remodeling. However, the results are not uniform in all organs. Kumar et al. have found that it induces APO in the rat liver [162], while Sinha et al. [163] showed that thyroid hormone stimulates hepatic lipid catabolism via activation of autophagy.

Another promising drug is Bendavia which is an overall MITO protective agent: It has shown beneficial effect early post-MI in the dog [164]. Clinical results are not yet conclusive.

7.21 Chronic Treatment: Prevention of Remodeling

Although most efforts are directed at acute MI, the very important problem of REM characterized by cardiac enlargement and leading to CHF and death should not be underestimated. It is postulated that it occurs in 30% of anterior infarcts, despite primary angioplasty and the administration of the four main drugs, ACE inhibitors or angiotensin receptor blockers, aldosterone inhibitors, and β-blockers. Thus, a large number of drugs have been and are still being tried to prevent or reverse this process.

Gajarsa and Kloner gave a very pertinent review [165] (Table 7.2).

The authors describe extensively the benefits of β-blocker therapy, clarifying that β1 receptors induce hypertrophy and APO, while β2 receptor stimulation may be antiapoptotic, up to a year in the rat, but only with concominant β1 blockade. They also describe the beneficial anti-angiotensin-II and antialdosterone therapy. Both these substances induce APO and fibrosis.

The authors also describe attempts at MMP inhibition; the PREMIER [166] study in which a broad MMP inhibitor PG-116800 showed no effect in humans although it had been very efficacious experimentally. Thus, before further describing therapeutic attempts against post-MI REM and CHF, one must be reminded that in real life most of these patients already receive anti-adrenergic, anti-angiotensin, and anti-aldosterone treatment in their great majority.

Statins, although they possess anti-necrotic anti-inflammatory and anti-apoptotic qualities, have proven disappointing in HF trials as already described in Chap. 13 (REM).

Tousoulis et al. [167] describe the efforts at nitric oxide manipulation, with emphasis on sildenafil, an NO synthase transcription enhancer.

TNFα neutralization would be an obvious target. However, it was not successful in the RENEWAL and ATTACH trials [168, 169].

Another long-used drug, pentoxifylline, which modulates TNFα mRNA expression, has proven successful in a small trial [170].

Also, interleukin-1 blockade by anakinra prevented REM after MI, without evidence of impaired healing [171]. This family of drugs is being intensively studied.

The n-3 polyunsaturated fatty acids (PUFA) have been antiapoptotic in many studies; α-linolenic acid prevents APO in cardiomyopathic hamsters [172].

Kanamori et al. [173] found that resveratrol reverses REM in rat hearts with large, old myocardial infarctions through enhanced AUTO. Large clinical studies are lacking.

A drug which has been tried in patients with heart failure with preserved ejection fraction is relaxin. This agent decreases APO in the swine acute MI model while also decreasing N, and inflammation, and improving the cardiac index [174].

Valproic acid, a drug widely used in psychiatric treatment, has been shown to ameliorate post-MI REM in the rat, by HDAC inhibition [175].

MAO inhibitors have a strong MITO protective action and have been shown to exert anti-REM activity in pressure overload [176].

Table 7.2 Overview of therapeutic modalities for ventricular remodeling

	Therapeutic modality	Drug	Remodeling effects	Clinical effects	Evidence
Pharmacology therapy	Angiotensin-converting enzyme inhibitor	Captopril, enalapri1, trandolapril	↓ LV EDV ↓ LV EDS	↓ All-cause mortality	Randomized controlled trial (RCT); SAVE SOLVD TRACE
	Angiotensin II receptor blocker	Valsartan, candesartan	↓ LV EDV ↓ LV EDS	Mortality equivalent to ACE-I	RCT: VALIANT RESOLVD
	Direct renin inhibitor	Aliskiren	↓ Myocardial fibrosis in mice		
	Aldosterone inhibitor	Aldactone, eplerenone	↓ LV EDV ↓ LV EDS ∅ Change in ESV/EDV	↓ All-cause mortality	RCT: RALES EPHESUS
	Beta blocker	Metoprolol, Carvedilol	↓ LV EDV ↓ LV EDS	↓ All-cause mortality	RCT: CAPRICORN, MERIT-HF
Molecular/cellular therapy	Cell therapy	Bone marrow derived stem cells	↓ LV EDV ↓ LV EDS ↓ LV EF	↓ Death, re-infarction, re-vascularization	RCT: REPAIR AMI Non-randomized: BALANCE
	Matrix metalloproteinase inhibitor	(PG-116800)	∅ Effects		RCT: PREMIER
Device	Left ventricular assist device (LVAD)		↓ MMP expression ↓ Apoptosis ↑ Contractility		

Adapted by permission from Gajarsa and Kloner [165]

We have shown favorable results with rasagiline at 4 weeks post-MI in the rat [177].

Recently Unsöld et al. [178] have shown that melusin, a chaperone protein, improves post-MI remodeling.

Some other drugs to be considered are ranolazine which is emerging as an anti-ischemic drug. Erythropoietin has been very successful in the animal but has been disappointing in the human as already described.

This brings into focus the great variety of therapies available for therapy of post-MI REM. The review by Dorn [179] emphasizes that in ventricular REM all three modalities of CD are involved. Also it must be reminded that in the post-MI heart, three distinct zones have been delineated: the infarct, the border, and the remote zone. Each has distinct characteristics.

Thus the difficulty of managing post-MI REM can be readily appreciated, since treatments must be combined. Also, in the general spirit of this book, it must be stressed that pharmacological, interventional-surgical, device, and cell and gene therapy should not be considered exclusive but complementary.

7.22 MicroRNAs and Cell Death

MicroRNAs (miRs) are small (<22–23 nucleotides) noncoding RNA molecules. Skommer et al. [180] gave a detailed review in 2014.

They classify miRs as pro-apoptotic: miR17-92 cluster, miR-150, miR-320, miR-761, miR-195, miR-34α and anti-apoptotic: miR-133α, miR-21, miR-24, miR-30, miR-210, miR-199α, miR-149, miR-499, miR-145, miR-378.

Dong et al. [181] also give a detailed review (Table 7.3)

Tony et al. [182] describe that silencing of miR-208α attenuates doxorubicin-induced apoptosis. Wang et al. [183] found the same for 532–3p.

Skommer et al. [180] also describe that miR-30, miR-201, and miR-212/miR-132 reduce autophagy. Dong et al. [181] mention the role of many miRs in beneficial and harmful autophagy.

As regards necrosis, Skommer et al. [180] mention that only limited evidence exists; they state the same for necroptosis. Dong et al. [181] found that miR-155, miR-30b, and IncRNA-H19 are antinecrotic, while miR-874, miR-2861, and IncRNA-NRF promote necrosis, with crosstalk between the three types of death. The authors describe that in the future miR (ncRNA)-based therapy is still a hope.

IncRNAs are long (IncRNAs>200 nucleotides) and short (circ RNAs<200 nucleotides) noncoding RNAs. Data on their role on cell death are still limited.

Table 7.3 Summary of ncRNAs linked to apoptosis in CVDs

ncRNAs	Targets/CVDs	Pro- or antiapoptotic
miR-1	Bcl-2/ml	Promotes apoptosis
miR-133a	Caspase-9/MI	Inhibits apoptosis
miR-17-92 cluster	STAT3/MI, HF	Induces apoptosis
miR-21	Bcl-2/MI	Antiapoptotic
miR-30	P53/MI	Antiapoptotic
miR-199a	Hif1α, Sirt1/MI	Antiapoptotic
miR-320	Hsp20/MI	Proapoptotic
miR-149	Puma/MI	Decreases apoptosis
miR-761	Mff/MI	Promotes apoptosis
miR-499	Calcineurin/MI	Inhibits apoptosis
miR-214	Pten/MI	Antiapoptotic
miR-145	Bnip3/MI	Decreases apoptosis
miR-378	Caspase-3/MI	Antiapoptotic
miR-195	Sirt1/lipotoxic cardiomyopathy	Proapoptotic
miR-34a	Sirt1/coronary artery disease	Promotes apoptosis
miR-l84	Bcl-xL, Bcl-w/MI	Proapoptotic
iniR-140	Mfn1/MI	Induces apoptosis
miR-421	Pink1/MI	Promotes apoptosis
miR-324-5p	Mtfr1/MI	Antiapoptotic
miR-361	Phb1/MI	Proapoptotic
miR-20Ka	GATA4/DOX cardiotoxicity	Promotes apoptosis
miR-532-3p	ARC/DOX cardiotoxicity	Proapoptotic
LncRNA-CARL	miR-539, Phb2/MI	Inhibits apoptosis
CircRNA-HRCR	miR-223, arc/cardiac hypertrophy	Antiapoptotic

Reprinted with adaptation by permission from Dong et al. [181]

In conclusion, it is obvious that supplemental technologies incrementally used in CD prevention and reversal are expected to be incrementally important for the human. However, the continued importance of basic research findings is obvious.

Cell death plays a major role in cardiac development, homeostasis, and disease. There has been a gradual realization that the three main recognized modalities, necrosis, apoptosis, and autophagy, cannot be described as completely distinct entities, but some intermediate forms and significant cross talk have been recognized. Therapeutic approaches are constantly emerging. Indeed Gonzalez et al. in 2011 [184] had already shown that the three modalities of cell death share many common characteristics and represent an intensity of effect continuum (Fig. 7.2). Cell death constitutes a major component of ischemia/reperfusion injury and cardiac remodeling and a main target of cardiac conditioning.

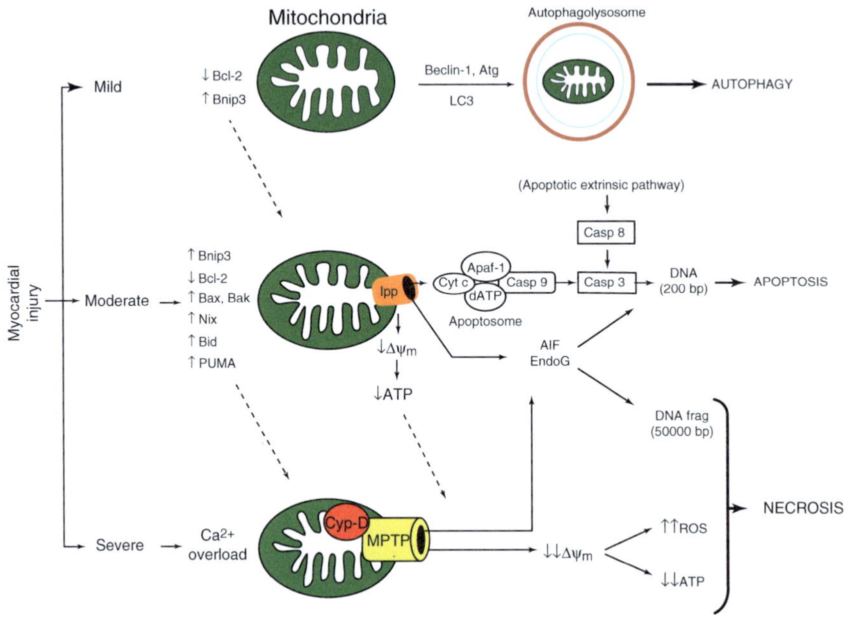

Fig. 7.2 Mechanisms and potential relationships among autophagy, apoptotic, and necrotic pathways. AIF, apoptosis-inducing factor; Apaf, apoptotic protease-activating factor; Atg, autophagy-related genes; ATP, adenosine triphosphate; Casp, caspase; Cyp D, cyclophilin D; Cyt c, cytochrome c; dATP, deoxyadenosine triphosphate; DNA, deoxyribonucleic acid; EndoG, endonuclease G; frag, fragmentation; Ipp, ion-permeable pore; MPTP, mitochondrial membrane transition pore; PUMA, p53 upregulated modulator of apoptosis; ROS, reactive oxygen species; ΔΨm, inner mitochondrial membrane potential. (Reproduced by permission from Gonzalez et al. [184])

References

1. Marín-García J. Cell death in the pathogenesis and progression of heart failure. Heart Fail Rev. 2016;21:117–21.
2. Galluzzi L, Maiuri MC, Vitale I, Zischka H, Castedo M, Zitvogel L, et al. Cell death modalities: classification and pathophysiological implications. Cell Death Differ. 2007;14:1237–43.
3. Kroemer G, Galluzzi L, Vandenabeele P, Abrams J, Alnemri ES, Baehrecke EH, et al. Classification of cell death: recommendations of the Nomenclature Committee on Cell Death 2009. Cell Death Differ. 2009;16:3–11.
4. Galluzzi L, Vitale I, Aaronson SA, Abrams JM, Adam D, Agostinis P, et al. Molecular mechanisms of cell death: recommendations of the Nomenclature Committee on Cell Death 2018. Cell Death Differ. 2018;25:486–541.
5. Fuchs Y, Steller H. Programmed cell death in animal development and disease. Cell. 2011;147:742–58.
6. Galluzzi L, Bravo-San Pedro JM, Kepp O, Kroemer G. Regulated cell death and adaptive stress responses. Cell Mol Life Sci. 2016;73:2405–10.
7. Whelan RS, Kaplinskiy V, Kitsis RN. Cell death in the pathogenesis of heart disease: mechanisms and significance. Annu Rev Physiol. 2010;72:19–44.

8. Majno G, Joris I. Apoptosis, oncosis, and necrosis. An overview of cell death. Am J Pathol. 1995;146:3–15.
9. Kostin S. Pathways of myocyte death: implications for development of clinical laboratory biomarkers. Adv Clin Chem. 2005;40:37–98.
10. Baines CP. The mitochondrial permeability transition pore and ischemia-reperfusion injury. Basic Res Cardiol. 2009;104:181–8.
11. Galluzzi L, Kepp O, Kroemer G. Mitochondrial regulation of cell death: a phylogenetically conserved control. Microb Cell. 2016;3:101–8.
12. Crompton M. Mitochondrial intermembrane junctional complexes and their role in cell death. J Physiol. 2000;529:11–21.
13. Dhanasekaran DN, Reddy EP. JNK signaling in apoptosis. Oncogene. 2008;27:6245–51.
14. Lemasters JJ, Theruvath TP, Zhong Z, Nieminen AL. Mitochondrial calcium and the permeability transition in cell death. Biochim Biophys Acta. 1787;2009:1395–401.
15. Hotchkiss RS, Strasser A, McDunn JE, Swanson PE. Cell death in disease. Mechanisms and emerging therapeutic concepts. N Engl J Med. 2009;361:1570–83.
16. Weiss JN, Korge P, Honda HM, Ping P. Role of the mitochondrial permeability transition in myocardial disease. Circ Res. 2003;93:292–301.
17. Pan X, Liu J, Nguyen T, Liu C, Sun J, Teng Y, et al. The physiological role of mitochondrial calcium revealed by mice lacking the mitochondrial calcium uniporter. Nature Cell Biol. 2013;15:1464–72. https://doi.org/10.1038/incb2868.
18. Susin SA, Lorenzo HK, Zamzami N, Marzo I, Snow BE, Brothers GM, et al. Molecular characterization of mitochondrial apoptosis-inducing factor. Nature. 1999;397:441–6.
19. Yang WS, Stockwell BR. Ferroptosis: death by lipid peroxidation. Trends Cell Biol. 2016;26:165–76.
20. Stockwell BR, Friedmann Angeli JP, Bayir H, Bush AI, Conrad M, Dixon SJ, et al. Ferroptosis: a regulated cell death nexus linking metabolism, redox biology, and disease. Cell. 2017;171:273–85.
21. Dixon SJ, Stockwell BR. The role of iron and reactive oxygen species in cell death. Nat Chem Biol. 2014;10:9–17.
22. Jorgensen I, Miao EA. Pyroptotic cell death defends against intracellular pathogens. Immunol Rev. 2015;265:130–42.
23. Cookson BT, Brennan MA. Pro-inflammatory programmed cell death. Trends Microbiol. 2001;9:113–4.
24. Shi J, Gao W, Shao F. Pyroptosis: gasdermin-mediated programmed necrotic cell death. Trends Biochem Sci. 2017;42:245–54.
25. Brough D, Rothwell NJ. Caspase-1-dependent processing of pro-interleukin-1beta is cytosolic and precedes cell death. J Cell Sci. 2007;120:772–81.
26. Franchi L, Eigenbrod T, Muñoz-Planillo R, Nuñez G. The inflammasome: a caspase-1-activation platform that regulates immune responses and disease pathogenesis. Nat Immunol. 2009;10:241–7.
27. Yang J, Zhao Y, Shao F. Non-canonical activation of inflammatory caspases by cytosolic LPS in innate immunity. Curr Opin Immunol. 2015;32:78–83.
28. Fatokun AA, Dawson VL, Dawson TM. Parthanatos: mitochondrial-linked mechanisms and therapeutic opportunities. Br J Pharmacol. 2014;171:2000–16.
29. David KK, Andrabi SA, Dawson TM, Dawson VL. Parthanatos, a messenger of death. Front Biosci (Landmark Ed). 2009;14:1116–28.
30. Overholtzer M, Mailleux AA, Mouneimne G, Normand G, Schnitt SJ, King RW, et al. A nonapoptotic cell death process, entosis, that occurs by cell-in-cell invasion. Cell. 2007;131:966–79.
31. Sun Q, Luo T, Ren Y, Florey O, Shirasawa S, Sasazuki T, et al. Competition between human cells by entosis. Cell Res. 2014;24:1299–310.
32. Clark SR, Ma AC, Tavener SA, McDonald B, Goodarzi Z, Kelly MM, et al. Platelet TLR4 activates neutrophil extracellular traps to ensnare bacteria in septic blood. Nat Med. 2007;13:463–9.

33. Feuerstein G, Ruffolo RR Jr, Yue TL. Apoptosis and congestive heart failure. Trends Cardiovasc Med. 1997;7:249–55.
34. Nishimura Y, Lemasters JJ. Glycine blocks opening of a death channel in cultured hepatic sinusoidal endothelial cells during chemical hypoxia. Cell Death Differ. 2001;8:850–8.
35. Gottlieb RA, Burleson KO, Kloner RA, Babior BM, Engler RL. Reperfusion injury induces apoptosis in rabbit cardiomyocytes. J Clin Invest. 1994;94:1621–18.
36. Garcia-Dorado D, Ruiz-Meana M, Inserte J, Rodriguez-Sinovas A, Piper HM. Calcium-mediated cell death during myocardial reperfusion. Cardiovasc Res. 2012;94:168–80.
37. Zong WX, Thompson CB. Necrotic death as a cell fate. Genes Dev. 2006;20:1–15.
38. Luke CJ, Pak SC, Askew YS, Naviglia TL, Askew DJ, Nobar SM, et al. An intracellular serpin regulates necrosis by inhibiting the induction and sequelae of lysosomal injury. Cell. 2007;130:1108–19.
39. Laster SM, Wood JG, Gooding LR. Tumor necrosis factor can induce both apoptic and necrotic forms of cell lysis. J Immunol. 1988;141:2629–34.
40. Syntichaki P, Xu K, Driscoll M, Tavernarakis N. Specific aspartyl and calpain proteases are required for neurodegeneration in C. elegans. Nature. 2002;419:939–44.
41. Kajstura J, Cheng W, Reiss K, Clark WA, Sonnenblick EH, Krajewski S, et al. Apoptotic and necrotic myocyte cell deaths are independent contributing variables of infarct size in rats. Lab Investig. 1996;74:86–107.
42. Clarke PG. Developmental cell death: morphological diversity and multiple mechanisms. Anat Embryol (Berl). 1990;181:195–213.
43. Pedrozo Z, Torrealba N, Fernández C, Gatica D, Toro B, Quiroga C, et al. Cardiomyocyte ryanodine receptor degradation by chaperone-mediated autophagy. Cardiovasc Res. 2013;98:277–85.
44. Lavandero S, Chiong M, Rothermel BA, Hill JA. Autophagy in cardiovascular biology. J Clin Invest. 2015;125:55–64.
45. Glick D, Barth S, Macleod KF. Autophagy: cellular and molecular mechanisms. J Pathol. 2010;221:3–12.
46. Wang ZV, Ferdous A, Hill JA. Cardiomyocyte autophagy: metabolic profit and loss. Heart Fail Rev. 2013;18:585–94.
47. Dhesi P, Tehrani F, Fuess T, Schwarz ER. How does the heart (not) die? The role of autophagy in cardiomyocyte homeostasis and cell death. Heart Fail. 2015;15:15–21.
48. Gottlieb RA, Mentzer RM Jr. Autophagy: an affair of the heart. Heart Fail Rev. 2013;18:575–84.
49. Tannous P, Zhu H, Johnstone JL, Shelton JM, Rajasekaran NS, Benjamin IJ, et al. Autophagy is an adaptive response in desmin-related cardiomyopathy. Proc Natl Acad Sci U S A. 2008;105:9745–50.
50. Maloyan A, Sayegh J, Osinska H, Chua BH, Robbins J. Manipulation of death pathways in desmin-related cardiomyopathy. Circ Res. 2010;106:1524–32.
51. Zhu WZ, Wang SQ, Chakir K, Yang D, Zhang T, Brown JH, et al. Linkage of beta1-adrenergic stimulation to apoptotic heart cell death through protein kinase A-independent activation of Ca^{2+}/calmodulin kinase II. J Clin Invest. 2003;111:617–25.
52. Ferdous A, Battiprolu PK, Ni YG, Rothermel BA, Hill JA. FoxO, autophagy, and cardiac remodeling. J Cardiovasc Transl Res. 2010;3:355–64.
53. Cao DJ, Jiang N, Blagg A, Johnstone JL, Gondalia R, Oh M, et al. Mechanical unloading activates FoxO3 to trigger Bnip3-dependent cardiomyocyte atrophy. J Am Heart Assoc. 2013;2(2):e000016. https://doi.org/10.1161/JAHA.113.000016.
54. Zhang J, Ney PA. Role of BNIP3 and NIX in cell death, autophagy, and mitophagy. Cell Death Differ. 2009;16:939–46.
55. Feng CC, Lin CC, Lai YP, Chen TS, Marthandam Asokan S, Lin JY, et al. Hypoxia suppresses myocardial survival pathway through HIF-1α-IGFBP-3-dependent signaling and enhances cardiomyocyte autophagic and apoptotic effects mainly via FoxO3a-induced BNIP3 expression. Growth Factors. 2016;34:73–86.

56. Liu C, Xue R, Wu D, Wu L, Chen C, Tan W, et al. REDD1 attenuates cardiac hypertrophy via enhancing autophagy. Biochem Biophys Res Commun. 2014;454:215–20.
57. Jin HO, Hong SE, Kim JH, Choi HN, Kim K, An S, et al. Sustained overexpression of Redd1 leads to Akt activation involved in cell survival. Cancer Lett. 2013;336:319–24.
58. Aits S, Jäättelä M. Lysosomal cell death at a glance. J Cell Sci. 2013;126:1905–12.
59. Plotegher N, Duchen MR. Mitochondrial dysfunction and neurodegeneration in lysosomal storage disorders. Trends Mol Med. 2017;23:116–34.
60. Kurz T, Terman A, Gustafsson B, Brunk UT. Lysosomes and oxidative stress in aging and apoptosis. Biochim Biophys Acta. 1780;2008:1291–303.
61. Yamashima T. Hsp70.1 and related lysosomal factors for necrotic neuronal death. J Neurochem. 2012;120:477–94.
62. Zhao M, Antunes F, Eaton JW, Brunk UT. Lysosomal enzymes promote mitochondrial oxidant production, cytochrome c release and apoptosis. Eur J Biochem. 2003;270:3778–86.
63. Yuan XM, Li W, Dalen H, Lotem J, Kama R, Sachs L, et al. Lysosomal destabilization in p53-induced apoptosis. Proc Natl Acad Sci U S A. 2002;99:6286–91.
64. Schuler M, Green DR. Mechanisms of p53 dependent apoptosis. Biochem Soc Trans. 2001;29:684–8.
65. Kung G, Konstantinidis K, Kitsis RN. Programmed necrosis, not apoptosis, in the heart. Circ Res. 2011;108:1017–36.
66. Konstantinidis K, Whelan RS, Kitsis RN. Mechanisms of cell death in heart disease. Arterioscler Thromb Vasc Biol. 2012;32:1552–62.
67. Proskuryakov SY, Konoplyannikov AG, Gabai VL. Necrosis: a specific form of programmed cell death? Exp Cell Res. 2003;283:1–16.
68. Linkermann A, Green DR. Necroptosis. N Engl J Med. 2014;370:455–65.
69. Karch J, Molkentin JD. Regulated necrotic cell death: the passive aggressive side of Bax and Bak. Circ Res. 2015;116:1800–9.
70. Nikoletopoulou V, Markaki M, Palikaras K, Tavernarakis N. Crosstalk between apoptosis, necrosis and autophagy. Biochim Biophys Acta. 1833;2013:3448–59.
71. Skulachev VP. Bioenergetic aspects of apoptosis, necrosis and mitoptosis. Apoptosis. 2006;11:473–85.
72. Micheau O, Tschopp J. Induction of TNF receptor I-mediated apoptosis via two sequential signaling complexes. Cell. 2003;114:181–90.
73. Xia P, Liu Y, Cheng Z. Signaling pathways in cardiac myocyte apoptosis. Biomed Res Int. 2016;2016:9583268.
74. Galluzzi L, Bravo-San Pedro JM, Vitale I, Aaronson SA, Abrams JM, Adam D, et al. Essential versus accessory aspects of cell death: recommendations of the NCCD 2015. Cell Death Differ. 2015;22:58–73.
75. Copetti T, Bertoli C, Dalla E, Demarchi F, Schneider C. p65/RelA modulates BECN1 transcription and autophagy. Mol Cell Biol. 2009;29:2594–608.
76. Vanden Berghe T, Linkermann A, Jouan-Lanhouet S, Walczak H, Vandenabeele P. Regulated necrosis: the expanding network of non-apoptotic cell death pathways. Nat Rev Mol Cell Biol. 2014;15:135–47.
77. Levin S, Bucci TJ, Cohen SM, Fix AS, Hardisty JF, LeGrand EK, et al. The nomenclature of cell death: recommendations of an ad hoc Committee of the Society of Toxicologic Pathologists. Toxicol Pathol. 1999;27:484–90.
78. Takemura G, Maruyama R, Goto K, Kanamori H, Tsujimoto A, Minatoguchi S, et al. Fate of isolated adult cardiomyocytes undergoing starvation-induced autophagic degeneration. Autophagy. 2009;5:90–2.
79. Kostin S. Types of cardiomyocyte death and clinical outcomes in patients with heart failure. J Am Coll Cardiol. 2011;57:1532–4.
80. Vigliano CA, Cabeza Meckert PM, Diez M, Favaloro LE, Cortés C, Fazzi L, et al. Cardiomyocyte hypertrophy, oncosis, and autophagic vacuolization predict mortality in idiopathic dilated cardiomyopathy with advanced heart failure. J Am Coll Cardiol. 2011;57:1523–31.

81. Piek A, de Boer RA, Silljé HH. The fibrosis-cell death axis in heart failure. Heart Fail Rev. 2016;21:199–211.
82. Zeisberg EM, Tarnavski O, Zeisberg M, Dorfman AL, McMullen JR, Gustafsson E, et al. Endothelial-to-mesenchymal transition contributes to cardiac fibrosis. Nat Med. 2007;13:952–61.
83. Chaanine AH, Jeong D, Liang L, Chemaly ER, Fish K, Gordon RE, et al. JNK modulates FOXO3a for the expression of the mitochondrial death and mitophagy marker BNIP3 in pathological hypertrophy and in heart failure. Cell Death Dis. 2012;3:265.
84. Nagoshi T, Matsui T, Aoyama T, Leri A, Anversa P, Li L, et al. PI3K rescues the detrimental effects of chronic Akt activation in the heart during ischemia/reperfusion injury. J Clin Invest. 2005;115:2128–38.
85. Schwartzbauer G, Robbins J. The tumor suppressor gene PTEN can regulate cardiac hypertrophy and survival. J Biol Chem. 2001;276:35786–93.
86. Muraski JA, Rota M, Misao Y, Fransioli J, Cottage C, Gude N, et al. Pim-1 regulates cardiomyocyte survival downstream of Akt. Nat Med. 2007;13:1467–75.
87. Liu J, Mao W, Ding B, Liang CS. ERKs/p53 signal transduction pathway is involved in doxorubicin-induced apoptosis in H9c2 cells and cardiomyocytes. Am J Physiol Heart Circ Physiol. 2008;295(5):H1956–65.
88. Shao Z, Bhattacharya K, Hsich E, Park L, Walters B, Germann U, et al. c-Jun N-terminal kinases mediate reactivation of Akt and cardiomyocyte survival after hypoxic injury in vitro and in vivo. Circ Res. 2006;98:111–8.
89. Saurin AT, Martin JL, Heads RJ, Foley C, Mockridge JW, Wright MJ, et al. The role of differential activation of p38-mitogen-activated protein kinase in preconditioned ventricular myocytes. FASEB J. 2000;14:2237–46.
90. Kasahara T, Koguchi E, Funakoshi M, Aizu-Yokota E, Sonoda Y. Antiapoptotic action of focal adhesion kinase (FAK) against ionizing radiation. Antioxid Redox Signal. 2004;4:3. https://doi.org/10.1089/15230860260196290.
91. Sedgerab LM, McDermott MF. TNF and TNF-receptors: from mediators of cell death and inflammation to therapeutic giants – past, present and future. Elsevier. 2014;25:453–72.
92. Hamid T, Guo SZ, Kingery JR, Xiang X, Dawn B, Prabhu SD. Cardiomyocyte NF-κB p65 promotes adverse remodelling, apoptosis, and endoplasmic reticulum stress in heart failure. Cardiovasc Res. 2011;89:129–38.
93. Maier HJ, Schips TG, Wietelmann A, Krüger M, Brunner C, Sauter M, et al. Cardiomyocyte-specific IκB kinase (IKK)/NF-κB activation induces reversible inflammatory cardiomyopathy and heart failure. Proc Natl Acad Sci U S A. 2012;109:11794–9.
94. Shin SY, Kim T, Lee HS, Kang JH, Lee JY, Cho KH, et al. The switching role of β-adrenergic receptor signalling in cell survival or death decision of cardiomyocytes. Nat Commun. 2014;5:5777.
95. Niu X, Watts VL, Cingolani OH, Sivakumaran V, Leyton-Mange JS, Ellis CL, et al. Cardioprotective effect of beta-3 adrenergic receptor agonism: role of neuronal nitric oxide synthase. J Am Coll Cardiol. 2012;59:1979–87.
96. O'Connell TD, Jensen BC, Baker AJ, Simpson PC. Cardiac alpha1-adrenergic receptors: novel aspects of expression, signaling mechanisms, physiologic function, and clinical importance. Pharmacol Rev. 2013;66:308–33.
97. Klainguti M, Aigner S, Kilo J, Eppenberger HM, Mandinova A, Aebi U, et al. Lack of nuclear apoptosis in cardiomyocytes and increased endothelin-1 levels in a rat heart model of myocardial stunning. Basic Res Cardiol. 2000;95:308–15.
98. Kajstura J, Cigola E, Malhotra A, Li P, Cheng W, Meggs LG, et al. Angiotensin II induces apoptosis of adult ventricular myocytes in vitro. J Mol Cell Cardiol. 1997;29:859–70.
99. Germack R, Griffin M, Dickenson JM. Activation of protein kinase B by adenosine A1 and A3 receptors in newborn rat cardiomyocytes. J Mol Cell Cardiol. 2004;37:989–99.
100. Germack R, Dickenson JM. Adenosine triggers preconditioning through MEK/ERK1/2 signalling pathway during hypoxia/reoxygenation in neonatal rat cardiomyocytes. J Mol Cell Cardiol. 2005;39:429–42.

101. Liu Q, Chen X, Macdonnell SM, Kranias EG, Lorenz JN, Leitges M, et al. Protein kinase C{alpha}, but not PKC{beta} or PKC{gamma}, regulates contractility and heart failure susceptibility: implications for ruboxistaurin as a novel therapeutic approach. Circ Res. 2009;105:194–200.
102. Little GH, Saw A, Bai Y, Dow J, Marjoram P, Simkhovich B, et al. Critical role of nuclear calcium/calmodulin-dependent protein kinase IIdeltaB in cardiomyocyte survival in cardiomyopathy. J Biol Chem. 2009;284:24857–68.
103. Zhu W, Woo AY, Yang D, Cheng H, Crow MT, Xiao RP. Activation of CaMKIIdeltaC is a common intermediate of diverse death stimuli-induced heart muscle cell apoptosis. J Biol Chem. 2007;282:10833–9.
104. MacDonnell SM, Weisser-Thomas J, Kubo H, Hanscome M, Liu Q, Jaleel N, et al. CaMKII negatively regulates calcineurin-NFAT signaling in cardiac myocytes. Circ Res. 2009;105:316–25.
105. Zhivotovsky B, Orrenius S. Calcium and cell death mechanisms: a perspective from the cell death community. Cell Calcium. 2014;50:211–21.
106. Hajnóczky G, Davies E, Madesh M. Calcium signaling and apoptosis. Biochem Biophys Res Commun. 2003;304:445–54.
107. Vafiadaki E, Arvanitis DA, Pagakis SN, Papalouka V, Sanoudou D, Kontrogianni-Konstantopoulos A, et al. The anti-apoptotic protein HAX-1 interacts with SERCA2 and regulates its protein levels to promote cell survival. Mol Biol Cell. 2009;20:306–18.
108. Zhao W, Waggoner JR, Zhang ZG, Lam CK, Han P, Qian J, et al. The anti-apoptotic protein HAX-1 is a regulator of cardiac function. Proc Natl Acad Sci U S A. 2009;106:20776–81.
109. Cokkinos DV. Mechanisms and modalities of cell death in translational cardiovascular research. Cham: Springer; 2015. p. 253–78.
110. Timmers L, Paster Kamp G, de Hoog VC, Arslan F, Appleman Y, de Kleijn DPV. The innate immune response in reperfused myocardium. Cardiovasc Res. 2012;94:276–83.
111. Oka T, Hikoso S, Yamaguchi O, Taneike M, Takeda T, Tamai T, et al. Mitochondrial DNA that escapes from autophagy causes inflammation and heart failure. Nature. 2012;485:251–5. https://doi.org/10.1038/nature10992.
112. Christia P, Frangogiannis NG. Targeting inflammatory pathways in myocardial infarction. Eur J Clin Investig. 2013;43:986–95.
113. Abraham E, Arcaroli J, Carmody A, Wang H, Tracey KJ. HMG-1 as a mediator of acute lung inflammation. J Immunol. 2000;165:2950–4.
114. Obeid M, Tesniere A, Ghiringhelli F, Fimia GM, Apetoh L, Perfettini JL, et al. Calreticulin exposure dictates the immunogenicity of cancer cell death. Nat Med. 2007;13:54–61.
115. Elliott MR, Chekeni FB, Trampont PC, Lazarowski ER, Kadl A, Walk SF, et al. Nucleotides released by apoptotic cells act as a find-me signal to promote phagocytic clearance. Nature. 2009;461:282–6.
116. Scaffidi P, Misteli T, Bianchi ME. Release of chromatin protein HMGB1 by necrotic cells triggers inflammation. Nature. 2002;418:191–5.
117. Sistigu A, Yamazaki T, Vacchelli E, Chaba K, Enot DP, Adam J, et al. Cancer cell-autonomous contribution of type I interferon signaling to the efficacy of chemotherapy. Nat Med. 2014;20:1301–9.
118. Chiba S, Baghdadi M, Akiba H, Yoshiyama H, Kinoshita I, Dosaka-Akita H, et al. Tumor-infiltrating DCs suppress nucleic acid-mediated innate immune responses through interactions between the receptor TIM-3 and the alarmin HMGB1. Nat Immunol. 2012;13:832–42.
119. Vacchelli E, Ma Y, Baracco EE, Sistigu A, Enot DP, Pietrocola F, et al. Chemotherapy-induced antitumor immunity requires formyl peptide receptor 1. Science. 2015;350:972–8.
120. Aachoui Y, Sagulenko V, Miao EA, Stacey KJ. Inflammasome-mediated pyroptotic and apoptotic cell death, and defense against infection. Curr Opin Microbiol. 2013;16:319–26.
121. Yellon DM, Hausenloy DJ. Myocardial reperfusion injury. N Engl J Med. 2007;357:1121–35.
122. Dutta P, Courties G, Wei Y, Leuschner F, Gorgatov R, Robbins C, et al. Myocardial infarction accelerates atherosclerosis. Nature. 2012;487:325–9.

123. Nicolaou P, Rodriguez P, Ren X, Zhou X, Qian J, Sadayappan S, et al. Inducible expression of active protein phosphatase-1 inhibitor-1 enhances basal cardiac function and protects against ischemia/reperfusion injury. Circ Res. 2009;104:1012–20.
124. Murphy E, Steenbergen C. Mechanisms underlying acute protection from cardiac ischemia-reperfusion injury. Physiol Rev. 2008;88:581–609.
125. Ong SB, Gustafsson AB. New roles for mitochondria in cell death in the reperfused myocardium. Cardiovasc Res. 2012;94:190–6.
126. Park JL, Lucchesi BR. Mechanisms of myocardial reperfusion injury. Ann Thorac Surg. 1999;68:1905–2012.
127. Eltzsching HK, Eckle T. Ischemia and reperfusion from mechanism to translation. Nature Med. 2011;17:1393–401.
128. Matsui Y, Takagi H, Qu X, Abdellatif M, Sakoda H, Asano T, et al. Distinct roles of autophagy in the heart during ischemia and reperfusion: roles of AMP-activated protein kinase and Beclin 1 in mediating autophagy. Circ Res. 2007;100:914–22.
129. Azad MB, Chen Y, Henson ES, Cizeau J, McMillan-Ward E, Israels SJ, et al. Hypoxia induces autophagic cell death in apoptosis-competent cells through a mechanism involving BNIP3. Autophagy. 2008;4:195–204.
130. Mani K, Kitsis RN. Myocyte apoptosis: programming ventricular remodelling. J Am Coll Cardiol. 2003;41:761–4.
131. Sam F, Sawyer DB, Chang DL, Eberli FR, Ngoy S, Jain M, et al. Progressive left ventricular remodeling and apoptosis late after myocardial infarction in mouse heart. Am J Physiol Heart Circ Physiol. 2000;279:H422–8.
132. Palojoki E, Saraste A, Eriksson A, Pulkki K, Kallajoki M, Voipio-Pulkki LM, et al. Cardiomyocyte apoptosis and ventricular remodeling after myocardial infarction in rats. Am J Phys. 2001;280:H2726–31.
133. Abbate A, Biondi-Zoccai GG, Baldi A. Pathophysiologic role of myocardial apoptosis in post-infarction left ventricular remodeling. J Cell Physiol. 2002;193:145–53.
134. Marín-García J, Goldenthal MJ, Damle S, Pi Y, Moe GW. Regional distribution of mitochondrial dysfunction and apoptotic remodeling in pacing-induced heart failure. J Card Fail. 2009;15:700–8.
135. Dent MR, Tappia PS, Dhalla NS. Gender differences in apoptotic signaling in heart failure due to volume overload. Apoptosis. 2010;15:499–510.
136. Sun M, Chen M, Dawood F, Zurawska U, Li JY, Parker T, et al. Tumor necrosis factor-alpha mediates cardiac remodeling and ventricular dysfunction after pressure overload state. Circulation. 2007;115:1398–407.
137. Ueno M, Kakinuma Y, Yuhki K, Murakoshi N, Iemitsu M, Miyauchi T, Yamaguchi I. Doxorubicin induces apoptosis by activation of caspase-3 in cultured cardiomyocytes in vitro and rat cardiac ventricles in vivo. J Pharmacol Sci. 2006;101:151–8.
138. Kajstura J, Cheng W, Sarangarajan R, Li P, Li B, Nitahara JA, et al. Necrotic and apoptotic myocyte cell death in the aging heart of Fischer 344 rats. Am J Phys. 1996;271:H1215–28.
139. Olivetti G, Giordano G, Corradi D, Melissari M, Lagrasta C, Gambert SR, et al. Gender differences and aging: effects on the human heart. J Am Coll Cardiol. 1995;26:1068–79.
140. Shirakabe A, Ikeda Y, Sciarretta S, Zablocki DK, Sadoshima J. Aging and autophagy in the heart. Circ Res. 2016;118:1563–76.
141. Kawai C, Matsumori A. Dilated cardiomyopathy update: infectious-immune theory revisited. Heart Fail Rev. 2013;18:703–14.
142. Brunner S, Theiss HD, Leiss M, Grabmaier U, Grabmeier J, Huber B, et al. Enhanced stem cell migration mediated by VCAM-1/VLA-4 interaction improves cardiac function in virus-induced dilated cardiomyopathy. Basic Res Cardiol. 2013;108:388.
143. Abbate A, Sinagra G, Bussani R, Hoke NN, Merlo M, Varma A, et al. Apoptosis in patients with acute myocarditis. Am J Cardiol. 2009;104:995–1000.
144. Zhang P, Cox CJ, Alvarez KM, Cunningham MW. Cutting edge: cardiac myosin activates innate immune responses through. TLRs J Immunol. 2009;183:27–31.

145. Knaapen MW, Davies MJ, De Bie M, Haven AJ, Martinet W, Kockx MM. Apoptotic versus autophagic cell death in heart failure. Cardiovasc Res. 2001;51:304–12.
146. Park M, Shen YT, Gaussin V, Heyndrickx GR, Bartunek J, Resuello RR, et al. Apoptosis predominates in nonmyocytes in heart failure. Am J Phys. 2009;297:H785–91.
147. Hausenloy DJ, Bøtker HE, Condorelli G, Ferdimandly P, Grurcia-Dorado D, Heusch G, et al. Translating cardioprotection for patient benefit: position paper from the Working Group of Cellular Biology of the Heart of the European Society of Cardiology. Cardiovasc Res. 2013;98:7–22.
148. Hausenloy DJ, Garcia-Dorado D, Bøtker HE, Davidson SM, Downey J, Engel FB, et al. Novel targets and future strategies for acute cardioprotection: Position Paper of the European Society of Cardiology Working Group on Cellular Biology of the Heart. Cardiovasc Res. 2017;113:564–85.
149. Piot C, Croisille P, Staat P, Thibault H, Rioufol G, Mewton N, et al. Effect of cyclosporine on reperfusion injury in acute myocardial infarction. N Engl J Med. 2008;359:473–81.
150. Soha NR, Clement RT, Feng J, Liu Y, Bianchi C, Horvath EM, et al. The effects therapeutic sulfide on myocardial apoptosis in response to ischemia-reperfusion injury. Eur J Cardiothorac Surg. 2008;33:906–13.
151. Smith CC, Davidson SM, Lim SY, Simkin JC, Hothersall JS, Yellon DM. Necrostatin: a potential novel cardioprotective agent? Cardiovasc Drugs Ther. 2007;21:227–3.
152. Zhang L, Zhang L, Li YH, Zhang HY, Chen ML, Gao MM, et al. High-dose glucose-insulin-potassium treatment reduces myocardial apoptosis in patients with acute myocardial infarction. Eur J Clin Investig. 2005;35:164–70.
153. Ovize M, Thibault H, Przyklenk K. Myocardial conditioning: opportunities for clinical translation. Circ Res. 2013;113:439–50.
154. Yellon DM, Downey JM. Preconditioning the myocardium: from cellular physiology to clinical cardiology. Physiol Rev. 2003;83:1113–51.
155. Al-Amran FG. Apoptosis amelioration through hypothermic reperfusion in heart transplant. J Pharmacol Pharmacother. 2013;4:275–80.
156. Ramani R. Hypothermia for brain protection and resuscitation. Curr Opin Anaesthesiol. 2006;19:487–91.
157. Fiuza-Luces C, Delmiro A, Soares-Miranda L, González-Murillo A, Martínez-Palacios J, Ramírez M. Exercise training can induce cardiac autophagy at end-stage chronic conditions: insights from a graft-versus-host-disease mouse model. Brain Behav Immun. 2013;pii:S0889–1591(13)00538-2. https://doi.org/10.1016/j.bbi.2013.11.007.
158. Tao R, Kim SH, Honbo N, Karliner JS, Alano CC. Minocycline protects cardiac myocytes against simulated ischemia–reperfusion injury by inhibiting poly (ADP-ribose) polymerase-1. J Cardiovasc Pharmacol. 2010;56:659–68.
159. Chen YF, Kobayashi S, Chen J, Redetzke RA, Said S, Liang Q, et al. Short term triiodo-L-thyronine treatment inhibits cardiac myocyte apoptosis in border area after myocardial infarction in rats. J Mol Cell Cardiol. 2008;44:180–7.
160. Pantos C, Mourouzis I, Saranteas T, Clavé G, Ligeret H, Noack-Fraissignes P, et al. Thyroid hormone improves postischaemic recovery of function while limiting apoptosis: a new therapeutic approach to support hemodynamics in the setting of ischaemia-reperfusion? Basic Res Cardiol. 2009;104:69–77.
161. Ferreyra C, Vargas F, Rodríguez-Gómez I, Pérez-Abud R, O'Valle F, Osuna A. Preconditioning with triiodothyronine improves the clinical signs and acute tubular necrosis induced by ischemia/reperfusion in rats. PLoS One. 2013;26:8:e74960. https://doi.org/10.1371/journal.pone.0074960.
162. Kumar A, Sinha RA, Tiwari M, Singh R, Koji T, Manhas N, et al. Hyperthyroidism induces apoptosis in rat liver through activation of death receptor-mediated pathways. J Hepatol. 2007;46:888–98.
163. Sinha RA, You SH, Zhou J, Siddique MM, Bay BH, Zhu X, et al. Thyroid hormone stimulates hepatic lipid catabolism via activation of autophagy. J Clin Invest. 2012;122:2428–38.

164. Sabbah HN, Wang M, Zhang K, Gupta RC, Rastogi S. Long-term therapy with Bendavia (MTP-131), a novel mitochondria-targeting peptide, improves left ventricular systolic function in dogs with chronic heart failure in dogs with chronic heart failure. European Society of Cardiology Congress Amsterdam, 31 August- 4 September 2013.
165. Gajarsa JJ, Kloner RA. Left ventricular remodeling in the post-infarction heart: a review of cellular, molecular mechanisms, and therapeutic modalities. Heart Fail Rev. 2011;16:13–21.
166. Hudson MP, Armstrong PW, Ruzyllo W, Brum J, Cusmano L, Krzeski P, et al. Effects of selective matrix metalloproteinase inhibitor (PG-116800) to prevent ventricular remodeling after myocardial infarction: results of the PREMIER (Prevention of Myocardial Infarction Early Remodeling) trial. J Am Coll Cardiol. 2006;48:15–20.
167. Tousoulis D, Papageorgiou N, Briasoulis A, Androulakis E, Charakida M, Tsiamis E, et al. Conflicting effects of nitric oxide and oxidative stress in chronic heart failure: potential therapeutic strategies. Heart Fail Rev. 2012;17:65–79.
168. Mann DL, McMurray JJ, Packer M, Swedberg K, Borer JS, Colucci WS, et al. Targeted anticytokine therapy in patients with chronic heart failure: results of the Randomized Etanercept Worldwide Evaluation (RENEWAL). Circulation. 2004;109:1594–602.
169. Chung ES, Packer M, Lo KH, Fasanmade AA, Willerson JT, Anti-TNF Therapy Against Congestive Heart Failure Investigators. Randomized, double-blind, placebo-controlled, pilot trial of infliximab, a chimeric monoclonal antibody to tumor necrosis factor-alpha, in patients with moderate-to-severe heart failure: results of the anti-TNF Therapy Against Congestive Heart Failure (ATTACH) trial. Circulation. 2003;107:3133–40.
170. Sliwa K, Woodiwiss A, Candy G, Badenhorst D, Libhaber C, Norton G, et al. Effects of pentoxifylline on cytokine profiles and left ventricular performance in patients with decompensated congestive heart failure secondary to idiopathic dilated cardiomyopathy. Am J Cardiol. 2002;90:1118–22.
171. Abbate A, Van Tassell BW, Biondi-Zoccai G, Kontos MC, Grizzard JD, Spillman DW, et al. Effects of interleukin-1 blockade with anakinra on adverse cardiac remodeling and heart failure after acute myocardial infarction [from the Virginia Commonwealth University-Anakinra Remodeling Trial (2) (VCU-ART2) pilot study]. Am J Cardiol. 2013;111:1394–400.
172. Carotenuto F, Minieri M, Monego G, Fiaccavento R, Bertoni A, Sinigaglia F, et al. A diet supplemented with ALA-rich flaxseed prevents cardiomyocyte apoptosis by regulating caveolin-3 expression. Cardiovasc Res. 2013;100:422–31.
173. Kanamori H, Takemura G, Goto K, Tsujimoto A, Ogino A, Takeyama T, et al. Resveratrol reverses remodeling in hearts with large, old myocardial infarctions through enhanced autophagy-activating AMP kinase pathway. Am J Pathol. 2013;182:701–13.
174. Di Lascio G, Harmelin G, Targetti M, Nanni C, Bianchi G, Gasbarri T, et al. Cellular retrograde cardiomyoplasty and relaxin therapy for postischemic myocardial repair in a rat model. Tex Heart Inst J. 2012;39:488–99.
175. Lee TM, Lin MS, Chang NC. Inhibition of histone deacetylase on ventricular remodeling in infarcted rats. Am J Phys. 2007;293:H968–77.
176. Kaludercic N, Carpi A, Menabò R, Di Lisa F, Paolocci N. Monoamine oxidases (MAO) in the pathogenesis of heart failure and ischemia/reperfusion injury. Biochim Biophys Acta. 1813;2011:1323–32.
177. Varela A, Mavroidis M, Katsimpoulas M, Sfiroera I, Kappa N, Mesa A, et al. The neuroprotective agent Rasagiline mesylate attenuates cardiac remodeling after experimental myocardial infarction. ESC Heart Fail. 2017;4:331–40.
178. Unsöld B, Kaul A, Sbroggiò M, Schubert C, Regitz-Zagrosek V, Brancaccio M, et al. Melusin protects from cardiac rupture and improves functional remodelling after myocardial infarction. Cardiovasc Res. 2014;101:97–107.
179. Dorn GW 2nd. Apoptotic and non-apoptotic programmed cardiomyocyte death in ventricular remodelling. Cardiovasc Res. 2009;81:465–73.
180. Skommer J, Rana I, Marques FZ, Zhu W, Du Z, Charchar FJ. Small molecules, big effects: the role of microRNAs in regulation of cardiomyocyte death. Cell Death Dis. 2014;5:e1325.

181. Dong Y, Liu C, Zhao Y, Ponnusamy M, Li P, Wang K. Role of noncoding RNAs in regulation of cardiac cell death and cardiovascular diseases. Cell Mol Life Sci. 2018;75:291–300.
182. Tony H, Yu K, Qiutang Z. MicroRNA-208a silencing attenuates doxorubicin induced myocyte apoptosis and cardiac dysfunction. Oxidative Med Cell Longev. 2015;2015:597032.
183. Wang JX, Zhang XJ, Feng C, Sun T, Wang K, Wang Y, et al. MicroRNA-532-3p regulates mitochondrial fission through targeting apoptosis repressor with caspase recruitment domain in doxorubicin cardiotoxicity. Cell Death Dis. 2015;6:e1677.
184. González A, Ravassa S, Beaumont J, López B, Díez J. New targets to treat the structural remodeling of the myocardium. J Am Coll Cardiol. 2011;58:1833–43.

Chapter 8
Healing of Myocardial Infarction

Nikolaos Papageorgiou and Dimitris Tousoulis

8.1 Introduction

Myocardial infarction (MI) and the resulting loss of myocardial contractility are the major causes of *heart failure* (HF). The bigger the infarct size, the worst the prognosis, and this also depends on the infarcted region [1, 2]. *Remodelling* is a strong predictor and closely associated to arrhythmias and sudden cardiac death [3, 4]. Loss of viable myocardium is progressive, while the infarcted region can expand after that loss.

Although healing of a wound and investigation of possible relevant mechanisms have been an ongoing research target through the years, whether these apply to myocardial wound healing remains unknown.

There are factors identified and possibly contributing to infarct healing. Reperfusion can limit the infarct size by preventing loss of viable myocardium but also by an additional beneficial effect on healing [5]. Moreover, mechanical stress can result in infarct expansion [6]. Other factors including age, sex, neurohumoral factors and drugs have been proposed to help as well. To date, there is limited data on genetic or acquired general healing deficiency which can promote infarct expansion.

In the present chapter, we critically review the role of specific factors which potentially influence infarct healing.

N. Papageorgiou
Electrophysiology Department, Barts Heart Centre, St. Bartholomew's Hospital, London, UK

1st Cardiology Department, Hippokration Hospital, Athens University Medical School, Athens, Greece

D. Tousoulis (✉)
1st Cardiology Department, Hippokration Hospital, Athens University Medical School, Athens, Greece

D. V. Cokkinos (ed.), *Myocardial Preservation*,
https://doi.org/10.1007/978-3-319-98186-4_8

8.2 Pathophysiology of Healing After Myocardial Infarction

Cardiac healing and repair following myocardial ischaemia start with an inflammatory phase during which the necrotic myocardium is replaced with granulation tissue, followed by a fibrogenic phase which leads in scar tissue formation.

Healing relies on recruitment as well as activation of myeloid cells particularly *monocytes*, which contribute to resorption of cellular debris and apoptotic cells, degradation of extracellular matrix components, regulation of granulation tissue formation and *neoangiogenesis*, mediated by cytokines, proteases and growth factors (Table 8.1) [6–8].

Although there is detailed histological analysis of the cellular composition of the healing infarct over time in experimental models of MI, so far there is only little understanding of the complex processes in the infarcted area where different subtypes of cells interact in a time-dependent manner with the tissue and promote wound healing.

The formation of new blood vessels is a critical event in infarct healing and requires well-coordinated interactions between endothelial cells, vascular smooth muscle cells and the extracellular matrix in response to angiogenic mediators [6].

During the healing process, fibroblasts proliferate and differentiate into contractile myofibroblasts acquiring smooth muscle features, which secrete large amounts of extracellular proteins [9]. Deposition of extracellular matrix is an essential step of infarct repair and for structural integrity of the infarcted myocardium and prevention of LV rupture. Disorganized collagen matrix renders the scar less resistant to distension, resulting in an increased wall stress and infarct thinning/chamber dilation. On the contrary, fibroblast proliferation and differentiation to myofibroblasts

Table 8.1 Ventricular dysfunction during remodelling

Mechanism	Changes	Results
Cell death	(+) Apoptosis (+) Necrosis	(−) Myocyte
Oxidative stress	(+) NADPH oxidase (+) Catecholamine degradation (+) Xanthine oxidase (+) Antioxidant systems	(+) Metalloproteinase activation (+) Apoptosis
Inflammation	(−) Adaptive response dysfunction	(+) Inflammatory cytokines (+) Macrophage
Calcium transport	(−) L-type calcium channels (−) Ryanodine (+) Calsequestrin (−) Calmodulin	(−) Calcium in systole (+) Calcium in diastole
Neurohormonal activation	(+) Renin–angiotensin–aldosterone system	(+) Cell death (+) Oxidative stress (+) Inflammation (+) Metalloproteinases and fibroblasts

+ increase/induce, – decrease/suppress

in distal areas of the infarct site result in excessive deposition of extracellular matrix proteins and significant increase in myocardial stiffness, resulting to diastolic dysfunction and heart failure. *Fibrosis* reduces myocyte oxygen, coronary reserve and enhances ischaemia.

8.3 Risk Factors Related to Myocardial Fibrosis and Necrosis

Acute MI is the result of several risk factors. Most of these risk factors are lifestyle related and other to gender related. The main risk factors related to myocardial fibrosis and necrosis are the following.

8.3.1 Type 2 Diabetes

Type 2 diabetes is associated with increased risk of coronary artery disease (CAD). The risk of CAD in subjects with diabetes is nearly doubled when looking at men and women together [10]. This seems to be an effect of impaired endothelial function, increased levels of free fatty acids, subclinical inflammation, changes in adipokines and changes in thrombosis/fibrinolysis [11]. Women with diabetes have a larger relative risk of CAD compared to men [10–12]. The underlying cause for this is still under investigation [12–14]. Interestingly, it has been shown that hormone replacement therapy is associated with increased risk of CAD in female with diabetes, while increased or decreased risk was not seen in nondiabetic females [15]. Despite these data, hormone replacement does not seem to explain all of the risk in CAD diabetic females [16]. The prevalence of diabetes type 2 has been increasing in the last decades as an effect of increasing survival rates, and since it takes many years to develop, it is highly possible that an increase in its incidence is yet to come [17–20].

8.3.2 Hypertension

Hypertension is associated with CAD in both men and women and the risk rises gradually with increasing blood pressure [21–24]. This risk increase with increasing blood pressure does not only refer to subjects with hypertension but also to those with normal blood pressure [21–25]. Studies have shown that history of hypertension is associated with an almost doubled risk of acute MI [24]. Whereas tendencies towards similar gender differences have been seen before with regard to the risk of CAD [26] and cardiovascular disease [25], there is overlapping in the confidence intervals while confounders might apply [26]. Women have been found to have a more gradual risk increase of cardiovascular mortality with regard to increasing blood pressure, in contrast to men where only very high levels showed a significant risk increase [27]. The effect of hypertensions on the risk of CAD is mostly an effect of different mechanisms leading to vascular remodelling [20]. Noradrenaline and adrenaline do not only increase arterial resistance but may have detrimental effects on the cardiomyocytes [19]. The risk of myocardial injury from a relative decrease in oxygen supply might also be a consequence of blood pressure damage to the heart that reduces the ability to respond to increased demands [19].

8.3.3 Dyslipidaemia

High levels of low-density lipoprotein (LDL) cholesterol have been associated with increased risk of CAD in both men and women [28–30]. Increased risk of CAD in both the two genders correlated with low levels of high-density lipoprotein (HDL) cholesterol. However, the risk increase seems to be higher in women than in men [28, 31]. The apolipoprotein B/apolipoprotein A1 ratio has been found to be a better predictor than LDL/HDL ratio [29]. Several studies have shown that triglycerides are associated with increased risk of CAD [32–34]. Although questions have been raised as to whether this relation is independent of other risk factors [35], triglycerides seem to be an independent risk factor for CAD in several occasions [36] including non-CAD populations [36]. Moreover, there is evidence of an inverse association between triglycerides and HDL cholesterol [36], as this has been demonstrated in several studies of patients with metabolic syndrome.

8.3.4 Metabolic Syndrome

It has been found that metabolic syndrome is associated with increased risk of CAD and cardiovascular disease in several studies [37, 38]. This risk seems to be higher in women compared to men [38, 39]. This is in agreement to the greater effect on CAD and cardiovascular disease in female with risk factors such as type 2 diabetes [12] and abdominal obesity [40], hypertension [26] and dyslipidaemia [28]. However, it is still debatable whether the syndrome itself imposes greater risk or its individual components [41, 42].

8.3.5 Smoking

It is well established that smoking is one of the most important risk factors for acute MI [24]. The detrimental effects of smoking on the cardiovascular system are mediated by promotion of vasomotor dysfunction, atherogenesis and thrombosis [43].

Free radical-mediated oxidative stress seems to play a major role [43]. On a recent meta-analysis [44], it was found that women had a 25% higher adjusted risk of CAD compared to men. The reasons for this gender difference are not clear, but one hypothesis is that a greater amount of toxic agents are extracted in women than in men from the same quantity of cigarettes smoked [44].

8.4 Factors Associated with Myocardial Healing

The acute phase of healing starts immediately after the reduction of blood flow at the site of the occlusion, and it is characterized by myocyte necrosis, apoptosis, increased inflammatory process and thinning and expansion of the infarct (Fig. 8.1). Cytokines and chemokines recruit neutrophils and macrophages to clear the infarct area of necrotic *myocytes* and extracellular matrix debris. Studies have shown that the acute phase lasts for around 5–7 days. Thereafter, the injured myocardium enters the granulation and early remodelling phase, where new fibrous tissue starts to form after suppression of inflammation. After a period of around 20 days, mature collagen has been deposited and organized into a scar, but the late remodelling phase continues for weeks to months with a progressive reduction of the ventricular function especially in the context of a big infarct.

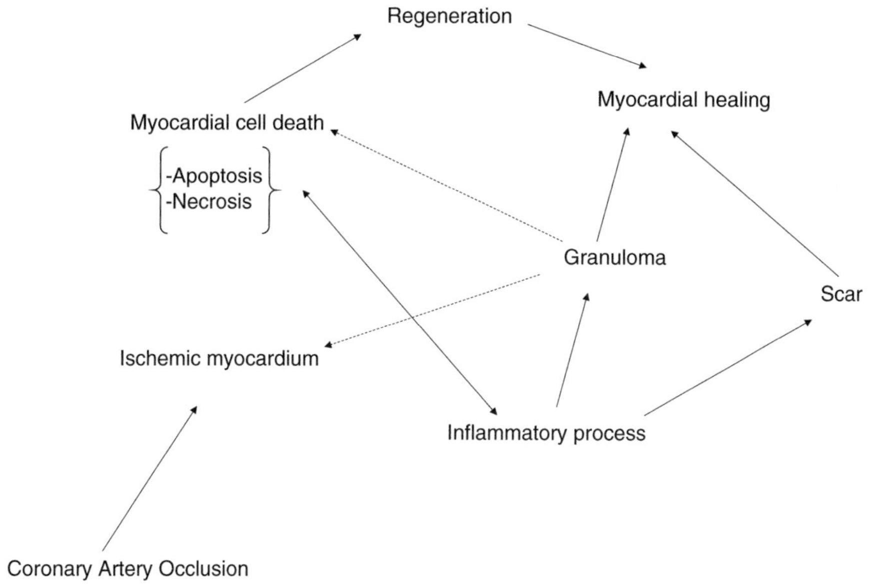

Fig. 8.1 Events associated with healing after acute myocardial infarction

8.4.1 The Role of Inflammatory Process

Pro-inflammatory cytokines and chemokines exert several effects on the myocardium in addition to attracting leukocytes to the infarct region. Matrix metalloproteinase (MMP) activity induced by increased inflammatory process can also result in ventricular rupture [45, 46], while chronic inflammation is associated with severe left ventricular (LV) remodelling [46, 47] and heart failure [47].

The post-MI inflammatory response affects the infarct size, but also the remaining perfused area of the LV. Chemokines such as macrophage inflammatory proteins (MIP)-1α and1β and monocyte chemoattractant protein (MCP)-1 are significantly increased. Enhanced expression of such molecules has direct effects on cardiomyocytes.

Cytokines have an impact on myocardial cell survival of the infarcted myocardium, contributing to mechanisms which induce or inhibit apoptosis. Interestingly, even individual cytokines can provide both survival and death signals, and the balance between them defines the cell's future. In experimental model, tumour necrosis factor (TNF) receptor knockout mice presented with larger infarct sizes and increased myocyte apoptosis compared to wild-type controls, suggesting a protective role for TNF at the healing phase [48]. Signal transduction upon binding of Interleukin-6 (IL-6) to its receptor activates pathways including phosphatidylinositol-3 kinase (PI3K) [49], which provides cytoprotective signals.

On the contrary, chemokines attract leukocytes in the infarct region. The CXC chemokines contains neutrophil chemoattractants, while the CC enroll mononuclear cells [50]. Increased neutrophil accumulation has been found in ruptured as compared to non-ruptured infarcts [51], suggesting a potential detrimental effect of neutrophils on myocardial injury/damage.

8.4.2 The Role of Matrix Metalloproteinases

MMPs are responsible for degrading the proteins of the extracellular matrix (ECM) by necrotic myocytes, a process that is essential before the fragments can be accessed and phagocytosed during the healing process. MMPs and tissue inhibitors of metalloproteinases (TIMPs) play an important role in cardiac pathophysiology [52–54], with TIMP-1 and MMP-2 and MMP-9 having an active involvement during acute MI (Table 8.2).

Of note, MMPs require cleavage by serine proteases to become active [60]. One of those is plasmin, which its activators such as urokinase and tPA as well as inhibitors like plasminogen activator inhibitor 1 (PAI-1) that contributes in the plasminogen system [61].

MMP-2 or MMP-9 gene deletion prevents ventricular rupture, as does gene transfer of TIMP-1. Ventricular rupture is a consequence of excessive infarct expansion [4], originally described as thinning and elongation of the infarct that could not

Table 8.2 Matrix metalloproteinases subgroups and their role in heart failure post-myocardial infarction

MMPs	Levels in HF	Role in HF
MMP-1 [55]	(−)	Unknown role in remodelling
MMP-2 [55, 56]	(+) In DCM (unchanged) in ICM	MMP-2 animals have prolonged survival, decreased LV rupture and decreased LV dilatation
MMP-3 [55, 57]	Increased in DCM, unchanged in ICM	LV rupture is unchanged after experimental MI in MMP-3
MMP-9 [55, 57–59]	Increased	MMP-9 animals have improved cardiac remodelling and decreased left ventricular rupture after experimental MI

MMP matrix metalloproteinases, (−) reduced, (+) increased, *LV* left ventricle, *DMC* dilated cardiomyopathy, *ICM* ischaemic cardiomyopathy, *MI* myocardial infarction

be explained by additional myocyte necrosis [62]. Histological examination demonstrated that myocyte bundles slipping relative to each other are responsible for this result [63]. The expansion of infarct starts within 24 h [63] and continues through the acute phase until extensive collagen deposition has taken place. This is during a period when the wall of the ventricle is vulnerable to mechanical deformation [64].

In experimental models, increased MMP-9 activity has been found within 24 h of the onset of ischaemia, mainly in neutrophils [65], and continues to increase 72 h post-MI. MMP-9 activity decreases after this point, while MMP-2 activity increases after 96 h and remains elevated for at least 2–4 weeks [65]. Macrophages, fibroblasts and myocytes are major sources of MMP-2 [66].

8.4.3 *The Role of Apoptosis*

Cell future depends on the balance between multiple competing signals. One of the best-studied pathways leading to apoptosis is the death receptor pathway 50, which includes TNF signalling. This pathway involves the activation of Fas by binding of its ligand (Fas ligand), which involved in cell death post-MI. Even so, Fas activation has been associated to induction of a transcription factor associated with hypertrophy [67]. Apoptosis can also be initiated in a mitochondrial-dependent manner. Irrespectively of the mechanism of activation, whether the apoptotic cascade goes on or is prevented could be subject to regulation by the Bcl-2 proteins family, growth factors such as IGF-1.

It has been demonstrated that in ischaemia/reperfusion, apoptosis is more pronounced than necrosis and also in the surrounding area of the infarct [68]. Decrease in apoptosis shortly after MI has been found to improve cardiac function and reduce adverse remodelling. Therefore, targeting apoptosis has emerged as potential therapeutic target.

8.4.4 *Oxidative Stress*

Reactive oxygen species may be produced by several sources in the myocardium, such as NADPH oxidase system and other enzymes including cytochrome P450, xanthine oxidase, and lipoxygenase, as well as catecholamine degradation. In normal conditions, there is a balance between reactive oxygen species production and antioxidant substances.

There is evidence suggesting an association between cardiac remodelling and oxidative stress as a result of increased reactive oxygen species production and decreased antioxidant defence. This can result into lipid peroxidation, DNA damage, proliferation of fibroblasts, activation of metalloproteinases and induction of apoptosis [69–71].

8.5 Candidate Factors Potentially Beneficial for Healing

Myocardial infarct develops during hours, remains ischaemic if there is no option of reperfusion and is also associated with stress of rhythmic cardiac contraction. The paracrine and autocrine milieu is potentially quite different between cutaneous and cardiac tissues. However, several similar steps of healing may be observed in wounds and appear to be general characteristics of healing. As an example of this, synthesis of collagen is downregulated in skin fibroblasts of patients with varicosis [72]. Such fibroblasts isolated from ulcers are characterized by reduced ability to synthesize collagen and particularly in states of hypoxia [73]. Therefore, apart from confounding environmental factors, a genetic defect is hypothesized to transmit varicose vein pathology, a systemic biochemical defect of the ECM [72]. The skin has been defined as a window on heritable disorders of connective tissue [74]. A number of factors meet the requirements of a potential general healing factor.

Secretory leukocyte protease inhibitor (SLPI) [75] regulates the synthesis of intracellular enzymes and the production of monocyte matrix metalloproteinases. In experimental model of SLPI knockout mice, these were characterized by wound-healing defects, more likely due to ongoing inflammation and inability to generate matrix. It has been shown expression of SLPI in the heart and in heart failure. However, the function of SLPI in healing of the infarct wound remains unclear.

Osteopontin, another protein, interacts with integrins and the CD44 receptor. It seems that it can potentially contribute to cell adhesion and signalling [76] and interact with fibronectin and collagen [77]. Its deficiency results in disorganization of the collagen matrix [78] suggesting a role in wound healing. Osteopontin deficiency also results in increased expansion of the infracted segment and decreased collagen accumulation [79]. Secreted protein acidic and rich in cysteine (SPARC) is an extracellular glycoprotein expressed in proliferating cells, and it is involved in ECM interaction. These can regulate cell adhesion, proliferation and migration [80]. SPARCs are expressed in the myocardium and enhanced with isoproterenol treatment [81].

However, the role of SPARCs in cardiac healing remains to be evaluated. Factor XIII may be also involved in several cross-link reactions which form and stabilize the fibrin network as well as modulating intestinal epithelial wound healing in vitro [82] and stabilizing bone defects in models of diabetes [83]. It also accelerates healing in diabetic foot [84]. So far, research on its role in healing myocardium is insufficient.

8.6 Therapeutic Approaches

Several strategies to promote wound healing and regeneration after AMI are under development (Table 8.3). Such therapeutic approaches aim to preserve ventricular function by increasing tissue repair after ischaemia/reperfusion.

8.6.1 Ischaemia/Reperfusion: A Challenging Concept

Ischaemia reperfusion is a very useful tool in the acute setting of MI, as the reopening of an occluded coronary artery is vital [94, 95]. Early research focused on agents that would render myocardial cells more resistant to the detrimental effects of ischaemia and reperfusion [96]. *Cardioprotection* encompasses the regulation of cellular events during ischaemia/reperfusion to reduce myocardial cell death [96]. Ischaemic conditioning strategies such as pre-and post-conditioning have been largely investigated in both animal and human studies. However, there is still difficulty in translating experimental results into a heterogeneous population of patients. Continuous research has led to the development of cardioprotective strategies, focusing on epigenetic regulation, limitation of cell necrosis and apoptosis, stem cell regeneration and gene therapy [97]. Among the mechanisms through which postischaemic myocardial damage has been shown to occur, mitochondrial dysfunction is a key step. In this context, a potential cardioprotective effect of intracoronary administration of 4-chlorodiazepam in animal models has been found [98],

Table 8.3 Heart failure drugs and their effect on healing

Drugs	Effect on remodelling	Effect on fibrosis	Effect on cytokines	Effect on MMPs
ACE-I [85, 86]	+	–	–	–
B-blocker [87, 88]	+	–	–	Unknown
MRAs [89]	+	–	Unknown	–
Endothelin antagonists [90]	Conflicting	–	–	–
Statins [91–93]	+	–	–	Conflicting results

MRAs mineralocorticoid receptor antagonists, *ACE* angiotensin-converting enzyme inhibitors, *MMPs* matrix metalloproteinases, + protective or positive/increase, – not protective or negative/reduce

therefore implicating a therapeutic role of intracoronary infusion of this agent in myocardial infraction [98]. In addition, studies have reported that platelet-rich plasma (PRP), which is rich in growth factors, can have a role in the healing of the ischaemic myocardium [99–102]. Significant Factor XIII amounts exist in platelets and have been found to play a role in the different steps of the reparative process, the formation of the three-dimensional fibrin meshwork. Finally, it is essential in stem cell recruitment, neoangiogenesis and collagen deposit, therefore playing a major role at the intersection of several pathways involved in myocardial healing [103].

8.6.2 Cell Therapy

Many randomized, controlled trials have used bone marrow cell (BMCs) to treat the culprit coronary artery during the first week of reperfusion. It has been shown that BMCs can reduce the infarct size and improve left ventricular systolic function [104].

In the CADUCEUS study [105], endomyocardial biopsies were placed into culture to expand 'cardiosphere-derived cells' (CDCs). These cells were then infused into the infarct-related artery a few months after MI resulting to smaller scar sizes and improved regional contractility at 6 months.

Initially, transplantation of BMCs is characterized by release of paracrine factors. Paracrine factors produced by BMCs support wound healing by acting on multiple target cells in the infarct wound [106, 107]. It is also possible that paracrine factors may activate endogenous cardiomyocyte progenitors to promote cardiac regeneration [108].

Human-induced *pluripotent stem cells* (iPSCs) can be expanded in mass culture to yield the cell numbers required for potential clinical applications [109]. Data have demonstrated that human embryonic stem cell-derived cardiomyocytes transplant could result in stable grafts that couple with existing cardiomyocytes in the infarct zone and improve systolic function [110]. Moreover, direct reprogramming of scar fibroblasts into cardiomyocytes may be another approach to heal the infarcted myocardium [111, 112].

8.6.3 Protein-Based Therapy

Wound healing involves intercellular interaction through secreted proteins. Therapeutic application of recombinant proteins seems very promising to provide an alternative option to support healing after acute MI.

Previous studies investigating the therapeutic potential of granulocyte colony-stimulating factor or erythropoietin have not been very promising [113, 114]. On the contrary studies on animal models have been more encouraging and potentially support healing. As such, application of follistatin-like 1 or thymosin β4 have been found to reduce infarct size in animals with reperfused MI by reducing reperfusion injury and inflammation [115, 116]. Fibroblast growth factor 9 promotes angiogenesis in the infarct zone, therefore stimulating adaptive cardiomyocyte hypertrophy [117]. In addition, intravenous administration of the matrix-interacting protein TSG-6 was found to decrease inflammation and infarct size in animal model [118]. Stem cell factor increases the recruitment of progenitor cells to the infarcted area and promotes cardiomyocyte cell cycle activity resulting in reduced infarct size and left ventricular remodelling [119].

There are different approaches of protein-based therapies aiming to maintain therapeutic concentrations of protein in the infarct area for significant time. Given that, studies have tried to fuse the cytokine or the growth factor of interest with a peptide or protein that will be attracted to the infarct wound after systemic delivery [120–122]. Other approaches fuse cytokines or growth factors with polyethylene glycol polymer chains (PEGylation) or with large non-functional polypeptides (XTENylation) to increase their plasma half-lives [123]. There is also another approach by engineering growth factor mutants that are resistant to protease and therefore remain more stable in plasma [124].

8.6.4 MicroRNA-Based Therapies

Over the last decade, *microRNAs* (miRNAs, miR-) have emerged as important modulators in cardiovascular disease. miRNAs are non-coding RNAs that inhibit the expression of specific mRNA targets. Expression levels of multiple miRs change in a time-dependent manner after acute MI [125]. miRNAs up or downregulation provides an extra layer of regulation controlling important aspects of wound healing, including cardiomyocyte survival and scar formation [126]. Therapies based on anti-miRs or miRNA mimetics are currently developed to suppress pathological miRNAs or to increase the levels of protective miRNAs [127]. Anti-miRs are taken up by a variety of tissues and prevent the function of their relative miRNAs. miRNA-based therapies affect families of genes under the control of the target miRNA [127]. Despite the encouraging results, there is still way to go for miR-based therapies to be applied into the clinic practice.

8.7 Critical Approach and Future Perspectives

Interpretation of the results of clinical studies is difficult due to several confounding variables such as different infarct size, gender, age and other factors. Ageing alters the inflammatory response in myocardial injury, while the infarct size is a critical determinant of remodelling in acute MI patient.

With regard to the new anti-inflammatory strategies, the scepticism relies on the fact that an intact immune system is required, whereas prolonged immune activation may also trigger detrimental effects that drive disease progression.

What is challenging, that immunosuppressive agents have to limit detrimental innate immune effects during the acute phase of healing, while these need to maintain and stimulate relevant innate immune mechanisms.

It has become evident that the pathophysiology of MI-associated HF is complex, while the healing process is very challenging. Studies on molecular signalling pathways continue to investigate new and more attractive targets for gene therapy. Research has identified endogenous small RNAs that specifically suppress the expression of target genes. Some of these small RNAs are actually downregulated after MI.

Specific delivery of exogenous small RNA and microRNAs into infarcted areas may be a promising approach for gene therapy. Furthermore, cell therapy appears a new attractive approach to achieve or promote myocardial healing. Myocyte regeneration has been difficult, and the mild beneficial effects shown in studies may be the result of angiogenesis, which in turn can be more easily achieved with the use of virus vectors. Nevertheless, the next phase of gene therapy for myocardial healing will make sufficient progress once more effective gene transfer vectors and methods of delivery are available.

8.8 Conclusion

Post-myocardial infarction healing has been studied extensively and importantly the role of major biological processes such as inflammation, apoptosis and MMP activity. Studies have shown that interventions aiming to reduce the activity of inflammation and MMPs must carefully consider the timing of inhibition as myocardial healing has specific characteristics.

The processes mentioned above can also be important in the late remodelling phase if the infarct is large, and acute interventions that reduce the severity of the initial response to injury may also attenuate ventricular remodelling.

Improved therapeutic approaches are required to improve healing process and prevent adverse cardiac remodelling which results in increased mortality. However, the healing process is highly complex and needs an in-depth understanding of the pathophysiological processes. Novel therapeutic approaches include progenitor cell therapy, miRNA modulation and interference with the inflammatory and fibrotic response. Despite the very exciting results deriving from experimental models, those approaches still need to prove their clinical utility.

References

1. Pfeffer JM, Pfeffer MA, Fletcher PJ, Braunwald E. Progressive ventricular remodeling in rat with myocardial infarction. Am J Phys. 1991;260:H1406–14.
2. Gaudron P, Kugler I, Hu K, Bauer W, Eilles C, Ertl G. Time course of cardiac structural, functional and electrical changes in asymptomatic patients after myocardial infarction: their inter-relation and prognostic impact. J Am Coll Cardiol. 2001;38:33–40.

3. Holmes JW, Yamashita H, Waldman LK, Covell JW. Scar remodelling and transmural deformation after infarction in the pig. Circulation. 1994;90:411–20.
4. Hochman JS, Choo H. Limitation of myocardial infarct expansion by reperfusion independent of myocardial salvage. Circulation. 1987;75:299–306.
5. Gaudron P, Hu K, Schamberger R, Budin M, Walter B, Ertl G. Effect of endurance training early or late after coronary artery occlusion on left ventricular remodeling, hemodynamics, and survival in rats with chronic transmural myocardial infarction. Circulation. 1994;89:402–12.
6. Dobaczewski M, Gonzalez-Quesada C, Frangogiannis NG. The extracellular matrix as a modulator of the inflammatory and reparative response following myocardial infarction. J Mol Cell Cardiol. 2010;48:504–11.
7. Frangogiannis NG. The immune system and cardiac repair. Pharmacol Res. 2008;58:88–111.
8. Kempf T, Zarbock A, Widera C, Butz S, Stadtmann A, Rossaint J, et al. GDF-15 is an inhibitor of leukocyte integrin activation required for survival after myocardial infarction in mice. Nat Med. 2011;17:581–8.
9. Brown RD, Ambler SK, Mitchell MD, Long CS. The cardiac fibroblast: therapeutic target in myocardial remodeling and failure. Annu Rev Pharmacol Toxicol. 2005;45:657–87.
10. The Emerging Risk Factor Collaboration. Diabetes mellitus, fasting blood glucose concentration, and risk of vascular disease: a collaborative meta-analysis of 102 prospective studies. Lancet. 2010;375:2215–22.
11. Laakso M. Cardiovascular disease in type 2 diabetes from population to man to mechanisms. The Kelly West award lecture 2008. Diabetes Care. 2010;33:442–9.
12. Huxley R, Barzi F, Woodward M. Excess risk of fatal coronary heart disease associated with diabetes in men and women: meta-analysis of 37 prospective cohort studies. BMJ. 2006;332:73–8.
13. Kanaya AM, Grady D, Barrett-Connor E. Explaining the sex difference in coronary heart disease mortality among patients with type 2 diabetes mellitus. Arch Intern Med. 2002;162:1737–45.
14. Rivellese AA, Riccardi G, Vaccaro O. Cardiovascular risk in women with diabetes. Nutr Metab Cardiovasc Dis. 2010;20:474–80.
15. Løkkegaard E, Pedersen AT, Heitmann BL, Jovanovic Z, Keiding N, Hundrup YA, et al. Relation between hormone replacement therapy and ischaemic heart disease in women: prospective observational study. BMJ. 2003;326:426–30.
16. Barrett-Connor E, Cohn BA, Wingard DL, Edelstein SL. Why is diabetes mellitus a stronger risk factor for fatal ischemic heart disease in women than in men? The Rancho Bernardo Study. JAMA. 1991;265:627–31.
17. Psaltopoulou T, Hatzis G, Papageorgiou N, Androulakis E, Briasoulis A, Tousoulis D. Socioeconomic status and risk factors for cardiovascular disease: impact of dietary mediators. Hell J Cardiol. 2017;58:32–42.
18. Guidelines Subcommittee. 1999 World Health Organization – international society of hypertension guidelines for the management of hypertension. J Hypertens. 1999;17:151–83.
19. Labarthe DR. Epidemiology and prevention of cardiovascular diseases: a global challenge. Gaithersburg: Aspen Publishers, Inc.; 1998.
20. Staessen JA, Wang J, Bianchi G, Birkenhäger WH. Essential hypertension. Lancet. 2003;361:1629–41.
21. Lewington S, Clarke R, Qizilbash N, Peto R, Collins R, Prospective Studies Collaboration. Age-specific relevance of usual blood pressure and vascular mortality: a meta-analysis of individual data for one million adults in 61 prospective studies. Lancet. 2002;360:1903–13.
22. Lawes CM, Rodgers A, Bennett DA, Parag V, Suh I, Ueshima H, et al. Blood pressure and cardiovascular disease in the Asia Pacific region. J Hypertens. 2003;21:707–16.
23. MacMahon S, Peto R, Cutler J, Collins R, Sorlie P, Neaton J. Blood pressure, stroke, and coronary heart disease. Part 1. Prolonged differences in blood pressure: prospective observational studies corrected for the regression dilution bias. Lancet. 1990;335:765–74.
24. Yusuf S, Hawken S, Ôunpuu S, Dans T, Avezum A, Lanas F, et al. Effect of potentially modifiable risk factors associated with myocardial infarction in 52 countries (the INTERHEART study): case-control study. Lancet. 2004;364:937–52.

25. Vasan RS, Larson MG, Leip EP, Evans JC, O'Donnell CJ, Kannel WB, et al. Impact of high-normal blood pressure on the risk of cardiovascular disease. N Engl J Med. 2001;345: 1291–7.
26. Selmer R. Blood pressure and twenty-year mortality in the city of Bergen, Norway. Am J Epidem. 1992;136:428–40.
27. Carlsson AC, Theobald H, Hellenius M-L, Wändell PE. Cardiovascular and total mortality in men and women with different blood pressure levels – a 26-year follow-up. Blood Press. 2009;18:105–10.
28. Wilson PWF, D'Agostino RB, Levy D, Belanger AM, Silbershatz H, Kannel WB. Prediciton of coronary heart disease using risk factor categories. Circulation. 1998;97:1837–47.
29. Sniderman AD, Junger I, Holme I, Aastveit A, Walldius G. Errors that result from using the TC/HDL C ratio rather than the apoB/apoA-1 ratio to identify the lipoprotein-related risk of vascular disease. J Intern Med. 2006;259:455–61.
30. National cholesterol education program (NCEP) expert panel on detection, evaluation, and treatment of high blood cholesterol in adults (Adult Treatment Panel III). Third report of the national cholesterol education program (NCEP) expert panel on detection, evaluation, and treatment of high blood cholesterol in adults (Adult Treatment Panel III) final report. Circulation. 2002;106:3143–421.
31. Pilote L, Dasgupta K, Guru V, Humphries KH, McGrath J, Norris C, et al. A comprehensive view of sex-specific issues related to cardiovascular disease. CMAJ. 2007;176:S1–S44.
32. Langsted A, Freiberg JJ, Tybjærg-Hansen A, Schnohr P, Jensen GB, Nordestgaard BG. Nonfasting cholesterol and triglycerides and association with risk of myocardial infarction and total mortality: the Copenhagen City Heart Study with 31 years of follow-up. J Intern Med. 2011;270:65–75.
33. Austin MA, Hokanson JE, Edwards KL. Hypertriglyceridemia as a cardiovascular risk factor. Am J Cardiol. 1998;81:7B–12B.
34. Hokanson JE, Austin MA. Plasma triglyceride level is a risk factor for cardiovascular disease independent of high-density lipoprotein cholesterol level: a meta-analysis of population-based prospective studies. J Cardiovasc Risk. 1996;3:213–9.
35. Avins AL, Neuhaus JM. Do triglycerides provide meaningful information about heart disease risk? Arch Int Med. 2000;160:1937–44.
36. Morrison A, Hokanson JE. The independent relationship between triglycerides and coronary heart disease. Vasc Health Risk Manag. 2009;5:89–95.
37. Ford ES. Risk for all-cause mortality, cardiovascular disease, and diabetes associated with the metabolic syndrome. Diabetes Care. 2005;28:1769–78.
38. Hunt KJ, Resendez RG, Williams K, Haffner SM, Stern MP. National cholesterol education program versus world health organization: metabolic syndrome in relation to all-cause and cardiovascular mortality in the San Antonio Heart Study. Circulation. 2004;110:1251–7.
39. Bentley-Lewis R, Koruda K, Seely EW. The metabolic syndrome in women. Nat Clin Pract Endocrinol Metab. 2007;3:696–704.
40. Canoy D, Boekholdt M, Wareham N, Luben R, Welch A, Bingham S. Body fat distribution and risk of coronary heart disease in men and women in the European prospective investigation into Cancer and nutrition in Norfolk cohort: a population-based prospective study. Circulation. 2007;16:2933–43.
41. Kahn R, Buse J, Ferrannini E, Stern M. The metabolic syndrome: time for a critical appraisal. Joint statement from the American Diabetes Association and European Association for the Study of Diabetes. Diabetologia. 2005;48:1684–99.
42. Reaven GM. The metabolic syndrome: time to get off the merry-go-round? J Intern Med. 2011;269:127–36.
43. Ambrose JA, Barua RS. The pathophysiology of cigarette smoking and cardiovascular disease. An update. J Am Coll Cardiol. 2004;43:1731–7.
44. Huxley RR, Woodward M. Cigarette smoking as a risk factor for coronary heart disease in women compared with men: a systematic review and meta-analysis of prospective cohort studies. Lancet. 2011;378:1297–305.

45. Horie H, Takahashi M, Minai K, Izumi M, Takaoka A, Nozawa M, et al. Long-term beneficial effect of late reperfusion for acute anterior myocardial infarction with percutaneous transluminal coronary angioplasty. Circulation. 1998;98:2377–82.
46. Sadanandan S, Buller C, Menon V, Dzavik V, Terrin M, Thompson B, et al. The late open artery hypothesis–a decade later. Am Heart J. 2001;142:411–21.
47. Abbate A, Bussani R, Biondi-Zoccai GG, Rossiello R, Silvestri F, Baldi F, et al. Persistent infarct-related artery occlusion is associated with an increased myocardial apoptosis at postmortem examination in humans late after an acute myocardial infarction. Circulation. 2002;106:1051–4.
48. Aikawa Y, Rohde L, Plehn J, Greaves SC, Menapace F, Arnold MO, et al. Regional wall stress predicts ventricular remodeling after anteroseptal myocardial infarction in the healing and early afterload reducing trial (HEART): an echocardiography-based structural analysis. Am Heart J. 2001;141:234–42.
49. Cheung PY, Sawicki G, Wozniak M, Wang W, Radomski MW, Schulz R. Matrix metalloproteinase-2 contributes to ischemia reperfusion injury in the heart. Circulation. 2000;101:1833–9.
50. Bettencourt-Dias M, Mittnacht S, Brockes JP. Heterogeneous proliferative potential in regenerative adult newt cardiomyocytes. J Cell Sci. 2003;116:4001–9.
51. Freude B, Masters TN, Robicsek F, Fokin A, Kostin S, Zimmermann R, et al. Apoptosis is initiated by myocardial ischemia and executed during reperfusion. J Mol Cell Cardiol. 2000;32:197–208.
52. Piccinni MP, Giudizi MG, Biagiotti R, Beloni L, Giannarini L, Sampognaro S, et al. Progesterone favors the development of human T helper cells producing Th2-type cytokines and promotes both IL-4 production and membrane CD30 expression in established Th1 cell clones. J Immunol. 1995;155:128–33.
53. Ashcroft GS, Dodsworth J, van Boxtel E, Tarnuzzer RW, Horan MA, Schultz GS, et al. Estrogen accelerates cutaneous wound healing associated with an increase in TGF-beta1 levels. Nat Med. 1997;3:1209–15.
54. Haynes MP, Sinha D, Russell KS, Collinge M, Fulton D, Morales-Ruiz M, et al. Membrane estrogen receptor engagement activates endothelial nitric oxide synthase via the PI3-kinase-Akt pathway in human endothelial cells. Circ Res. 2000;87:677–82.
55. Wozniak G, Noll T, Bott U, Hehrlein FW. Factor XIII: experimental and clinical results in diabetic foot ulcer. Zentralbl Chir. 1999;124(Suppl 1):73–7.
56. Spinale FG, Coker ML, Heung LJ, Bond BR, Gunasinghe HR, Etoh T, et al. A matrix metalloproteinase induction/activation system exists in the human left ventricular myocardium and is upregulated in heart failure. Circulation. 2000;102:1944–9.
57. Hayashidani S, Tsutsui H, Ikeuchi M, Shiomi T, Matsusaka H, Kubota T, et al. Targeted deletion of MMP-2 attenuates early LV rupture and late remodeling after experimental myocardial infarction. Am J Physiol Heart Circ Physiol. 2003;285:H1229–35.
58. Heymans S, Luttun A, Nuyens D, Theilmeier G, Creemers E, Moons L, et al. Inhibition of plasminogen activators or matrix metalloproteinases prevents cardiac rupture but impairs therapeutic angiogenesis and causes cardiac failure. Nat Med. 1999;5:1135–42.
59. Ducharme A, Frantz S, Aikawa M, Rabkin E, Lindsey M, Rohde LE, et al. Targeted deletion of matrix metalloproteinase-9 attenuates left ventricular enlargement and collagen accumulation after experimental myocardial infarction. J Clin Invest. 2000;106:55–62.
60. Ashcroft GS, Horan MA, Ferguson MW. Aging is associated with reduced deposition of specific extracellular matrix components, an upregulation of angiogenesis, and an altered inflammatory response in a murine incisional wound healing model. J Invest Dermatol. 1997;108:430–7.
61. Binko J, Murphy TV, Majewski H. 17Beta-oestradiol enhances nitric oxide synthase activity in endothelium-denuded rat aorta. Clin Exp Pharmacol Physiol. 1998;25:120–7.
62. Zdrojewski T, Gaudron P, Whittaker P, Poelzl S, Schiemann J, Hu K, et al. Ventricular remodeling after myocardial infarction and effects of ACE inhibition on hemodynamics and scar formation in SHR. Cardiovasc Pathol. 2002;11:88–93.

63. Ichihara S, Senbonmatsu T, Price E Jr, Ichiki T, Gaffney FA, Inagami T. Targeted deletion of angiotensin II type 2 receptor caused cardiac rupture after acute myocardial infarction. Circulation. 2002;106:2244–9.
64. Phillips MI, Kagiyama S. Angiotensin II as a pro-inflammatory mediator. Curr Opin Investig Drugs. 2002;3:569–77.
65. Maggioni AP, Maseri A, Fresco C, Franzosi MG, Mauri F, Santoro E, et al. Age-related increase in mortality among patients with first myocardial infarctions treated with thrombolysis. The investigators of the GruppoItaliano per lo Studio dellaSopravvivenzanell'Infarto Miocardico (GISSI-2). N Engl J Med. 1993;329:1442–8.
66. Vaccarino V, Parsons L, Every NR, Barron HV, Krumholz HM. Sexbased differences in early mortality after myocardial infarction. National registry of myocardial infarction 2 participants. N Engl J Med. 1999;341:217–25.
67. Podesser BK, Siwik DA, Eberli FR, Sam F, Ngoy S, Lambert J, et al. ET(A)-receptor blockade prevents matrix metalloproteinase activation late postmyocardial infarction in the rat. Am J Physiol Heart Circ Physiol. 2001;280:H984–91.
68. Scherrer-Crosbie M, Ullrich R, Bloch KD, Nakajima H, Nasseri B, Aretz HT, et al. Endothelial nitric oxide synthase limits left ventricular remodeling after myocardial infarction in mice. Circulation. 2001;104:1286–91.
69. Sawyer DB, Siwik DA, Xiao L, Pimentel DR, Singh K, Colucci WS. Role of oxidative stress in myocardial hypertrophy and failure. J Mol Cell Cardiol. 2002;34(4):379–88.
70. Giordano FJ. Oxygen, oxidative stress, hypoxia, and heart failure. J Clin Invest. 2005;115(3):500–8.
71. Munzel T, Gori T, Keaney JF Jr, Maack C, Daiber A. Pathophysiological role of oxidative stress in systolic and diastolic heart failure and its therapeutic implications. Eur Heart J. 2015;36(38):2555–64.
72. Yamasaki K, Edington HD, McClosky C, Tzeng E, Lizonova A, Kovesdi I, et al. Reversal of impaired wound repair in iNOS deficient mice by topical adenoviral-mediated iNOS gene transfer. J Clin Invest. 1998;101:967–71.
73. Sansilvestri-Morel P, Rupin A, Jaisson S, Fabiani JN, Verbeuren TJ, Vanhoutte PM. Synthesis of collagen is dysregulated in cultured fibroblasts derived from skin of subjects with varicose veins as it is in venous smooth muscle cells. Circulation. 2002;106:479–83.
74. Herrick SE, Ireland GW, Simon D, McCollum CN, Ferguson MW. Venous ulcer fibroblasts compared with normal fibroblasts show differences in collagen but not fibronectin production under both normal and hypoxic conditions. J Invest Dermatol. 1996;106:187–93.
75. Holbrook KA, Byers PH. Skin is a window on heritable disorders of connective tissue. Am J Med Genet. 1989;34:105–21.
76. Seemuller U, Arnhold M, Fritz H, Wiedenmann K, Machleidt W, Heinzel R, et al. The acid-stable proteinase inhibitor of human mucous secretions (HUSI-I, antileukoprotease). Complete amino acid sequence as revealed by protein and cDNA sequencing and structural homology to whey proteins and Red Sea turtle proteinase inhibitor. FEBS Lett. 1986;199:43–8.
77. Denhardt DT, Guo X. Osteopontin: a protein with diverse functions. FASEB J. 1993;7:1475–82.
78. Mukherjee BB, Nemir M, Beninati S, Cordella-Miele E, Singh K, Chackalaparampil I, et al. Interaction of osteopontin with fibronectin and other extracellular matrix molecules. Ann N Y AcadSci. 1995;760:201–12.
79. Liaw L, Birk DE, Ballas CB, Whitsitt JS, Davidson JM, Hogan BL. Altered wound healing in mice lacking a functional osteopontin gene (spp1). J Clin Invest. 1998;101:1468–78.
80. Trueblood NA, Xie Z, Communal C, Sam F, Ngoy S, Liaw L, et al. Exaggerated left ventricular dilation and reduced collagen deposition after myocardial infarction in mice lacking osteopontin. Circ Res. 2001;88:1080–7.
81. Lane TF, Sage EH. The biology of SPARC, a protein that modulates cell-matrix interactions. FASEB J. 1994;8:163–73.
82. Masson S, Arosio B, Luvara G, Gagliano N, Fiordaliso F, Santambrogio D, et al. Remodelling of cardiac extracellular matrix during beta-adrenergic stimulation: upregulation of SPARC in the myocardium of adult rats. J Mol Cell Cardiol. 1998;30:1505–14.

83. Cario E, Goebell H, Dignass AU. Factor XIII modulates intestinal epithelial wound healing in vitro. Scand J Gastroenterol. 1999;34:485–90.
84. El-Hakim IE. The effect of fibrin stabilizing factor (F.XIII) on healing of bone defects in normal and uncontrolled diabetic rats. Int J Oral Maxillofac Surg. 1999;28:304–8.
85. Fraccarollo D, Bauersachs J, Kellner M, Galuppo P, Ertl G. Cardioprotection by long-term ET(A) receptor blockade and ACE inhibition in rats with congestive heart failure: mono-versus combination therapy. Cardiovasc Res. 2002;54:85–94.
86. Fraccarollo D, Galuppo P, Hildemann S, Christ M, Ertl G, Bauersachs J, et al. J Am Coll Cardiol. 2003;42:1666–73.
87. Prabhu SD, Chandrasekar B, Murray DR, Freeman GL. Betaadrenergic blockade in developing heart failure: effects on myocardial inflammatory cytokines, nitric oxide, and remodeling. Circulation. 2000;101:2103–9.
88. Wei S, Chow LT, Sanderson JE. Effect of carvedilol in comparison with metoprolol on myocardial collagen postinfarction. J Am Coll Cardiol. 2000;36:276–81.
89. Silvestre JS, Heymes C, Oubenaissa A, Robert V, Aupetit-Faisant B, Carayon A, et al. Activation of cardiac aldosterone production in rat myocardial infarction: effect of angiotensin II receptor blockade and role in cardiac fibrosis. Circulation. 1999;99:2694–701.
90. Fraccarollo D, Galuppo P, Bauersachs J, Ertl G. Collagen accumulation after myocardial infarction: effects of ETA receptor blockade and implications for early remodeling. Cardiovasc Res. 2002;54:559–67.
91. Rosenson RS, Tangney CC, Casey LC. Inhibition of proinflammatory cytokine production by pravastatin. Lancet. 1999;353:983–4.
92. Hayashidani S, Tsutsui H, Shiomi T, Suematsu N, Kinugawa S, Ide T, et al. Fluvastatin, a 3-hydroxy-3-methylglutaryl coenzyme a reductase inhibitor, attenuates left ventricular remodeling and failure after experimental myocardial infarction. Circulation. 2002;105:868–73.
93. Tiefenbacher CP, Kapitza J, Dietz V, Lee CH, Niroomand F. Reduction of myocardial infarct size by fluvastatin. Am J Physiol Heart Circ Physiol. 2003;285:H59–64.
94. Whittle J, Conigliaro J, Good CB, Kelley ME, Skanderson M. Understanding of the benefits of coronary revascularization procedures among patients who are offered such procedures. Am Heart J. 2007 Oct;154(4):662–8.
95. Fröhlich GM, Meier P, White SK, Yellon DM, Hausenloy DJ. Myocardial reperfusion injury: looking beyond primary PCI. Eur Heart J. 2013 Jun;34(23):1714–22.
96. Kren L, Meluzin J, Pavlovsky Z, Mayer J, Kala P, Groch L, et al. Experimental model of myocardial infarction: histopathology and reperfusion damage revisited. Pathol Res Pract. 2010;206(9):647–50.
97. Sluijter JP, Condorelli G, Davidson SM, Engel FB, Ferdinandy P, Hausenloy DJ, et al. Nucleus of the European Society of Cardiology Working Group Cellular Biology of the Heart. Novel therapeutic strategies for cardioprotection. Pharmacol Ther. 2014;144(1):60–70.
98. Tsamatsoulis M, Kapelios CJ, Katsaros L, Vakrou S, Sousonis V, Sventzouri S, et al. Cardioprotective effects of intracoronary administration of 4-chlorodiazepam in small and large animal models of ischemia-reperfusion. Int J Cardiol. 2016 Dec 1;224:9095.
99. Spartalis E, Tomos P, Moris D, Athanasiou A, Markakis C, Spartalis MD, et al. Role of platelet-rich plasma in ischemic heart disease: an update on the latest evidence.World. J Cardiol. 2015 Oct 26;7(10):665–70.
100. Mishra A, Velotta J, Brinton TJ, Wang X, Chang S, Palmer O, et al. RevaTenplatelet-rich plasma improves cardiac function after myocardial injury. Cardiovasc Revasc Med. 2011;12(3):158–63.
101. Li XH, Zhou X, Zeng S, Ye F, Yun JL, Huang TG, et al. Effects of intramyocardial injection of platelet-rich plasma on the healing process after myocardial infarction. Coron Artery Dis. 2008 Aug;19(5):363–70.
102. Wehberg KE, Answini G, Wood D, Todd J, Julian J, Ogburn N, et al. Intramyocardial injection of autologous platelet-rich plasma combined with transmyocardial revascularization. Cell Transplant. 2009;18(3):353–9.
103. Gemmati D, Zeri G, Orioli E, Mari R, Moratelli S, Vigliano M, et al. Factor XIII-A dynamics in acute myocardial infarction: a novel prognostic biomarker? Thromb Haemost. 2015;114(1):123–32.

104. Jeevanantham V, Butler M, Saad A, Abdel-Latif A, Zuba-Surma EK, Dawn B. Adult bone marrow cell therapy improves survival and induces long-term improvement in cardiac parameters: a systematic review and meta-analysis. Circulation. 2012;126:551–68.
105. Makkar RR, Smith RR, Cheng K, Malliaras K, Thomson LE, Berman D, et al. Intracoronary cardiosphere-derived cells for heart regeneration after myocardial infarction (CADUCEUS): a prospective, randomised phase 1 trial. Lancet. 2012;379:895–904.
106. Gnecchi M, Zhang Z, Ni A, Dzau VJ. Paracrine mechanisms in adult stem cell signalling and therapy. Circ Res. 2008;103:1204–19.
107. Korf-Klingebiel M, Kempf T, Sauer T, Brinkmann E, Fischer P, Meyer GP, et al. Bone marrow cells are a rich source of growth factors and cytokines: implications for cell therapy trials after myocardial infarction. Eur Heart J. 2008;29:2851–8.
108. Loffredo FS, Steinhauser ML, Gannon J, Lee RT. Bone marrow-derived cell therapy stimulates endogenous cardiomyocyte progenitors and promotes cardiac repair. Cell Stem Cell. 2011;8:389–98.
109. Zweigerdt R, Olmer R, Singh H, Haverich A, Martin U. Scalable expansion of human pluripotent stem cells in suspension culture. Nat Protoc. 2011;6:689–700.
110. Shiba Y, Fernandes S, Zhu WZ, Filice D, Muskheli V, Kim J, et al. Human ES-cell-derived cardiomyocytes electrically couple and suppress arrhythmias in injured hearts. Nature. 2012;489:322–5.
111. Qian L, Huang Y, Spencer CI, Foley A, Vedantham V, Liu L, et al. In vivo reprogramming of murine cardiac fibroblasts into induced cardiomyocytes. Nature. 2012;485:593–8.
112. Song K, Nam YJ, Luo X, Qi X, Tan W, Huang GN, et al. Heart repair by reprogramming non-myocytes with cardiac transcription factors. Nature. 2012;485:599–604.
113. Zohlnhofer D, Dibra A, Koppara T, de Waha A, Ripa RS, Kastrup J, et al. Stem cell mobilization by granulocyte colony-stimulating factor for myocardial recovery after acute myocardial infarction: a meta-analysis. J Am Coll Cardiol. 2008;51:1429–37.
114. Najjar SS, Rao SV, Melloni C, Raman SV, Povsic TJ, Melton L, et al. Intravenous erythropoietin in patients with ST-segment elevation myocardial infarction: REVEAL: a randomized controlled trial. JAMA. 2011;305:1863–72.
115. Ogura Y, Ouchi N, Ohashi K, Shibata R, Kataoka Y, Kambara T, et al. Therapeutic impact of follistatin-like 1 on myocardial ischemic injury in preclinical models. Circulation. 2012;126:1728–38.
116. Hinkel R, El-Aouni C, Olson T, Horstkotte J, Mayer S, Muller S, et al. Thymosin beta4 is an essential paracrine factor of embryonic endothelial progenitor cell mediated cardioprotection. Circulation. 2008;117:2232–40.
117. Korf-Klingebiel M, Kempf T, Schluter KD, Willenbockel C, Brod T, Heineke J, et al. Conditional transgenic expression of fibroblast growth factor 9 in the adult mouse heart reduces heart failure mortality after myocardial infarction. Circulation. 2011;123:504–14.
118. Lee RH, Pulin AA, Seo MJ, Kota DJ, Ylostalo J, Larson BL, et al. Intravenous hMSCs improve myocardial infarction in mice because cells embolized in lung are activated to secrete the anti-inflammatory protein TSG-6. Cell Stem Cell. 2009;5:54–63.
119. Yaniz-Galende E, Chen J, Chemaly ER, Liang L, Hulot JS, McCollum L, et al. Stem cell factor gene transfer promotes cardiac repair after myocardial infarction via in situ recruitment and expansion of c-kit+ cells. Circ Res. 2012;111:1434–45.
120. He W, Zhang L, Ni A, Zhang Z, Mirotsou M, Mao L, et al. Exogenously administered secreted frizzled related protein 2 (Sfrp2) reduces fibrosis and improves cardiac function in a rat model of myocardial infarction. Proc Natl Acad Sci USA. 2010;107:21110–5.
121. Jarvinen TA, Ruoslahti E. Target-seeking antifibrotic compound enhances wound healing and suppresses scar formation in mice. Proc Natl Acad Sci USA. 2010;107:21671–6.
122. Ziegler M, Elvers M, Baumer Y, Leder C, Ochmann C, Schonberger T, et al. The bispecific SDF1-GPVI fusion protein preserves myocardial function after transient ischemia in mice. Circulation. 2012;125:685–96.

123. Schellenberger V, Wang CW, Geething NC, Spink BJ, Campbell A, To W, et al. A recombinant polypeptide extends the in vivo half-life of peptides and proteins in a tunable manner. Nat Biotechnol. 2009;27:1186–90.
124. Kanki S, Segers VF, Wu W, Kakkar R, Gannon J, Sys SU, et al. Stromal cell-derived factor-1 retention and cardioprotection for ischemic myocardium. Circ Heart Fail. 2011;4:509–18.
125. D'Alessandra Y, Pompilio G, Capogrossi MC. MicroRNAs and myocardial infarction. Curr Opin Cardiol. 2012;27:228–35.
126. Roy S, Sen CK. MiRNA in innate immune responses: novel players in wound inflammation. Physiol Genomics. 2011;43:557–65.
127. van Rooij E, Olson EN. MicroRNA therapeutics for cardiovascular disease: opportunities and obstacles. Nat Rev Drug Discov. 2012.

Chapter 9
Myocardial Stunning

Dennis V. Cokkinos

9.1 General Considerations [1]

This phenomenon represents a nonlethal complication of ischemia, when by definition this is reversed by reperfusion. The definition as given by Braunwald and Kloner [1] in 1982 is still being used today:

> "Delayed recovery of regional myocardial contractile function after reperfusion, despite the absence of reversible damage and despite restoration of normal flow."

It must be remembered that at this time restoration of blood flow after an acute myocardial infarction was just becoming a reality while wide application of thrombolysis and primary angioplasty was yet to follow. Actually the first laboratory observation of STUN comes from the team of Vatner [2]:

These investigators found that in conscious dogs, regional myocardial dysfunction persisted for 3 h after 5 min temporary coronary occlusion. Interestingly, if the duration of occlusion was increased to 15 min, this depression persisted for more than 6 h. These authors also described that electrocardiographic changes resolved more promptly.

Further studies followed with similar results [3–5].

As Bolli and Marban point out in a pertinent review in 1999 [6], an essential element of STUN is that no reversible damage is produced and that the dysfunction is not caused by a primary defect or deficit of myocardial perfusion, which in the clinical setting means that the dysfunctional myocardium is subtended by normal or near-normal flow [7].

Kloner et al. in 1998 [8] from the proceedings of a workshop of the National Heart, Lung, and Blood Institute pointed out that the manifestation of STUN could

D. V. Cokkinos (✉)
Heart and Vessel Department, Biomedical Research Foundation,
Academy of Athens - Gregory Skalkeas, Athens, Greece
e-mail: dcokkinos@bioacademy.gr

D. V. Cokkinos (ed.), *Myocardial Preservation*,
https://doi.org/10.1007/978-3-319-98186-4_9

be summarized as follows: Both clinically and experimentally STUN can be seen under the following circumstances:

(a) After a reversible application of ischemia, not longer than 20 min in a dog [5].
  The findings in humans with the applications of intermittent occlusion during the course of percutaneous coronary angioplasty (PTCA) will be discussed later on.
(b) After repeated brief interruptions of coronary flow. A caveat to this phenomenon is that multiple ischemic episodes can either cause hibernation as will be discussed in the corresponding chapter, or preconditioning [9].
(c) In some cases in the dog, with flow interruption >20 min but <3 h, most of the myocardium has reversible dysfunction [10, 11].

Verani et al. [12] have shown that systolic and diastolic dysfunction may persevere for up to 24 h [12].

Clinically, this phenomenon can occur in the human in the case of "aborted" myocardial infarction which was described in the previous chapter.

(d) After stress tests either with exercise or dobutamine in the human, as will be discussed later.
(e) After the application of cardioplegia either in animal models, mostly dogs and pigs, but also during open heart surgery in humans.

In more detail, STUN has been described in the following clinical settings:

9.1.1 At Percutaneous (PTCA)

These results come from early applications of the technique, at which longer inflation-occlusion times were used. Thus, Serruys et al. [13] found that after 4–6 inflations of a total duration of 252 s, regional dysfunction occurred which was restored to normal.

Sheiban et al. [14] found that inflations up to 5–7 min were followed by myocardial dysfunction for up to 24–26 h.

As regards diastolic dysfunction, Wijns et al. [15] also found that it was also affected.

9.1.2 Angina Pectoris

Here unstable angina is mainly described. Thus, Nixon et al. in 1982 [16] described persistent cardiac dysfunction after unstable angina episodes with 2D echocardiography.

de Feyter et al. [17] and Renkin et al. [18] found similar results; notably in their pts, eventual angioplasty improved these results. Bolli et al. [19] also reported myocardial dysfunction lasting up to days after unstable angina.

Tamaki et al. [20] using an ambulatory radionuclide detector found dysfunction after ischemic events, during everyday activities.

Of course, nowadays the diagnosis of unstable angina versus that of non-ST elevation myocardial infarction is made with troponin assay which was not available during these earlier studies.

Another type of unstable angina which comes close to experimental studies is Prinzmetal's angina caused by coronary arterial spasm when it occurs in pts with normal coronary arteries [21]. Interestingly, after episodes of Prinzmetal's angina, a persistent decrease of adrenergic receptors has been found, as evidenced by defects of MIBG scintigraphy [22].

9.1.3 Acute Myocardial Infarction

The problem of myocardial necrosis is discussed in the chapter on ischemia reperfusion injury. What has been noted since the early applications of intracoronary infusion of streptokinase in 1981 [22] was that myocardial regional function improved not right after the drug administration but within 1–10 days, even within 16 days according to Stack et al. [23]. This gradual improvement has been associated with the resolution of myocardial ST.

Further observations have been contributed by Schmidt et al. [24] who stress that after an acute myocardial infarction subjected to intracoronary thrombolysis, the initial regional improvement was slow but was accelerated after 3 days up to 6 months. Bourdillon et al. [25] reported different results: The greater improvement was seen at the first 3 days, with less improvement afterward.

In these cases, as discussed by A. Kokkinos [26], it is difficult to assess if further myocardial function improvement is hampered by the residual coronary stenosis which is not improved by thrombolysis. Actually, Sheehan [27] have found the degree of residual stenosis was a determining factor for the resolution of STUN.

However, similar findings were seen early on with primary angioplasty, with improvement of diastolic filling within 7 days after an acute infarct [28].

In this clinical context, the early laboratory findings of Reimer and Jennings are important [29]. They described that cells displaying properties of "stunned" myocardium, located mainly in the subepicardium and mid-myocardium, have been salvaged and gradually show improved contractility [30, 31].

9.1.4 Exercise-Induced Ischemia

Bolli and Marban [6] describe stunning after exercise-induced ischemia. Before discussing the role of coronary arterial stenosis in this process, they mention that STUN can be produced after exercise in dogs and left ventricular hypertrophy in the absence of any coronary stenosis [32].

Obviously, in this case, the inappropriate increase in myocardial mass makes its satisfactory perfusion difficult to achieve. This has actually been shown by exercise thallium 201 scintigraphy [33]; in a similar way prolonged recovery after exercise has been found in pts with idiopathic dilated cardiomyopathy [34].

A wide array of data has been given for exercise-induced STUN in pts with coronary artery disease.

Among the earliest studies, Robertson et al. [35] studied pts with more 2D echocardiography and found longer dysfunction times in pts with more than one-vessel disease, persisting for around 30 min or more.

Kloner et al. [36] found similar results with Tl^{99} sestamibi; transient wall motion abnormality was greater with severe ischemia. Rinaldi et al. [37] found both systolic and diastolic dysfunction after exercise and postulated that STUN may persist for up to 60 min.

Sustained diastolic dysfunction was also seen after the exercise by Fragasso et al. [38]. STUN was also recorded with radionuclide ventriculography by the groups of Schneider et al. [39] and Vatterott et al. [40].

However, STUN is not caused only by exercise. Tsoukas et al. [41] from the group of P. Nihoyannopoulos found that after dobutamine stress test, systolic dysfunction was seen during stress and regressed after 15–20–25 min in pts with one-, two-, and three-vessel disease, respectively. Interestingly, dysfunction persisted after regression of electrocardiographic changes.

Camici et al. [42] used PET to assess STUN after treadmill exercise. They found persistence uptake of 18FDG after regression of ischemia. In this context, the time course of STUN can be different as well as its differentiation from hibernation according to the histologic technique which is described by Kloner and Jennings [43].

9.1.5 Stunning in Other Conditions

It has been well described that atrial STUN can be seen after the electric cardioversion of atrial fibrillation, which can actually persist for days and can cause embolic phenomena and acute pulmonary edema [44–48].

Our group some years ago showed that angiotensin receptor blockers could diminish this phenomenon [49].

Apart from atrial STUN, Fung et al. [50] have shown that cardioversion could cause ventricular dysfunction.

Three more interesting manifestations of STUN have emerged over the last years:

9.2 Hemodialysis

Since 2007 Selby and McIntyre [51] have described that acute cardiac dysfunction can occur during dialysis.

Zuidema and Dellsperger [52] give a detailed report.

They noted that at multivariate analysis age, predialysis troponin T levels, hypotension during hemodialysis, and ultrafiltration volumes independently predicted STUN.

Apart from other factors which in common contribute to the cause of STUN, in hemodialysis additional considerations should be mentioned.

Thus, increased volume loss by ultrafiltration may produce hemoconcentration with microcirculatory shear stress and reduced perfusion. In fact, Mclytyre et al. [53] have shown that STUN during hemodialysis is associated with an acute reduction in global and segmental myocardial blood flow.

9.3 Sepsis

It is another cause of reversible cardiac dysfunction.

Most probably, acute sepsis causes cardiac dysfunction, among others through the β-adrenergic pathway [54].

Similarly, lipopolysaccharide infusion can cause transient myocardial dysfunction in the human [55].

9.4 Takotsubo Cardiomyopathy

This has been widely studied over the last years.

Actually, Guaricci et al. [56] in a recent review place it in the description of myocardial STUN. The name of the syndrome comes from the Japanese, meaning octopus trap because of the peculiar shape with apical ballooning which the heart acquires in the majority of cases.

Other names given are "broken heart syndrome." The European Society of Cardiology lists it as unclassified cardiomyopathy [57].

The syndrome is characterized by striking left ventricular dysfunction which emerges in response to mental stress. As causative factors, catecholamine-mediated STUN, multivessel coronary vasospasm, and microvascular dysfunction are enumerated [58, 59].

In supraphysiological doses, epinephrine can, according to Paur et al. [60], manifest negative inotropic effects: β2-adrenergic receptors activate the inhibitory adenylate cycle (cAMP) G protein.

The apical ballooning which characterizes the majority of cases is ascribed to the much greater (tenfold) sympathetic intervention of the left ventricular apex as compared to the base [61].

It is interesting that Paur et al. [60] in an animal model showed that epinephrine and not norepinephrine could induce the Takotsubo syndrome; they postulate that the latter has a lower affinity to β2-adrenergic receptors.

It must be remembered that this syndrome had been described under another term but with a similar picture. Neurogenic STUN was seen in acute cerebral episodes [62] and subarachnoid hemorrhage [63].

Dawson [64] also gives a very recent review on Takotsubo cardiomyopathy, stressing that although typically the syndrome occurs with normal coronary arteries, incidental coronary artery disease has been found; also the possible influence of norepinephrine and dopamine has been postulated [65].

The same author [64] describes the sequelae of the cardiomyopathic episode, in that the follow-up of pts demonstrating this syndrome is not innocent, resembling that of a classical myocardial infarction [66, 67].

In the same vein, over many years, cardiomyopathy has been described in pheochromocytoma [68].

In a very recent editorial, Tofield [69] describes the creation of a global international Takotsubo registry and reminds that even great and sudden joy can trigger a similar picture. He mentions that pheochromocytoma no longer excludes the presence of the syndrome and that coronary artery disease is not considered an exclusion criterion.

Here it must be stressed that as in many other, already described, cases of STUN, it cannot be ascertained if during transient dysfunction cardiomyocyte death does not occur.

The above-described categories of STUN give another concept of STUN, that under certain circumstances of increased oxygen needs (tachycardia, increased contractility), coronary flow is not adequate to support tissue needs and hypoxia-driven dysfunction ensues. This may be further compounded by vasoconstriction.

9.4.1 Thyroid Disorders

In the chapter on cardiac remodeling, the beneficial actions of thyroid hormones on the myocardial are described. However, hyperthyroidism itself can cause myocardial STUN [70].

Cocaine use can cause acute heart failure. This may be ascribed to the decrease of uptake of norepinephrine by the heart and spleen, thus allowing free epinephrine to activate the adrenergic receptors [71].

According to Guaricci et al. [56], the mitochondria may be involved in this process, and cocaine can promote apoptotic pathways, Fas-dependent and mitochondria-dependent.

9.4.2 Tachycardia Induced Cardiomyopathy

This type of reversible heart failure has been described since many years [72, 73]. It is usually reversible when tachycardia is converted or ablated, but residual dysfunction may persist; here it must be reminded that this type of arrhythmia often occurs in abnormal hearts [74].

However, incessant tachycardia can cause dysfunction even in normal hearts.

9.4.3 Mechanisms: Pathophysiology of Stunning

As Guaricci et al. [56] point out, multiple hypotheses exist. Kim et al. [75] also gave a detailed review some years ago. Most authors agree that two hypotheses exist which are not mutually exclusive [76].

The first is overexpression of free oxygen radicals (ROS). Kloner and Jennings [77] in 2001 described the "oxyradical hypothesis" based on an initial series of experiments by Roberto Bolli's group [78], according to which 50% to 70% of the STUN effect is due to an explosive increase of ROS, during the first reperfusion minutes. Bolli and Marban [6] point out that differences as regards production of ROS and severity of STUN are greater in open chest as compared to conscious dogs, due to artifacts in the former model. Indeed, increase of the production of ROS was subsequently verified in the conscious dog model within 15 min coronary occlusion [79, 80, 82].

According to Bolli and Marban [6], the exact source of oxyradical production is not clear. In the rat and canine models, xanthine oxidase may be a major source [80, 81].

However, they point out that antioxidants decrease STUN in rabbits [83] and pigs [84] in which xanthine oxidase activity is very low. Also, according to Bolli and Marban [6], antioxidants can diminish post-global ischemia in isolated hearts [84].

However, in various models with the use of superoxide dismutase and catalase, results have been conflicting [6, 85].

Sekili et al. [80] postulate that the hydroxyl radical (-OH) may be the main mediator of STUN. Also they propose that NO released during reperfusion can react with superoxide to produce peroxynitrite [86].

Additionally Kloner and Jennings [43] propose that ROS can react with proteins, phospholipids, and thiols. Bolli and Marban [6] also describe that ROS "attack" the sarcolemma, interfering with its calcium transport and Ca2+ ATPase activity [80].

They also inhibit Na + K + ATPase [87], thus resulting in sodium overload with consequent activation of the Na + Ca + exchange activity [86] and calcium overload. Bolli and Marban [6] stress the "calcium hypothesis," which they propose includes three distinct possible mechanisms: decreased responsiveness of the contractile proteins to Ca2+, Ca2+ overload, and excitation-contraction uncoupling due to sarcoplasmic reticulum dysfunction. It is postulated that ROS can be the case of Ca2+ overload [88].

In the stunned myocardium, Bolli and Marban [6] point out that there is agreement that Ca2+ availability is not limited to the stunned myocardium but the main problem may be a reduction of maximal Ca2+ activated force.

Additionally, Guaricci et al. [56] point out that Ca2+ overload may activate proteases such as calpain I, which results in troponin I degradation and contractile dysfunction [89].

These effects may be prevented with the calpain inhibitor calpastatin [90].

Here it must be repeated that it is not proven that in STUN, no cardiomyocyte death is produced. Actually Guaricci et al. [56] point out that inflammation apoptosis may be involved [91].

This brings into question the finding that serum troponin is elevated in cases in which cardiomyocyte death is not probable, such as exercise-induced ischemia as our group has recently shown [92] and in heart failure [93]. It is postulated that this increase in the periphery altered myocardial membrane permeability [92–94] or micronecrosis [95] or myocardial fibrosis [96].

9.5 Stunning After Cardiac Surgery

One aspect of ST already referred to must be again discussed; STUN may protect the heart through dysfunction to prevent cell death. It is reminded that in the chapter on conditioning, inhibition of the contractile apparatus is a main feature of its induction of cardioprotection.

9.5.1 Genomics of Protection in STUN

Depré and Vatner [97] give a detailed account. They estimate that many genes that were upregulated in the stunned myocardium are involved in growth mechanisms, such as ATF-3, CAPP, elongation factors, H11 kinase, endonexin, and P311. Additional factors are:

9.5.2 Cytoprotection

αβ-Crystallin; HSP20, 27, and 70; and AMP-activated protein kinase

9.5.3 Anti-apoptosis

PAI-1 and 2, inhibitor of apoptosis (IAP), and early growth factor

9.5.4 Therapeutic Aspects

It was already been discussed that catecholamines when given acutely can decrease the myocardial dysfunction associated with STUN [7]; however long term, they are well-known to be deleterious. Levosimendan, a calcium-sensitizing agent, can be beneficial in acute and chronic heart failure [98, 99].

Old drugs discussed in the chapter on ischemia reperfusion injury especially β-blockers can obviously be applicable to STUN prevention. Also, limiting the severity and duration of ischemia can diminish STUN. Moreover, late preconditioning has been shown to prevent STUN.

Efforts at decreasing postischemic contractile dysfunction are being proposed [100] for many years [101].

More details are given in the chapter on ischemia reperfusion injury.

In conclusion, STUN occurs in many stressful situations especially in the setting of reversible myocardial ischemia. It is characterized by transient systolic and diastolic dysfunction which may in some cases jeopardize the myocardium and tilt the tables toward acute heart failure. Its main causes are ROS overproduction and Ca^{2+} overload, noxious processes which can be interconnected through causative mechanisms. Early correction is the best way to prevent or diminish it together with other widely employed cardioprotective measures, including late preconditioning.

References

1. Braunwald E, Kloner RA. The stunned myocardium: prolonged, postischemic ventricular dysfunction. Circulation. 1982;66:1146–9.
2. Heyndrickx GR, Millard RW, McRitchie RJ, Maroko PR, Vatner SF. Regional myocardial functional and electrophysiological alterations after brief coronary artery occlusion in conscious dogs. J Clin Invest. 1975;56:978–85.
3. Weiner JM, Astein CS, Arthur JH, Pirzada FA, Hood WB Jr. Persistence of myocardial injury following brief periods of coronary occlusion. Cardiovasc Res. 1976;10:678–86.
4. Kloner RA, Ellis SG, Lange R, Braunwald E. Studies of experimental coronary artery reperfusion. Effects on infarct size, myocardial function, biochemistry, ultrastructure and microvascular damage. Circulation. 1983;68:I8–15.
5. Bolli R, Zhu WX, Thornby JI, O'Neill PG, Roberts R. Time course and determinants of recovery of function after reversible ischemia in conscious dogs. Am J Phys. 1988;254:H102–14.
6. Bolli R, Marbán E. Molecular and cellular mechanisms of myocardial stunning. Physiol Rev. 1999;79:609–34.
7. Bolli R. Myocardial 'stunning' in man. Circulation. 1992;86:1671–91.
8. Kloner RA, Bolli R, Marban E, Reinlib L, Braunwald E. Medical and cellular implications of stunning, hibernation, and preconditioning: an NHLBI workshop. Circulation. 1998;97:1848–67.
9. Cohen MV, Downey JM. Myocardial stunning in dogs: preconditioning effect and influence of coronary collateral flow. Am Heart J. 1990;120:282–91.
10. Lavallee M, Cox D, Patrick TA, Vatner SF. Salvage of myocardial function by coronary artery reperfusion 1, 2, and 3 hours after occlusion in conscious dogs. Circ Res. 1983;53:235–47.
11. Bush LR, Buja LM, Samowitz W, Rude RE, Wathen M, Tilton GD, et al. Recovery of left ventricular segmental function after long-term reperfusion following temporary coronary occlusion in conscious dogs. Comparison of 2- and 4-hour occlusions. Circ Res. 1983;53:248–63.
12. Verani MS, Bolli R, Tadros S, Myers ML, Borges Neto S, Jain A, et al. Dissociation between global and regional systolic and diastolic ventricular function during coronary occlusion and reperfusion. Heart J. 1987;114:687–95.
13. Serruys PW, Wijns W, van den Brand M, Meij S, Slager C, Schuurbiers JC, et al. Left ventricular performance, regional blood flow, wall motion, and lactate metabolism during transluminal angioplasty. Circulation. 1984;70:25–36.
14. Sheiban I, Tonni S, Marini A, Trevi G. Clinical and therapeutic implications of chronic left ventricular dysfunction in coronary artery disease. Am J Cardiol. 1995;75:23E–30E.

15. Wijns W, Serruys PW, Slager CJ, Grimm J, Krayenbuehl HP, Hugenholtz PG, et al. Effect of coronary occlusion during percutaneous transluminal angioplasty in humans on left ventricular chamber stiffness and regional diastolic pressure-radius relations. J Am Coll Cardiol. 1986;7:455–63.
16. Nixon JV, Brown CN, Smitherman TC. Identification of transient and persistent segmental wall motion abnormalities in patients with unstable angina by two-dimensional echocardiography. Circulation. 1982;65:1497–503.
17. de Feyter PJ, Suryapranata H, Serruys PW, Beatt K, van den Brand M, Hugenholtz PG. Effects of successful percutaneous transluminal coronary angioplasty on global and regional left ventricular function in unstable angina pectoris. Am J Cardiol. 1987;60:993–7.
18. Renkin J, Wijns W, Ladha Z, Col J. Reversal of segmental hypokinesis by coronary angioplasty in patients with unstable angina, persistent T wave inversion, and left anterior descending coronary artery stenosis. Additional evidence for myocardial stunning in humans. Circulation. 1990;82:913–21.
19. Bolli R, Hartley CJ, Rabinovitz RS. Clinical Relevance of Myocardial Stunning. In: Opie LH, editor. Stunning, hibernating and calcium in myocardial ischemia and reperfusion: Kluver Academic publishers; 1992. p. 56–82.
20. Tamaki N, Yasuda T, Moore RH, Gill JB, Boucher CA, Hutter AM Jr, et al. Continuous monitoring of left ventricular function by an ambulatory radionuclide detector in patients with coronary artery disease. J Am Coll Cardiol. 1988;12:669–79.
21. Mathias P, Kerin NZ, Blevins RD, Cascade P, Rubenfire M. Coronary vasospasm as a cause of stunned myocardium. Am Heart J. 1987;113:383–5.
22. Sakata K, Miura F, Sugino H, Saegusa T, Shirotani M, Yoshida H, et al. Assessment of regional sympathetic nerve activity in vasospastic angina: analysis of iodine 123-labeled metaiodobenzylguanidine scintigraphy. Am Heart J. 1997;133:484–9.
23. Stack RS, Phillips HR 3rd, Grierson DS, Behar VS, Kong Y, Peter RH, et al. Functional improvement of jeopardized myocardium following intracoronary streptokinase infusion in acute myocardial infarction. J Clin Invest. 1983;72:84–95.
24. Schmidt WG, Sheehan FH, von Essen R, Uebis R, Effert S. Evolution of left ventricular function after intracoronary thrombolysis for acute myocardial infarction. Am J Cardiol. 1989;63:497–502.
25. Bourdillon PD, Broderick TM, Williams ES, Davis C, Dillon JC, Armstrong WF, et al. Early recovery of regional left ventricular function after reperfusion in acute myocardial infarction assessed by serial two-dimensional echocardiography. Am J Cardiol. 1989;63:641–6.
26. Kokkinos AD. Investigation of cardioprotection induced by ischemic preconditioning in ischemic heart which have been subjected to an initial ischemic episode PhD. Thesis Athens; 2002, p. 19–22.
27. Sheehan FH, Mathey DG, Schofer J, Dodge HT, Bolson EL. Factors that determine recovery of left ventricular function after thrombolysis in patients with acute myocardial infarction. Circulation. 1985;71:1121–8.
28. Williamson BD, Lim MJ, Buda AJ. Transient left ventricular filling abnormalities (diastolic stunning) after acute myocardial infarction. Am J Cardiol. 1990;66:897–903.
29. Reimer KA, Jennings RB. The "wavefront phenomenon" of myocardial ischemic cell death. II. Transmural progression of necrosis within the framework of ischemic bed size (myocardium at risk) and collateral flow. Lab Investig. 1979;40:633–44.
30. Ellis SG, Henschke CI, Sandor T, Wynne J, Braunwald E, Kloner RA. Time course of functional and biochemical recovery of myocardium salvaged by reperfusion. J Am Coll Cardiol. 1983;1:1047–55.
31. Theroux P, Ross J Jr, Franklin D, Kemper WS, Sasayama S. Coronary arterial reperfusion. III. Early and late effects on regional myocardial function and dimensions in conscious dogs. Am J Cardiol. 1976;38:599–606.
32. Hittinger L, Shannon RP, Kohin S, Manders WT, Kelly P, Vatner SF. Exercise-induced subendocardial dysfunction in dogs with left ventricular hypertrophy. Circ Res. 1990;66:329–43.

33. Emmett L, Magee M, Freedman SB, Van der Wall H, Bush V, Trieu J, et al. The role of left ventricular hypertrophy and diabetes in the presence of transient ischemic dilation of the left ventricle on myocardial perfusion SPECT images. J Nucl Med. 2005;46:1596–601.
34. Tanabe Y, Takahashi M, Hosaka Y, Ito M, Ito E, Suzuki K. Prolonged recovery of cardiac output after maximal exercise in patients with chronic heart failure. J Am Coll Cardiol. 2000;35:1228–36.
35. Robertson WS, Feigenbaum H, Armstrong WF, Dillon JC, O'Donnell J, McHenry PW. Exercise echocardiography: a clinically practical addition in the evaluation of coronary artery disease. J Am Coll Cardiol. 1983;2:1085–91.
36. Kloner RA, Allen J, Cox TA, Zheng Y, Ruiz CE. Stunned left ventricular myocardium after exercise treadmill testing in coronary artery disease. Am J Cardiol. 1991;68:329–34.
37. Rinaldi CA, Linka AZ, Masani ND, Avery PG, Jones E, Saunders H, et al. Randomized, double-blind crossover study to investigate the effects of amlodipine and isosorbide mononitrate on the time course and severity of exercise-induced myocardial stunning. Circulation. 1998;98:749–56.
38. Fragasso G, Benti R, Sciammarella M, Rossetti E, Savi A, Gerundini P, et al. Symptom-limited exercise testing causes sustained diastolic dysfunction in patients with coronary disease and low effort tolerance. J Am Coll Cardiol. 1991;17:1251–15.
39. Schneider RM, Weintraub WS, Klein LW, Seelaus PA, Agarwal JB, Helfant RH. Rate of left ventricular functional recovery by radionuclide angiography after exercise in coronary artery disease. Am J Cardiol. 1986;57:927–32.
40. Vatterott PJ, Hanley PC, Mankin HT, Gibbons RJ. The divergent recovery of ST-segment depression and radionuclide angiographic indicators of myocardial ischemia. Am J Cardiol. 1990;66:296–301.
41. Tsoukas A, Ikonomidis I, Cokkinos P, Nihoyannopoulos P. Significance of persistent left ventricular dysfunction during recovery after dobutamine stress echocardiography. J Am Coll Cardiol. 1997;30:621–6.
42. Camici P, Araujo LI, Spinks T, Lammertsma AA, Kaski JC, Shea MJ, et al. Increased uptake of 18F-fluorodeoxyglucose in postischemic myocardium of patients with exercise-induced angina. Circulation. 1986;74:81–8.
43. Kloner RA, Jennings RB. Consequences of brief ischemia: stunning, preconditioning, and their clinical implications: part 2. Circulation. 2001;104:3158–67.
44. Harjai K, Mobarek S, Abi-Samra F, Gilliland Y, Davison N, Drake K, et al. Mechanical dysfunction of the left atrium and the left atrial appendage following cardioversion of atrial fibrillation and its relation to total electrical energy used for cardioversion. Am J Cardiol. 1998;81:1125–9.
45. Fatkin D, Kuchar DL, Thorburn CW, Feneley MP. Transesophageal echocardiography before and during direct current cardioversion of atrial fibrillation: evidence for "atrial stunning" as a mechanism of thromboembolic complications. J Am Coll Cardiol. 1994;23:307–16.
46. Jordaens L, Missault L, Germonpré E, Callens B, Adang L, Vandenbogaerde J, et al. Delayed restoration of atrial function after conversion of atrial flutter by pacing or electrical cardioversion. Am J Cardiol. 1993;71:63–7.
47. Dabek J, Gasior Z, Monastyrska-Cup B, Jakubowski D. Cardioversion and atrial stunning. Pol Merkur Lekarski. 2007;22:224–8.
48. Antonielli E, Pizzuti A, Dogliani S, Stasi M, Bassignana A, Doronzo B. Absence of left atrial stunning after cardioversion of recent-onset atrial fibrillation in patients at low-stroke risk. Eur J Emerg Med. 2017;24:217–23.
49. Dagres N, Karatasakis G, Panou F, Athanassopoulos G, Maounis T, Tsougos E, et al. Pretreatment with Irbesartan attenuates left atrial stunning after electrical cardioversion of atrial fibrillation. Eur Heart J. 2006;27:2062–8.
50. Fung KC, Tan HC, Kritharides L. Acute reductions in ventricular myocardial tissue velocities after direct current cardioversion of atrial fibrillation. J Am Soc Echocardiogr. 2003;16:656–63.

51. Selby NM, McIntyre CW. The acute cardiac effects of dialysis. Semin Dial. 2007;20:220–8.
52. Zuidema MY, Dellsperger KC. Myocardial stunning with hemodialysis: clinical challenges of the cardiorenal patient. Cardiorenal Med. 2012;2:125–33.
53. McIntyre CW, Burton JO, Selby NM, Leccisotti L, Korsheed S, Baker CS, et al. Hemodialysis-induced cardiac dysfunction is associated with an acute reduction in global and segmental myocardial blood flow. Clin J Am Soc Nephrol. 2008;3:19–26.
54. Suzuki T, Suzuki Y, Okuda J, Kurazumi T, Suhara T, Ueda T, et al. Sepsis-induced cardiac dysfunction and β-adrenergic blockade therapy for sepsis. J Intensive Care. 2017;5:22.
55. Suffredini AF, Fromm RE, Parker MM, Brenner M, Kovacs JA, Wesley RA, et al. The cardiovascular response of normal humans to the administration of endotoxin. N Engl J Med. 1989;321:280–7.
56. Guaricci AI, Bulzis G, Pontone G, Scicchitano P, Carbonara R, Rabbat M, et al. Current interpretation of myocardial stunning. Trends Cardiovasc Med. 2018;28:263–71.
57. Lyon AR, Bossone E, Schneider B, Sechtem U, Citro R, Underwood SR, et al. Current state of knowledge on Takotsubo syndrome: a Position Statement from the Taskforce on Takotsubo Syndrome of the Heart Failure Association of the European Society of Cardiology. Eur J Heart Fail. 2016;18:8–27.
58. Williams R, Arri S, Prasad A. Current Concepts in the Pathogenesis of Takotsubo Syndrome. Heart Fail Clin. 2016;12:473–84.
59. Boland TA, Lee VH, Bleck TP. Stress-induced cardiomyopathy. Crit Care Med. 2015;43:686–93.
60. Paur H, Wright PT, Sikkel MB, Tranter MH, Mansfield C, O'Gara P, et al. High levels of circulating epinephrine trigger apical cardiodepression in a β2-adrenergic receptor/Gi-dependent manner: a new model of Takotsubo cardiomyopathy. Circulation. 2012;126:697–706.
61. Lyon AR, Rees PS, Prasad S, Poole-Wilson PA, Harding SE. Stress (Takotsubo) cardiomyopathy – a novel pathophysiological hypothesis to explain catecholamine-induced acute myocardial stunning. Nat Clin Pract Cardiovasc Med. 2008;5:22–9.
62. Murthy SB, Shah S, Venkatasubba Rao CP, Suarez JI, Bershad EM. Clinical characteristics of myocardial stunning in acute stroke. J Clin Neurosci. 2014;21:1279–82.
63. Sugimoto K, Inamasu J, Hirose Y, Kato Y, Ito K, Iwase M, et al. The role of norepinephrine and estradiol in the pathogenesis of cardiac wall motion abnormality associated with subarachnoid hemorrhage. Stroke. 2012;43:1897–903.
64. Dawson DK. Acute stress-induced (takotsubo) cardiomyopathy. Heart. 2018;104:96–102.
65. Wittstein IS, Thiemann DR, Lima JA, Baughman KL, Schulman SP, Gerstenblith G, et al. Neurohumoral features of myocardial stunning due to sudden emotional stress. N Engl J Med. 2005;352:539–48.
66. Templin C, Ghadri JR, Diekmann J, Napp LC, Bataiosu DR, Jaguszewski M, et al. Clinical Features and Outcomes of Takotsubo (Stress) Cardiomyopathy. N Engl J Med. 2015;373:929–38.
67. Tornvall P, Collste O, Ehrenborg E, Järnbert-Petterson H. A case-control study of risk markers and mortality in takotsubo stress cardiomyopathy. J Am Coll Cardiol. 2016;67:1931–6.
68. Varghese RT, John AM, Paul TV. Catecholamine induced cardiomyopathy in pheochromocytoma. Indian J Endocrinol Metab. 2013;17:733–5.
69. Tofield A. Connecting the pieces of Takotsubo 'broken heart'. Eur Heart J. 2018;39:2021–2.
70. Pereira N, Parisi A, Dec GW, Choo J, Hajjar R, Gordon PC. Myocardial stunning in hyperthyroidism. Clin Cardiol. 2000;23:298–300.
71. Schwartz BG, Rezkalla S, Kloner RA. Cardiovascular effects of cocaine. Circulation. 2010;122:2558–69.
72. Cruz FE, Cheriex EC, Smeets JL, Atié J, Peres AK, Penn OC, et al. Reversibility of tachycardia-induced cardiomyopathy after cure of incessant supraventricular tachycardia. J Am Coll Cardiol. 1990;16:739–44.
73. Tanaka R, Spinale FG, Crawford FA, Zile MR. Effect of chronic supraventricular tachycardia on left ventricular function and structure in newborn pigs. J Am Coll Cardiol. 1992;20:1650–60.

74. Spinale FG, Holzgrefe HH, Mukherjee R, Arthur SR, Child MJ, Powell JR, et al. LV and myocyte structure and function after early recovery from tachycardia-induced cardiomyopathy. Am J Phys. 1995;268:H836–47.
75. Kim SJ, Depre C, Vatner SF. Novel mechanisms mediating stunned myocardium. Heart Fail Rev. 2003;8:143–53.
76. Pantos C, Mourouzis I, Cokkinos DV. Myocardial ischemia. Basic concepts. In: Myocardial Ischemia. p. 11–76.
77. Kloner RA, Jennings RB. Consequences of brief ischemia: stunning, preconditioning, and their clinical implications: part 1. Circulation. 2001;104:2981–9.
78. Bolli R, Patel BS, Jeroudi MO, Lai EK, McCay PB. Demonstration of free radical generation in "stunned" myocardium of intact dogs with the use of the spin trap alpha-phenyl N-tert-butyl nitrone. J Clin Invest. 1988;82:476–85.
79. Li XY, McCay PB, Zughaib M, Jeroudi MO, Triana JF, Bolli R. Demonstration of free radical generation in the "stunned" myocardium in the conscious dog and identification of major differences between conscious and open-chest dogs. J Clin Invest. 1993;92:1025–41.
80. Sekili S, McCay PB, Li XY, Zughaib M, Sun JZ, Tang L, et al. Direct evidence that the hydroxyl radical plays a pathogenetic role in myocardial "stunning" in the conscious dog and demonstration that stunning can be markedly attenuated without subsequent adverse effects. Circ Res. 1993;73:705–23.
81. Charlat MI, O'Neill PG, Egan JM, Abernethy DR, Michael LH, Myers ML, et al. Evidence for a pathogenetic role of xanthine oxidase in the "stunned" myocardium. Am J Phys. 1987;252:H566–77.
82. Xia Y, Zweier JL. Substrate control of free radical generation from xanthine oxidase in the postischemic heart. J Biol Chem. 1995;270:18797–803.
83. Tang X-L, Rizvi AN, Qiu Y, et al. Evidence that the hydroxyl radical triggers late preconditioning against myocardial stunning in conscious rabbits. Circulation. 1997;96(Suppl I):I–255.
84. Sun JZ, Tang XL, Park SW, Qiu Y, Turrens JF, Bolli R. Evidence for an essential role of reactive oxygen species in the genesis of late preconditioning against myocardial stunning in conscious pigs. J Clin Invest. 1996;97:562–76.
85. Shlafer M, Kane PF, Kirsh MM. Superoxide dismutase plus catalase enhances the efficacy of hypothermic cardioplegia to protect the globally ischemic, reperfused heart. J Thorac Cardiovasc Surg. 1982;83:830–9.
86. Ishida H, Genka C, Hirota Y, Hamasaki Y, Nakazawa H. Distinct roles of peroxynitrite and hydroxyl radical in triggering stunned myocardium-like impairment of cardiac myocytes in vitro. Mol Cell Biochem. 1999;198:31–8.
87. Renlund DG, Gerstenblith G, Lakatta EG, Jacobus WE, Kallman CH, Weisfeldt ML. Perfusate sodium during ischemia modifies post-ischemic functional and metabolic recovery in the rabbit heart. J Mol Cell Cardiol. 1984;16:795–801.
88. Corretti MC, Koretsune Y, Kusuoka H, Chacko VP, Zweier JL, Marban E. Glycolytic inhibition and calcium overload as consequences of exogenously generated free radicals in rabbit hearts. J Clin Invest. 1991;88:1014–25.
89. Van Eyk JE, Murphy AM. The role of troponin abnormalities as a cause for stunned myocardium. Coron Artery Dis. 2001;12:343–7.
90. Gao WD, Liu Y, Mellgren R, Marban E. Intrinsic myofilament alterations underlying the decreased contractility of stunned myocardium. A consequence of Ca2+–dependent proteolysis? Circ Res. 1996;78:455–65.
91. Anselmi A, Abbate A, Girola F, Nasso G, Biondi-Zoccai GG, Possati G, et al. Myocardial ischemia, stunning, inflammation, and apoptosis during cardiac surgery: a review of evidence. Eur J Cardiothorac Surg. 2004;25:304–11.
92. Pipikos T, Kapelouzou A, Tsilimigras DI, Fostinis Y, Pipikou M, Theodorakos A, et al. Stronger correlation with myocardial ischemia of highsensitivity troponin T than other biomarkers. J Nucl Cardiol. 2018. https://doi.org/10.1007/s12350-018-1199-6.

93. Januzzi JL Jr, Filippatos G, Nieminen M, Gheorghiade M. Troponin elevation in patients with heart failure: on behalf of the third Universal Definition of Myocardial Infarction Global Task Force: Heart Failure Section. Eur Heart J. 2012;33:2265–71.
94. Eisen A, Bonaca MP, Jarolim P, Scirica BM, White HD, Tendera M, et al. High-sensitivity troponin I in stable patients with atherosclerotic disease in the TRA 2°P – TIMI 50 trial. Clin Chem. 2017;63:307–15.
95. Ahmed W, Schlett CL, Uthamalingam S, Truong QA, Koenig W, Rogers IS, et al. Single resting hsTnT level predicts abnormal myocardial stress test in acute chest pain patients with normal initial standard troponin. JACC Cardiovasc Imaging. 2013;6:72–82.
96. Seydelmann N, Liu D, Krämer J, Drechsler C, Hu K, Nordbeck P, et al. High-sensitivity troponin: a clinical blood biomarker for staging cardiomyopathy in fabry disease. J Am Heart Assoc. 2016;5(6). pii: e002839.
97. Depre C, Vatner SF. Cardioprotection in stunned and hibernating myocardium. Heart Fail Rev. 2007;12:307–17.
98. García González MJ, Domínguez RA. Pharmacologic treatment of heart failure due to ventricular dysfunction by myocardial stunning: potential role of levosimendan. Am J Cardiovasc Drugs. 2006;6:69–75.
99. García-González MJ, Domínguez-Rodríguez A, Ferrer-Hita JJ. Utility of levosimendan, a new calcium sensitizing agent, in the treatment of cardiogenic shock due to myocardial stunning in patients with ST-elevation myocardial infarction: a series of cases. J Clin Pharmacol. 2005;45:704–8.
100. Sun JZ, Tang XL, Knowlton AA, Park SW, Qiu Y, Bolli R. Late preconditioning against myocardial stunning. An endogenous protective mechanism that confers resistance to postischemic dysfunction 24 h after brief ischemia in conscious pigs. J Clin Invest. 1995;95:388–403.
101. Gross GJ, Kersten JR, Warltier DC. Mechanisms of postischemic contractile dysfunction. Ann Thorac Surg. 1999;68:1898–904.

Chapter 10
Myocardial Hibernation

Dennis V. Cokkinos

Myocardial hibernation (HIB) plays a major role in current efforts to manage heart failure in patients with chronic ischemic heart disease.

This interesting term was first used by Diamond et al. [1] who described that in chronically ischemic and dysfunctional myocardium contractility could be increased by post extrasystolic potentiation by atrial stimulation. Subsequently, it was introduced and greatly popularized by Rahimtoola in a seminal article [2] in 1989. He gave the following description:

Hibernation is a state of persistently impaired myocardial and left ventricular (LV) function at rest due to reduced coronary blood flow that can be partially or completely restored to normal if the myocardial oxygen supply/ demand relationship is favorably altered, either by improving blood flow and/or reducing demand. According to the results of several types of studies, especially PET studies with fludexyglucose, the cardiac contractile tissue is still alive but depressed because the arterial flow is decreased. Moreover it can regain contractility if arterial flow is restored.

As a very distinguished triad of reviewers [3], suggest the term has been adapted from the animal kingdom, although seasonal plants can be postulated to hibernate in winter. It is called perennation or dormancy according to Wikipedia.

Thus the reduction of myocardial contractility is perceived as an adaptation to counteract the energy deficit, with the consequence of maintaining myocardial integrity and viability [4].

D. V. Cokkinos (✉)
Heart and Vessel Department, Biomedical Research Foundation,
Academy of Athens - Gregory Skalkeas, Athens, Greece
e-mail: dcokkinos@bioacademy.gr

D. V. Cokkinos (ed.), *Myocardial Preservation*,
https://doi.org/10.1007/978-3-319-98186-4_10

Stephen Vatner's group [5] studied an animal model of natural hibernation, the woodchucks in winter. These authors describe that in mammalian hibernation body functions are down-regulated during winter so survival can be effected in cold exposure and decreased energy (food) availability [6].

They found, as already mentioned in the chapter on conditioning, that hibernation and conditioning share many commonly regulated genes [7]. However, they [6] stress that some genes involved in conditioning (both first and second window), such as the adenosine A2B receptor, iNOS and COX2 were not upregulated in the woodchucks during winter. Additionally, they found that the CREB protein network is activated in the woodchuck but not involved in conditioning. CREB is involved in cell proliferation, differentiation, adaptation, survival and decrease of apoptosis [8] through upregulation of Bcl-2 [9].

In a simpler but interesting observation, Laske et al. [10] recorded the heart rate and corresponding activity of an adult female black bear during 6 years with an implanted monitor. At hibernation she had 22–25 beats per minute versus 95 in the summer. Birthing in January was marked by a transient increase in heart rate. Yan et al. [5] also point out very pertinently that in the human paradigm, coronary flow is emphatically reduced while it is normal in the hibernating animal. Braunwald and Rutherford [11] very early stressed the need for revascularization in order to reverse dysfunction.

Both Heusch and Schulz [12] and Ross [13] point out that there exists short and long term HIB.

Obviously, short-term HIB is difficult to differentiate from "stunning" pathophysiologically, although of course the mechanisms are different. Thus, Heusch and Schultz [12] in their Table 1 give the following characteristics which differentiate the two types of HIB:

10.1 Short-Term HIB Characteristics [12]

- Perfusion – contraction imbalance.
- Recovery of contractile function during reperfusion.
- Recovery of metabolic parameters during persistent ischemia.
- Recruitable inotropic reserve but at the expense of metabolic recovery.

The authors enlarge on this last item stressing that the increase of contractility during inotropic stimulation renews the supply demand imbalance caused by noxious sequelae (possible course towards cell injury). In the chapters on conditioning and stunning it is stressed that contractile apparatus inhibition is a key cardioprotective mechanism. Before discussing the long-term form, it must be remembered, and this is the "leitmotif" of this book, that in the clinical setting, a patient with significant stenosis of one or more coronary arteries can undergo an acute myocardial infarct, with myocardial loss coursing toward remodeling and heart failure, conditioning, stunning, or hibernation.

10.2 Long Term HIB

It is characterized by:

- A decrease in the number of myofibrils and increased collagen deposition.

Here it is stressed that HIB is a key element of cardiac remodeling as described in the respective chapter.

- Recovery of contractile function during reperfusion. This is a key feature of HIB, in that after myocardial flow is restored, cardiac function is expected to improve. Thus, the question of viability looms extremely important.

This chapter will focus mainly on long-term HIB because this form has the greater clinical consequences and because a separate chapter is devoted to myocardial stunning. This state implies an important stenosis of a vessel subtending a large area of myocardial area, i. e. multiple stenoses or left anterior artery stenosis.

Many animal studies have suggested that when a coronary stenosis reaches more than 70% of the lumen, no reactive hyperemia can be seen, i. e. coronary flow reserve is lost [14–16].

Camici and Rimoldi [17] give a detailed review of myocardial blood flow in pts with HIB.

These authors stress that hibernating myocardium is characterized by impaired coronary flow reserve. They also reiterate the evidence that repetitive ischemic stunning in pts may lead to a chronic stage of myocardial dysfunction characteristic of HIB, which may be in the other side of the coin with stunning.

Here however, the importance of regional coronary blood flow should be stressed. Gallagher et al. [18] have shown that there exists a linear relationship between systolic wall thickening and subendocardial or transmural flow but not epicardial flow.

According to Ross [13] critical residual metabolic flow levels for the maintenance of viability are 50% for total myocardial mass and 25% for subendocardial flow in the pig.

Schulz and Heusch [19] point out the need for repeated measurements of coronary blood flow.

Kloner et al. [20] in an important Workshop 20 years ago postulate that anaerobic metabolism exists in HIB, which maintains viability, although Ferrari [21] points out that the main element of levels of energy production during ischemia leading to HIB is the early diminution of high energy phosphate bonds. Creatinine phosphate decreases faster than ATP, resulting into an increase of inorganic phosphates and a decrease of pH, with decrease of cardiac contractility and diminution of oxidative mitochondrial injury. However, Flameng et al. [22] by studying biopsy samples with dysfunctional but viable myocardium found a normal ratio of ADP to ATP and creatine phosphate concentration.

Heusch et al. [3] in the aforementioned review describe the course of myocardial metabolism towards HIB. They describe again that during ischemia the recovery of the early disturbance of substrate and energy metabolism is parallel to the decrease of contractility; this restores myocardial energy balance. They also describe that in a swine model during the production of ischemia under anesthesia, early disturbances gradually return to normal during 180 min of sustained moderate ischemia [23]. They repeat that the most convincing explanation for the already mentioned restoration of creatine phosphate content and the energy change of ATP is the downregulation of energy demand through the decrease of contractility. However, they describe a different picture in chronic HIB. Thus in swine with 3 months' coronary stenosis there is a matched reduction in myocardial flow and function but importantly a reduction of myocardial oxygen consumption and lack of lactate extraction [24].

An increase of glucose extraction is a key element [25, 26].

Interestingly, in pigs with chronic coronary stenosis and chronic reduction in both myocardial flow and contractility, ATP and creatine phosphate contents were normal [27].

Heusch et al. [3] also describe studies in humans. Thus, preservation of ^{18}FDG uptake in areas with hypoperfusion and hypocontractility are predictive of recovery after revascularization [28–31]. These findings are in accordance with the clinical use of ^{18}FDG in myocardial viability studies which will be described subsequently.

According to Wiggers et al. [32] in humans, areas of myocardium with reversibility had a normal lactate and ATP production; fibrosis as a replacement mechanism was not evident. According to Heusch et al. [3] this may be the key difference from the results of Vogt et al. [33] also in humans, who found increased lactate and decreased ATP and creatine phosphate [33].

Studies with PET using C-11 acetate, an index of oxidative metabolism, showed that acetate clearance was reduced in regions with chronic HIB [34].

This reduction was largely related to the decreased blood flow.

Moreover in hibernating but viable myocardium in patients with an old infarct, low-dose dobutamine infusion was associated with an increase of inotropic reserve, together with an upregulation of acetate clearance [35].

According to Heusch et al. [3] in chronic HIB, the main characteristic is preservation of metabolic activity, with parallel preservation of cardiomyocyte integrity.

Glycogen content is also increased; according to Depré et al. [36]; these changes are analogous to the fetal heart changes.

Ng et al. [37] used acoustic microscopy to study hibernating myocardium; acoustic microscopy of normal cardiomyocytes showed intracellular linear echoes suggestive of myofibrils; cardiomyocytes of hibernating myocardium revealed absence of myofibrils and dense intracellular echoes that corresponded to glycogen accumulation on optical microscopy.

Reduced myofibrillar content and increased glycogen content was seen by Gunning et al. [38] with electron microscopy. Significantly, these authors found that the mean myocyte glycogen content is analogous to contractile reserve. This will be further discussed.

Borgers [39] remarks that glycogen occupies 2% of the cell volume in the adult but 30% in the fetal heart; a similar picture is seen in HIB which corresponds to a survival state with cells poor in contractile filaments but rich in glycogen.

Ausma et al. [40] in left ventricular biopsies from 21 pts with chronic HIB found that 27% of cardiomyocytes were characterized as hibernating because of a reduced number of myofibrils and increased glycogen content, suggestive of dedifferentiation rather than degeneration or apoptosis.

Here it must be mentioned that reduced expression of the glycogen synthase kinase 3β has been found in chronically hibernating myocardium, which may be responsible not only for the observed increased glycogen deposits, but also is an antisurvival kinase [41].

These findings bring into focus two key questions:

(a) Does HIB represent a return to the fetal phenotype, which, as described in the corresponding chapter is ischemia resistant?

Indeed, this is discussed by Borgers [39] who remarks that the adaptation to the fetal phenotype is a program of cell survival. The author points out, that the adoption of the fetal phenotype is also seen in the infarct border zones, end stage dilated cardiomyopathy, and atrial fibrillation [42]. Dispersyn et al. [42] in chronic hibernating myocardium (28 pts) found no apoptosis, or Bcl-2, p53 or PCNA changes in dedifferentiated myocardium; they postulate that HIB may be a prelude to apoptosis but not actually indicative of cell death.

Thijssen et al. [43] in a hibernation swine model found that with the transition to hibernating myocardium desmin, cardiotin and titin were globally reduced. They described that this model represents an expression of cardiac remodeling.

Indeed Dispersyn et al. [42] described cardiomyocyte remodeling in chronic ischemia and hibernation.

(b) Does cell death occur in HIB?

The appearance of myofibrillar loss has already been described [37, 38].

In this aspect Timolati et al. [44] by studying long-term cultured adult cardiomyocytes exposed to doxorubicin conclude that myofibrillar damage contributes to contractile dysfunction prior to cell death. Thus most of the available evidence points out that in HIB no appreciable cell death exists.

Heusch et al. [3] in the Table 3 of their review give some pertinent morphological features of chronic hibernation, i. e.

- Loss of myofiaments, sarcoplasmic reticulum, connexin 43.
- Numerous small doughnut-like mitochondria.
- Disorganization of the cytoskeleton.
- Sequestration of cellular particles in the extracellular space, indicative of fibrosis.

Thus, if some previous reports of minimal patchy necrosis in pigs [45, 46] together with no necrosis but patchy fibrosis [26, 27, 47] and evidence of patchy subendocardial apoptosis [46, 48] are seen, one has to agree that the role of cell death in HIB is speculative [49]; this reminds that clinical viability as will be further described, is the key to the definition of HIB.

Indeed, chronic HIB creates an antiapoptotic and cytoprotective pattern of genes such as the inhibitor of apoptosis protein, HSP70 [50].

Additionally, overexpression of inducible NO synthase (iNOS) and cyclooxygenase has been found in humans [51].

Depré et al. [52] have further described genomics of survival in myocardial HIB. Apart from those already mentioned [50] they mention genes promoting cardiomyocyte growth and survival such as H11 kinase and HIF1-1, which stimulates glucose metabolism by increasing expression of glucose transporter (GLUT1) and angiogenesis through VEGF1. They also describe novel genes, which are gene products that do not recall any known sequence in public databases; they differentiate them from unknown genes, which are characterized in other tissues but whose role in the heart has not yet been determined.

In this context, Heusch et al. [3] point out that the aforementioned iNOS and cyclooxygenase 2 do not only affect survival, but also point out to the existence of inflammation. In a chronic model in the mouse with repetitive ischemia reperfusion episodes chemokine expression was increased, together with macrophage infiltration [53]. Also in humans, recruitment of mononuclears and increase of MCP- 1 was seen [54], together with an overexpression of TNFα [55].

Same findings have emerged from a microembolisation model [56]. On the other side, HIB may be associated with some protective mechanisms. Thus it induces immune unresponsiveness (anergy) [57]; TNFα production in response to LPS is reduced in peritoneal macrophages from hibernating animals even under normothermic conditions [58].

Some other characteristic features of chronic HIB relevant to the human must be mentioned:

A heterogeneous impairment of norepinephrine uptake is seen in a pig model [59], with altered adrenergic receptor density in humans [60] Canty et al. [61] have shown that the swine model of HIB is vulnerable to sudden death due to ventricular tachycardia degenerating into fibrillation; characteristically in these animals, infarcts were infrequent and small. This has very robust clinical implication in the human: pts with hibernating myocardium must be protected from arrhythmias while revascularization is being contemplated.

Finally, in chronic HIB, reduced calcium responsiveness is manifested by reduced maximal contractile response [62] to calcium. Importantly, SERCA-2, phospholamban and the Na^+ – Ca^{2+} exchanger were not reduced at 4–6 weeks, but they were reduced at 3 months [63].

In human myocardium with HIB no changes were seen [64]; many of the mechanisms have already been discussed in stunning.

Thus, many studies [3, 6] bring into focus another universal protective mechanism, preconditioning or conditioning [3].

HIB and conditioning have 2 major features in common:

(a) They represent important survival mechanisms
(b) They can be triggered by a brief period of myocardial ischemia followed by reperfusion.

However, it is clear that despite the advantageous mechanisms that it employs, the hibernating heart is in a precarious situation. Cardiac dysfunction is present, since as it already has been stated, HIB and cardiac remodeling go together.

Sudden death due to ventricular arrhythmias is a threat, and myocardial loss is imminent, i. e. the hibernating heart may sleep to death [39].

It is obvious that the heart must reclaim its normal blood supply and this can be effected by revascularization.

Another consideration of HIB should be taken into account: Dispersyn et al. [42] have described that it can be caused not only by chronic myocardial ischemia. They have shown this in goats with pacing-induced chronic atrial fibrillation. They showed the already described cardiomyocyte dedifferentiation but not apoptosis.

10.3 Assessment of Myocardial Viability

The question of viability detection remains extremely important [31].

A very detailed review is given by Camici et al. [65].

Grewirtz and Dilsizian [66] also give more details in a more recent review.

10.3.1 Dobutamine Stress Echocardiography

The "biphasic response", i. e. an initial improvement with deterioration of contractility of viable segments with higher doses of dobutamine (up to 40 μg/kg/min) together with atropine administration defines viable segments with great accuracy.

The technique can be supplemented with employment of myocardial contrast, i. e. microbubbles with a diameter smaller than red blood cells. Contrast material not only accurately delineates the left ventricular cavity, but also depicts an intact microvasculature, indicative of viability of the corresponding segment [65–68].

Contrast use confers higher sensitivity but results into lower specificity. The technique recently is supplemented by the addiction of tissue doppler imaging techniques [69–71].

10.3.2 Single-Photon Emission Tomography (SPECT)

The main compounds used are based on:

(a) Tl201. It depends on regional myocardial blood flow and also on cardiomyocyte (sarcolemmal) membrane integrity. The most widely used protocol to investigate viability is to administer the compound at the end of exercise or adenosine/dipyridamole injection and image the myocardium 4 h later. If the exercise

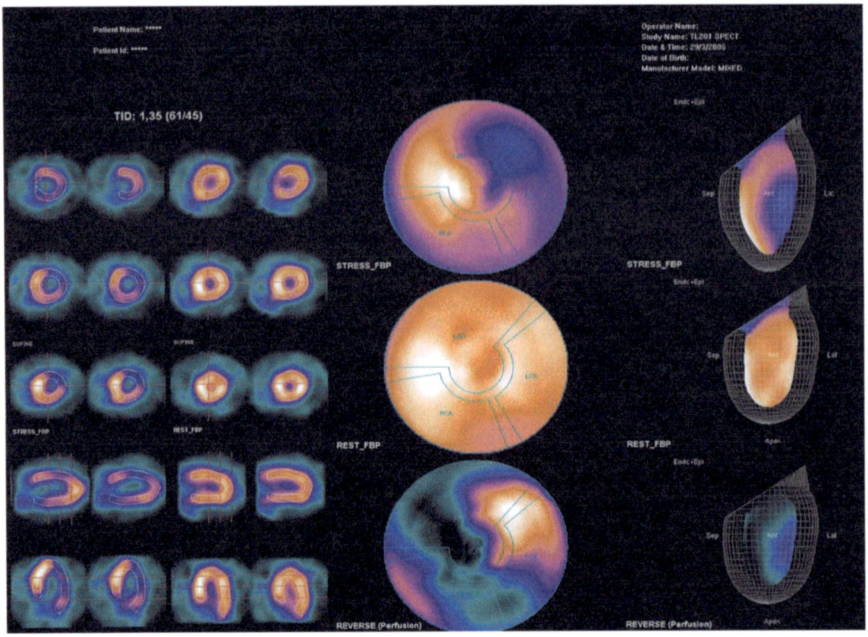

Fig. 10.1 Thallium 201 stress imaging during adenosine and post reinjection 4 h post stress imaging mid cavity slices in the short, vertical and horizontal long axes are displayed during stress (1st, 3nd and fifth rows) and post reinjection of 1 mCi of Thallium −201 (2nd, fourth and sixth rows) Completely reversible defects in anterior, antero-lateral, lateral and posterolateral wall. Also transient dilation of LV cavity. (Courtesy of Maria Koutelou MD, Nuclear Medicine Dept, Onassis Cardiac Surgery Center 3-7-2018.)

defect has disappeared it is ascribed to ischemia. If it persists, a small additional dose of isotope is given and the myocardium is scanned again 4–24 h later. If the defect has disappeared or diminished, this portion of the myocardium is considered to be viable [72, 73] (Fig. 10.1). A modification is to administer nitrates.

Tc 99 m compounds; sestamibi and tetrofosmin are the ones more commonly used. Since Tc 99 does not redistribute as Tl201 does, they must be given repeatedly [74].

Both isotopes can be used as gated SPECT to detect both viability and function [75], by recording ejection fraction and regional motion reversibility [76]. SPECT has higher sensitivity but lower specificity than stress echo to predict reversibility of segmental dysfunction, although this can be improved by gating [74].

10.3.3 Positron Emission Tomography (PET)

The main isotope used is ^{18}FDG (fludeoxyglucose) which images glucose uptake by the myocardium. For research purposes it was given together with NH13, which measures myocardial blood flow. If ^{18}FDG uptake is maintained or increased while perfusion is decreased, a flow/metabolism missmatch is indicative of viable myocardium [77].

In current clinical practice ^{18}FDG is given alone since NH13 requires a cyclotron on site. The technique detects switches of metabolism to glucose away from free fatty acid use [28, 78].

PET is considered as the gold standard for the detection of viability. However, in real life it is less used than stress echo and:

10.3.4 *Cardiovascular Magnetic Resonance*

It can be used with dobutamine stress [79]. Gadolinium chelated contrast agents are used to delineate perfusion defects, microvascular obstruction and fibrotic tissue [80].

Importantly, these agents do not penetrate into cardiomyocytes with intact membranes but persist in scarred or infarcted tissue, which appears bright [81]. Thus "bright is dead" (Fig. 10.2). Camici et al. [65] in their Table 1 provide an assessment of the diagnostic accuracy of the aforementioned nuclear techniques:

10.4 Performance of Imaging Techniques [82]

SPECT techniques give sensitivities up to 80%, with specificities of around 80–90%.

Stress echo gives lower sensitivities (65–76%) but high enough specificities (68–89%), while PET has 81% sensitivity and around 65% specificity. In general stress echo has superior specificity. CMR has sensitivities around 81–86% and specificities around 92% [80].

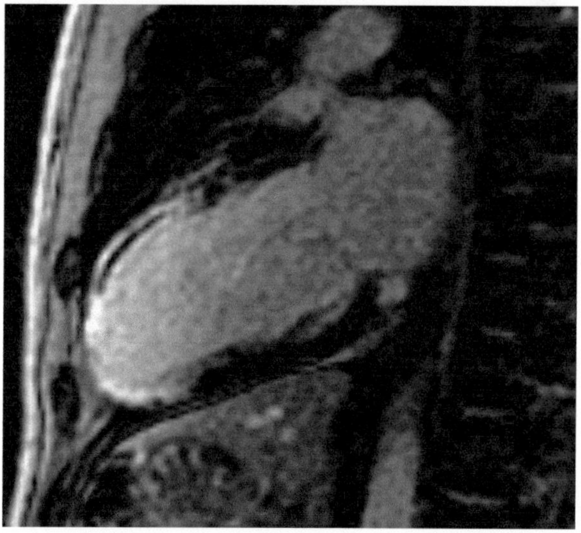

Fig. 10.2 Extensive antero-apical myocardial infarction (white area). The black area within the white area represents microvascular obstruction. Only the basal part of the anterior wall and the inferior wall are viable. (Courtesy of Sophie Mavrogeni MD, Cardiology Dept, Onassis Cardiac Surgery Center)

Because the selection of the right patient for revascularization can be a difficult decision, this author agrees in principle and in practice with the multimodal approach proposed by Bax et al. [83], who propose sequential testing with Tl201 SPECT and stress echo. I propose a stress dobutamine echo first with measurement of left anterior descending coronary flow reserve with adenosine since the question of viability most commonly arises with large anterior infarcts. If viability is found to exist, I propose revascularization. If the result is negative or ambiguous, I add Tl201 stress redistribution - reinjection. In any way, it must be held in mind that for contractility improvement to occur, ≥20% of the LV myocardium must be found to be viable [84, 85].

Before the impact of revascularization on the improvement of myocardial dysfunction is described, some more techniques proposed by Gewirtz and Dilsizian [66] are given, based on molecular mechanisms.

They propose the following targets:

- The myocyte compartment
- To image perfusion:
- With PET: Water-O15, NH-13, Rubidium-82, FDG-18 flupiridaz.
- With SPECT: Tl201, Tc99 sestamibi and tetrofosmin
- With MRI: Gadolinium
- With CT: Contrast injection

10.4.1 Metabolism

Glucose: ^{18}FDG, fatty acids: C-11 palmitate, oxidative metabolism: C-11 acetate, ischemic memory: I-123-BMIPP, lipid microbubbles targeting P-selectin. Inorganic phosphate metabolism (oxidative phosphorylation): 31-PMRS.

It must be noted that many of the above tracers are still in the research stage but are mentioned in this book because they represent a signaling pathway which must be known.

10.4.2 Myocardial Function

Echocardiography, CMR, ECG-gated SPECT or PET.

10.4.3 Cell Death

Necrosis: Tc99m pyrophosphate.
Apoptosis: SPECT: Tc99m annexin-V.
MRI: Ferromagnetic- labeled annexin-V, Annexin-V- coated gadolinium liposomes.

10.4.4 Renin-Angiotensin System

Labelled angiotensin- connecting- enzyme inhibitors (captopril, lisnopril, zofenoprilat).

Angiotensin II type 1 receptor inhibitors: Labeled losartan.

Interstitial space CMR: Gadolinium contrast.

Cardiac microvasculature: PET blood flow, contrast echocardiography, CMR with gadolinium contrast.

10.5 Deciding on Revascularization

The vital question remains: how these viability detection techniques can guide revascularization with the aim of improving left ventricular function.

Camici et al. [65] give a very lucid account. They mention several studies which show a LVEF improvement of ≥5% after revascularization in ≈60% of patients, with a range from 38% to 88%.

This wide range shows how important is to accurately detect viability. Underwood et al. [86] give a meta-analysis which actually shows that only pts with viability can have an increase in LVEF. Camici et al. [65] stress that the recovery of the viable myocardium can take up to 14 months [85]. This obviously depends on the amount of injury that the hibernating but viable myocardium has suffered which cannot always be measured accurately. However Bax et al. point out that in the majority of studies a follow-up of 2–6 months was noted [87]. However, these data raise another very important question: Is contractility improvement translated into improved survival? In a meta-analysis of 24 nonrandomized studies which between 1992 and 1999 included 3088 pts with a LVEF ≤40%, an association of revascularization and improved survived [31] was seen especially in those with the worst function. No improvement was seen in pts without viability.

To further study the effect of vascularization on viability, Camici et al. [65] pooled information from 14 nonrandomized trials conducted between 1998 and 2006 in which Kaplan-Meier survival curves were reported.

A trend for survival was seen with vascularization versus medical treatment, only in pts with viability.

Bourque et al. [88] from a meta-analysis of 9 relevant studies with 1244 pts found a markedly reduced but statistically significant interaction between viability status and treatment allocation .

Fath-Ordoubadi et al. [89] studied 24 consecutive pts with hibernating myocardium who were subjected to coronary angioplasty. Cardiac function improved significantly as regards LVEF and PTCA involved territory.

It is obvious that dilating a LAD stenosis is expected to produce a greater improvement. The already mentioned impact of the extent of viability on the improvement of left ventricular function has already been discussed. Desideri et al. [90] found that the risk of death with medical treatment is significantly increased if the viable tissues exceeds 20% the left ventricle, together with the existence of LBBB.

Another question is how long one should wait after viability is diagnosed. It seems that shorter times (≤30 days) are associated with lower mortality [91] Tarakji et al. [92] found that early vascularization (within 6 months) may be associated with reduced mortality.

The above postulations underwent a considerable shaking of confidence when the results of the STICH trial were published in 2011 [93]. They enrolled 1212 pts with or without bypass surgery; altogether 601 underwent evaluation for presence or absence of viability as assessed with SPECT, stress dobutamine echo, or both; of these, 298 were randomized to medical treatment plus revascularization vs 303 who received only medical therapy. There was no significant interaction between viability status and treatment. Moreover, the presence of viability was associated with lower mortality at a follow-up of 5.1 years. However after adjustment of other significant baseline prognostic variables in a multivariable model, this difference was no longer significant. Many issues have been voiced in discussion of these results. Two commentaries are worth presenting:

Perrone - Fillardi and Pinto [94] discuss the results of the previous meta-analysis by Allman et al. [31] stressing that their conclusions were endorsed by the European Society of Cardiology and the European Association for Cardiothoracic Surgery, as stated in their Guidelines [95]. Perrone - Fillardi and Pinto [94] voice many reservations on the methodology of the STICH trial, pointing out that there was no description of LVEF or LV volume changes. They also comment on the very low mortality of STICH pts with viable myocardium undergoing only medical therapy, only 7%/ year as compared to 15%/ year in the Allman [31] meta-analysis. Thus, we may be "victims" of our medical treatment success. They concluded that the STICH trial does not close the door, but will influence the planning of subsequent trials on this subject.

Shah et al. [96] in a review on the same subject discuss 2 more small prospective trial randomized trials, the Heart Failure Revascularization Trial (HEART) [97], and the PET and recovery results PARR-2 [98], both of which were neutral.

However some comments are necessary: In the HEART study [97] only 138 of the planned 800pts were enrolled. Of the 69pts assigned to invasive therapy only 45 had revascularization. These numbers are too small to give meaningful results. In the PARR-2 [98] trial, 25% of pts did not adhere to recommended management based on PET findings. Although the overall result was not significant, pts with a higher PET viability underwent revascularization to a higher degree. In their Fig. 7, survival was better in the "adherence to PET" group, previous bypass surgery had a significant association with the outcome at 300 days. The authors remark that there is potential value for ^{18}FDG PET, particularly in a high risk patient population.

Another point worth pointing out is that in STICH more than 85% of pts were taking the "big 4" medications (β- blockers, ACE inhibitors or angiotensin receptor blockers, statins, aspirin).

Shah et al. [96] also raised some interesting questions, especially what constitutes "benefit" from therapy. Specifically in their Fig. 10.1 they give a good pathway diagram and in their Fig. 3 the various ways expressing response to therapy, both from the clinical (improved exercise capacity, quality of life, survival) and imaging viewpoint segmental, recovery, global functional recovery.

Of course an entity must be reiterated, reverse remodeling. Many points with this discussion can be found in the chapter on cardiac remodeling. It has already been stressed that HIB is the basis of many cases of REM. However as can be seen from Fig. 10.1 of Shah et al. [96], by the time scar has been formed, as can be found in many cases of REM, a stage beyond cell death detections has been reached.

In conclusion, HIB is seen in many pts with severe coronary stenosis subtending a large area of the myocardium, usually with LAD lesions These patients usually have a previous myocardial infarction: In the STICH trial the overall incidence of a previous infarct was 80% with 75–78% in those with viability vs 93–96% in those without. Usually pts have a LVEF ≤35%. In these patients a viability test from those already enumerated should be carried out and revascularization (bypass surgery or interventional procedure) carried out although some second thoughts have arisen from recent randomized trials.

Probably the best candidates are those with more than 25% of their left ventricular myocardium detected as being viable, by any available technique.

References

1. Diamond GA, Forrester JS, deLuz PL, Wyatt HL, Swan HJ. Post-extrasystolic potentiation of ischemic myocardium by atrial stimulation. Am Heart J. 1978;95:204–9.
2. Rahimtoola SH. The hibernating myocardium. Am Heart J. 1989;117:211–21.
3. Heusch G, Schulz R, Rahimtoola SH. Myocardial hibernation: a delicate balance. Am J Physiol Heart Circ Physiol. 2005;288:H984–99.
4. Heusch G. Hibernating myocardium. Physiol Rev. 1998;78:1055–85.
5. Yan L, Kudej RK, Vatner DE, Vatner SF. Myocardial ischemic protection in natural mammalian hibernation. Basic Res Cardiol. 2015;110:9.
6. Carey HV, Andrews MT, Martin SL. Mammalian hibernation: cellular and molecular responses to depressed metabolism and low temperature. Physiol Rev. 2003;83:1153–81.
7. Murphy E. Primary and secondary signaling pathways in early preconditioning that converge on the mitochondria to produce cardioprotection. Circ Res. 2004;94:7–16.
8. Mayr B, Montminy M. Transcriptional regulation by the phosphorylation-dependent factor CREB. Nat Rev Mol Cell Biol. 2001;2:599–609.
9. Freeland K, Boxer LM, Latchman DS. The cyclic AMP response element in the Bcl-2 promoter confers inducibility by hypoxia in neuronal cells. Brain Res Mol Brain Res. 2001;92:98–106.
10. Laske TG, Iaizzo PA, Garshelis DL. Six Years in the Life of a Mother Bear - The Longest Continuous Heart Rate Recordings from a Free-Ranging Mammal. Sci Rep. 2017;7:40732.
11. Braunwald E, Rutherford JD. Reversible ischemic left ventricular dysfunction: evidence for the "hibernating myocardium". J Am Coll Cardiol. 1986;8:1467–70.
12. Heusch G, Schulz R. Characterization of hibernating and stunned myocardium. Eur Heart J. 1997;18(Suppl D):D102–10.
13. Ross J Jr. Myocardial perfusion-contraction matching. Implications for coronary heart disease and hibernation. Circulation. 1991;83:1076–83.
14. Goldstein RA, Kirkeeide RL, Demer LL, Merhige M, Nishikawa A, Smalling RW, et al. Relation between geometric dimensions of coronary artery stenoses and myocardial perfusion reserve in man. J Clin Invest. 1987;79:1473–8.
15. Uren NG, Melin JA, De Bruyne B, Wijns W, Baudhuin T, Camici PG. Relation between myocardial blood flow and the severity of coronary-artery stenosis. N Engl J Med. 1994;330:1782–8.

16. Voudris V, Manginas A, Vassilikos V, Koutelou M, Kantzis J, Cokkinos DV. Coronary flow velocity changes after intravenous dipyridamole infusion: measurements using intravascular Doppler guide wire. A documentation of flow inhomogeneity. J Am Coll Cardiol. 1996;27:1148–55.
17. Camici PG, Rimoldi OE. Myocardial blood flow in patients with hibernating myocardium. Cardiovasc Res. 2003;57:302–11.
18. Gallagher KP, Matsuzaki M, Osakada G, Kemper WS, Ross J Jr. Effect of exercise on the relationship between myocardial blood flow and systolic wall thickening in dogs with acute coronary stenosis. Circ Res. 1983;52:716–29.
19. Schulz R, Heusch G. Hibernating myocardium. Heart. 2000;84:587–94.
20. Kloner RA, Bolli R, Marban E, Reinlib L, Braunwald E. Medical and cellular implications of stunning, hibernation, and preconditioning: an NHLBI workshop. Circulation. 1998;97:1848–67.
21. Ferrari R. Pathophysiological vs biochemical ischaemia: a key to transition from reversible to irreversible damage. Eur Heart J Suppl. 2001;3(Suppl C):C2–C10.
22. Flameng W, Vanhaecke J, Van Belle H, Borgers M, De Beer L, Minten J. Relation between coronary artery stenosis and myocardial purine metabolism, histology and regional function in humans. J Am Coll Cardiol. 1987;9:1235–42.
23. Fedele FA, Gewirtz H, Capone RJ, Sharaf B, Most AS. Metabolic response to prolonged reduction of myocardial blood flow distal to a severe coronary artery stenosis. Circulation. 1988;78:729–35.
24. Fallavollita JA, Malm BJ, Canty JM Jr. Hibernating myocardium retains metabolic and contractile reserve despite regional reductions in flow, function, and oxygen consumption at rest. Circ Res. 2003;92:48–55.
25. Fallavollita JA, Logue M, Canty JM Jr. Stability of hibernating myocardium in pigs with a chronic left anterior descending coronary artery stenosis: absence of progressive fibrosis in the setting of stable reductions in flow, function and coronary flow reserve. J Am Coll Cardiol. 2001;37:1989–95.
26. Fallavollita JA, Perry BJ, Canty JM Jr. 18F-2-deoxyglucose deposition and regional flow in pigs with chronically dysfunctional myocardium. Evidence for transmural variations in chronic hibernating myocardium. Circulation. 1997;95:1900–9.
27. McFalls EO, Baldwin D, Palmer B, Marx D, Jaimes D, Ward HB. Regional glucose uptake within hypoperfused swine myocardium as measured by positron emission tomography. Am J Phys. 1997;272:H343–9.
28. Gerber BL, Ordoubadi FF, Wijns W, Vanoverschelde JL, Knuuti MJ, Janier M, et al. Positron emission tomography using(18)F-fluoro-deoxyglucose and euglycaemic hyperinsulinaemic glucose clamp: optimal criteria for the prediction of recovery of post-ischaemic left ventricular dysfunction. Results from the European Community Concerted Action Multicenter study on use of(18)F-fluoro-deoxyglucose Positron Emission Tomography for the Detection of Myocardial Viability. Eur Heart J. 2001;22:1691–701.
29. Knuesel PR, Nanz D, Wyss C, Buechi M, Kaufmann PA, von Schulthess GK, et al. Characterization of dysfunctional myocardium by positron emission tomography and magnetic resonance: relation to functional outcome after revascularization. Circulation. 2003;108:1095–100.
30. Vanoverschelde JL, Depré C, Gerber BL, Borgers M, Wijns W, Robert A, et al. Time course of functional recovery after coronary artery bypass graft surgery in patients with chronic left ventricular ischemic dysfunction. Am J Cardiol. 2000;85:1432–9.
31. Allman KC, Shaw LJ, Hachamovitch R, Udelson JE. Myocardial viability testing and impact of revascularization on prognosis in patients with coronary artery disease and left ventricular dysfunction: a meta-analysis. J Am Coll Cardiol. 2002;39:1151–8.
32. Wiggers H, Noreng M, Paulsen PK, Bøttcher M, Egeblad H, Nielsen TT, et al. Energy stores and metabolites in chronic reversibly and irreversibly dysfunctional myocardium in humans. J Am Coll Cardiol. 2001;37:100–8.

33. Vogt AM, Elsässer A, Nef H, Bode C, Kübler W, Schaper J. Increased glycolysis as protective adaptation of energy depleted, degenerating human hibernating myocardium. Mol Cell Biochem. 2003;242:101–7.
34. Vanoverschelde JL, Wijns W, Depré C, Essamri B, Heyndrickx GR, Borgers M, et al. Mechanisms of chronic regional postischemic dysfunction in humans. New insights from the study of noninfarcted collateral-dependent myocardium. Circulation. 1993;87:1513–23.
35. Hata T, Nohara R, Fujita M, Hosokawa R, Lee L, Kudo T, et al. Noninvasive assessment of myocardial viability by positron emission tomography with 11C acetate in patients with old myocardial infarction. Usefulness of low-dose dobutamine infusion. Circulation. 1996;94:1834–341.
36. Depré C, Tomlinson JE, Kudej RK, Gaussin V, Thompson E, Kim SJ, et al. Gene program for cardiac cell survival induced by transient ischemia in conscious pigs. Proc Natl Acad Sci U S A. 2001;98:9336–41.
37. Ng DW, Sathish S, Khan A, Chandrasoma P, Wijns W, Chandraratna PA. Identification of hibernating myocardium by acoustic microscopy. Ultrasound Med Biol. 2004;30:693–6.
38. Gunning MG, Kaprielian RR, Pepper J, Pennell DJ, Sheppard MN, Severs NJ, et al. The histology of viable and hibernating myocardium in relation to imaging characteristics. J Am Coll Cardiol. 2002;39:428–35.
39. Borgers M. Hibernating myocardium: Programmed cell survival or programmed cell death? Exp Clin Cardiol. 2002;7:69–72.
40. Ausma J, Thoné F, Dispersyn GD, Flameng W, Vanoverschelde JL, Ramaekers FC, et al. Dedifferentiated cardiomyocytes from chronic hibernating myocardium are ischemia-tolerant. Mol Cell Biochem. 1998;186:159–68.
41. Kim SJ, Peppas A, Hong SK, Yang G, Huang Y, Diaz G, et al. Persistent stunning induces myocardial hibernation and protection: flow/function and metabolic mechanisms. Circ Res. 2003;92:1233–9.
42. Dispersyn GD, Ausma J, Thoné F, Flameng W, Vanoverschelde JL, Allessie MA, et al. Cardiomyocyte remodelling during myocardial hibernation and atrial fibrillation: prelude to apoptosis. Cardiovasc Res. 1999;43:947–57.
43. Thijssen V, Borgers M, Lenders MH, Ramaekers FC, Suzuki G, Palka B, et al. Temporal and spatial variations in structural protein expression during the progression from stunned to hibernating myocardium. Circulation. 2004;110:3313–21.
44. Timolati F, Anliker T, Groppalli V, Perriard JC, Eppenberger HM, Suter TM, et al. The role of cell death and myofibrillar damage in contractile dysfunction of long-term cultured adult cardiomyocytes exposed to doxorubicin. Cytotechnology. 2009;61:25–36.
45. Chen C, Ma L, Dyckman W, Santos F, Lai T, Gillam LD, et al. Left ventricular remodeling in myocardial hibernation. Circulation. 1997;96(9 Suppl):II-46–50.
46. Chen C, Ma L, Linfert DR, Lai T, Fallon JT, Gillam LD, et al. Myocardial cell death and apoptosis in hibernating myocardium. J Am Coll Cardiol. 1997;30:1407–12.
47. Mills I, Fallon JT, Wrenn D, Sasken H, Gray W, Bier J, et al. Adaptive responses of coronary circulation and myocardium to chronic reduction in perfusion pressure and flow. Am J Phys. 1994;266:H447–57.
48. Lim H, Fallavollita JA, Hard R, Kerr CW, Canty JM Jr. Profound apoptosis-mediated regional myocyte loss and compensatory hypertrophy in pigs with hibernating myocardium. Circulation. 1999;100:2380–6.
49. Heusch G. What are underlying mechanisms of myocardial hibernation? Dialogues Cardiovasc Med. 1997;2:79–83.
50. Depré C, Kim SJ, John AS, Huang Y, Rimoldi OE, Pepper JR, et al. Program of cell survival underlying human and experimental hibernating myocardium. Circ Res. 2004;95:433–40.
51. Baker CS, Dutka DP, Pagano D, Rimoldi O, Pitt M, Hall RJ, et al. Immunocytochemical evidence for inducible nitric oxide synthase and cyclooxygenase-2 expression with nitrotyrosine formation in human hibernating myocardium. Basic Res Cardiol. 2002;97:409–15.

52. Depre C, Vatner SF. Cardioprotection in stunned and hibernating myocardium. Heart Fail Rev. 2007;12:307–17.
53. Dewald O, Frangogiannis NG, Zoerlein M, Duerr GD, Klemm C, Knuefermann P, et al. Development of murine ischemic cardiomyopathy is associated with a transient inflammatory reaction and depends on reactive oxygen species. Proc Natl Acad Sci U S A. 2003;100:2700–5.
54. Frangogiannis NG, Shimoni S, Chang SM, Ren G, Shan K, Aggeli C, et al. Evidence for an active inflammatory process in the hibernating human myocardium. Am J Pathol. 2002;160:1425–33.
55. Kalra DK, Zhu X, Ramchandani MK, Lawrie G, Reardon MJ, Lee-Jackson D, et al. Increased myocardial gene expression of tumor necrosis factor-alpha and nitric oxide synthase-2: a potential mechanism for depressed myocardial function in hibernating myocardium in humans. Circulation. 2002;105:1537–40.
56. Thielmann M, Dörge H, Martin C, Belosjorow S, Schwanke U, van De Sand A, et al. Myocardial dysfunction with coronary microembolization: signal transduction through a sequence of nitric oxide, tumor necrosis factor-alpha, and sphingosine. Circ Res. 2002;90:807–13.
57. Prendergast BJ, Freeman DA, Zucker I, Nelson RJ. Periodic arousal from hibernation is necessary for initiation of immune responses in ground squirrels. Am J Physiol Regul Integr Comp Physiol. 2002;282:R1054–62.
58. Novoselova EG, Kolaeva SG, Makar VR, Agaphonova TA. Production of tumor necrosis factor in cells of hibernating ground squirrels Citellus undulatus during annual cycle. Life Sci. 2000;67:1073–80.
59. Luisi AJ Jr, Fallavollita JA, Suzuki G, Canty JM Jr. Spatial inhomogeneity of sympathetic nerve function in hibernating myocardium. Circulation. 2002;106:779–81.
60. Shan K, Bick RJ, Poindexter BJ, Nagueh SF, Shimoni S, Verani MS, et al. Altered adrenergic receptor density in myocardial hibernation in humans: A possible mechanism of depressed myocardial function. Circulation. 2000;102:2599–606.
61. Canty JM Jr, Suzuki G, Banas MD, Verheyen F, Borgers M, Fallavollita JA. Hibernating myocardium: chronically adapted to ischemia but vulnerable to sudden death. Circ Res. 2004;94:1142–9.
62. Bito V, Heinzel FR, Weidemann F, Dommke C, van der Velden J, Verbeken E, et al. Cellular mechanisms of contractile dysfunction in hibernating myocardium. Circ Res. 2004;94:794–801.
63. Fallavollita JA, Jacob S, Young RF, Canty JM Jr. Regional alterations in SR Ca(2+)-ATPase, phospholamban, and HSP-70 expression in chronic hibernating myocardium. Am J Phys. 1999;277:H1418–28.
64. Lüss H, Schäfers M, Neumann J, Hammel D, Vahlhaus C, Baba HA, et al. Biochemical mechanisms of hibernation and stunning in the human heart. Cardiovasc Res. 2002;56:411–21.
65. Camici PG, Prasad SK, Rimoldi OE. Stunning, hibernation, and assessment of myocardial viability. Circulation. 2008;117:103–14.
66. Gewirtz H, Dilsizian V. Myocardial Viability: Survival Mechanisms and Molecular Imaging Targets in Acute and Chronic Ischemia. Circ Res. 2017;120:1197–212.
67. Hayat SA, Senior R. Contrast echocardiography for the assessment of myocardial viability. Curr Opin Cardiol. 2006;21:473–8.
68. Ragosta M, Camarano G, Kaul S, Powers ER, Sarembock IJ, Gimple LW. Microvascular integrity indicates myocellular viability in patients with recent myocardial infarction. New insights using myocardial contrast echocardiography. Circulation. 1994;89:2562–9.
69. Hoffmann R, Altiok E, Nowak B, Heussen N, Kühl H, Kaiser HJ, et al. Strain rate measurement by doppler echocardiography allows improved assessment of myocardial viability inpatients with depressed left ventricular function. J Am Coll Cardiol. 2002;39:443–9.
70. Thibault H, Derumeaux G. Assessment of myocardial ischemia and viability using tissue Doppler and deformation imaging: the lessons from the experimental studies. Arch Cardiovasc Dis. 2008;101:61–8.
71. McLean DS, Anadiotis AV, Lerakis S. Role of echocardiography in the assessment of myocardial viability. Am J Med Sci. 2009;337:349–54.

72. Ling LH, Christian TF, Mulvagh SL, Klarich KW, Hauser MF, Nishimura RA, et al. Determining myocardial viability in chronic ischemic left ventricular dysfunction: a prospective comparison of rest-redistribution thallium 201 single-photon emission computed tomography, nitroglycerin-dobutamine echocardiography, and intracoronary myocardial contrast echocardiography. Am Heart J. 2006;151:882–9.
73. Naruse H, Kondo T, Arii T, Morita M, Ohyanagi M, Iwasaki T, et al. Comparative accuracy of various Tl-201 reinjection imaging protocols to detect myocardial viability. Ann Nucl Med. 1996;10:119–26.
74. Sciagrà R, Pellegri M, Pupi A, Bolognese L, Bisi G, Carnovale V, et al. Prognostic implications of Tc-99 m sestamibi viability imaging and subsequent therapeutic strategy in patients with chronic coronary artery disease and left ventricular dysfunction. J Am Coll Cardiol. 2000;36:739–45.
75. Sciagrà R, Imperiale A, Antoniucci D, Migliorini A, Parodi G, Comis G, et al. Relationship of infarct size and severity versus left ventricular ejection fraction and volumes obtained from 99mTc-sestamibi gated single-photon emission computed tomography in patients treated with primary percutaneous coronary intervention. Eur J Nucl Med Mol Imaging. 2004;31:969–74.
76. Tillisch J, Brunken R, Marshall R, Schwaiger M, Mandelkern M, Phelps M, et al. Reversibility of cardiac wall-motion abnormalities predicted by positron tomography. N Engl J Med. 1986;314:884–8.
77. Auerbach MA, Schöder H, Hoh C, Gambhir SS, Yaghoubi S, Sayre JW, et al. Prevalence of myocardial viability as detected by positron emission tomography in patients with ischemic cardiomyopathy. Circulation. 1999;99:2921–16.
78. Ferrannini E, Santoro D, Bonadonna R, Natali A, Parodi O, Camici PG. Metabolic and hemodynamic effects of insulin on human hearts. Am J Phys. 1993;264:E308–E3015.
79. Bree D, Wollmuth JR, Cupps BP, Krock MD, Howells A, Rogers J, et al. Low-dose dobutamine tissue-tagged magnetic resonance imaging with 3-dimensional strain analysis allows assessment of myocardial viability in patients with ischemic cardiomyopathy. Circulation. 2006;114(1 Suppl):I33–6.
80. Kim RJ, Wu E, Rafael A, Chen EL, Parker MA, Simonetti O, et al. The use of contrast-enhanced magnetic resonance imaging to identify reversible myocardial dysfunction. N Engl J Med. 2000;343:1445–53.
81. Judd RM, Wagner A, Rehwald WG, Albert T, Kim RJ. Technology insight: assessment of myocardial viability by delayed-enhancement magnetic resonance imaging. Nat Clin Pract Cardiovasc Med. 2005;2:150–8.
82. Elfigih I, Henein MY. Non-invasive imaging in detecting myocardial viability: Myocardial function versus perfusion. Int J Cardiol Heart Vasc. 2014;5:51–6.
83. Bax JJ, Maddahi J, Poldermans D, Elhendy A, Schinkel A, Boersma E, et al. Preoperative comparison of different noninvasive strategies for predicting improvement in left ventricular function after coronary artery bypass grafting. Am J Cardiol. 2003;92:1–4.
84. Hanekom L, Jenkins C, Jeffries L, Case C, Mundy J, Hawley C, et al. Incremental value of strain rate analysis as an adjunct to wall-motion scoring for assessment of myocardial viability by dobutamine echocardiography: a follow-up study after revascularization. Circulation. 2005;112:3892–900.
85. Bax JJ, Maddahi J, Poldermans D, Elhendy A, Cornel JH, Boersma E, et al. Sequential (201) Tl imaging and dobutamine echocardiography to enhance accuracy of predicting improved left ventricular ejection fraction after revascularization. J Nucl Med. 2002;43:795–802.
86. Underwood SR, Bax JJ, vom Dahl J, Henein MY, Knuuti J, van Rossum AC, et al. Imaging techniques for the assessment of myocardial hibernation. Report of a Study Group of the European Society of Cardiology. Eur Heart J. 2004;25:815–36.
87. Bax JJ, Visser FC, Poldermans D, Elhendy A, Cornel JH, Boersma E, et al. Time course of functional recovery of stunned and hibernating segments after surgical revascularization. Circulation. 2001;104(12 Suppl 1):I314–8.

88. Bourque JM, Hasselblad V, Velazquez EJ, Borges-Neto S, O'connor CM. Revascularization in patients with coronary artery disease, left ventricular dysfunction, and viability: a meta-analysis. Am Heart J. 2003;146:621–7.
89. Fath-Ordoubadi F, Beatt KJ, Spyrou N, Camici PG. Efficacy of coronary angioplasty for the treatment of hibernating myocardium. Heart. 1999;82:210–6.
90. Desideri A, Cortigiani L, Christen AI, Coscarelli S, Gregori D, Zanco P, et al. The extent of perfusion-F18-fluorodeoxyglucose positron emission tomography mismatch determines mortality in medically treated patients with chronic ischemic left ventricular dysfunction. J Am Coll Cardiol. 2005;46:1264–9.
91. Bax JJ, Schinkel AF, Boersma E, Rizzello V, Elhendy A, Maat A, et al. Early versus delayed revascularization in patients with ischemic cardiomyopathy and substantial viability: impact on outcome. Circulation. 2003;108(Suppl 1):II39–42.
92. Tarakji KG, Brunken R, McCarthy PM, Al-Chekakie MO, Abdel-Latif A, Pothier CE, et al. Myocardial viability testing and the effect of early intervention in patients with advanced left ventricular systolic dysfunction. Circulation. 2006;113:230–7.
93. Bonow RO, Maurer G, Lee KL, Holly TA, Binkley PF, Desvigne-Nickens P, et al. Myocardial viability and survival in ischemic left ventricular dysfunction. N Engl J Med. 2011;364:1617–25.
94. Perrone-Filardi P, Pinto FJ. Looking for myocardial viability after a STICH trial: not enough to close the door. J Nucl Med. 2012;53:349–52.
95. Wijns W, Kolh P, Danchin N, Di Mario C, Falk V, Folliguet T, et al. Guidelines on myocardial revascularization. Eur Heart J. 2010;31:2501–55.
96. Shah BN, Khattar RS, Senior R. The hibernating myocardium: current concepts, diagnostic dilemmas, and clinical challenges in the post-STICH era. Eur Heart J. 2013;34:1323–36.
97. Cleland JG, Calvert M, Freemantle N, Arrow Y, Ball SG, Bonser RS, et al. The Heart Failure Revascularisation Trial (HEART). Eur J Heart Fail. 2011;13:227–33.
98. Beanlands RS, Nichol G, Huszti E, Humen D, Racine N, Freeman M, et al. F-18-fluorodeoxyglucose positron emission tomography imaging-assisted management of patients with severe left ventricular dysfunction and suspected coronary disease: a randomized, controlled trial (PARR-2). J Am Coll Cardiol. 2007;50:2002–12.

Chapter 11
The Fetal Phenotype

Dennis V. Cokkinos

11.1 Re-Emergence of the Fetal Gene Program

This aspect is already mentioned many times, in cardiac hypertrophy and cardiac remodeling, and also in cardiac regeneration.

The response of the myocardium to any type of stress is the return of the fetal phenotype and a suppression of the adult myocardial phenotype. The features of this switch have been very well described by Taegtmeyer et al. [1] and Swynghedauw [2].

The main characteristics of this change are given below:

11.1.1 Metabolic Aspects

It should be remembered that the fetal heart functions in a low oxygen milieu, and metabolically depends on carbohydrates, mainly lactate and glucose for ATP synthesis with only limited utilization of long chain fatty acid oxidation [3].

Only 24 h after birth, a shift occurs from carbohydrate to fatty acid oxidation. The fetal cardiomyocyte's volume consists of glycogen up to 30% [4], while in the adult heart glycogen occupies up to 2% of the cardiomyocyte volume. Genetic ablation of glycogen synthase in mice results in 90% perinatal mortality accompanied by cardiac malformations [5]. It must be remembered, that glycogen content in the rodents is lower them in the human [6].

D. V. Cokkinos (✉)
Heart and Vessel Department, Biomedical Research Foundation,
Academy of Athens - Gregory Skalkeas, Athens, Greece
e-mail: dcokkinos@bioacademy.gr

D. V. Cokkinos (ed.), *Myocardial Preservation*,
https://doi.org/10.1007/978-3-319-98186-4_11

It must also be remembered that ischemic preconditioning, a protective intervention, is followed by a decrease in cardiomyocyte glycogen [7], parallel to ischemia time, a finding referred to by many authors.

In the early postnatal period plasma glycogen also increases; while insulin levels fall [8] in parallel fatty acid oxidation starts.

The substrate change in the heart is associated with the action of PPAR-α (peroxisome proliferator- activated receptor alpha) and its coactivator, PGC-1α, which controls fatty acid uptake and oxidation.PGC-1α also promotes mitochondrial biogenesis; the fetal heart has fewer mitochondria and their activities are lower [9].

It should be remembered that T3 which is necessary for maturation of the heart, also promotes mitochondrial biogenesis [10].

The fetal heart is also dependent on the cytosolic NADH glycolytic pathways, which decrease post-natally [11].

These changes according to Rajabi et al. [12], can be explained by the environmental changes to which the fetal heart is exposed: During gestation it is exposed to a hypoxic environment, receiving a continuous maternal supply of carbohydrates and aminoacids, which ceases after birth, and the heart is obliged to oxidize fatty acids.

The authors underline that in disease this ability to shift from the glycolytic to the fatty acid oxidation is lost [13], with a decrease in "metabolic flexibility".

As already discussed in the chapter on cardiac remodeling, the change observed in the contactile sarcomeric proteins is characteristic of the fetal pattern [2]. The general pattern is a decrease of the "fetal" βMHC and an increase of the "adult type" aMHC after birth.

However a great variability within this pattern exists. Thus, in small animals i. e. mice and rats with a fast heart rate, the heart contains up to 90% αMHC, specifically the V1 form (a a). The intermediate size experimental animals, guinea pigs and rabbits express the α β form (V1 and V2) while V3 (β β)......(bovine and human hearts) contain very little V1. These percentages apply to the ventricular myocardium [14].

According to Krenz and Robins [15], transgenic mice overexpressing βMHC are at a disadvantage under isoproterenol stress. They postulate that the increase in βMHC maybe a maladaptive response.

Danzi et al. [16] state that rat atrial myocytes express predominantly α-MHC protein and a smaller amount of β-MHC, similar to that of the adult ventricle.

However, Fuller et al. [17] in a canine HF model produced by prolonged RV pacing found significantly increased levels of βMHC in the right atria and right atria appendage and ventricle as compared to controls; they were not increased in the left ventricle. However, it must be noted that basal (control) percentages were much lower in the atria (20–30%) as compared to the ventricles (80–95%).

Narolska et al. [18] found that force development in ventricular tissue was 5 times more economical but nine times slower than in atrial tissue. They found significant linear correlations between MHC isoform composition, ATP consumption and rate of force development. The α-MHC isoform has the highest ATPase activity, while the β-MHC the lowest contractile activity [19].

Here it must be underlined that βMHC is actually decreased in the failing heart but the βMHC-β/α-MHC is increased due to a greater decrease of αMHC [20].

The importance of the decrease of αMHC was highlighted by Reiser et al. [21] who showed that even a small diminution of its levels decreases cardiac contractility and output.

These changes in MHC concentration are governed by thyroid hormones, which promote αMHC overexpression and underexpression of βMHC [22].

Another contractile protein which exhibits significant changes is human skeletal α- actin

In the fetal and neonatal stage α-skeletal actin predominates, but in the adult myocardium the α- cardiac actin is expressed [23].

Titin isoforms also undergo important changes, with the fetal myocardium expressing a greater proportion of compliant isoforms, which are replaced by adult isoforms later [24].

11.1.2 ANP, BNP Expression

The atrial natriuretic peptide is expressed in the transition from the fetal to the adult heart and increases again when there is a return to the fetal phenotype [25].

These changes may reflect on the whole the expression of a protected phenotype in the fetal heart. This is well expressed by the work of Taegtmeyer's group [1, 12]. These authors describe that the metabolic signals act as regulators of a coordinated cardiac stress response. This stress has many expressions such as pressure and volume overload, unloading, tachycardia, altered conduction- pacing, ischemia, remodeling hypothyroidism and diabetes mellitus. Many of these stressors have been shown to be inter-related.

Cameron and Elmers [25] give a very detailed review in 2003. They remind that the atrial factor was purified and sequences in 1984 [26], followed by the identification of family of natriuretic peptics with diuretic, natriuretic, vasorelaxant and antiproliferative effects. ANP and brain natriuretic peptide (BNP) are secreted by the atria and ventricles respectively in the adult heart; they act through binding to the natriuretic peptide receptor, resulting in the generation of the second messenger cGMP.

In the adult heart, as already described, ANP mRNA is mostly expressed in the atrium, while its levels in the left ventricle are very low [27]. In the fetal rodent ventricles and in humans, ANP levels, are higher than in the adult [28, 29]. The same has been reported for BNP [30, 31].

Thus, it can be said that in the embryonic heart in many species the ventricle is the predominant site of ANP and BNP secretion. Here it must be underlined that the third natriuretic peptide CNP has not been detected in mouse or human embryos [32].

These findings apply to the normal adult heart. In cardiac hypertrophy ventricular ANP production is reactivated [33]; the same happens after myocardial infarction [34] and in heart failure [35]; these instances all represent an indication of the fetal gene program return.

ANP suppresses proliferation of muscular smooth muscle cells [36], hypertrophy [37], and apoptosis [25, 38, 39]. Cox and Marsh [40] give a systematic review of fetal genes as biomarkers of cardiac hypertrophy and dysfunction.

In the paradigm of diabetic rodent models, they stress that levels of Serca-2 increase during fetal development and increase further through adulthood [41].

Cox and Marsh [40] also describe many transcription factors involved in the fetal program. Thus, GATA4 is highly expressed. Apart from being required for normal development of cardiac valves [42], it also activates the already mentioned α-MHC [43] and BNP [44].

Importantly, GATA4 contributes to β-MHC upregulation in aortic constriction cardiac hypertrophy [45].

The Nk2 homebox protein NKX2–5/CSX is upregulated in fetal development; it requires GATA4 to be expressed [46].

Its re-expression is a seen in heart failure models [47]. MEF2 also regulates fetal gene expression; HAND 1/2 is also highly expressed in the fetal heart [48].

Cox and Marsh [40] also point out that experimentally induced diabetes (streptozotocin) was associated with reduced cardiac weight but diet-induced or genetic models were associated with cardiac hypertrophy. They showed a wide variation of fetal gene expression which is confounded by the various diabetogenic methods. They also point out that while in pathologic hypertrophy glycolytic metabolism is a characteristic feature [49], the diabetic heart is almost exclusively reliant on fatty acid oxidation [50].

However, Rajabi et al. [12] point out that a closer association of the diabetic heart to the fetal pattern exists, as regards MHC and GLUT and c-myc and c-fos activation isoform changes [51].

Rajabi et al. [12] also stress a very interesting aspect of the return to the fetal gene program: Protection of the stressed heart, in analogy to the danger of the fetal heart when it loses its blood supply, and that glycogen increase is associated with increased survival in anoxia [52], and that it preserves Ca^{2+} hemostasis and cell survival [53, 54].

Additionally, the switch of intracellular free glucose to glycogen protects cardiomyocyte proteins against glycosylation and glucotoxicity [54].

Here it should be remembered that glycogen content is increased in the hibernating myocardium [55], which is "protected" as described in the corresponding chapter.

Also, according to the same authors [12] hypocontractility, as caused by Serca-2 down-regulation is an energy conserving mechanism. Actually, ischemic preconditioning (Chap. 14) is characterized by a decrease in contractility.

It has already been noted that T3 promotes biogenesis of the mitochondria. Hypothyroid hearts typically undergo fetal program expression [56]. The failing-remodeling heart is characterized by tissue hypothyroidism [57].

Rajabi et al. [12] point out that at the same level of stress, survival is greater in the fetal than the adult heart. Another aspect linked to the fetal pattern is that upregulation of the largely cardioprotective Akt also raises glycogen levels [58].

Also, phosphorylation of GLUT4 by Akt increases glucose uptake and inhibits apoptosis [59, 60].

Rajabi et al. [12] also imply that nutrient deprivation can activate autophagy. Here it must be pointed out that the fetal heart program has certain disadvantages. Thus, in Chap. 14 It is described that according to some authors the fetal heart cannot be preconditioned [61, 62].

Awad et al. have noted [63] what in rats ischemic preconditioning develops within 7 days from birth [57].

Also, we have shown what the hypothyroid heart is protected against ischemia but cannot be further preconditioned [64].

Dirkx et al. [65] give a very extensive review on regulation of fetal gene expression in heart failure. In addition to those mentioned already, they describe the following:

Nuclear factor of activated T-cells (NFAT) which in the postnatal myocardium regulates "fetal genes" BNP including while dominant negative NFAT reduces ANF. It also regulates various microRNAs the role of which will be discussed later.

Myocyte enhancer factor 2 (Mef 2), which is identified with the promoter regions of some fetal and cardiac genes, including αMHC, skeletal α-actin 1 and Serca-2. Its depletion inhibits cardiac hypertrophy, fibrosis and fetal gene activation in response to pressure overload.

GATA- binding proteins, whose overexpression induces hypertrophic remodeling in the adult heart [66].

Cardiac homeobox transcription Factor Csx/NKX2–5, in transgenic mice with fetal gene expression and cardiac hypertrophy remodeling.

SMAD (small mother against decapentoplegic) family In the adult heart this family regulates fibrosis, apoptosis and hypertrophic remodelling.

11.1.3 Serum Response Factor (SRF)

In the adult heart, its cardiac-specific overexpression results in dilated cardiomyopathy. It also associates with the already mentioned GATA 4 and NKX2–5 which regulate hypertrophic response in the adult heart [67].

Also, its cardiac-specific overexpression downregulates mR-1, miR-133α and regulates miR-21, which are involved in hypertrophic REM.

Dirkx et al. [65] also referred to the epigenetic control of the fetal gene program. They mention the following:

Histone aceryltransferases (HATs), of which p300 and the CREB- binding protein, which in the adult heart are associated with cardiac hypertrophic REM [68].

11.1.4 Histone Deacetylases (HDACs)

This is a large family consisting of four classes, which catalyse the removal of the acetylgroup from histone residues. Kee et al. give a good account [69]:

They are divided in 4 classes [70]:

Class I consists of 1, 2, 3 and 8, and they are associated with pathological myocardial hypertrophy.

Class IIa suppresses cardiac hypertrophy while the role of class IIb which consists of 6 and 10 is not well proven.

Class III are a certain family which are cardioprotective; the effects of Class IV [71] is not proven yet. Accordingly, some HDAC inhibitors may inhibit cardiac hypertrophy [70, 71].

Accordingly, in the chapter on cardiac remodeling valproic acid has been found to decrease post infarct remodeling in the rat [72]. HDACs also regulate fibrosis [73] and apoptosis [74].

11.2 The Role of microRNAs

miR-1 and miR-133 are co- expressed. After aortic constriction in the mouse miR-1 is downregulated.

Overexpression of miR-133 suppresses hypertrophic growth decreased expression of both miR-1 and 133 were observed in mouse and human models of cardiac hypertrophy. Also, treatment with an antagomir antagonising miR-133 caused marked and sustained cardiac hypertrophy.

miR208 deficient mice are resistant to hypertrophic REM, fibrosis and fetal activation. Also,miR-208α over expression induces cardiac hypertrophy [75–77].

miR-9 has also been described as antihypertrophic, and miR-195 is associated with re-activation of the fetal gene program [65]. Another consideration must be given: the fetal phenotype as produced in hybernation [78] and heart failure [79] is a form of dedifferantiation for cells to regenerate they must first be dedifferentiated [80]. Teleologically it can be postulated that the fetal heart prepears for regeneration [81, 82].

Finally, the very experienced group of Taegtmeyer et al. [80–82] point out that the unloaded heart undergoes atrophic remodeling. Unexpectedly, the atrophic-like the hypertrophic heart- is associated with the fetal program. Taegtmeyer [80] shows similarities and differences among hypertrophy, atrophy, and diabetes (Fig. 11.1).

In conclusion, the fetal pattern represents the adaptation of the -adult- heart to a stressful situation in order to conserve its integrity, since it has an energy and contractile energy expenditure sparing effect. It seen in the hypertrophic remodeling and diabetic process, but also in the unloaded- atrophic heart.

For cells to regenerate, they must first be de-differentiated [79]. Teleologically it can be postulated that the fetal heart is a preparation for regeneration.

	Hypertrophy	Atrophy	Diabetes
Contractile proteins			
α-MHC	↓	↓	↓
β-MHC	↑	↑	↑
Cardiac α-actin	↓	↓	↓
Skeletal α-actin	↑	↑	↑
Ion pumps			
α_2 Na/K-ATPase	↓	↓	↓
SERCA 2a	↓	↓	↓
Metabolic proteins			
GLUT4	↓	↓	↓
GLUT1	=	=	↓
Muscle CPT-1	↓	↓	=
Liver CPT-1	=	=	=
mCK	↓	↓	↓
PPARα	↓	↓	↓
PDK4	↓	↓	↑
MCD	↓	↓	↑
UCP2	↓	↓	=
UCP3	↓	↓	↓
Protooncogenes			
c-fos	↑	↑	↓

Fig. 11.1 Coordinated transcriptional responses of the heart in hypertrophy, atrophy, and diabetes. Reproduced with permission from Taegtmeyer [80]

References

1. Taegtmeyer H, Sen S, Vela D. Return to the fetal gene program: a suggested metabolic link to gene expression in the heart. Ann N Y Acad Sci. 2010;1188:191–8.
2. Swynghedauw B. Molecular mechanisms of myocardial remodeling. Physiol Rev. 1999;79:215–62.
3. Bartelds B, Knoester H, Smid GB, Takens J, Visser GH, Penninga L, et al. Perinatal changes in myocardial metabolism in lambs. Circulation. 2000;102:926–31.
4. Navaratnam V. Heart muscle: Vetrastructural studies Cambridge. New York: University Press; 1987. referred in 1.
5. Pederson BA, Chen H, Schroeder JM, Shou W, DePaoli-Roach AA, Roach PJ. Abnormal cardiac development in the absence of heart glycogen. Mol Cell Biol. 2004;24:7179–87.
6. Van der Vusse GJ, Reneman RS. Glycogen and lipids endogeneous substances. In: Drake-Holland A-J, MIM N, editors. Cardiac metabolism. New York: Willey; 1983. p. 215–37.
7. Barbosa V, Sievers RE, Zaugg CE, Wolfe CL. Preconditioning ischemia time determines the degree of glycogen depletion and infarct size reduction in rat hearts. Am Heart J. 1996;131:224–30.
8. Girard J, Ferré P, Pégorier JP, Duée PH. Adaptations of glucose and fatty acid metabolism during perinatal period and suckling-weaning transition. Physiol Rev. 1992;72:507–62.
9. Goodwin CW, Mela L, Deutsch C, Forster RE, Miller LD, Kelivoria-Papadopoulos M. Development and adaptation of heart mitochondrial respiratory chain function in fetus and in newborn. Adv Exp Med Biol. 1976;75:713–9.
10. Weitzel JM, Iwen KA, Seitz HJ. Regulation of mitochondrial biogenesis by thyroid hormone. Exp Physiol. 2003;88:121–8.
11. Scholz TD, Koppenhafer SL. tenEyck CJ, Schutte BC. Ontogeny of malate-aspartate shuttle capacity and gene expression in cardiac mitochondria. Am J Phys. 1998;274:C780–8.

12. Rajabi M, Kassiotis C, Razeghi P, Taegtmeyer H. Return to the fetal gene program protects the stressed heart: a strong hypothesis. Heart Fail Rev. 2007;12:331–43.
13. Taegtmeyer H, Golfman L, Sharma S, Razeghi P, van Arsdall M. Linking gene expression to function: metabolic flexibility in the normal and diseased heart. Ann N Y Acad Sci. 2004;1015:202–13.
14. Morkin E. Regulation of myosin heavy chain genes in the heart. Circulation. 1993;87:1451–60.
15. Krenz M, Robbins J. Impact of beta-myosin heavy chain expression on cardiac function during stress. J Am Coll Cardiol. 2004;44:2390–7.
16. Danzi S, Klein S, Klein I. Differential regulation of the myosin heavy chain genes alpha and beta in rat atria and ventricles: role of antisense RNA. Thyroid. 2008;18:761–8.
17. Fuller GA, Bicer S, Hamlin RL, Yamaguchi M, Reiser PJ. Increased myosin heavy chain-beta with atrial expression of ventricular light chain-2 in canine cardiomyopathy. J Card Fail. 2007;13:680–6.
18. Narolska NA, van Loon RB, Boontje NM, Zaremba R, Penas SE, Russell J, et al. Myocardial contraction is 5-fold more economical in ventricular than in atrial human tissue. Cardiovasc Res. 2005;65:221–9.
19. Gustafson TA, Bahl JJ, Markham BE, Roeske WR, Morkin E. Hormonal regulation of myosin heavy chain and alpha-actin gene expression in cultured fetal rat heart myocytes. J Biol Chem. 1987;262:13316–22.
20. Razeghi P, Young ME, Alcorn JL, Moravec CS, Frazier OH, Taegtmeyer H. Metabolic gene expression in fetal and failing human heart. Circulation. 2001;104:2923–31.
21. Reiser PJ, Portman MA, Ning XH, Schomisch MC. Human cardiac myosin heavy chain isoforms in fetal and failing adult atria and ventricles. Am J Physiol Heart Circ Physiol. 2001;280:H1814–20.
22. Morkin E. Control of cardiac myosin heavy chain gene expression. Microsc Res Tech. 2000;50:522–31.
23. Schwartz K, Boheler KR, de la Bastie D, Lompre AM, Mercadier JJ. Switches in cardiac muscle gene expression as a result of pressure and volume overload. Am J Phys. 1992;262:R364–9.
24. Lahmers S, Wu Y, Call DR, Labeit S, Granzier H. Developmental control of titin isoform expression and passive stiffness in fetal and neonatal myocardium. Circ Res. 2004;94:505–13.
25. Cameron VA, Ellmers LJ. Natriuretic peptides during development of the fetal heart and circulation. Endocrinology. 2003;144:2191–4.
26. Kangawa K, Matsuo H. Purification and complete amino acid sequence of alpha-human atrial natriuretic polypeptide (alpha-hANP). Biochem Biophys Res Commun. 1984;118:131–9.
27. Ruskoaho H. Atrial natriuretic peptide: synthesis, release, and metabolism. Pharmacol Rev. 1992;44:479–602.
28. Takahashi T, Allen PD, Izumo S. Expression of A-, B-, and C-type natriuretic peptide genes in failing and developing human ventricles. Correlation with expression of the ca(2+)-ATPase gene. Circ Res. 1992;71:9–17.
29. Gardner DG, Hedges BK, Wu J, LaPointe MC, Deschepper CF. Expression of the atrial natriuretic peptide gene in human fetal heart. J Clin Endocrinol Metab. 1989;69:729–37.
30. Hersey RM, Nazir MA, Whitney KD, Klein RM, Sale RD, Hinton DA, et al. Atrial natriuretic peptide in heart and specific binding in organs from fetal and newborn rats. Cell Biochem Funct. 1989;7:35–41.
31. Cameron VA, Aitken GD, Ellmers LJ, Kennedy MA, Espiner EA. The sites of gene expression of atrial, brain, and C-type natriuretic peptides in mouse fetal development: temporal changes in embryos and placenta. Endocrinology. 1996;137:817–24.
32. Scott JN, Jennes L. Distribution of atrial natriuretic factor in fetal rat atria and ventricles. Cell Tissue Res. 1987;248:479–81.
33. Day ML, Schwartz D, Wiegand RC, Stockman PT, Brunnert SR, Tolunay HE, et al. Ventricular atriopeptin. Unmasking of messenger RNA and peptide synthesis by hypertrophy or dexamethasone. Hypertension. 1987;9:485–91.

34. Cameron VA, Rademaker MT, Ellmers LJ, Espiner EA, Nicholls MG, Richards AM. Atrial (ANP) and brain natriuretic peptide (BNP) expression after myocardial infarction in sheep: ANP is synthesized by fibroblasts infiltrating the infarct. Endocrinology. 2000;141:4690–7.
35. Luchner A, Stevens TL, Borgeson DD, Redfield M, Wei CM, Porter JG, et al. Differential atrial and ventricular expression of myocardial BNP during evolution of heart failure. Am J Phys. 1998;274:H1684–9.
36. Abell TJ, Richards AM, Ikram H, Espiner EA, Yandle T. Atrial natriuretic factor inhibits proliferation of vascular smooth muscle cells stimulated by platelet-derived growth factor. Biochem Biophys Res Commun. 1989;160:1392–6.
37. Horio T, Nishikimi T, Yoshihara F, Matsuo H, Takishita S, Kangawa K. Inhibitory regulation of hypertrophy by endogenous atrial natriuretic peptide in cultured cardiac myocytes. Hypertension. 2000;35:19–24.
38. Wu CF, Bishopric NH, Pratt RE. Atrial natriuretic peptide induces apoptosis in neonatal rat cardiac myocytes. J Biol Chem. 1997;272:14860–6.
39. Kuhn M, Holtwick R, Baba HA, Perriard JC, Schmitz W, Ehler E. Progressive cardiac hypertrophy and dysfunction in atrial natriuretic peptide receptor (GC-A) deficient mice. Heart. 2002;87:368–74.
40. Cox EJ, Marsh SA. A systematic review of fetal genes as biomarkers of cardiac hypertrophy in rodent models of diabetes. PLoS One. 2014;9:e92903.
41. Periasamy M, Bhupathy P, Babu GJ. Regulation of sarcoplasmic reticulum Ca2+ ATPase pump expression and its relevance to cardiac muscle physiology and pathology. Cardiovasc Res. 2008;77:265–73.
42. Rivera-Feliciano J, Lee KH, Kong SW, Rajagopal S, Ma Q, Springer Z, et al. Development of heart valves requires Gata4 expression in endothelial-derived cells. Development. 2006;133:3607–18.
43. Molkentin JD, Kalvakolanu DV, Markham BE. Transcription factor GATA-4 regulates cardiac muscle-specific expression of the alpha-myosin heavy-chain gene. Mol Cell Biol. 1994;14:4947–57.
44. Maitra M, Schluterman MK, Nichols HA, Richardson JA, Lo CW, Srivastava D, et al. Interaction of Gata4 and Gata6 with Tbx5 is critical for normal cardiac development. Dev Biol. 2009;326:368–77.
45. Hasegawa K, Lee SJ, Jobe SM, Markham BE, Kitsis RN. Cis-acting sequences that mediate induction of beta-myosin heavy chain gene expression during left ventricular hypertrophy due to aortic constriction. Circulation. 1997;96:3943–53.
46. Lien CL, Wu C, Mercer B, Webb R, Richardson JA, Olson EN. Control of early cardiac-specific transcription of Nkx2-5 by a GATA-dependent enhancer. Development. 1999;126:75–84.
47. Azakie A, Fineman JR, He Y. Myocardial transcription factors are modulated during pathologic cardiac hypertrophy in vivo. J Thorac Cardiovasc Surg. 2006;132:1262–71.
48. Thattaliyath BD, Firulli BA, Firulli AB. The basic-helix-loop-helix transcription factor HAND2 directly regulates transcription of the atrial naturetic peptide gene. J Mol Cell Cardiol. 2002;34:1335–44.
49. Kolwicz SC Jr, Tian R. Glucose metabolism and cardiac hypertrophy. Cardiovasc Res. 2011;90:194–201.
50. Chess DJ, Stanley WC. Role of diet and fuel overabundance in the development and progression of heart failure. Cardiovasc Res. 2008;79:269–78.
51. Depre C, Young ME, Ying J, Ahuja HS, Han Q, Garza N, et al. Streptozotocin-induced changes in cardiac gene expression in the absence of severe contractile dysfunction. J Mol Cell Cardiol. 2000;32:985–96.
52. Dawes GS, Mott JC, Shelley HJ. The importance of cardiac glycogen for the maintenance of life in foetal lambs and newborn animals during anoxia. J Physiol. 1959;146:516–38.
53. Depré C, Vanoverschelde JL, Melin JA, Borgers M, Bol A, Ausma J, et al. Structural and metabolic correlates of the reversibility of chronic left ventricular ischemic dysfunction in humans. Am J Phys. 1995;268:H1265–75.

54. Taegtmeyer H. Glycogen in the heart--an expanded view. J Mol Cell Cardiol. 2004;37:7–10.
55. Kim SJ, Peppas A, Hong SK, Yang G, Huang Y, Diaz G, et al. Persistent stunning induces myocardial hibernation and protection: flow/function and metabolic mechanisms. Circ Res. 2003;92:1233–9.
56. Kinugawa K, Minobe WA, Wood WM, Ridgway EC, Baxter JD, Ribeiro RC, et al. Signaling pathways responsible for fetal gene induction in the failing human heart: evidence for altered thyroid hormone receptor gene expression. Circulation. 2001;103:1089–94.
57. Pantos C, Mourouzis I, Saranteas T, Paizis I, Xinaris C, Malliopoulou V, et al. Thyroid hormone receptors alpha1 and beta1 are downregulated in the post-infarcted rat heart: consequences on the response to ischaemia-reperfusion. Basic Res Cardiol. 2005;100:422–32.
58. Matsui T, Li L, Wu JC, Cook SA, Nagoshi T, Picard MH, et al. Phenotypic spectrum caused by transgenic overexpression of activated Akt in the heart. J Biol Chem. 2002;277:22896–901.
59. Gottlob K, Majewski N, Kennedy S, Kandel E, Robey RB, Hay N, et al. Inhibition of early apoptotic events by Akt/PKB is dependent on the first committed step of glycolysis and mitochondrial hexokinase. Genes Dev. 2001;15:1406–18.
60. Majewski N, Nogueira V, Robey RB, Hay N. Akt inhibits apoptosis downstream of BID cleavage via a glucose-dependent mechanism involving mitochondrial hexokinases. Mol Cell Biol. 2004;24:730–40.
61. Baker JE, Holman P, Gross GJ. Preconditioning in immature rabbit hearts: role of KATP channels. Circulation. 1999;99:1249–54.
62. Baker EJ, Boerboom LE, Olinger GN, Baker JE. Tolerance of the developing heart to ischemia: impact of hypoxemia from birth. Am J Phys. 1995;268:H1165–73.
63. Awad WI, Shattock MJ, Chambers DJ. Ischemic preconditioning in immature myocardium. Circulation. 1998;98:II206–13.
64. Mourouzis I, Dimopoulos A, Saranteas T, Tsinarakis N, Livadarou E, Spanou D, et al. Ischemic preconditioning fails to confer additional protection against ischemia-reperfusion injury in the hypothyroid rat heart. Physiol Res. 2009;58:29–38.
65. Dirkx E, da Costa Martins PA, De Windt LJ. Regulation of fetal gene expression in heart failure. Biochim Biophys Acta. 1832;2013:2414–24.
66. Liang Q, De Windt LJ, Witt SA, Kimball TR, Markham BE, Molkentin JD. The transcription factors GATA4 and GATA6 regulate cardiomyocyte hypertrophy in vitro and in vivo. J Biol Chem. 2001;276:30245–302453.
67. Sepulveda JL, Vlahopoulos S, Iyer D, Belaguli N, Schwartz RJ. Combinatorial expression of GATA4, Nkx2-5, and serum response factor directs early cardiac gene activity. J Biol Chem. 2002;277:25775–257782.
68. Gusterson RJ, Jazrawi E, Adcock IM, Latchman DS. The transcriptional co-activators CREB-binding protein (CBP) and p300 play a critical role in cardiac hypertrophy that is dependent on their histone acetyltransferase activity. J Biol Chem. 2003;278:6838–47.
69. Kee HJ, Bae EH, Park S, Lee KE, Suh SH, Kim SW, et al. HDAC inhibition suppresses cardiac hypertrophy and fibrosis in DOCA-salt hypertensive rats via regulation of HDAC6/HDAC8 enzyme activity. Kidney Blood Press Res. 2013;37:229–39.
70. Gregoretti IV, Lee YM, Goodson HV. Molecular evolution of the histone deacetylase family: functional implications of phylogenetic analysis. J Mol Biol. 2004;338:17–31.
71. Eom GH, Cho YK, Ko JH, Shin S, Choe N, Kim Y, et al. Casein kinase-2α1 induces hypertrophic response by phosphorylation of histone deacetylase 2 S394 and its activation in the heart. Circulation. 2011;123:2392–403.
72. Lee TM, Lin MS, Chang NC. Inhibition of histone deacetylase on ventricular remodeling in infarcted rats. Am J Physiol Heart Circ Physiol. 2007;293:H968–77.
73. Kee HJ, Kook H. Krüppel-like factor 4 mediates histone deacetylase inhibitor-induced prevention of cardiac hypertrophy. J Mol Cell Cardiol. 2009;47:770–80.
74. Ma P, Pan H, Montgomery RL, Olson EN, Schultz RM. Compensatory functions of histone deacetylase 1 (HDAC1) and HDAC2 regulate transcription and apoptosis during myocyte development. Proc Natl Acad Sci U S A. 2012;109:E481–9.

75. Sayed D, Hong C, Chen IY, Lypowy J, Abdellatif M. MicroRNAs play an essential role in the development of cardiac hypertrophy. Circ Res. 2007;100:416–24.
76. Carè A, Catalucci D, Felicetti F, Bonci D, Addario A, Gallo P, et al. MicroRNA-133 controls cardiac hypertrophy. Nat Med. 2007;13:613–8.
77. Dispersyn GD, Geuens E, Ver Donck L, Ramaekers FC, Borgers M. Adult rabbit cardiomyocytes undergo hibernation-like dedifferentiation when co-cultured with cardiac fibroblasts. Cardiovasc Res. 2001;51:230–40.
78. Szibor M, Pöling J, Warnecke H, Kubin T, Braun T. Remodeling and dedifferentiation of adult cardiomyocytes during disease and regeneration. Cell Mol Life Sci. 2014;71:1907–16.
79. Jopling C, Sleep E, Raya M, Martí M, Raya A, Izpisúa Belmonte JC. Zebrafish heart regeneration occurs by cardiomyocyte dedifferentiation and proliferation. Nature. 2010;464:606–9.
80. Taegtmeyer H. From fetal to fatal. In: Cokkinos DV, Pantos C, Heusch G, Taegtmeyer H, editors. Myocardial ischemia. New York: Springer; 2006. p. 1–9.
81. Razeghi P, Taegtmeyer H. Cardiac remodeling: UPS lost in transit. New York. Circ Res. 2005;97:964–6.
82. Baskin KK, Taegtmeyer H. Taking pressure off the heart: the ins and outs of atrophic remodelling. Cardiovasc Res. 2011;90:243–50.

Chapter 12
Cardiac Remodeling: The Course Toward Heart Failure – I. General Concepts

Dennis V. Cokkinos

A definition of cardiac remodeling REM is first attempted.

First, some general definitions should be given. Thus, Swynghedauw [1] in a seminal review described that in REM unfavorable changes emerge which result in the rearrangement of normal cardiac structures.

Sutton and Sharpe [2] describe it as changes in the structure, shape, size, and function of LV.

A similar definition is given in a consensus statement regulated by Cohn et al. [3]. Pfeffer and Braunwald [4] describe it as a progressive dilation of the LV cavity. Here it must be underlined that the term "dilation" is currently used rather than "dilatation."

These geometric changes are initially considered as "adaptive": Thus, increases in wall thickness as described in the chapter on ventricular hypertrophy contribute to a decrease of LV wall stress [5].

Also, an increase in end-diastolic volume preserves the stroke volume, according to Starling's law. However, these changes eventually become "maladaptive" [6].

Although in the strict sense of the word REM can be used to define all types of hypertrophy, even concentric, it is more widely used to describe LV cavity enlargement. It will be used in this sense from now on.

To ensure homogeneity in reporting results, common quantitative definitions should be employed.

As already stressed, REM is characterized by an increase of LV end-diastolic volume. Actually it was first described by McKay et al. [7] in 1986, as an increase by 20% of the LV end-diastolic volume index. In this early report, such an increase was seen in 11/25 of patients with an anterior infarct but only in 6/15 of patients

D. V. Cokkinos (✉)
Heart and Vessel Department, Biomedical Research Foundation,
Academy of Athens - Gregory Skalkeas, Athens, Greece
e-mail: dcokkinos@bioacademy.gr

D. V. Cokkinos (ed.), *Myocardial Preservation*,
https://doi.org/10.1007/978-3-319-98186-4_12

with an inferior infarct. This definition is also being used in large studies such as the AMICI trial [8] and by Savoye et al. [9] and Bolognese et al. [10]; in a study of the effects of primary angioplasty and in a chronic failure cohort [11], it was found to adversely affect survival.

An LVEDV increase of 20% was also associated with a worse prognosis in the VALIANT study [12]. However, the LVESV is also being used, as in a study on the effect of ivabradine [13].

Interestingly, LVESV was also predictive of post-infarct course in the GUSTO-I trial [14, 15].

In the aforementioned VALIANT trial, LVESV was equally predictive of a worse prognosis [12].

White et al. [16] also had previously found, using contrast ventriculography, that LVESV is the better predictor for survival.

If smaller volumes are employed to describe outcomes in LV REM, better results have been reported [17]; here it must be pointed out that reperfusion therapy, either by thrombolysis or primary PCI, has practically eliminated the evolution toward a typical LV aneurysm.

Obviously, these measurements are needed to arrive at a homogeneity of result recording. However, as Bhatt et al. recently observed [18], a general consensus emerges that larger LV volumes are consistently related to poor clinical outcomes.

The author believes that continuous measurements are more representative than one measurement at a single point, usually 4–8 weeks post-MI, but agrees with the need of uniformity in reporting.

The same holds true in the reporting of a “reverse REM” which in general signifies a decrease of LV volumes after an intervention. Here, more agreement can be seen, since the majority of researchers agree on a >10% decrease of LVESV [19–21].

Kramer et al. compared various echocardiographic indices in the assessment of mortality after drug or device therapy [21].

In this study they included 30 mortality trials of 25 drug device therapies which comprised 69,766 patients with a median follow-up (FU) of 6 months. They found practically similar odds ratio correlations for death as regards LVEF ($r = -0.51$), LVEDD ($r = 0.44$), and LVESD ($r = 0.48$).

12.1 Causes of LV REM

Burchfield et al. [23] give a detailed review on the mechanisms of this phenomenon.

They mention that coronary artery disease (CAD) is a leading cause of HF-rEF and REM as the result of an antecedent MI. This will be subsequently discussed in detail.

However as shown in Table 12.1, many other causes can lead to REM.

Table 12.1 The main causes of cardiac remodeling

Previous large myocardial infarction
Cardiomyopathy, dilated and hypertrophic
Hypertension
Valvular disease (aortic stenosis and regurgitation, mitral regurgitation)
Antineoplastic agent chemotherapy, environmental pollution
Diabetes mellitus type 1 or 2
Morbid obesity
Genetic diseases (cardiomyopathies, cardiac defects)
Arrhythmias
Tachycardiomyopathy, multiple extrasystoles
Conduction defects
LBBB
Right ventricular stimulation

12.2 Hypertension

According to the American Heart Association statistics of 2013 [24], hypertension is still the most important risk factor for HF. This has not changed in more recent statistics.

In this case concentric hypertrophy occurs, as described in the corresponding chapter. It must be stressed that hypertension is now being treated in a more effective way than previously. Consequently, it does not commonly lead to LV cavity dilation any longer. However, it must be remembered that the very interesting entity of heart failure with preserved ejection fraction (HFpEF) is mainly seen in hypertensive patients who in their majority do not have cardiac dilation but increased wall thickness and diastolic pressures together with slow LV relaxation and increased stiffness. It is more prevalent in the elderly hypertensive females with a higher body mass [25]. Borlaug [26] remarks that there is heterogeneity in EF, with values above 45% having better outcomes.

12.3 Valvular Heart Disease

Aortic stenosis leads to pressure overload and concentric hypertrophy. Nowadays, with both surgical and interventional replacement advances, LV dilation is seen very rarely.

On the contrary, eccentric hypertrophy which corresponds to REM due to diastolic or systolic LV enlargement is commonly seen in both mitral and aortic regurgitation. There has been much discussion whether pressure overload is more benign than volume overload. Correction of regurgitation is advised before appreciable LV dilation occurs (LVEDD not above 70 mm in aortic or LVESD above 55 mm in mitral regurgitation). No such limits are offered for aortic stenosis.

However, in the experimental setting, some different opinions have been expressed. Thus, Toischer et al. [29] postulate that experimentally produced volume overload is considered more benign than pressure overload. Chemaly et al. [30] with the aid of cardiac magnetic tomography have found that volume overload causes less fibrosis than pressure overload.

Dilated cardiomyopathy is by definition characterized by cardiac dilation which entails REM. Interrupting the vicious cycle of the dilation begetting dilation has been the rationale of volume reduction surgery which however has fallen into disuse, the last report being in 2005 [31].

A corollary to this effort would be the earliest possible therapy which will be subsequently described to interrupt this cycle. In the term of dilated cardiomyopathy, many genetically determined causes of cardiac dysfunction are included.

Interestingly, in hypertrophic cardiomyopathy (HCM), a small percentage (5–10%) of patients manifests with time a course toward cardiac dilation, i.e., REM [33]. They have a poorer prognosis.

Cardiac dysfunction caused by chemotherapy for neoplastic disease represents a cause of REM [34, 35].

Diabetes mellitus types I and II can be accompanied by cardiac dysfunction not related to ischemic heart disease. The same has been described for morbid obesity [36].

Rhythm disturbances offer a very interesting paradigm. Thus, tachycardiomyopathy was described many years ago in cases of supraventricular arrhythmias followed by rapid ventricular response.

Actually, when these cases were initially described, it was difficult to determine which caused the other, the arrhythmia or the cardiac dysfunction.

Unrecognized or untreated hyperthyroidism with atrial fibrillation often causes such a picture.

Frequent premature ventricular contraction (more than 30% of the total cardiac beats/day) can cause cardiac dysfunction and dilation which regresses when they are eliminated by ablation [39].

Left bundle branch block or pacing from the right ventricle has been associated with cardiac dysfunction and dilation. Braunschweig [40] uses the term "dyssynchronopathy" to describe this finding.

Therapy with resynchronization can produce very significant results [41], as will be described in the next chapter.

However, as Burchfield et al. [23] point out, cardiac REM currently mainly concerns ischemic heart disease.

Finally, the athlete's heart is a very interesting paradigm. The LVEDV can increase significantly, but the stroke volume is increased, and the LVEF remains normal. Also the molecular characteristics of pathologic hypertrophy are not seen. More is described in the chapter on cardiac hypertrophy.

12.4 Post-myocardial Infarction REM

This is the most common cause of REM. According to Fraccarollo et al. [43], REM after an MI can be divided into stages.

The first is loss of cardiac myocytes, due either to necrosis, apoptosis, or also possibly autophagy, as described in the chapters on cell death and ischemia reperfusion injury.

The clinical statistics are quite interesting: with all modern intervention, specifically primary angioplasty and employment of currently recommended drugs, REM is seen in up to 30% of anterior infarcts [9] as seen in the REVE (REmodelage VEntriculaire) study group.

Papadopoulos et al. [44] found a similar ratio as well as Galiuto et al. in the AMICI trial [8]. Masci et al. [45] reported that in infarcts undergoing primary PCI, 30% of the anterior infarcts manifested REM vs 17% of inferior.

By hospital discharge, Giannuzzi et al. [46] reported that of non-anterior infarcts only, 19% had developed an increase of the LVDVI >20%; this occurred in 38% of the anterior infarcts.

These data are not surprising or unexpected. REM depends on the size of the infarct. The left anterior descending artery invariably perfuses a greater cardiac mass than the circumflex or the right coronary artery [47].

These authors [48] have described that to reduce REM the myocardial infarct size needs to be reduced to <20% in the rat. Again in the rat, an infarct size >40% of the LV is critical [49].

Miura and Miki [48] pertinently point out that rat hearts tolerate myocardial loss better than humans, in whom a 40% loss is fatal. In the aforementioned study by Masci et al. [45] by CMR at 1 week, anterior infarcts caused a nonreversible cardiomyocyte loss of 14% vs 9% of inferior ones.

Apart from the size of the infarct, which is a main factor, the following factors can affect the extent of REM: many of these are given in Fig. 12.1 of Bhatt et al. [18].

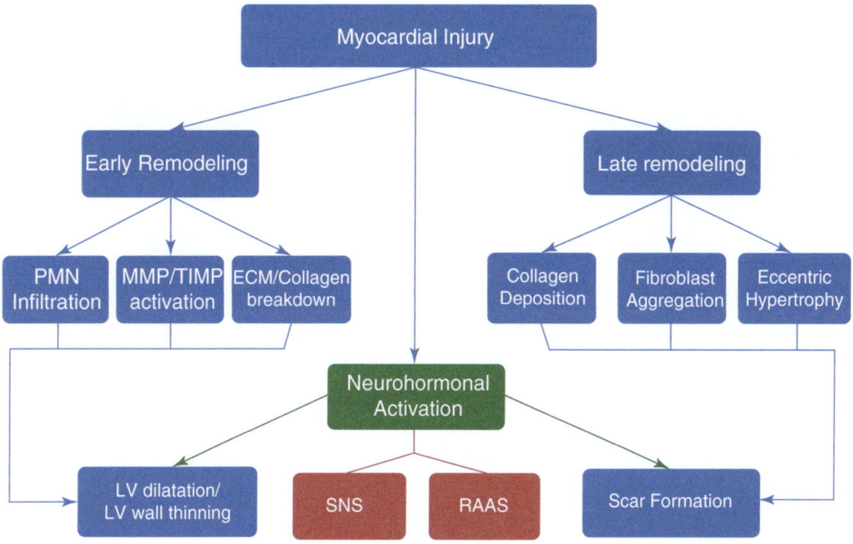

Fig. 12.1 Major interactions between cellular, extracellular, and neurohormonal components in the development of adverse post-MI cardiac remodeling. (Reprinted by permission from Bhatt et al. [18])

12.5 Age

Both human and animal studies showed that aged individuals manifest greater REM [50].

However, Ennezat et al. [51] on behalf of the REVE investigators did not find that age was associated with REM increase (overall around 30%) after an inaugural anterior MI.

As regards polymorphisms, Bauters et al. [52] found 14 polymorphisms in 3 different systems (RAS, adrenergic, and metalloproteinases) which did not affect REM; actually, more than 50 polymorphisms have been implicated in REM [53, 54].

Diabetes mellitus is also associated with greater REM, clinically [55] and experimentally [56].

The same holds true for hypercholesterolemia and hypertension [57, 58].

Smoking increases REM [58] through multiple mechanisms, such as mitogen-activated protein kinase activation, hypertension, increased oxidative stress, impaired NO bioavailability, and endothelial dysfunction experimentally [59, 60].

Interestingly, in a very recent study, hypertrophy decreased post-MI REM due to infarct expansion in mice [61].

12.6 Mechanisms of REM

The initial mechanism is mechanical. According to Hill and Olson [6], the loss of function of a myocardial segment results in dilation and overwork of the initially normally contracting myocardial segments, thus causing "stretch," and with deleterious consequences; this stretch engenders fibrosis via a mechanotransduction process [59].

The molecular processes underlying the influence of mechanotransduction have been recently described [63].

According to Chemaly et al. [30], the process of REM after an AMI represents a combination of both types of overload, pressure, and volume. A main determinant of REM is the expansion of myocardium around the necrotic core of the myocardium, the border zone (BOR) [61–65].

Expansion can occur within the first day of AMI. The importance of the BOR as regards the various molecular processes is described further Zornoff et al. giving a detailed account [66].

They described that in normal hearts both the systolic and diastolic tensions are at the maximum value at the midventricle, intermediate at the base, and lowest at the apex. In REM and after the aforementioned expansion, they describe that the ventricle loses its elliptical form and becomes spherical; in this case in the apical parietal level, in which the tension also is increased. Additionally, diastolic parietal tension increases more than the systolic.

Clarke et al. [67] have given a detailed description of the natural history of the LVEF in patients with HF.

They found that patients with previous MI were more likely to evolve from HFpEF to HFrEF, at a study period of ~360 days. Interestingly, they found that patients with hypertension were more likely to revert from HFrEF to HFpEF, underlying the importance of treating hypertension. Women were more likely to retain their HFpEF status; this was also seen with β-blocker, angiotensin converting enzyme inhibitor (ACEI), or angiotensin receptor blocker (ARB) therapy.

These mechanical disturbances set in motion a series of biochemical, metabolic, and molecular changes.

A main determinant in the emergence of the fetal phenotype is very thoroughly described by Swynghedauw [1]. This is further described in the respective chapter where the main characteristics of the fetal phenotype are given in Chap. 11. Apart from these, some significant changes should be stressed.

Tissue hypothyroidism is a main characteristic of REM, with a decrease of TRβ1 and an initial increase of TRα1 which, however in the absence of tissue T3, acts as an aporeceptor [68], at 2–15 weeks post-infarct, before also decreasing especially in the border zone at 34 weeks [69] according to studies from our group.

We have also found that this tissue hypothyroidism is more pronounced in diabetic rat hearts [56].

Also, in patients after an initial MI, we have found that low serum T3 is associated with a lower possibility of LVEF improvement [70].

However, before further proceeding with the description of molecular changes, the main culprit leading to REM, cell death (CD), is further described in the respective chapter.

Thus, the degree of ongoing apoptosis (APO) leading to cardiomyocyte loss and eventual REM should be adequately stressed.

Data given by Abbate et al. [71] are very pertinent.

The cellular apoptotic rate was calculated in 14 patients who died within 2 months (12–34 days) after an AMI. This rate was significantly correlated with the emergence of progressive REM, both in the infarct and also in the unaffected areas; it was also associated with post-MI symptoms. Seventy-one percent of patients had a large MI (more than 30% of the LV wall circumference). This report gives the important information that apoptosis also occurs in the remote "unaffected" region and is correlated with REM.

The same authors [72] also studied post-MI patients and found that apoptosis, although occurring at a very low rate, can be seen for up to 3–8 months after an initial MI and is a main determinant of the emergence of HF.

Elsässer et al. [73] studied 14 patients with clinical hibernation undergoing surgical myocardial revascularization by intraoperative biopsies from the area designated as hibernating, which could be correlated with the border zone, at 6–12 weeks post-infarct. They found apoptosis to be increased in 5/14 of their patients.

Similar results have emerged experimentally.

Thus, Palojoki et al. [74] found increased apoptosis in rats for up to 12 weeks in the border zone in the animals developing LV dilation.

In an experimental mole of HF caused by coronary microembolization [75], a 20-fold greater apoptosis is found in the border zone for up to 4 months.

In an older study, Misao et al. [76] studied 27 human hearts, 15 after an old MI (>1 month).The pro-apoptotic protein Bax was overexpressed in 83% of hearts with an old MI. The shortest period for Bax overexpression was 14 days, and the longest was 10 years.

In rats developing HF after an experimental MI (unpublished data), we found increased apoptosis in the border zone for up to 34 months. This corresponds to 20 years in man. Here, a caveat must be mentioned. The role of autophagy in HF, as also described in the chapter on cell death, is less clear. Interestingly, Yang et al. [77] found that autophagy restoration protects against REM in experimental hypertension.

The various experiments in animals have been carried out with either permanent or reversible occlusion of the culprit artery. The same holds true for human studies. Many older studies had probably included patients without reperfusion.

Currently, very few patients with an AMI are left without either thrombolysis, primary PCI, or both. The importance of opening the occluded artery will be discussed later. However, almost 20 years ago, Michael et al. [78] had shown that with similar experimental MI sizes, permanent occlusion was associated with greater expansion and mortality.

Early studies on thrombolysis showed that it decreases LV wall motion abnormalities [79, 80] with a smaller LVESV and LVEDV at 6 months.

Late post-infarct artery patency is also associated with decreased mortality and LV function [80, 81].

The same can be seen when TIMI flow is considered: <TIMI2 flow is associated with the worst clinical outcomes [82].

Baseline viability is a strong predictor of late REM occurrence [83].

12.7 Important Changes in Molecular Mechanisms

Calcium cycling is a very important mechanism underlying cardiac function but also indirect structure. A full account was given by Haghighi et al. [84].

Zornoff et al. [66] very pertinently point out that calcium transport through the sarcoplasmic reticulum is an active, multifunctional complex which involves the membrane system but also intracellular systems such as the L-type channels, ryanodine, and calsequestrin which regulate the amount of calcium involved in cardiac contraction.

Thus SERCA-2 (sarcoplasmic/endoplasmic reticulum calcium ATPase 2) and specifically its α-isoform present in cardiomyocytes [86] are definitely reduced during the course toward heart failure [85–87].

The progressive decrease of SERCA-2 according to Zarain-Herzberg et al. [87] may lead to the activation of the low-affinity mitochondrial Ca2+ uniporter and an increase in the mitochondrial Ca2+ uptake especially in the SR-mitochondrial junction, ultimately resulting into the disruption of the mitochondrial membrane potential and activation of the mPTP leading to apoptosis.

Sari et al. [88] have also found that inhibition of SERCA-2 (by thapsigargin) promotes apoptosis.

We have also found (unpublished observation) that the SERCA-2/phospholamban ratio decreases during the course of experimentally induced HF.

This suggests a slower cytosolic Ca2+ decay on the beat-to-beat basis, which may lead to the activation of the low-affinity mitochondrial Ca2+ uniporter and an increase in mitochondrial Ca2+ uptake. Efforts toward increasing mitochondrial SERCA-2 are described in the "gene therapy" chapter.

Also, Akt decreases during the course toward HF [89, 90].

An Akt increase is usually associated with physiological growth [91]. It is also cardioprotective [92].

Stress-signaling kinases (p38MAPK, JNK) are also increased during the emergence of HF. They are prohypertrophic and pro-apoptotic [93–95].

12.7.1 Changes in Myosin Heavy Chains

These are also discussed in detail in Chap. 11 on the return to the fetal phenotype. Briefly the αMHC isoform has the highest ATPase activity [1].

β-adrenergic receptor (BAR) changes:

The concentration of 2 main receptors differs: β1 are far more abundant; β1 cause more readily REM than β2 receptors. β1ARs decrease while β2 increase the cytosolic Ca2+ [96, 97].

The role of β3ARs is recently being investigated. Briefly they are cardioprotective [98].

12.8 Renin-Angiotensin-Aldosterone System (RAAS)

The role of this system is also debated during REM. It causes, as discussed, hypertrophy and increase of fibrosis, increased vessel permeability, and metalloproteinase activation, vasoconstriction, and water retention, together with an increase in oxidative stress and a direct cytotoxic effect [99, 100].

12.9 Fibrosis

Excessive extracellular matrix (ECM) deposition is a main and possibly indispensable feature of pathological REM, occurring through the action of cardiac fibroblasts, which under stress produce increased mostly collagen I and III and fibronectin [101].

Fibroblasts are the most abundant cell types in the myocardium and are derived from resident fibroblasts, adult epicardial cells undergoing endothelial-to-mesenchymal transition. Here it must be reminded that CMCs represent about 1/3 of all cells in the myocardium, although they occupy 2/3 of the myocardial volume [102–104]. They can also [105] be derived from circulating, collagen-secreting bone marrow-derived cells.

Fedak et al. [106] devote an extensive review on this subject.

They describe that ECM is composed of fibrillar collagen, elastin, microfibrillar proteins, proteoglycans, and adhesive proteins such as laminin and fibronectin. They stress that ECM is not just an inert scaffold but also creates an active microenvironment for cell signaling. Composition of the ECM can influence the phenotype of cardiomyocytes [107] and increase both proliferation [108] and hypertrophy [109].

Additionally, deficient cell-ECM interactions can cause apoptosis-anoikis [110].

As regards actual ECM composition, Fedak et al. [106] remind that the myocardium contains less elastin than the great vessels.

As regards proteoglycans, according to Weber [111], they may contribute to "lubricating" the myocardial space for contraction and sequester growth factors and other proteins for cellular signaling.

Apart from the actual abundance of collagen, its composition is very important. Type I collagen is found to be up to 85% in the normal heart. It has very high tensile strength. Type III collagen is less rigid and confers elasticity. In end stage, changes in favor of collagen I are found, although definite picture is absent [112].

Apart from the collagen abundance and isoforms, reduction of cross-linking is associated with LV dilation [113].

Collagen is not a static element. It is estimated that it has a turnover of 0.6% per day [114].

This continuous turnover is influenced by the interplay of collagen breakdown proteins – metalloproteinases – and their tissue inhibitors.

12.10 Metalloproteinases

These are zinc-dependent enzymes, in every stage of tissue – and cardiovascular – evolution.

Fedak et al. [106] mentioned in 2005 that there exist at least 20–25 known MMP species. They are generally classified into four groups, based on their specificity for matrix components such as collagenases (MMP-1 and MMP-13), gelatinases (MMP-2 and MMP-9), stromelysin (MMP-3), and membrane-type MMPs (MT1-MMP). The latter are a novel class situated on the extracellular side of the membrane.

The majority of the MMPs are constitutively expressed but are also highly inducible, especially in HF [115].

ECM remodeling by the various MMPs can alter its signaling capacity including collagen degradation products. ADAMs (a disintegrin and metalloproteinase) are a novel class of enzymes which simultaneously degrade ECM and activate key biopeptides in the interstitial microenvironment [116].

Thus, they can modify cell-cell and cell-matrix interactions via integrin receptors.

MMPs are synthesized in the myocardium; as already mentioned, they are elevated in HF.

They are believed to be produced by both fibroblasts and the mast cells [117].

Their action is generally detrimental and associated with REM process both after an experimental MI [118] and in dilated human cardiomyopathy [119].

Mutant mice with decreased MMP expression have less REM as reviewed by Fedak et al. [106]. The same has been seen after administration of MMP inhibitors [120].

12.11 MMP Inhibitors

Dixon and Spinale [121] also discuss the role of the proteolytic enzymes such as MMPs in REM. The early stages that they discuss will be further described in the chapters on cell death and ischemia reperfusion injury. They describe that in the later phases, ECM changes can be found within all myocardial regions: within the actual MI region, the newly forming scar tissue is followed by persistent proteolysis and remains unstable and prone to expansion due to deformation from intracavitary LV stresses [122, 123], even without a new infarct.

Civitarese et al. [124] also describe that integrins influence fibroblast morphology, adhesion, and collagen REM. They also mediate CMC development. They stress that inappropriate formation of disorganized fibrillar collagen is characteristic of diabetic and idiopathic dilated cardiomyopathy. Integrins also mediate hypertrophy by their activation through mechanotransduction and adrenergic stimulation.

Importantly, certain cytokines such as TNF-α are involved in the increase of MMP activity [125].

Exerting an action opposite to MMPs, are TIMPs (tissue inhibitors of metalloproteinases). TIMPs are also involved in ECM turnover [126].

Four types of TIMPs have been identified: 1–4. They are all expressed in normal human myocardium, and they may contribute to REM, although findings may not be completely consistent. Thus, TIMP-1 has been found to be decreased in IRI cardiac dysfunction [127–129].

Others have, however, found that both TIMP-1 and TIMP-2 are elevated in REM.

Li et al. [129] have shown that TIMP-1 and TIMP-3 are reduced in the failing human heart mRNA and protein as well as TMP-4 (protein level) while TIMP-2 was not changed.

TIMP-3 is highly expressed in the human heart and is reduced in HF.

These findings demonstrate the very complex interaction of various factors on ECM turnover in HF and REM [130].

12.12 Remote Region Fibrosis

An ongoing question concerns the extent of fibrosis in the region remote region from the infarct regions. Some authors claim that it does not practically increase [131].

In the region remote from the infarct area, most researchers believe that it exists but is much less than in the infarct area [132, 133, 134].

According to Dixon and Spinale [121], a differential expression of MMPs has been found in various regions of post-MI myocardium.

Wilson et al. [135] examining sheep myocardium 8 weeks post-MI found an increase of MMP-8, MMP-13, and MT1-MNP by more than 300% in the MI region and the border zone, while MMP-1 and MMP-9 were unchanged in the remote region but decreased in the MI region and border zone, in which MMP-2 increased. When TIMPs were examined, again differential expressions were found: TIMP-4 decreased by 50% in the MI region, while TIMP-1, TIMP-2, and TIMP-3 levels were undetected in this region.

According to Dixon and Spinale [121], these findings signify the difficulty of employing MMP and TIMP therapy in the clinical arena.

The association of fibrosis with inflammation has already been mentioned. Inflammation within its various expressions has acquired a major significance in post-MI REM in recent years.

12.13 Inflammation

Burchfield et al. [23] give a brief mention of this very important process. They underline that in ventricular REM, many inflammatory molecules and pathways are activated such as the complement system [136], T-cells [137], and formation of autoantibodies [138], which have been reported.

Hofmann and Franz [139] give a very detailed account of the T-cells in MI.

They underline that the main organ for their generation is the thymus; its resolution, starting in childhood, coincides with an age-associated decline in T-cell receptor diversity and the evolution of highly differentiated peripheral memory T-cells within an "aged" T-cell compartment. This memory is strongly modulated by various chronic virus infections, especially *Cytomegalovirus* (CMV). This includes an expansion of the effector memory CD4+ (which identifies antigen) and CD8+ (which identifies cytotoxic T-cells) compartment [140].

During the course of adaptive immune responses, naive T-cells have to recognize their antigens; additional stimuli are required for their activation (T-cell priming).

Natural CD4+ regulatory T-cells constitute an anti-inflammatory immune-regulatory subset.

The principles of T-cell migration are very complex. Thus, according to Hofmann and Franz [139], memory T-cells in their peripheral compartment upon antigen recognition undertake proliferation and effector function execution. They enter the lymph nodes either from the affected lymphatics or from the blood and exit via the thoracic duct which drains to the blood.

T-cell recognition of antigens leads to their migration and retention in secondary lymphoid organs from where they are recruited to sites of inflammation [141].

These processes are strongly influenced by chemokine receptors. Specifically, CCR4 and OXCR3 promote the T cells' preference for homing to the myocardium [142].

Hofmann and Franz [139] also point out that recirculating T-cells contain only a very small portion of disease-specific cells. They further provide an account of the role of T-cells in various myocardial injury-associated patterns:

Acute coronary syndromes. These are very well analyzed by Ammirati et al. [143].

In ischemia reperfusion injury (IRI), CD4+ but not CD8+ T-cell depletion in mice showed a decrease in infarct size [144].

However, T-regulatory cells can contribute against the emergence of IRI. Thus, endogenous adenosine signaling can offset the injurious action of CD4+ T-cells. Additionally, CD4+ cells rapidly accumulate in murine hearts following IR [145].

This recruitment, according to recent data, is correlated with microvascular obstruction [146].

Hofmann et al. [147] also postulate that CD8+ memory T-cell subsets are entrapped in the coronary microcirculation early after reperfusion. These authors further describe the role of lymphocytes in non-reperfused MI. They mention their murine experiments [152], according to which both conventional effector CD4+ T-regulatory cells and Fixp3+ T-regulatory cells infiltrate the myocardium within a few days after an MI. Depletion of CD4+ T-regulatory cells induced a preferential M1-like phenotype, whereas their activation induced a M2-like phenotype inducing the expression of arginase-1, interleukin-13, osteopontin, and TGF-β [153], which all involve ECM formation.

Hofmann and Frantz [139] also discuss experimental evidence on the role of CD8+ T-cells. They have been described in the peri-infarct zone of rats 7 days after MI [154].

They [139] ascribe to these cells an infarct size-reducing capacity. They also conclude by noting indications that while, in the acute phase, CD4+ T-cells aggravate IRI, in the long-term, they may be required for proper healing. The role of inflammation is continuous.

Wang and Frangogiannis [150] discuss its role in the repair of the infected myocardium. They reiterate that for descriptive purposes the reparative response following MI can be divided into three distinct but overlapping phases: the inflammatory, the proliferative, and the maturation phases. These processes are also described in the chapter on healing of the myocardium.

Acute sudden necrosis of CMCs activates the innate immune system. Necrotic CMCs, as also described in the chapter on cardiomyocyte death release endogenous "danger" signals, the DAMPs (damage-associated molecular patterns) [151].

In this group are included high-mobility group box-1 (HMGβ1), heat shock proteins (HsPs), ATP, and matrix fragments [152].

DAMPs signal through the activation of Toll-like receptors (TLRs).

12.14 Role of the Complement

This system has a central role in the innate immune response. It can be activated by the release of subcellular substances such as cardiolipin. Its inhibition has therapeutic potential. As Wang and Frangogiannis [150] point out, although very favorable results have been reported in experimental studies, clinical data have shown no consistent benefit [153].

12.15 Toll-like receptors (TLRs)

The generation of reactive oxygen species (ROS) activation can activate the immune system and trigger cytokine and chemokine release partly through NF-kβ activation [154].

NF-kB is central in the role of TLR signaling. TLR-2, TLR-3, and TLR-4 play an important role in post-MI inflammation. Thus, TLR-2 mediates maladaptive REM and impairs cardiac function [160].

A similar action is ascribed to TLR-4 [156].

TLR-3 also can aggravate ischemia reperfusion injury [158].

TLRs, complement activation, and ROS activate the transcription factor NF-kβ, which trigger cytokine, chemokine, and adhesion molecule expression in the ischemic myocardium. Although most data suggest noxious action, cytoprotective responses have also been reported [158].

12.16 Chemokine and Cytokine Induction

Chemokines are involved in the post-MI inflammatory response [159, 160].

A very well-studied chemokine is MCP-1 (monocyte chemoattractant protein), which recruits mononuclear cells but also has angiogenic and arteriogenic healing actions and increases ECM synthesis [161] increasing myofibroblast accumulation in healing infarcts [163].

12.17 Cytokines

They are stimulated by TLR signaling, ROS generation and NF-kβ activation, both, as Wang and Frangogiannis point out [56], in resident and blood-derived cells.

The best studied cytokine is IL-1 which has diverse actions. It can stimulate synthesis of other cytokines, chemokines, growth factors, and adhesion molecules and leukocyte recruitment [164].

It is a central mediator in the post-MI inflammatory response. It also promotes ECM degradation [165].

TNF-α (tumor necrosis factor-α) is released early post-MI [166] and is a key mediator of the pro-inflammatory response.

12.18 The Cellular Immune Response

Neutrophils are recruited early in the infarct site. They release oxidants and proteases and phagocytose dead cells and debris. Migration of the neutrophils to the infarcted area requires the activation of many stages of a specific cascade, which induces through various ways the involvement of various adhesion molecules.

Their capture by the endothelium involves members of the selectin family. As they roll on the endothelium, they adhere more firmly to the endothelial cells through integrin activation [167].

Activated integrins interact with endothelial ICAM-1 (intercellular adhesion molecule) to ensure firmer adhesion; after this step, transmigration occurs, again dependent on various adhesion molecules. Experimentally, integrin inhibition has given very good results [168]; however clinical results have not been equally satisfactory [169].

12.19 Monocytes-Macrophages

As described by Wang and Frangogiannis [150] and shown by Nahrendorf et al. [170], subpopulations of these cells are sequentially recruited in the infarct zone.

Chemokines play an important role, together with TGF-β (transforming growth factor-β) and free radicals. These cells are predominantly derived from the bone marrow; additionally they are mobilized from the spleen [171]. Their activation further induces atherosclerotic signaling [172].

In the clinical setting, Emami et al. [173] have shown by ^{18}FDG-PET imaging that bone marrow and spleen activation predicts future events.

The recruited monocytes may differentiate into macrophages; various stimulating factors are involved in the process, such as macrophage colony-stimulating factor (M-CSF) and the granulocyte-macrophage colony-stimulating factor (GM-CSF) [174].

Apart from their scavenging role, the activated macrophages also produce growth factors and cytokines which stimulate healing and angiogenesis but also exacerbate REM through MMPs.

12.20 The Mast Cell

Mast cells are originated from pluripotent progenitor cells of the bone marrow. After migration to the myocardium, they release pro-inflammatory mediators which trigger the cytokine reaction cascade, especially histamine and TNF-α [175].

12.21 Proliferative Healing Phase

Again this process is described in the corresponding chapter. Corrective balance between cessation of inflammation and phagocytic removal is crucial for healing to begin. Receptors have been found which in effect serve as a molecular trap to remove cytokines or chemokines from their local microenvironment and antagonize their action. These are generally termed "stop" signals.

The role of TLRs has already been described. Their activity may physiologically antagonize members of the IRAK family (interleukin-1 receptor-associated kinase) which also limits IL-1 inflammatory activity, thus inhibiting ECM degradation [176].

Wang and Frangogiannis [150] comment on various additional mediators.

They consider TGF-β as a "master switch." It suppresses cytokine and chemokine synthesis and mediates ECM-preserving actions. It is predominantly upregulated in the border zone [177].

GDF-15 which will be discussed later as a biomarker also belongs to the TGF super family; it counteracts chemokine-triggered integrin activation, thus limiting leukocyte adhesion. It is also a proliferative factor [178].

12.22 IL-10: A Protective Interleukin

This cytokine has strong anti-inflammatory properties; it is expressed by activated Th2 lymphocytes and macrophages infiltrating the infarct zone [179].

It also promotes MMP-1 production [180].

Wang and Frangogiannis [150] also stress the beneficial effect of angiogenesis for infarct healing.

According to Cochain et al. [181], factors stimulating vascular formation are basic fibroblast growth factor (BFGF), vascular endothelial growth factor (VEGF), and also HIF-1α (hypoxia-inducible factor). They stress that not one factor can promote adequate angiogenesis and that combinations including stem/progenitor cells are essential.

The above authors [150, 181] describe the importance of the maturation phase, in which further fibrosis is inhibited as fibroblasts become quiescent and infarct vasculature matures. Importantly they describe that new vessel coated by "pericytes" are derived from the pertinent vessels [182].

After an AMI as Schirone et al. [183] point out in a recent review, chronic inflammation in the remodeling heart reduces ATP and phosphocreatine concentration and impairs mitochondrial carbohydrate metabolism and fatty acid oxidation [184].

Inflammatory cytokines also interfere with SERCA-2α [185].

Recently, Westman et al. [186] very pertinently point out that inflammation is a main driver for post-MI REM. They mention the term inflammasome [187].

Importantly, they mention that this complex is assembled in response to damage- or pathogen-associated molecular patterns and activates caspase-1. In accordance with the aforementioned work by Wang and Frangogiannis [150], they designate days 0 to 3 as comprising the pro-inflammatory phase and days 2–7 as comprising the proliferative phase. Thus neutrophils predominate on day 0, macrophages from day 3, and dendritic cells and lymphocytes by day 6.

They also mention the possible role of chronic infection, which poses an incremental risk of AMI and death [188]. However, they can only postulate that it could have an effect on LV REM. They also mention that the aforementioned risk factor for LV REM (smoking, hyperlipidemia, obesity, and diabetes) also affect inflammation.

12.23 Oxidative Stress

The continuous role of oxidative stress has already been described in the inflammatory phase.

This is a key element of most processes leading to REM. Opie et al. [189] describe that many factors involved in REM such as angiotensin II, TNF-α, and mechanical stress promote the formation of ROS. They point out that high ROS production can contribute to the course toward HF through hypertrophy [190] and fibrosis [191].

Zornoff et al. [66] point out that ROS can derive from mitochondrial electron transporters, NADPH oxidase system, cyclooxygenase activity, cytochrome P450, glucose oxidase, xanthine oxidase, lipoxygenase, and catecholamine degradation [192, 193].

Mitochondrial ROS are physiologically generated, but at high concentrations, they damage their DNA adversely alter energy production [194] through the mitochondrial transport chain which is used to generate a protein gradient for ATP synthesis according to Turrens [195].

Mitochondrial-induced REM is mediated by the activation of ERK 1/2 [196].

Inhibition of ROS by glutathione peroxidase has been shown to reduce REM after an MI [197].

Additionally, aldehyde dehydrogenase 2 (ALDH 2) which detoxifies myocardial reactive aldehydes produced by oxidative stress reduces post-MI REM [198].

12.24 Metabolic Remodeling

The energy starvation process contributes to maladaptive REM, which promotes HF, as reviewed recently by Peterzan et al. [199].

It must be reminded that in HF regardless of species or etiology, the total creatine pool is consistently reduced. Creatine transporter activity is also reduced, leading to a fall in creatine which predates the fall in ATP [200].

However, it seems that creatine must be depleted by about 86% before affecting resting contractile function, and phosphocreatine activity suppressed by more than 74% before contractile reserve is diminished [201].

12.25 Other Factors Involved in REM

Protein kinase C mechanisms

Newton et al. [202] have recently given a very detailed review.

They raise the postulation that PKC inhibitors may be suitable for treating HF or IRI. They reiterate that there are nine PKC genes.

Conventional PKCs (α,β,γ) are activated by diacylglycerol (DAG) and Ca2+; novel PKCs (δ,ε,θ,η) are not activated by Ca2+, and atypical PKCs (ζ, λ/I) are not regulated by second messengers.

They describe which PKCs are involved in heart disease.

PKCα is the most abundantly expressed in CMCs [203].

PKCα overexpression (adenoviral-meditated) induces hypertrophy in cultured neonatal ventricular CMCs [204].

Subsequent studies showed that this isoenzyme primarily decreases contractility. Thus, enhanced contractility in PKCαKO mice confers protection against transverse aortic constriction-induced HF, as shown by Braz et al. [204, 205] who showed that PKCα regulates cardiac contraction by phosphorylating inhibitor-1, a negative regulator of protein phosphatase-1 (PP-1). A decrease in inhibitor-1 phosphorylation in PKCαKO mice leads to a decrease in PP-1 activity, an increase in phospholamban phosphorylation, and an enhanced SERCA-2 activity and contractility.

PKCβ may contribute to cardiac growth and/or pathological REM, although Newton et al. [202] offer many conflicting views beyond the scope of this review.

As regards the novel isoenzymes, their action can be summarized as follows:

- Activated PKCε localizes in the mitochondria where it phosphorylates elements of mitochondrial IPC signaling, leading to cardioprotection [206].
- PKCδ activation contributes to IRI, by decreasing pH and ATP production, increasing ROS accumulation, inhibiting Akt, and increasing apoptosis [207, 208].
- Calpains are described in the chapter on cell death. Their role on REM is reviewed by Letavernier et al. [209].

12.26 Chronic Ischemia-Hypoxia Hypothesis

Peers [210] has given a very pertinent Brown Prize Lecture in 2002 [204] stressing the effect of chronic hypoxia on ROS production, inflammation, and subsequent cell death. Revascularization is the main way to reverse hypoxia.

12.27 MicroRNAs

These ubiquitous oligonucleotides are involved in every cellular aspect, including the myocardium. Their role in REM has been described by many authors [43, 211–217]. Fraccarollo et al. [43] showed that miRNAs are involved in many processes in various tissues (Fig. 12.2).

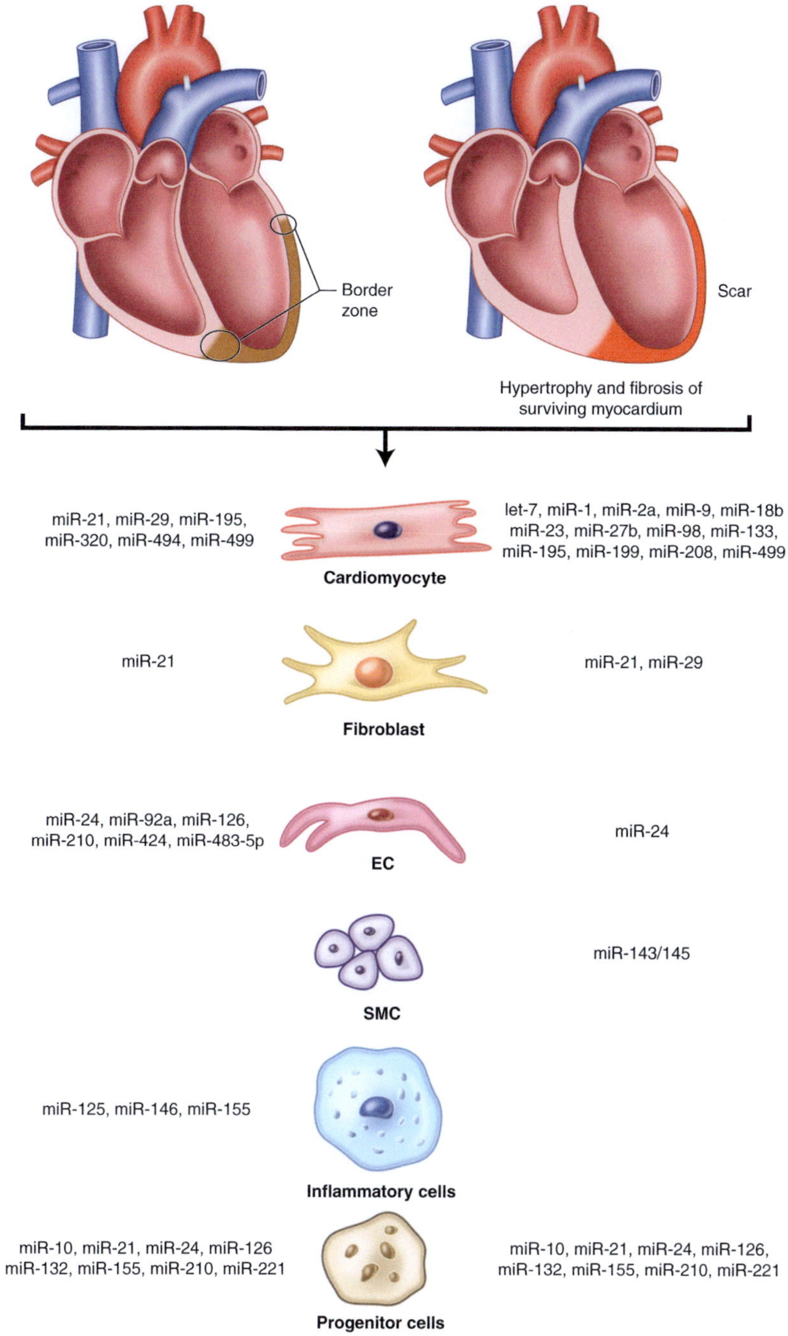

Fig. 12.2 miRNAs as potential targets to modulate cardiac healing and remodeling during/after myocardial ischemia with putative assignment to cell types. (Left) miRNAs regulated early during hypoxia and healing processes mainly confined to the infarct and border zones: (right) miRNAs involved in the chronic remodeling process of hypertrophy and fibrosis of the surviving myocardium. See text for details. EC endothelial cell, SMC smooth muscle cell. (Reproduced with permission from Fraccarollo et al. [43])

Recently, Garikipati et al. [218] showed that miR375 inhibition attenuates post-MI inflammation, apoptosis, and REM in mice. The same was shown for miR-34 by Bernardo et al. [219].

Van Rooij et al. [220] give a signature pattern of stress-responsive microRNAs that can evoke cardiac hypertrophy and heart failure.

More data are given in the next chapter regarding therapy of cardiac remodeling.

In conclusion, chronic cardiac remodeling is a distinct maladaptive entity leading to cardiac dysfunction, heart failure, and death. Cardiomyocyte cell death by apoptosis is a premium mover; chronic hypoxia and inflammation also participate.

References

1. Swynghedauw B. Molecular mechanisms of myocardial remodeling. Physiol Rev. 1999;79:215–62.
2. Sutton MG, Sharpe N. Left ventricular remodeling after myocardial infarction: pathophysiology and therapy. Circulation. 2000;27(101):2981–8.
3. Cohn JN, Ferrari R, Sharpe N. Cardiac remodeling--concepts and clinical implications: a consensus paper from an international forum on cardiac remodeling. Behalf of an International Forum on Cardiac Remodeling. J Am Coll Cardiol. 2000;35:569–82.
4. Pfeffer MA, Braunwald E. Ventricular remodeling after myocardial infarction. Experimental observations and clinical implications. Circulation. 1990;81:1161–72.
5. Grossman W, Jones D, McLaurin LP. Wall stress and patterns of hypertrophy in the human left ventricle. J Clin Invest. 1975;56:56–64.
6. Hill JA, Olson EN. Cardiac plasticity. N Engl J Med. 2008;358:1370–80.
7. McKay RG, Pfeffer MA, Pasternak RC, Markis JE, Come PC, Nakao S, et al. Left ventricular remodeling after myocardial infarction: a corollary to infarct expansion. Circulation. 1986;74:693–702.
8. Galiuto L, Garramone B, Scarà A, Rebuzzi AG, Crea F, La Torre G, et al. The extent of microvascular damage during myocardial contrast echocardiography is superior to other known indexes of post-infarct reperfusion in predicting left ventricular remodeling: results of the multicenter AMICI study. J Am Coll Cardiol. 2008;51:552–9.
9. Savoye C, Equine O, Tricot O, Nugue O, Segrestin B, Sautière K, et al. Left ventricular remodeling after anterior wall acute myocardial infarction in modern clinical practice (from the REmodelage VEntriculaire [REVE] study group). Am J Cardiol. 2006;98:1144–9.
10. Bolognese L, Neskovic AN, Parodi G, Cerisano G, Buonamici P, Santoro GM, et al. Left ventricular remodeling after primary coronary angioplasty: patterns of left ventricular dilation and long-term prognostic implications. Circulation. 2002;106:2351–7.
11. Lee TH, Hamilton MA, Stevenson LW, Moriguchi JD, Fonarow GC, Child JS, et al. Impact of left ventricular cavity size on survival in advanced heart failure. Am J Cardiol. 1993;72:672–6.
12. Solomon SD, Skali H, Anavekar NS, Bourgoun M, Barvik S, Ghali JK, et al. Changes in ventricular size and function in patients treated with valsartan, captopril, or both after myocardial infarction. Circulation. 2005;111:3411–9.
13. Tardif JC, O'Meara E, Komajda M, Böhm M, Borer JS, Ford I, et al. Effects of selective heart rate reduction with ivabradine on left ventricular remodelling and function: results from the SHIFT echocardiography substudy. Eur Heart J. 2011;32:2507–15.
14. Migrino RQ, Young JB, Ellis SG, White HD, Lundergan CF, Miller DP, et al. End-systolic volume index at 90 to 180 minutes into reperfusion therapy for acute myocardial infarction is a strong predictor of early and late mortality. The Global Utilization of Streptokinase and

t-PA for Occluded Coronary Arteries (GUSTO)-I Angiographic Investigators. Circulation. 1997;96:116–21.
15. Mann DL, Bogaev R, Buckberg GD. Cardiac remodelling and myocardial recovery: lost in translation? Eur J Heart Fail. 2010;12:789–96.
16. White HD, Norris RM, Brown MA, Brandt PW, Whitlock RM, Wild CJ. Left ventricular end-systolic volume as the major determinant of survival after recovery from myocardial infarction. Circulation. 1987;76:44–51.
17. Cokkinos DV, Belogianneas C. Left ventricular remodelling: a problem in search of solutions. Eur Cardiol Rev. 2016;11:29–35.
18. Bhatt AS, Ambrosy AP, Velazquez EJ. Adverse remodeling and reverse remodeling after myocardial infarction. Curr Cardiol Rep. 2017;19:71. https://doi.org/10.1007/s11886-017-0876-4.
19. Yu CM, Bleeker GB, Fung JW, Schalij MJ, Zhang Q, van der Wall EE, et al. Left ventricular reverse remodeling but not clinical improvement predicts long-term survival after cardiac resynchronization therapy. Circulation. 2005;112:1580–6.
20. Funaro S, La Torre G, Madonna M, Galiuto L, Scarà A, Labbadia A, et al. Incidence, determinants, and prognostic value of reverse left ventricular remodelling after primary percutaneous coronary intervention: results of the Acute Myocardial Infarction Contrast Imaging (AMICI) multicenter study. Eur Heart J. 2009;30:566–75.
21. Hessel MH, Bleeker GB, Bax JJ, Henneman MM, den Adel B, Klok M, et al. Reverse ventricular remodelling after cardiac resynchronization therapy is associated with a reduction in serum tenascin-C and plasma matrix metalloproteinase-9 levels. Eur J Heart Fail. 2007;9:1058–63.
22. Kramer DG, Trikalinos TA, Kent DM, Antonopoulos GV, Konstam MA, Udelson JE. Quantitative evaluation of drug or device effects on ventricular remodeling as predictors of therapeutic effects on mortality in patients with heart failure and reduced ejection fraction: a meta-analytic approach. J Am Coll Cardiol. 2010;56:392–406.
23. Burchfield JS, Xie M, Hill JA. Pathological ventricular remodeling: mechanisms: part 1 of 2. Circulation. 2013;128:388–400.
24. Go AS, Mozaffarian D, Roger VL, Benjamin EJ, Berry JD, Borden WB, et al. Heart disease and stroke statistics--2013 update: a report from the American Heart Association. Circulation. 2013;127:e6–e245.
25. Borlaug BA, Paulus WJ. Heart failure with preserved ejection fraction: pathophysiology, diagnosis, and treatment. Eur Heart J. 2011;32:670–9.
26. Borlaug BA. Defining HFpEF: where do we draw the line? Eur Heart J. 2016;37:463–5.
27. Tribouilloy C, Grigioni F, Avierinos JF, Barbieri A, Rusinaru D, Szymanski C, et al. Survival implication of left ventricular end-systolic diameter in mitral regurgitation due to flail leaflets a long-term follow-up multicenter study. J Am Coll Cardiol. 2009;54:1961–8.
28. Vahanian A. ESC guidelines Desk Reference ESC Committee for Practice Guidelines. p. 181–94. 2010.
29. Toischer K, Rokita AG, Unsöld B, Zhu W, Kararigas G, Sossalla S, et al. Differential cardiac remodeling in preload versus afterload. Circulation. 2010;122:993–1003.
30. Chemaly ER, Kang S, Zhang S, McCollum L, Chen J, Bénard L, et al. Differential patterns of replacement and reactive fibrosis in pressure and volume overload are related to the propensity for ischaemia and involve resistin. J Physiol. 2013;591:5337–55.
31. Koyama T, Nishina T, Ono N, Sakakibara Y, Nemoto S, Ikeda T, et al. Early and mid-term results of left ventricular volume reduction surgery for dilated cardiomyopathy. J Card Surg. 2005;20:S39–42.
32. Seidman JG, Seidman C. The genetic basis for cardiomyopathy: from mutation identification to mechanistic paradigms. Cell. 2001;104:557–67.
33. Hamada T, Kubo T, Kitaoka H, Hirota T, Hoshikawa E, Hayato K, et al. Clinical features of the dilated phase of hypertrophic cardiomyopathy in comparison with those of dilated cardiomyopathy. Clin Cardiol. 2010;33:E24-8.
34. Segura AM, Radovancevic R, Demirozu ZT, Frazier OH, Buja LM. Anthracycline treatment and ventricular remodeling in left ventricular assist device patients. Tex Heart Inst J. 2015;42:124–30.

35. Zhao Y, McLaughlin D, Robinson E, Harvey AP, Hookham MB, Shah AM, et al. Nox2 NADPH oxidase promotes pathologic cardiac remodeling associated with Doxorubicin chemotherapy. Cancer Res. 2010;70:9287–97. https://doi.org/10.1158/0008-5472.CAN-10-2664.
36. Harmancey R, Wilson CR, Taegtmeyer H. Adaptation and maladaptation of the heart in obesity. Hypertension. 2008;52:181–7.
37. Fenelon G, Wijns W, Andries E, Brugada P. Tachycardiomyopathy: mechanisms and clinical implications. Pacing Clin Electrophysiol. 1996;19:95–106.
38. Martin CA, Lambiase PD. Pathophysiology, diagnosis and treatment of tachycardiomyopathy. Heart. 2017;103:1543–52. https://doi.org/10.1136/heartjnl-2016-310391.
39. Ban JE, Park HC, Park JS, Nagamoto Y, Choi JI, Lim HE, et al. Electrocardiographic and electrophysiological characteristics of premature ventricular complexes associated with left ventricular dysfunction in patients without structural heart disease. Europace. 2013;15:735–41.
40. Braunschweig F. When cardiac function dangles on a thread of conduction: dyssynchronopathy in patients with left bundle branch block. J Am Coll Cardiol. 2013;61:1096–8.
41. Gold MR, Daubert C, Abraham WT, Ghio S, St John Sutton M, Hudnall JH, et al. The effect of reverse remodeling on long-term survival in mildly symptomatic patients with heart failure receiving cardiac resynchronization therapy: results of the REVERSE study. Heart Rhythm. 2015;12:524–30.
42. Maron BJ. Distinguishing hypertrophic cardiomyopathy from athlete's heart physiological remodelling: clinical significance, diagnostic strategies and implications for preparticipation screening. Br J Sports Med. 2009;43:649–56.
43. Fraccarollo D, Galuppo P, Bauersachs J. Novel therapeutic approaches to post-infarction remodelling. Cardiovasc Res. 2012;94:293–303.
44. Papadopoulos CE, Karvounis HI, Giannakoulas G, Karamitsos TD, Efthimiadis GK, Parharidis GE. Predictors of left ventricular remodeling after reperfused acute myocardial infarction. Am J Cardiol. 2007;99:1024–5.
45. Masci PG, Ganame J, Francone M, Desmet W, Lorenzoni V, Iacucci I, et al. Relationship between location and size of myocardial infarction and their reciprocal influences on post-infarction left ventricular remodelling. Eur Heart J. 2011;32:1640–8.
46. Giannuzzi P, Temporelli PL, Bosimini E, Gentile F, Lucci D, Maggioni AP, et al. Heterogeneity of left ventricular remodeling after acute myocardial infarction: results of the Gruppo Italiano per lo Studio della Sopravvivenza nell'Infarto Miocardico-3 Echo Substudy. Am Heart J. 2001;141:131–8.
47. University of Minnesota. Atlas of human cardiac anatomy.
48. Miura T, Miki T. Limitation of myocardial infarct size in the clinical setting: current status and challenges in translating animal experiments into clinical therapy. Basic Res Cardiol. 2008;103:501–13.
49. Minicucci MF, Azevedo PS, Martinez PF, Lima AR, Bonomo C, Guizoni DM, et al. Critical infarct size to induce ventricular remodeling, cardiac dysfunction and heart failure in rats. Int J Cardiol. 2011;151:242–3.
50. Jelani A, Jugdutt BI. STEMI and heart failure in the elderly: role of adverse remodeling. Heart Fail Rev. 2010;15:513–21.
51. Ennezat PV, Lamblin N, Mouquet F, Tricot O, Quandalle P, Aumégeat V, et al. The effect of ageing on cardiac remodelling and hospitalization for heart failure after an inaugural anterior myocardial infarction. Eur Heart J. 2008;29:1992–9.
52. Bauters C, Lamblin N, Ennezat PV, Mycinski C, Tricot O, Nugue O, et al. A prospective evaluation of left ventricular remodeling after inaugural anterior myocardial infarction as a function of gene polymorphisms in the renin-angiotensin-aldosterone, adrenergic, and metalloproteinase systems. Am Heart J. 2007;153:641–8.
53. Timmers L, van Keulen JK, Hoefer IE, Meijs MF, van Middelaar B, den Ouden K, et al. Targeted deletion of nuclear factor kappaB p50 enhances cardiac remodeling and dysfunction following myocardial infarction. Circ Res. 2009;104:699–706.
54. Palmer BR, Devereaux CL, Dhamrait SS, Mocatta TJ, Pilbrow AP, Frampton CM, et al. The common G-866A polymorphism of the UCP2 gene and survival in diabetic patients following myocardial infarction. Cardiovasc Diabetol. 2009;8:31.

55. Walker AM, Patel PA, Rajwani A, Groves D, Denby C, Kearney L, et al. Diabetes mellitus is associated with adverse structural and functional cardiac remodelling in chronic heart failure with reduced ejection fraction. Diab Vasc Dis Res. 2016;13:331–40.
56. Cokkinos DV, Pantos C. Type 1 diabetes impairs compensatory response after myocardial infarction; role of tissue hypothyroidism and effects of thyroid hormone administration. Bull Acad Natl Med. 2011;195:151–64. discussion 164-5
57. Maczewski M, Maczewska J, Duda M. Hypercholesterolaemia exacerbates ventricular remodelling after myocardial infarction in the rat: role of angiotensin II type 1 receptors. Br J Pharmacol. 2008;154:1640–8.
58. Kudo H, Kai H, Kajimoto H, Koga M, Takayama N, Mori T, et al. Exaggerated blood pressure variability superimposed on hypertension aggravates cardiac remodeling in rats via angiotensin II system-mediated chronic inflammation. Hypertension. 2009;54:832–8.
59. Gu L, Pandey V, Geenen DL, Chowdhury SA, Piano MR. Cigarette smoke-induced left ventricular remodelling is associated with activation of mitogen-activated protein kinases. Eur J Heart Fail. 2008;10:1057–64.
60. Talukder MA, Johnson WM, Varadharaj S, Lian J, Kearns PN, El-Mahdy MA, et al. Chronic cigarette smoking causes hypertension, increased oxidative stress, impaired NO bioavailability, endothelial dysfunction, and cardiac remodeling in mice. Am J Physiol Heart Circ Physiol. 2011;300:H388–96.
61. Iismaa SE, Li M, Kesteven S, Wu J, Chan AY, Holman SR, et al. Cardiac hypertrophy limits infarct expansion after myocardial infarction in mice. Sci Rep. 2018;8:6114.
62. Humphrey JD, Dufresne ER, Schwartz MA. Mechanotransduction and extracellular matrix homeostasis. Nat Rev Mol Cell Biol. 2014;15:802–12.
63. Swynghedauw B. Darwinian evolution and cardiovascular remodeling. Heart Fail Rev. 2016;21:795–802.
64. Hochman JS, Bulkley BH. Expansion of acute myocardial infarction: an experimental study. Circulation. 1982;65:1446–50.
65. Richardson WJ, Holmes JW. Why Is Infarct Expansion Such an Elusive Therapeutic Target? J Cardiovasc Transl Res. 2015;8:421–30.
66. Zornoff LA, Paiva SA, Duarte DR, Spadaro J. Ventricular remodeling after myocardial infarction: concepts and clinical implications. Arq Bras Cardiol. 2009;92:150–64.
67. Clarke CL, Grunwald GK, Allen LA, Barón AE, Peterson PN, Brand DW, et al. Natural history of left ventricular ejection fraction in patients with heart failure. Circ Cardiovasc Qual Outcomes. 2013;6:680–6.
68. Pantos C, Mourouzis I, Xinaris C, Kokkinos AD, Markakis K, Dimopoulos A, et al. Time-dependent changes in the expression of thyroid hormone receptor alpha 1 in the myocardium after acute myocardial infarction: possible implications in cardiac remodelling. Eur J Endocrinol. 2007;156:415–24.
69. Pantos C, Mourouzis I, Galanopoulos G, Gavra M, Perimenis P, Spanou D, et al. Thyroid hormone receptor alpha1 downregulation in postischemic heart failure progression: the potential role of tissue hypothyroidism. Horm Metab Res. 2010;42:718–24.
70. Lymvaios I, Mourouzis I, Cokkinos DV, Dimopoulos MA, Toumanidis ST, Pantos C. Thyroid hormone and recovery of cardiac function in patients with acute myocardial infarction: a strong association? Eur J Endocrinol. 2011;165:107–14.
71. Abbate A, Biondi-Zoccai GG, Bussani R, Dobrina A, Camilot D, Feroce F, et al. Increased myocardial apoptosis in patients with unfavorable left ventricular remodeling and early symptomatic post-infarction heart failure. J Am Coll Cardiol. 2003;41:753–60.
72. Abbate A, Biondi-Zoccai GG, Baldi A. Pathophysiologic role of myocardial apoptosis in post-infarction left ventricular remodeling. J Cell Physiol. 2002;193:145–53.
73. Elsässer A, Vogt AM, Nef H, Kostin S, Möllmann H, Skwara W, et al. Human hibernating myocardium is jeopardized by apoptotic and autophagic cell death. J Am Coll Cardiol. 2004;43:2191–9.
74. Palojoki E, Saraste A, Eriksson A, Pulkki K, Kallajoki M, Voipio-Pulkki LM, et al. Cardiomyocyte apoptosis and ventricular remodeling after myocardial infarction in rats. Am J Physiol Heart Circ Physiol. 2001;280:H2726–31.

75. Anversa P, Olivetti G, Capasso JM. Cellular basis of ventricular remodeling after myocardial infarction. Am J Cardiol. 1991;68:7D–16D.
76. Misao J, Hayakawa Y, Ohno M, Kato S, Fujiwara T, Fujiwara H. Expression of bcl-2 protein, an inhibitor of apoptosis, and Bax, an accelerator of apoptosis, in ventricular myocytes of human hearts with myocardial infarction. Circulation. 1996;94:1506–12.
77. Yang L, Gao JY, Ma J, Xu X, Wang Q, Xiong L, et al. Cardiac-specific overexpression of metallothionein attenuates myocardial remodeling and contractile dysfunction in l-NAME-induced experimental hypertension: Role of autophagy regulation. Toxicol Lett. 2015;237:121–32.
78. Michael LH, Ballantyne CM, Zachariah JP, Gould KE, Pocius JS, Taffet GE, et al. Myocardial infarction and remodeling in mice: effect of reperfusion. Am J Phys. 1999;277:H660–8.
79. Touchstone DA, Beller GA, Nygaard TW, Tedesco C, Kaul S. Effects of successful intravenous reperfusion therapy on regional myocardial function and geometry in humans: a tomographic assessment using two-dimensional echocardiography. J Am Coll Cardiol. 1989;13:1506–13.
80. Simes RJ, Topol EJ, Holmes DR Jr, White HD, Rutsch WR, Vahanian A, et al. Link between the angiographic substudy and mortality outcomes in a large randomized trial of myocardial reperfusion. Importance of early and complete infarct artery reperfusion. GUSTO-I Investigators. Circulation. 1995;91:1923–8.
81. Ross AM, Coyne KS, Moreyra E, Reiner JS, Greenhouse SW, Walker PL, et al. Extended mortality benefit of early postinfarction reperfusion. GUSTO-I Angiographic Investigators. Global Utilization of Streptokinase and Tissue Plasminogen Activator for Occluded Coronary Arteries Trial. Circulation. 1998;97:1549–56.
82. Mehta RH, Harjai KJ, Cox D, Stone GW, Brodie B, Boura J, et al. Clinical and angiographic correlates and outcomes of suboptimal coronary flow inpatients with acute myocardial infarction undergoing primary percutaneous coronary intervention. J Am Coll Cardiol. 2003;42:1739–46.
83. Goel PK, Bhatia T, Kapoor A, Gambhir S, Pradhan PK, Barai S, et al. Left ventricular remodeling after late revascularization correlates with baseline viability. Tex Heart Inst J. 2014;41:381–8.
84. Haghighi K, Sanoudou D, Kranias E. In: Cokkinos DV, editor. Calcium Cycling Circuits in Cardiac Physiology and Pathophysiology in Introduction to Translational Cardiovascular Research. Cham: Springer; 2015. p. p205–15.
85. Currie S, Smith GL. Enhanced phosphorylation of phospholamban and downregulation of sarco/endoplasmic reticulum Ca2+ ATPase type 2 (SERCA 2) in cardiac sarcoplasmic reticulum from rabbits with heart failure. Cardiovasc Res. 1999;41:135–46.
86. Zarain-Herzberg A, Afzal N, Elimban V, Dhalla NS. Decreased expression of cardiac sarcoplasmic reticulum Ca(2+)-pump ATPase in congestive heart failure due to myocardial infarction. Mol Cell Biochem. 1996;163-164:285–90.
87. Hasenfuss G, Meyer M, Schillinger W, Preuss M, Pieske B, Just H. Calcium handling proteins in the failing human heart. Basic Res Cardiol. 1997;92(Suppl 1):87–93.
88. Sari FR, Watanabe K, Widyantoro B, Thandavarayan RA, Harima M, Kodama M, et al. Sex differences play a role in cardiac endoplasmic reticulum stress (ERS) and ERS-initiated apoptosis induced by pressure overload and thapsigargin. Cardiovasc Pathol. 2011;20:281–90.
89. Mourouzis I, Giagourta I, Galanopoulos G, Mantzouratou P, Kostakou E, Kokkinos AD, et al. Thyroid hormone improves the mechanical performance of the post-infarcted diabetic myocardium: a response associated with up-regulation of Akt/mTOR and AMPK activation. Metabolism. 2013;62:1387–93.
90. Adamopoulos S, Gouziouta A, Mantzouratou P, Laoutaris ID, Dritsas A, Cokkinos DV, et al. Thyroid hormone signalling is altered in response to physical training in patients with end-stage heart failure and mechanical assist devices: potential physiological consequences? Interact Cardiovasc Thorac Surg. 2013;17:664–8.
91. Kemi OJ, Ceci M, Wisloff U, Grimaldi S, Gallo P, Smith GL, et al. Activation or inactivation of cardiac Akt/mTOR signaling diverges physiological from pathological hypertrophy. J Cell Physiol. 2008;214:316–21.

92. Kim SJ, Abdellatif M, Koul S, Crystal GJ. Chronic treatment with insulin-like growth factor I enhances myocyte contraction by upregulation of Akt-SERCA2a signaling pathway. Am J Physiol Heart Circ Physiol. 2008;295:H130–5.
93. Dhanasekaran DN. Reddy EP.JNK signaling in apoptosis. Oncogene. 2008;27:6245–51.
94. Chaanine AH, Jeong D, Liang L, Chemaly ER, Fish K, Gordon RE, et al. JNK modulates FOXO3a for the expression of the mitochondrial death and mitophagy marker BNIP3 in pathological hypertrophy and in heart failure. Cell Death Dis. 2012;3:265.
95. Baines CP. Molkentin JD.STRESS signaling pathways that modulate cardiac myocyte apoptosis. J Mol Cell Cardiol. 2005;38:47–62.
96. Dorn GW. 2nd.Adrenergic pathways and left ventricular remodeling. J Card Fail. 2002;8(6 Suppl):S370–3.
97. Yang J, Liu Y, Fan X, Li Z, Cheng Y. A pathway and network review on beta-adrenoceptor signaling and beta blockers in cardiac remodeling. Heart Fail Rev. 2014;19:799–814.
98. Cannavo A, Koch WJ. Targeting β3-Adrenergic Receptors in the Heart: Selective Agonism and β-Blockade. J Cardiovasc Pharmacol. 2017;69:71–8.
99. Patten RD, Konstam MA. Ventricular remodeling and the renin angiotensin aldosterone system. Congest Heart Fail. 2000;6:187–92.
100. Morrone D, Marzilli M. Role of RAAS inhibition in preventing left ventricular remodeling in patients post myocardial infarction. Heart Metab. 2010;47:9–13.
101. Spinale FG. Myocardial matrix remodeling and the matrix metalloproteinases: influence on cardiac form and function. Physiol Rev. 2007;87:1285–342.
102. Zak R. Cell proliferation during cardiac growth. Am J Cardiol. 1973;31:211–9.
103. Zeisberg EM, Tarnavski O, Zeisberg M, Dorfman AL, McMullen JR, Gustafsson E, et al. Endothelial-to-mesenchymal transition contributes to cardiac fibrosis. Nat Med. 2007;13:952–61.
104. Iwano M, Plieth D, Danoff TM, Xue C, Okada H, Neilson EG. Evidence that fibroblasts derive from epithelium during tissue fibrosis. J Clin Invest. 2002;110:341–50.
105. Haudek SB, Xia Y, Huebener P, Lee JM, Carlson S, Crawford JR, et al. Bone marrow-derived fibroblast precursors mediate ischemic cardiomyopathy in mice. Proc Natl Acad Sci U S A. 2006;103:18284–9.
106. Fedak PW, Verma S, Weisel RD, Li RK. Cardiac remodeling and failure From molecules to man (Part II). Cardiovasc Pathol. 2005;14:49–60.
107. Simpson DG, Terracio L, Terracio M, Price RL, Turner DC, Borg TK. Modulation of cardiac myocyte phenotype in vitro by the composition and orientation of the extracellular matrix. J Cell Physiol. 1994;161:89–105.
108. Hornberger LK, Singhroy S, Cavalle-Garrido T, Tsang W, Keeley F, Rabinovitch M. Synthesis of extracellular matrix and adhesion through beta (1) integrins are critical for fetal ventricular myocyte proliferation. Circ Res. 2000;87:508–15.
109. Ross RS, Pham C, Shai SY, Goldhaber JI, Fenczik C, Glembotski CC, et al. Beta1 integrins participate in the hypertrophic response of rat ventricular myocytes. Circ Res. 1998;82:1160–72.
110. Ding B, Price RL, Goldsmith EC, Borg TK, Yan X, Douglas PS, et al. Left ventricular hypertrophy in ascending aortic stenosis mice: anoikis and the progression to early failure. Circulation. 2000;101:2854–62.
111. Weber KT. Cardiac interstitium in health and disease: the fibrillar collagen network. J Am Coll Cardiol. 1989;13:1637–52.
112. Marijianowski MM, Teeling P, Mann J, Becker AE. Dilated cardiomyopathy is associated with an increase in the type I/type III collagen ratio: a quantitative assessment. J Am Coll Cardiol. 1995;25:1263–72.
113. Woodiwiss AJ, Tsotetsi OJ, Sprott S, Lancaster EJ, Mela T, Chung ES, et al. Reduction in myocardial collagen cross-linking parallels left ventricular dilatation in rat models of systolic chamber dysfunction. Circulation. 2001;103:155–60.
114. Bonnin CM, Sparrow MP, Taylor RR. Collagen synthesis and content in right ventricular hypertrophy in the dog. Am J Phys. 1981;241:H708–13.
115. Nagase H, Woessner JF Jr. Matrix metalloproteinases. J Biol Chem. 1999;274:21491–4.

116. Schlöndorff J, Blobel CP. Metalloprotease-disintegrins: modular proteins capable of promoting cell-cell interactions and triggering signals by protein-ectodomain shedding. J Cell Sci. 1999;112:3603–17.
117. Chancey AL, Brower GL, Janicki JS. Cardiac mast cell-mediated activation of gelatinase and alteration of ventricular diastolic function. Am J Physiol Heart Circ Physiol. 2002;282:H2152–8.
118. Romanic AM, Burns-Kurtis CL, Gout B, Berrebi-Bertrand I, Ohlstein EH. Matrix metalloproteinase expression in cardiac myocytes following myocardial infarction in the rabbit. Life Sci. 2001;68:799–814.
119. Thomas CV, Coker ML, Zellner JL, Handy JR, Crumbley AJ 3rd, Spinale FG. Increased matrix metalloproteinase activity and selective upregulation in LV myocardium from patients with end-stage dilated cardiomyopathy. Circulation. 1998;97:1708–15.
120. Yarbrough WM, Mukherjee R, Brinsa TA, Dowdy KB, Scott AA, Escobar GP, et al. Matrix metalloproteinase inhibition modifies left ventricular remodeling after myocardial infarction in pigs. J Thorac Cardiovasc Surg. 2003;125:602–10.
121. Dixon JA, Spinale FG. Myocardial remodeling: cellular and extracellular events and targets. Annu Rev Physiol. 2011;73:47–68.
122. Zimmerman SD, Criscione J, Covell JW. Remodeling in myocardium adjacent to an infarction in the pig left ventricle. Am J Physiol Heart Circ Physiol. 2004;287:H2697–704.
123. MacKenna D, Summerour SR, Villarreal FJ. Role of mechanical factors in modulating cardiac fibroblast function and extracellular matrix synthesis. Cardiovasc Res. 2000;46:257–63.
124. Civitarese RA, Kapus A, McCulloch CA, Connelly KA. Role of integrins in mediating cardiac fibroblast-cardiomyocyte cross talk: a dynamic relationship in cardiac biology and pathophysiology. Basic Res Cardiol. 2017;112:116.
125. Li YY, McTiernan CF, Feldman AM. Proinflammatory cytokines regulate tissue inhibitors of metalloproteinases and disintegrin metalloproteinase in cardiac cells. Cardiovasc Res. 1999;42:162–72.
126. Vanhoutte D, Heymans S. TIMPs and cardiac remodeling: 'Embracing the MMP-independent-side of the family'. J Mol Cell Cardiol. 2010;48:445–53.
127. Baghelai K, Marktanner R, Dattilo JB, Dattilo MP, Jakoi ER, Yager DR, et al. Decreased expression of tissue inhibitor of metalloproteinase 1 in stunned myocardium. J Surg Res. 1998;77:35–9.
128. Tyagi SC, Kumar S, Voelker DJ, Reddy HK, Janicki JS, Curtis JJ. Differential gene expression of extracellular matrix components in dilated cardiomyopathy. J Cell Biochem. 1996;63:185–98.
129. Li YY, Feldman AM, Sun Y, McTiernan CF. Differential expression of tissue inhibitors of metalloproteinases in the failing human heart. Circulation. 1998;98:1728–34.
130. Fedak PW, Altamentova SM, Weisel RD, Nili N, Ohno N, Verma S, et al. Matrix remodeling in experimental and human heart failure: a possible regulatory role for TIMP-3. Am J Physiol Heart Circ Physiol. 2003;284:H626–34.
131. Hervas A, Ruiz-Sauri A, Gavara J, Monmeneu JV, de Dios E, Rios-Navarro C, et al. A Multidisciplinary Assessment of Remote Myocardial Fibrosis After Reperfused Myocardial Infarction in Swine and Patients. J Cardiovasc Transl Res. 2016;9:321–33.
132. Jellis C, Martin J, Narula J, Marwick TH. Assessment of nonischemic myocardial fibrosis. J Am Coll Cardiol. 2010;56:89–97.
133. Carrick D, Haig C, Rauhalammi S, Ahmed N, Mordi I, McEntegart M, et al. Pathophysiology of LV Remodeling in Survivors of STEMI: Inflammation, Remote Myocardium, and Prognosis. JACC Cardiovasc Imaging. 2015;8(7):779–89.
134. Biesbroek PS, Amier RP, Teunissen PFA, Hofman MBM, Robbers LFHJ, van de Ven PM, et al. Changes in remote myocardial tissue after acute myocardial infarction and its relation to cardiac remodeling: A CMR T1 mapping study. PLoS One. 2017;12:e0180115.

135. Wilson EM, Moainie SL, Baskin JM, Lowry AS, Deschamps AM, Mukherjee R, et al. Region- and type-specific induction of matrix metalloproteinases in post-myocardial infarction remodeling. Circulation. 2003;107:2857–63.
136. Aukrust P, Gullestad L, Lappegård KT, Ueland T, Aass H, Wikeby L, et al. Complement activation in patients with congestive heart failure: effect of high-dose intravenous immunoglobulin treatment. Circulation. 2001;104:1494–500.
137. Diwan A, Tran T, Misra A, Mann DL. Inflammatory mediators and the failing heart: a translational approach. Curr Mol Med. 2003;3:161–82.
138. Caforio AL, Mahon NG, Baig MK, Tona F, Murphy RT, Elliott PM, et al. Prospective familial assessment in dilated cardiomyopathy: cardiac autoantibodies predict disease development in asymptomatic relatives. Circulation. 2007;115:76–83.
139. Hofmann U, Frantz S. Role of T-cells in myocardial infarction. Eur Heart J. 2016;37:873–9.
140. Nikolich-Žugich J. Aging of the T cell compartment in mice and humans: from no naive expectations to foggy memories. J Immunol. 2014;193:2622–9.
141. von Andrian UH. Mackay CR.T-cell function and migration. Two sides of the same coin. N Engl J Med. 2000;343:1020–34.
142. Komarowska I, Coe D, Wang G, Haas R, Mauro C, Kishore M, et al. Hepatocyte Growth Factor Receptor c-Met Instructs T Cell Cardiotropism and Promotes T Cell Migration to the Heart via Autocrine Chemokine Release. Immunity. 2015;42:1087–99.
143. Ammirati E, Moroni F, Magnoni M, Camici PG. The role of T and B cells in human atherosclerosis and atherothrombosis. Clin Exp Immunol. 2015;179:173–87.
144. Yang Z, Day YJ, Toufektsian MC, Xu Y, Ramos SI, Marshall MA, et al. Myocardial infarct-sparing effect of adenosine A2A receptor activation is due to its action on CD4+ T lymphocytes. Circulation. 2006;114:2056–64.
145. Klingenberg R, Brokopp CE, Grivès A, Courtier A, Jaguszewski M, Pasqual N, et al. Clonal restriction and predominance of regulatory T cells in coronary thrombi of patients with acute coronary syndromes. Eur Heart J. 2015;36:1041–8.
146. Boag SE, Das R, Shmeleva EV, Bagnall A, Egred M, Howard N, et al. T lymphocytes and fractalkine contribute to myocardial ischemia/reperfusion injury in patients. J Clin Invest. 2015;125:3063–76.
147. Hofmann U, Beyersdorf N, Weirather J, Podolskaya A, Bauersachs J, Ertl G, et al. Activation of CD4+ T lymphocytes improves wound healing and survival after experimental myocardial infarction in mice. Circulation. 2012;125:1652–63.
148. Weirather J, Hofmann UD, Beyersdorf N, Ramos GC, Vogel B, Frey A, et al. Foxp3+ CD4+ T cells improve healing after myocardial infarction by modulating monocyte/macrophage differentiation. Circ Res. 2014;115:55–67.
149. Curato C, Slavic S, Dong J, Skorska A, Altarche-Xifró W, Miteva K, et al. Identification of noncytotoxic and IL-10-producing CD8+AT2R+ T cell population in response to ischemic heart injury. J Immunol. 2010;185:6286–93.
150. Wang J, Frangogiannis NG. In: Cokkinos DV, editor. Repair of the infarcted myocardium in Introduction to Translational Cardiovascular Research. Cham: Springer; 2015. p. 279–97.
151. Arslan F, de Kleijn DP, Pasterkamp G. Innate immune signaling in cardiac ischemia. Nat Rev Cardiol. 2011;8:292–300.
152. Frangogiannis NG. The immune system and the remodeling infarcted heart: cell biological insights and therapeutic opportunities. J Cardiovasc Pharmacol. 2014;63:185–95.
153. APEX AMI Investigators, Armstrong PW, Granger CB, Adams PX, Hamm C, Holmes D Jr, et al. Pexelizumab for acute ST-elevation myocardial infarction in patients undergoing primary percutaneous coronary intervention: a randomized controlled trial. JAMA. 2007;297:43–51.
154. Xuan YT, Tang XL, Banerjee S, Takano H, Li RC, Han H, et al. Nuclear factor-kappaB plays an essential role in the late phase of ischemic preconditioning in conscious rabbits. Circ Res. 1999;84:1095–109.

155. Shishido T, Nozaki N, Yamaguchi S, Shibata Y, Nitobe J, Miyamoto T, et al. Toll-like receptor-2 modulates ventricular remodeling after myocardial infarction. Circulation. 2003;108:2905–10.
156. Timmers L, Sluijter JP, van Keulen JK, Hoefer IE, Nederhoff MG, Goumans MJ, et al. Toll-like receptor 4 mediates maladaptive left ventricular remodeling and impairs cardiac function after myocardial infarction. Circ Res. 2008;102:257–64.
157. Lu C, Ren D, Wang X, Ha T, Liu L, Lee EJ, et al. Toll-like receptor 3 plays a role in myocardial infarction and ischemia/reperfusion injury. Biochim Biophys Acta. 1842;2014:22–31.
158. Gordon JW, Shaw JA, Kirshenbaum LA. Multiple facets of NF-kB in the heart: to be or not to NF-κB. Circ Res. 2011;108:1122–32.
159. Frangogiannis NG, Smith CW, Entman ML. The inflammatory response in myocardial infarction. Cardiovasc Res. 2002;53:31–47.
160. Frangogiannis NG. Chemokines in the ischemic myocardium: from inflammation to fibrosis. Inflamm Res. 2004;53:585–95.
161. Salcedo R, Ponce ML, Young HA, Wasserman K, Ward JM, Kleinman HK, et al. Human endothelial cells express CCR2 and respond to MCP-1: direct role of MCP-1 in angiogenesis and tumor progression. Blood. 2000;96:34–40.
162. Gharaee-Kermani M, Denholm EM, Phan SH. Costimulation of fibroblast collagen and transforming growth factor beta1 gene expression by monocyte chemoattractant protein-1 via specific receptors. J Biol Chem. 1996;271:17779–84.
163. Dewald O, Zymek P, Winkelmann K, Koerting A, Ren G, Abou-Khamis T, et al. CCL2/Monocyte Chemoattractant Protein-1 regulates inflammatory responses critical to healing myocardial infarcts. Circ Res. 2005;96:881–9.
164. Bujak M, Dobaczewski M, Chatila K, Mendoza LH, Li N, Reddy A, et al. Interleukin-1 receptor type I signaling critically regulates infarct healing and cardiac remodeling. Am J Pathol. 2008;173:57–67.
165. Saxena A, Chen W, Su Y, Rai V, Uche OU, Li N, et al. IL-1 induces proinflammatory leukocyte infiltration and regulates fibroblast phenotype in the infarcted myocardium. J Immunol. 2013;191:4838–48.
166. Frangogiannis NG, Lindsey ML, Michael LH, Youker KA, Bressler RB, Mendoza LH, et al. Resident cardiac mast cells degranulate and release preformed TNF-alpha, initiating the cytokine cascade in experimental canine myocardial ischemia/reperfusion. Circulation. 1998;98:699–710.
167. Middleton J, Patterson AM, Gardner L, Schmutz C, Ashton BA. Leukocyte extravasation: chemokine transport and presentation by the endothelium. Blood. 2002;100:3853–60.
168. Lefer DJ, Shandelya SM, Serrano CV Jr, Becker LC, Kuppusamy P, Zweier JL. Cardioprotective actions of a monoclonal antibody against CD-18 in myocardial ischemia-reperfusion injury. Circulation. 1993;88:1779–87.
169. Faxon DP, Gibbons RJ, Chronos NA, Gurbel PA, Sheehan F, HALT-MI Investigators. The effect of blockade of the CD11/CD18 integrin receptor on infarct size in patients with acute myocardial infarction treated with direct angioplasty: the results of the HALT-MI study. J Am Coll Cardiol. 2002;40:1199–204.
170. Nahrendorf M, Swirski FK, Aikawa E, Stangenberg L, Wurdinger T, Figueiredo JL, et al. The healing myocardium sequentially mobilizes two monocyte subsets with divergent and complementary functions. J Exp Med. 2007;204:3037–47.
171. Ismahil MA, Hamid T, Bansal SS, Patel B, Kingery JR, Prabhu SD. Remodeling of the mononuclear phagocyte network underlies chronic inflammation and disease progression in heart failure: critical importance of the cardiosplenic axis. Circ Res. 2014;114:266–82.
172. Dutta P, Courties G, Wei Y, Leuschner F, Gorbatov R, Robbins CS, et al. Myocardial infarction accelerates atherosclerosis. Nature. 2012;487:325–9.
173. Emami H, Singh P, MacNabb M, Vucic E, Lavender Z, Rudd JH, et al. Splenic metabolic activity predicts risk of future cardiovascular events: demonstration of a cardiosplenic axis in humans. JACC Cardiovasc Imaging. 2015;8:121–30.

174. Frangogiannis NG, Mendoza LH, Ren G, Akrivakis S, Jackson PL, Michael LH, et al. MCSF expression is induced in healing myocardial infarcts and may regulate monocyte and endothelial cell phenotype. Am J Physiol Heart Circ Physiol. 2003;285:H483–92.
175. Frangogiannis NG, Perrard JL, Mendoza LH, Burns AR, Lindsey ML, Ballantyne CM, et al. Stem cell factor induction is associated with mast cell accumulation after canine myocardial ischemia and reperfusion. Circulation. 1998;98:687–98.
176. Chen W, Saxena A, Li N, Sun J, Gupta A, Lee DW, et al. Endogenous IRAK-M attenuates postinfarction remodeling through effects on macrophages and fibroblasts. Arterioscler Thromb Vasc Biol. 2012;32:2598–608.
177. Dean RG, Balding LC, Candido R, Burns WC, Cao Z, Twigg SM, et al. Connective tissue growth factor and cardiac fibrosis after myocardial infarction. J Histochem Cytochem. 2005;53:1245–56.
178. Carrillo-García C, Prochnow S, Simeonova IK, Strelau J, Hölzl-Wenig G, Mandl C, et al. Growth/differentiation factor 15 promotes EGFR signalling, and regulates proliferation and migration in the hippocampus of neonatal and young adult mice. Development. 2014;141:773–83.
179. Frangogiannis NG, Mendoza LH, Lindsey ML, Ballantyne CM, Michael LH, Smith CW, et al. IL-10 is induced in the reperfused myocardium and may modulate the reaction to injury. J Immunol. 2000;165:2798–808.
180. Lacraz S, Nicod LP, Chicheportiche R, Welgus HG. Dayer JM.IL-10 inhibits metalloproteinase and stimulates TIMP-1 production in human mononuclear phagocytes. J Clin Invest. 1995;96:23182.
181. Cochain C, Channon KM, Silvestre JS. Angiogenesis in the infarcted myocardium. Antioxid Redox Signal. 2013;18:1100–13. 04-2310
182. Dobaczewski M, Akrivakis S, Nasser K, Michael LH, Entman ML, Frangogiannis NG. Vascular mural cells in healing canine myocardial infarcts. J Histochem Cytochem. 2004;52:1019–29.
183. Schirone L, Forte M, Palmerio S, Yee D, Nocella C, Angelini F, et al. A Review of the Molecular Mechanisms Underlying the Development and Progression of Cardiac Remodeling. Oxidative Med Cell Longev. 2017;2017:3920195.
184. Neubauer S. The failing heart--an engine out of fuel. N Engl J Med. 2007;356:1140–51.
185. Frati G, Schirone L, Chimenti I, Yee D, Biondi-Zoccai G, Volpe M, et al. An overview of the inflammatory signalling mechanisms in the myocardium underlying the development of diabetic cardiomyopathy. Cardiovasc Res. 2017;113:378–88.
186. Westman PC, Lipinski MJ, Torguson R. Waksman R.A comparison of cangrelor, prasugrel, ticagrelor, and clopidogrel in patients undergoing percutaneous coronary intervention: A network meta-analysis. Cardiovasc Revasc Med. 2017;18:79–85.
187. Schroder K, Tschopp J. The inflammasomes. Cell. 2010;140:821–32.
188. Rupprecht HJ, Blankenberg S, Bickel C, Rippin G, Hafner G, Prellwitz W, et al. Impact of viral and bacterial infectious burden on long-term prognosis in patients with coronary artery disease. Circulation. 2001;104:25–31.
189. Opie LH, Commerford PJ, Gersh BJ, Pfeffer MA. Controversies in ventricular remodelling. Lancet. 2006;36:356–67.
190. Sawyer DB, Siwik DA, Xiao L, Pimentel DR, Singh K, Colucci WS. Role of oxidative stress in myocardial hypertrophy and failure. J Mol Cell Cardiol. 2002;34:379–88.
191. Siwik DA, Pagano PJ, Colucci WS. Oxidative stress regulates collagen synthesis and matrix metalloproteinase activity in cardiac fibroblasts. Am J Physiol Cell Physiol. 2001;280:C53–60.
192. Takimoto E, Kass DA. Role of oxidative stress in cardiac hypertrophy and remodeling. Hypertension. 2007;49:241–8.
193. Giordano FJ. Oxygen, oxidative stress, hypoxia, and heart failure. J Clin Invest. 2005;115:500–8.
194. Burgoyne JR, Mongue-Din H, Eaton P, Shah AM. Redox signaling in cardiac physiology and pathology. Circ Res. 2012;111:1091–106.

195. Turrens JF. Mitochondrial formation of reactive oxygen species. J Physiol. 2003;552:335–44.
196. Dai DF, Johnson SC, Villarin JJ, Chin MT, Nieves-Cintrón M, Chen T, et al. Mitochondrial oxidative stress mediates angiotensin II-induced cardiac hypertrophy and Galphaq overexpression-induced heart failure. Circ Res. 2011;108:837–46.
197. Shiomi T, Tsutsui H, Matsusaka H, Murakami K, Hayashidani S, Ikeuchi M, et al. Overexpression of glutathione peroxidase prevents left ventricular remodeling and failure after myocardial infarction in mice. Circulation. 2004;109:544–9.
198. Gomes KM, Campos JC, Bechara LR, Queliconi B, Lima VM, Disatnik MH, et al. Aldehyde dehydrogenase 2 activation in heart failure restores mitochondrial function and improves ventricular function and remodelling. Cardiovasc Res. 2014;103:498–508.
199. Peterzan MA, Lygate CA, Neubauer S, Rider O. Metabolic remodelling in hypertrophied and failing myocardium: a review. Am J Physiol Heart Circ Physiol. 2017:ajpheart.00731.2016.
200. Shen W, Asai K, Uechi M, Mathier MA, Shannon RP, Vatner SF, et al. Progressive loss of myocardial ATP due to a loss of total purines during the development of heart failure in dogs: a compensatory role for the parallel loss of creatine. Circulation. 1999;100:2113–8.
201. Kapelko VI, Kupriyanov VV, Novikova NA, Lakomkin VL, Steinschneider AY, Severina MY, et al. The cardiac contractile failure induced by chronic creatine and phosphocreatine deficiency. J Mol Cell Cardiol. 1988;20:465–79.
202. Newton AC, Antal CE, Steinberg SF. Protein kinase C mechanisms that contribute to cardiac remodelling. Clin Sci (Lond). 2016;130:1499–510.
203. Hambleton M, Hahn H, Pleger ST, Kuhn MC, Klevitsky R, Carr AN, et al. Pharmacological- and gene therapy-based inhibition of protein kinase Calpha/beta enhances cardiac contractility and attenuates heart failure. Circulation. 2006;114:574–82.
204. Braz JC, Bueno OF, De Windt LJ, Molkentin JD. PKC alpha regulates the hypertrophic growth of cardiomyocytes through extracellular signal-regulated kinase1/2 (ERK1/2). J Cell Biol. 2002;156:905–19.
205. Braz JC, Gregory K, Pathak A, Zhao W, Sahin B, Klevitsky R, et al. PKC-alpha regulates cardiac contractility and propensity toward heart failure. Nat Med. 2004;10:248–54.
206. Dorn GW 2nd, Souroujon MC, Liron T, Chen CH, Gray MO, Zhou HZ, et al. Sustained in vivo cardiac protection by a rationally designed peptide that causes epsilon protein kinase C translocation. Proc Natl Acad Sci U S A. 1999;96:12798–803.
207. Murriel CL, Mochly-Rosen D. Opposing roles of delta and epsilonPKC in cardiac ischemia and reperfusion: targeting the apoptotic machinery. Arch Biochem Biophys. 2003;420:246–54.
208. Churchill EN, Mochly-Rosen D. The roles of PKCdelta and epsilon isoenzymes in the regulation of myocardial ischaemia/reperfusion injury. Biochem Soc Trans. 2007;35:1040–2.
209. Letavernier E, Zafrani L, Perez J, Letavernier B, Haymann JP, Baud L. The role of calpains in myocardial remodelling and heart failure. Cardiovasc Res. 2012;96:38–45.
210. Peers C. The G. L. Brown Prize Lecture. Hypoxic regulation of ion channel function and expression. Exp Physiol. 2002;87:413–22.
211. Topkara VK, Mann DL. Clinical applications of miRNAs in cardiac remodeling and heart failure. Per Med. 2010;7:531–48.
212. Kumarswamy R, Thum T. Non-coding RNAs in cardiac remodeling and heart failure. Circ Res. 2013;113:676–89.
213. Devaux Y, Vausort M, McCann GP, Kelly D, Collignon O, Ng LL, et al. A panel of 4 microRNAs facilitates the prediction of left ventricular contractility after acute myocardial infarction. PLoS One. 2013;8:e70644.
214. Devaux Y, Vausort M, McCann GP, Zangrando J, Kelly D, Razvi N, et al. MicroRNA-150: a novel marker of left ventricular remodeling after acute myocardial infarction. Circ Cardiovasc Genet. 2013;6:290–8.
215. Montgomery RL, Hullinger TG, Semus HM, Dickinson BA, Seto AG, Lynch JM, et al. Therapeutic inhibition of miR-208a improves cardiac function and survival during heart failure. Circulation. 2011;124:1537–47.

216. Kumarswamy R, Lyon AR, Volkmann I, Mills AM, Bretthauer J, Pahuja A, et al. SERCA2a gene therapy restores microRNA-1 expression in heart failure via an Akt/FoxO3A-dependent pathway. Eur Heart J. 2012;33:1067–75.
217. Wahlquist C, Jeong D, Rojas-Muñoz A, Kho C, Lee A, Mitsuyama S, et al. Inhibition of miR-25 improves cardiac contractility in the failing heart. Nature. 2014;508:531–5.
218. Garikipati VN, Verma SK, Jolardarashi D, Cheng Z, Ibetti J, Cimini M, et al. Therapeutic Inhibition of miR-375 Attenuates Post-MI Inflammatory Response and Left Ventricular Dysfunction via PDK-1-AKT Signaling Axis. Cardiovasc Res. 2017; https://doi.org/10.1093/cvr/cvx052.
219. Bernardo BC, Gao XM, Winbanks CE, Boey EJ, Tham YK, Kiriazis H, et al. Therapeutic inhibition of the miR-34 family attenuates pathological cardiac remodeling and improves heart function. Proc Natl Acad Sci U S A. 2012;109:17615–20.
220. van Rooij E, Sutherland LB, Liu N, Williams AH, McAnally J, Gerard RD, et al. A signature pattern of stress-responsive microRNAs that can evoke cardiac hypertrophy and heart failure. Proc Natl Acad Sci U S A. 2006;103:18255–60.

Chapter 13
Cardiac Remodeling: The Course Towards Heart Failure-II. Diagnostic and Therapeutic Approaches

Dennis V. Cokkinos

13.1 Diagnosis

The diagnosis of cardiac remodeling (REM) is constantly undergoing developments. It should not be forgotten that the very simple electrocardiogram (ECG) can offer a clue toward diagnostic REM. Thus, notching in the QRS complex after myocardial infarction (MI) is strongly suggestive of REM, with prospects for reverse remodeling after cardiac resynchronization therapy (CRT) [1]. Furthermore, the ECG is valuable in predicting success after CRT. Thus, a left bundle branch block (LBBB) pattern with a QRS duration of ≈150 ms is very strongly suggestive of success after synchronized pacing [2].

As expected, because of its ease of application, echocardiography (echo) is the technique most widely used to diagnose and follow the course of REM. Various measurements have been already referred to. Echo remains a very useful tool in experimental REM. In a recent rat study, Azevedo et al. [3] found many parameters predictive of REM at 6 mo, such as left atrial (LA) dilation, the left ventricular (LV) end-diastolic diameter (LVEDD), the LV end-systolic diameter (LVESD), the LV mass index (LVMI), the E-wave to A-wave ratio (E/A), and the isovolumic relaxation time adjusted for the heart rate (IVRT/HR).

In clinical studies, transthoracic echo (TTE) studies have shown that evolution toward REM can be seen quite early [4]. Migrino et al. [5] found that the LV end-systolic volume (LVESV) index by contrast ventriculography 90–180 min after thrombolysis was predictive of 6-month mortality. Of course, it must not be forgotten that in a much older study using LV contrast ventriculography 4–8 weeks post-MI in 60 patients, White et al. [6] found that at 78-month follow-up the end-systolic

D. V. Cokkinos (✉)
Heart and Vessel Department, Biomedical Research Foundation,
Academy of Athens - Gregory Skalkeas, Athens, Greece
e-mail: dcokkinos@bioacademy.gr

D. V. Cokkinos (ed.), *Myocardial Preservation*,
https://doi.org/10.1007/978-3-319-98186-4_13

volume (LVESV) had greater predictive volume than the end-diastolic volume (LVEDV) or the ejection fraction (EF).

Advances in echo are constant and numerous. Real-time three-dimensional (3D) imaging may give a better picture for selection for CRT [7]. Contrast echocardiography can also give better delineation of volume [8].

Great progress has been achieved with the introduction of various parameters of tissue Doppler. Thus, speckle tracking and LV strain can give very detailed information. Speckle tracking may also reliably image fibrosis.

Global longitudinal strain [9] adds useful information with regard to prediction of a course toward REM (observed in 25.5% of patients).

Finally, dyssynchronization evaluation may add prognostic information regarding progression to REM [9] and successful application of CRT [10, 11].

Microbubble imaging, as described by Yeh and Nihoyannopoulos [12], can aid molecular imaging of myocardial perfusion or in vivo detection of various molecular markers in animals, such as selectins, intercellular adhesion molecule 1 (ICAM-1), vascular cell adhesion molecule 1 (VCAM-1), integrins, von Willebrand factor, vascular endothelial growth factor receptor (VEGFR)– glycoprotein (GP) IIb/IIIa receptors, matrix metalloproteinases (MMPs), activated leukocytes, and others. It can be predicted that advances in various forms of echo will continue to occur.

13.1.1 Cardiac Magnetic Resonance Imaging

Cardiac magnetic resonance imaging (CMR) is increasingly being used in the evaluation of gene and cellular therapies. CMR may better delineate LV mass and volume [13]. CMR can also better image microvascular obstruction, which is an important predictor of REM, scar formation [14], and myocardial edema, and it can also distinguish between reversible and irreversible injury [14–16]. CMR has also been used to define REM, with very good area under the curve (AUC) values [17].

13.1.2 Radionuclide Imaging

Radionuclide imaging can be used to measure myocardial viability (VIA), which is a key factor to prompt the application of revascularization [18]. When extensive REM ensues, VIA may become of less pivotal importance, although no time limits have been set.

Assessment of late redistribution by single-photon emission computed tomography (SPECT) remains a valuable approach in comparison with other techniques [19].

More data are given in Chap. 10, which discusses myocardial hibernation. We believe that it can, up to a point, predict REM [20] as Berti et al. [21] have shown.

In 2011, Konstam et al. [22] discussed the various aforementioned techniques as being able to evaluate REM. They believe that the LV volume and perturbation of the normally elliptical LV chamber geometry are important factors. They also stress that REM determines future cardiac events and the course toward heart failure (HF).

The positron emission tomography (PET) approach is based on detection of a shift in myocardial perfusion energetics [22], as described in Chap.10 on myocardial hibernation. It has given an important impetus to investigating the molecular processes underlying REM as well, as described by Paschali et al. [23]. Also, Curley et al. [24] have published an excellent recent review.

The following processes can be investigated:

Myocardial perfusion: This is assessed using N-13 ammonia, rubidium-82 (Rb-82), and 015-water. N-13 enters cardiac myocytes (CMCs) also in proportion to blood flow, while Rb-82, which is a K+ analog, is taken up by CMCs in proportion to blood flow. Only the former two are approved by the US Food and Drug Administration (FDA).

Myocardial metabolism: Fluorodeoxyglucose (^{18}F-FDG), a glucose analog taken up by CMCs through glucose transporters (GLUTs) 1 and 4, is the one still mainly used. Palmitic acid and acetate labeled with carbon 11 (^{11}C) have not gained wide application.

Myocardial innervation: A gold standard for many years has been metaiodobenzylguanidine (MIBG). Its uptake is decreased in dysfunctional myocardium [25].

However, new agents are emerging, such as hydroxyephedrine (HED) and epinephrine (EPI) labeled with ^{11}C. The latter is being considered as a neuronal imaging tracer.

A newer MIBG analog, LM1195 labeled with ^{18}F, is being investigated, as is a radiolabeled β-receptor antagonist (GP12 177) and MQNβ, a muscarinic receptor agonist.

The use of these newer labeling agents is part of the general subject of molecular imaging.

Molecular Imaging

This notion has existed for many years, in the hope of noninvasively investigating cardiac structure and function without the need to revert to myocardial biopsy. In 2010, Dixon and Spinale [25] published an important review on this subject. At that time they pointed out certain domains and targets to investigate the post-MI REM process. If a synthesis of the above reviews is attempted, the following processes can be measured by SPECT, PET, CMR, ultrasound, and optical imaging.

Inflammation

- Extracellular matrix processes: Collagen, MMPs.
- Vasculature: Angiotensin, integrins, vascular endothelial growth factor (VEGF), smooth muscle cells (SMCs), actin.
- Growth/viability: Transforming growth factor-β (TGF-β), apoptotic markers, myofibroblasts.

Cell Death

- Apoptosis (annexin-V): Paschali et al. [23] and Bengel [26] give some further important insights into the subject of imaging agents.
- Renin–angiotensin aldosterone system [27, 28].
- Magnetic resonance imaging has also been used for molecular imaging. It has excellent temporal and spatial resolution but lower sensitivity than nuclear imaging. It utilizes two major imaging agents: gadolinium (Gd) and iron. Gd chelates are water soluble; they are distributed to the interstitial tissue but do not enter intact cells. They can image macrophages; thus a probe of myeloperoxidase (MPO) activity is being investigated [23, 29].

Biomarkers

Vasan [30] has written an excellent review on this topic. He refers to a National Institutes of Health (NIH) definition [31] according to which a biomarker (BM) is "a characteristic that is objectively measured and evaluated as an indicator of normal biological processes, pathogenic processes, or pharmacological responses to a therapeutic intervention" and defines various types of BM.

Currently, a large number of BMs are being used to investigate REM (Table 13.1). What must be pointed out is that many of them represent adaptive mechanisms against cell death, HF, ischemia, fibrosis, and inflammation. Thus, Zannad [32], in a 2014 editorial, also stresses the value of integrating BMs and imaging, in this case concerning fibrosis. He describes the pros and cons of echo and magnetic resonance imaging in assessing fibrosis and the use of plasma levels of by-products of collagen synthesis, as investigated by Ellims et al. [33].

The list is constantly growing; systems biology approaches identifying pathways related to ventricular post-MI dysfunction are being developed.

Thus, Azuaje et al. [34] report an integrative approach to identify pathways related to post-MI REM. They have found a diversity of pathway level perturbations. They obtained total RNA from 32 MI patients, extracted from whole blood cells by PAXgene™ technology.

Transcriptomic profiles were obtained using oligonucleotide microarrays representing 25,000 genes. A global "perturbation score" was calculated. Highly perturbed pathways included those implicated in antigen-dependent B-cell activation and synthesis of leucine. BM models were also integrated to increase prognostic performance.

Interestingly, Yang et al. [35] have also used a systems approach, which additionally identified the importance of β-adrenergic receptor signaling.

13.2 Therapy

With all currently employed techniques, REM occurs in around 30% of anterior MIs. In the Acute Myocardial Infarction Contrast Imaging (AMICI) trial an appreciable degree (39%) of reverse REM was found [36].

Table 13.1 Biomarkers in cardiac remodeling (REM)

Myocardial injury, apoptosis
(hs)TnI, TnT
CK-MB
Myosin light-chain kinase I
sFas
Heart-type fatty-acid protein
Cytochrome C
M 30 Neurohormonal axis activation
Norepinephrine
Angiotensin II, renin, aldosterone
Antidiuretic hormone/copeptin
Endothelin, prolactin
Stretch, myocardial stress
NT-proBNP, BNP, ANP forms
Proadrenomedullin
ST2, copeptin
GDF15
Extracellular matrix REM
MMPs, TIMPs
Galectin 3, cystatin C
Osteopontin, procollagen types I and III
Inflammation
(hs)CRP
Interleukins
TNF-α
Osteoprotegerin
MCP-1, GDF15
Proliferation and differentiation
Syndecan-1, syndecan-4
Oxidative stress
Malondialdehyde, myeloperoxidase
TBARs
Oxidized low-density lipoproteins
Superoxide dismutase
Glutathione forms
Total plasma polyphenols
Catalase
Thyroid hormones
FT3, FT4, rT3

ANP atrial natriuretic peptide, *BNP* brain natriuretic peptide, *CK* creatine kinase, *CRP* C-reactive protein, *GDF15* growth/differentiation factor 15, *hs* high-sensitivity, *FT3* free tri-iodothyronine, *FT4* free thyroxine, *MCP-1* monocyte chemoattractant protein 1, *MMP* matrix metalloproteinase, *NT* N-terminal, *rT3* reverse tri-iodothyronine, *sFas* soluble Fas, *ST2* interleukin 1 receptor-like 1, *TBAR* thiobarbituric acid reactive substance, *TIMP* tissue inhibitor of metalloproteinase, *TNF-α* tumor necrosis factor alpha, *TnI* troponin I, *TnT* troponin T

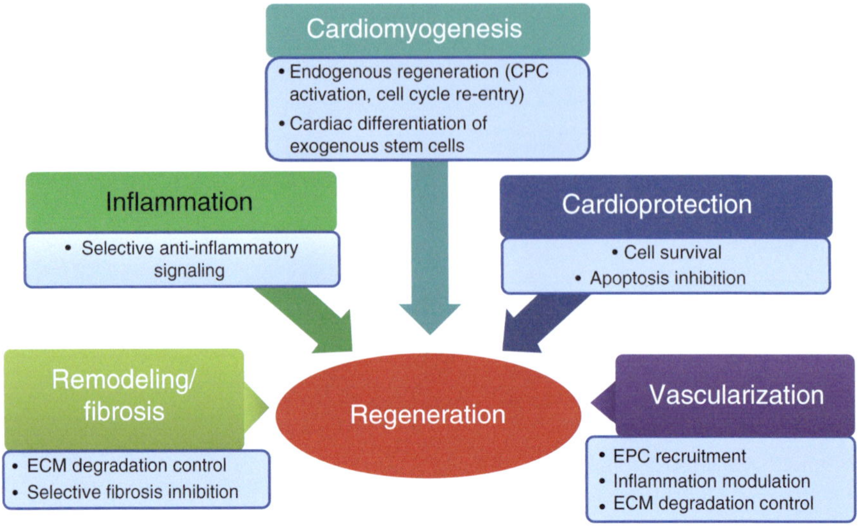

Fig. 13.1 Targets and goals of therapeutic strategies for myocardial regeneration. (Reproduced from Ruvinov et al. [38], with permission)

However, we should not only address post-MI REM. The course of many cardiomyopathies can be delayed by either pharmaceutical gene or cell therapy. It should be stressed that the two types of therapy are not mutually exclusive but complementary [37]. Also, device and CRT approaches have shown considerable progress.

The conclusions drawn from the data stress that therapy for REM should be combined and holistic. Ruvinov et al. [38] give a very detailed graph of this approach [3] in which cardioprotection, angiogenesis, anti-inflammatory, and antifibrotic treatment are combined with regeneration and cardiomyogenesis (Fig. 13.1).

It is very difficult to provide a logical sequence for the description of all of these modalities. For didactic reasons I will try to separate them into pharmaceutical, device, gene, and cell therapy, again stressing that all of these are complementary. In pharmaceutical therapy, conditioning and exercise can be included. Reperfusion, which is essential, can be achieved pharmaceutically (via thrombolysis) or mechanically (via percutaneous coronary intervention (PCI)). This combination is not unusual.

The most important element in preventing post-MI REM is earlier reperfusion, as described in the Chap. 6, on ischemia–reperfusion injury (IRI).

13.2.1 Adjunctive Therapy in Reperfusion with Primary Percutaneous Coronary Intervention

The number of drugs and procedures that have been tried is legion. However, the conclusions of the European Society of Cardiology (ESC) working group on the cellular biology of the heart in 2013 [39] are sobering: they state that there is currently no effective clinical therapy for protecting the heart against the detrimental effects of acute IRI. They note that 17 studies have been judged as negative, though 15 of these studies are described as promising. In these are included adenosine IGF-1, melatonin, intravenous (IV) metoprolol, insulin-like growth factor 1 (IGF-1), placement of an Impella device, nitric oxide (NO) donors, nitrate, sevoflurane, thymosin B4, mangafodipir, melatonin, Bendavia, and TRO40303. The last two are still under study. The same working group reached similar conclusions in 2017 [40]. The drugs considered to give positive results are described further such as metoprolol and cyclosporine-A.

Unfortunately, after the initial processing results reported by Newton et al. [41], the results of the much larger Does Cyclosporine Improve Clinical Outcome in ST Elevation Myocardial Infarction Patients (CIRCUS) trial, with 395 patients receiving the drug and 326 controls, were disappointing in that the drug did not prevent REM at 12 months [42]. The 6-month results of the Cyclosporine A in Reperfused Acute Myocardial Infarction (CYCLE) trial [43], with 267 patients receiving cyclosporine A and 203 controls, were equally disappointing. Many reasons have been given to explain these disappointing results [44], but it is difficult to see how another cyclosporine trial can be planned.

Other approaches showing positive results in cardioprotection were "conditioning" (or conditioning-mimetic) with cariporide, hypothermia, O_2 delivery, exenatide, and the old-timer glucose–insulin–potassium (GIK)—the Sodi-Pallares solution—which has been used since I was a cardiology fellow in the late 1960s.

Obviously, limiting infarct size is a very important aspect in alleviating the process of REM. However, efforts to reach that goal continue in the chronic phase, practically for life. Many reviews are available on this subject [3, 45–48].

The position paper from the ESC myocardial function working group also gives important insights into novel therapies [49]. This expert group offers the following goals: Improving myocardial function, preventing CMC death, angiogenesis, regulating interstitial REM.

Before embarking on the discussion of some agents commonly used in humans, an important caveat must be mentioned. If the innumerable reports on drug anti-REM therapy in experimental animals are taken into account, REM should not occur at all, since many of them have greatly blunted the course toward REM. However, rodent hearts handle infarct production better than human hearts do [50].

Moreover, in animal experiments usually one artery is occluded and the myocardium is otherwise normal; also, genetic polymorphisms are limited. This is in strong contrast to human cases of MI. Another point is that in animals only one drug is used at a time; in humans frequently at least four drugs are used in combination, i.e., β-blockers, angiotensin-converting-enzyme (ACE) inhibitors or angiotensin receptor blockers (ARBs), antialdosterone therapy, and statins. Thus, the exact contribution of each drug family is difficult to determine.

13.2.2 *Clinical Aspects of Pharmacological Therapy*

The main aspects are summarized in the following subsections.

13.2.2.1 Prevention of Cardiac Myocyte Death

The roles of continuing apoptosis and dysregulation of autophagy are described in the Chap. 7, which discusses cell death.

β-Blockers are antiapoptotic. It should be remembered that β1-adrenergic receptors are the most abundant ones in the myocardium [51, 52].

β2-receptors exert a protective effect on the heart [52, 53]. The β2-agonist clenbuterol is being used by the group of Sir Magdi Yacoub to wean patients off a left ventricular assist device (LVAD), as will be described further [54]. We have shown that clenbuterol increases cell growth [55].

The role of β3-receptors has recently been investigated. They may have an antiapoptotic effect [56].

Angiotensin-Converting-Enzyme Inhibitors and Angiotensin Receptor Blockers

Angiotensin II is a well-known inducer of CMC apoptosis [57, 58].

The above agents have, apart from their clinical beneficial results, also been shown experimentally to reduce apoptosis. Here, the findings of Albuquerque et al. [59] should be remembered: that many genetic polymorphisms influencing HF involve the Renin-Angiotensin-Aldosterone system. In rat experiments, no differences between ACE inhibitors and ARBs were seen with regard to post-MI REM [60].

A new combination therapy including the ARB valsartan and the neprilysin inhibitor sacubitril (LCZ 696) has been compared with enalapril [61]. It was associated with decreases in mortality, hospitalization for HF, symptoms, and physical limitation. This combination was previously shown to reduce myocardial fibrosis and hypertrophy, and to increase the EF in rats post-MI [62].

Inhibition of aldosterone by eplerenone also decreases REM [63]. Thus, more detailed study needs to be done on this subject, since this treatment is costly. In a substudy, eplerenone was found to improve collagen turnover [64].

Spironolactone improved REM in patients with dilated cardiomyopathy [65, 66]. Here some discrepant results should be mentioned. Early administration of spironolactone prevents REM in patients with a first anterior MI [67]. However, the findings of the recent Aldosterone Lethal Effects Blocked in Acute MI Treated With or Without Reperfusion to Improve Outcome and Survival at Six Months Follow-Up (ALBATROSS) trial [68] were a disappointment. This trial first used intravenous potassium canrenoate followed by oral spironolactone for 6 months in patients with MI without HF at the onset. Of these patients, 77% had ST-elevation MI (STEMI); 802 received spironolactone and 801 received standard treatment. The treatment failed to decrease worsening HF at 6 months, which occurred in only 5.6–5.9%. This can be construed as a negative effect against REM but could have been due to the patients' very good early EF (50%), which would be hard to improve further.

Statins

Statins are routinely used after MI and are regularly included in the "big 4" drugs. They have been shown to decrease IRI [69]. Thanks to their pleiotropic activity, they have also been shown to reduce inflammation, as displayed both by measurement of inflammatory markers in the Myocardial Ischemia Reduction with Aggressive Cholesterol Lowering (MIRACL) study [70] in patients and by magnetic resonance imaging in rats [71]. Statins are also reported to have antioxidant effects [72], decreasing reactive oxygen species (ROS) and apoptosis; they also activate adenosine triphosphate (ATP)–sensitive potassium (K^+ATP) channels [73]. However, in a trial in which 40 patients taking rosuvastatin 20–40 mg and 46 controls were included, Krum et al. [74] found no difference in REM, proinflammatory cytokine levels, and neurohumoral parameters in patients with chronic systolic HF. The effect of statins in HF has been addressed in many studies; in two large studies [75, 76] the results were neutral.

In an editorial, Kjekshus [77] postulates that by lowering cholesterol and stabilizing vulnerable plaques, statins may prevent future recurrent acute coronary syndromes (ACS), which could cause further CMC death and REM. This deduction was drawn from a very large meta-analysis conducted by Preiss et al. [78].

A question that has not been answered is whether the "big 4" drugs together can produce a more favorable result than one or two drugs given separately, or if an additional cardioprotective drug can exert a supplemental effect beyond that produced by the aforementioned combination.

Direct antiapoptotic interventions using pan-caspase inhibitors have been applied experimentally. Tarone et al. [49] raise the question as to whether they may shift the process from apoptosis to necrosis, although necrosis is scant in chronic HF (see Chap. 7, which discusses cell death). They mention the emergence of the concept of necroptosis. In this aspect the drug necrostatin-1 is being used. It is antiapoptotic and has already been used experimentally against post-IRI REM in mice [79, 80].

Letavernier et al. [81] have reviewed the role of calpains in REM and HF. Calpains are calcium-activated neutral cysteine proteases. They contribute to hypertrophy, inflammation, fibrosis, and cardiac dysfunction. They are also involved in IRI-related death. In IRI, Ca^{2+}-activated calpains hydrolyze proteins in the sarcolemma and skeleton, causing sarcolemmal injury and rupture, and promote myofibrillar degradation and loss of sarcomere structure [82]. However, calpains can also be cardioprotective in certain circumstances by contributing to myocardial repair [83]. Thus, their clinical application is far from established at present.

Neuregulin is involved in CMC regeneration. This action is mediated by the all-important cardioprotective phosphatidylinositol-3-kinase/protein kinase B (PI3K-Akt) and extracellular signal–regulated kinase 1 and 2 (ERK1/2) pathways [84]. In a recombinant form it is cardioprotective in rodent and canine models, and is being tried in humans [85, 86].

13.2.2.2 Attenuation of Proteotoxicity

This can be effected by molecular chaperones—heat shock proteins—and small ATP-independent heat shock proteins (HSPBs), with αβ-crystallin (HSPβ5) as a main representative. Also, HSPβ6 (HSP20) controls both CMC survival (via the Akt pathway) and contractility through the protein phosphatase-1 (pp1)–phospholamban–sarcoplasmic/endoplasmic reticulum calcium ATPase-2 (SERCA-2) axis [87].

Melusin also acts through the ERK1/2 PI3/AH pathways and exerts a cardioprotective action [88].

Ubiquitin ligases are acquiring importance as protective (anti-IRI, antihypertrophic) agents [89].

Protein kinases regulate CMC cell fate decisions. However, currently few therapies targeting them are emerging.

Sildenafil, an inhibitor of phosphodiesterase 5, protects against transverse aortic constriction (TAC)–induced REM [90]. In clinical HF this drug may induce reverse REM [91]. However, the drug was not successful in the Phosphodiesterase-5 Inhibition to Improve Clinical Status and Exercise Capacity in Heart Failure with Preserved Ejection Fraction (RELAX) trial in patients with HF with a preserved EF (HFpEF) [92].

NO donor findings are still not conclusive, but nitroxyl (HNO) produced by NO synthase (NOS) in vitro under oxidative or nitrosative stress [93] is being studied in animal and human studies. An oral endothelial NOS (eNOS) enhancer, AVE9488 [94], has been shown to improve REM after experimental MI.

13.2.2.3 Improvement in Cardiac Contractility

Improvement in contractility without overly increasing oxygen consumption or increasing cell death, such as occurs via excessive β1 stimulation, can produce a beneficial turn of events, since a decrease in cardiac size has many favorable effects. It must be remembered that β-adrenergic receptor (β-AR) signaling is downregulated in HF. Of course, excessive catecholaminergic stimulation increases CMC death. Thus, alternative methods for increasing contractility are being sought.

Manipulation of Sarcoplasmic/Endoplasmic Reticulum Calcium ATPase-2α

Notably, in HF, frequency-dependent SERCA-2α upregulation is absent. However, apart from thyroid hormones, which are discussed later, pharmacological approaches to SERCA-2α increase are not clinically available. Unfortunately, the Calcium Upregulation by Percutaneous Administration of Gene Therapy in Patients with Cardiac Disease (CUPID 2) trial [95], performed in a large number of patients (123 patients receiving active treatment versus 127 patients receiving placebo treatment) did not repeat the promising results of the first phase I/II trial in 39 patients [96].

Roger Hajjar [97] stresses that the transfection efficacy of SERCA-2α, a large molecule, is very low. Also, from the clinical aspect the amount of fibrosis in the myocardium of the patients to whom SERCA-2α is administered by intracoronary (IC) infusion must play a role. Again, as in the case of cyclosporine, the very unfavorable consequences of a negative trial are huge.

Cardiac Myosin Activators

One of the main representatives of this type of drug is omecamtiv mecarbil, which binds directly to the myosin catalytic domain and has yielded favorable results [98, 99]. A question arises from the finding that in high doses it may produce ischemia due to reduction of the diastolic phase. However, in the 20-week Chronic Oral

Study of Myosin Activation to Increase Contractility (COSMIC) trial, REM was improved [100].

Levosimendan

Levosimendan has been used for many years. Initially it was used in single-infusion protocols [101]. However, it is being successfully used in chronic (repeated or intermittent) infusions [102, 103]. Experimentally it reduces REM in pigs post-MI [104] and in hypertensive Dahl/Rapp rats [105].

Other Drugs

As already mentioned, the drugs being used experimentally are legion. Here, some of the most promising ones are described.

Ivabradine has been shown to favorably affect HF. In the echo substudy of the Systolic Heart Failure Treatment with the I_f Inhibitor Ivabradine trial (SHIFT) it decreased REM [106]. It may be a logical alternative in patients with HF in whom a decrease in the HR<70/min cannot be effected by β-blockers.

Metabolic Modulators

Metabolic modulators include insulinotropics and insulinomimetics.

Metformin has been very effective against REM in rats [107]. It has been found to attenuate fibrosis [108] in an experimental setting.

The new drug empagliflozin has given excellent clinical results in reducing mortality by 14% in diabetic patients [109]. It is currently being used in a large number of trials, and it is also providing impetus to study new mechanisms of HF. It has been shown to prevent systolic function worsening in an experimental model of pressure overload in nondiabetic mice [110]. Clinically, it was shown to improve LV mass in a subgroup in the same trial [111].

Ischemia Modifiers

Ranolazine has been used as an anti-ischemic agent. It exerts its action in combination with enalapril or metoprolol to prevent REM in dogs with HF [112]. It has been found to reverse the effects of serum- and glucocorticoid-regulated kinase 1 (SGK-1) [113].

Nicorandil is an anti-ischemic and conditioning mimetic drug used mostly against IRI. It has recently been found to decrease REM in a post-MI experimental model [114].

Histone Deacetylase Inhibitors

The histone deacetylase (HDAC) inhibitor family of drugs decreases hypertrophy. In the rat, valproic acid decreases REM [115]. It is commonly used in neurological diseases, which makes it an attractive agent.

Monoamine Oxidase Inhibitors

Monoamine oxidase inhibitors have been found to have distinct protective effects on mitochondrial integrity [116].

We have shown that a drug widely used in Parkinson's disease and Alzheimer disease—rasagiline [117]—decreased REM at 1 month post-MI in the rat.

Tetracyclines

Tetracyclines have been shown to increase SERCA-2α; also, they inhibit MMPs and are anti-apoptotic [118, 119].

Yabluchanskiy et al. [119] stress the potential effects of other MMP inhibitors. In a well planned clinical trial, doxycycline was found to decrease REM in post-MI patients with low residual coronary flow [120].

The antioxidant thioredoxin, which also increases Akt activation, has been used successfully in an experimental study [121].

Various antioxidants are continuously being tried, especially quercetin, resveratrol, and curcumin [122]. Resveratrol has been found to be equipotent to perindopril in attenuating post-MI REM in rats [123].

Nuclear Factor Erythroid 2–Related Factor 2 Activators

Nuclear factor erythroid 2–related factor 2 (Nrf-2), a regulator of cellular resistance to oxidants, is contained in plant-derived phytochemicals [124]. Sulforaphane has been found to reduce IRI and inflammation [125]. Their ease of administration makes these drugs attractive, but further data are needed.

Allopurinol is a very widely known and used drug. It decreases ROS while diminishing REM in the rat [126].

Similar cardioprotective effects have been observed with the newer uric acid–lowering agent flebuxostat in pressure overload hypertrophy [127].

Two disappointing failures of promising drugs should be mentioned. The mitochondrial protective drug MTP-131 did not improve REM in 118 patients undergoing primary PCI in the Evaluation of Myocardial Effects of Bendavia for Reducing Reperfusion Injury in Patients With Acute Coronary Events (EMBRACE STEMI) study [128]. Similar findings have been reported for TRO40303—also a mitochondrial protective agent [129].

Tarone et al. [49] also mention two other targets for which many drugs could be beneficial, as discussed in the following sections.

Antifibrotic Action

The role of fibrosis in REM has been extensively described. López et al. [130] describe that lysyl oxidase (LOX) inhibition could be an attractive target, since both LOX and myocardial stiffness are increased in animal models of HF and in the myocardium of patients with hypertension or HF. They also describe that experimentally the loop diuretic torasemide decreases LOX expression and improves LV function [131]. However in the Effect of a New Formulation of Torasemide (Prolonged Release) on Myocardial Fibrosis in Patients With Heart Failure (TORAFIC) trial, fibrosis in hypertensive patients was not decreased by either torasemide or furosemide [132].

Angiogenetic Therapy
The ESC working group on the cellular biology of the heart reports that many agents (VEGF family) have proved successful experimentally, as well as in phase I trials with recombinant human VEGF (rhVEGF), although the results of two clinical trials [133, 134] were disappointing; it stresses that efforts continue, and it mentions placental growth factor (PLGF) as a promising agent [135].

Erythropoietin
The neuro- and cardioprotective agent erythropoietin has given excellent results in experimental studies. However, in clinical trials it has failed to produce a benefit. Talan et al. [136] have discussed possible reasons for this discrepancy.

Hormones
Many hormones have been studied in REM. Growth hormone promotes proliferation of CMCs [137] but has been abandoned clinically.

Estradiol has been found to reduce apoptosis and oxidative stress experimentally [138]. Conversely, testosterone has shown anti-REM action in the rat [139].

Parathyroid hormone has shown very favorable results experimentally, increasing neovascularization (↑ VEGF) and decreasing thinning of the myocardium, scar extension, and border zone apoptosis [140].

In a parallel action, vitamin D supplementation has shown favorable results in mice after MI [141]. Rafacho et al. [142] have reported that vitamin D leads to decreased REM in rats exposed to smoking, together with a decrease in oxidative stress.

Two hormones involved in metabolism have also given encouraging experimental results. Adiponectin has cardioprotective and anti-inflammatory actions [143]. Ghrelin decreases cardiac sympathetic activity and has been shown to decrease REM in rats post-MI [144].

Thyroid Hormones
Our group has worked for many years on the subject of thyroid hormones. An account of the action of these hormones and their action against REM is given in a recent review [145]. Thus, they have been shown to prevent REM early (at 2 weeks) [146] and at 13 weeks post-MI in rats [147], and even to reverse REM late post-MI [148]. They have been shown to have favorable effects in diabetic post-MI rats [149]. These results have been replicated by other investigators in rabbits and rats [150–153]. Chen et al. [154] found that tri-iodothyronine (T3) inhibits apoptosis in the border zone through Akt upregulation. We have observed some interesting results concerning Akt overexpression in post-MI rats. We found [155] that higher than regularly employed doses of T3 increase Akt, mortality, and REM in rats 3 weeks after MI. It must be noted that Akt generally induces physiological hypertrophy and is cardioprotective [156], but high doses given chronically may increase fibrosis [157–159]. Rajagopalan and Gerdes [160] give a very

detailed review. In brief, they stress the following beneficial actions against REM: improvement in contractility but also relaxation, reduction of fibrosis, and improvement in metabolic function. They also stress the importance of the correct dose; T3 has been found to be important for mitochondrial biogenesis [161], but at high doses it depletes mitochondrial ATP production through an increase in oxidative stress [162, 163].

Chen et al. [164] followed up 5599 patients with a diagnosis of HF for 434 days. They found that both low thyroid-stimulating hormone (TSH) levels (<1.3 mIU/L) and high TSH levels (>3.6 mIU/L) were associated with increased mortality and cardiac-related hospitalization. We found similar results in patients post-MI: a lower triiodothyronine (T3) level was associated with lesser recovery of cardiac function [165].

Pingitore et al. [166] give a very detailed recent review on cardioprotection and thyroid hormones. They stress the antiapoptotic effects in both the acute and chronic phases of ischemic heart disease (IHD), and the induction of prosurvival pathways, including PI3K/Akt and the protein kinase C (PKC) signaling cascade, HSP70 and HSP27 upregulation, and p38MAPK suppression.

The same group of authors, in the Thyroid Hormone Replacement Therapy in ST Elevation Myocardial Infarction (THiRST) study [167], gave tailored doses of T3 to patients with low T3 serum levels after acute MI. They found a moderate but distinct improvement of REM by CMR.

Thyroid hormones can induce cardiac repair after acute MI [168]. According to Pantos et al. [169], this action may be exerted through the thyroid hormone receptor α1 (TRα1).

With regard to the role of thyroid hormones in cardiac regeneration, this is an open question because they induce myocardial differentiation, while (as described in the Chap. 16, which discusses regeneration) dedifferentiation is a requisite for regeneration. However, they may enhance regeneration through actions on progenitor cells. In this respect, Kubin et al. [170] have shown that oncostatin is a major mediator of REM and CMC dedifferentiation. They describe that it is a major factor for DEDIF (fetal pattern expression) and REM during acute MI or chronic idiopathic dilated cardiomyopathy (IDCM). Oncostatin treatment induced expression of progenitor cell markers and improved REM after MI but was detrimental in IDCM. They postulate that DEDIF initially protects stressed hearts but fails to support cardiac structure and function upon continued activation.

13.2.3 Nonpharmacological Nondevice Therapies

13.2.3.1 Exercise Rehabilitation

Garza et al. [171] give a very detailed review on exercise rehabilitation. They postulate that the improved function may be due to mitigation of the noxious action of the renin–angiotensin–aldosterone (RAAS) system, an improved balance between MMP-1 and tissue inhibitor of metalloproteinase (TIMP)-1, favorable myosin heavy chain (MHC) isoform switching, improved mitochondrial calcium handling, diminution of oxidative stress, and improved angiogenesis. Exercise training also decreases apoptosis in rats [172] and in skeletal muscle in patients [173]. It also reduces inflammation indices [174].

Apart from many experimental findings, Giannuzzi et al. [175], in the Exercise in Left Ventricular Dysfunction and Chronic Heart Failure (ELVD-CHF) trial, observed diminution of volumes and an increase in the left ventricular EF (LVEF) in 45 patients randomized to training, as compared with 45 controls.

Dubach et al. [176] reported similar results after exercise training in patients evaluated by CMR. In a meta-analysis of 812 patients with HF across 14 clinical trials, Haykowsky [177] also found favorable results.

We also found [178] that even in patients with end-stage HF in whom an LVAD has been applied, exercise training for 12–14 months improves the EF, serum and cardiac tissue T3, and cardiac Akt.

Since it is an easy and inexpensive modality, its importance is easy to appreciate.

13.2.3.2 Continuous Preconditioning

In the description of pathogenesis it was stated that in REM a long series of noxious processes is involved.

Wei et al. [179] reported that in rats, continued remote conditioning for 1 month post-MI improved REM. Currently, there are numerous trials examining this modality. More data are given in the Chap. 14, which discusses conditioning [180].

The place of revascularization, either interventional or surgical, is covered in Chap. 9, which discusses myocardial hibernation; also, the place of cell and gene therapy is described in the Chaps. 17 and 18.

13.2.4 Device Therapy

13.2.4.1 Electrical–Mechanical

It has already been stated that REM occurs after about 30% of anterior acute MIs. Some more data on these estimates should be given: in a study from the Kaiser Permanente Colorado Institute for Health Research [181], 2413 patients were followed for 44 years and 49.9% of them died. For patients with an initial diagnosis of HF with a reduced EF (HFrEF) after 5 years, there was a 13% probability that they would improve to HFpEF, a 31% probability that they would remain in HFrEF, and a 56% probability that they would die. Of this total group of patients, 872 (36%); had a previous MI. Significantly, in patients with a previous MI there was a hazard ratio of 1.75 for transition from HFrEF to HFpEF. When hypertension was taken into account, the hazard ratio for transition from HFpEF to HFrEF was 1.11 (p value not significant) while the hazard ratio for transition from HFrEF to HFpEF was 1.68, underlying the importance of therapy. No use of device therapy was reported in this study.

In a recent review, Bhatt et al. [4] listed some major therapeutic advances to stop adverse LV REM and promote reverse REM. CRT was included among them, but not device therapy.

Goldfinger and Nair [182], in a 2014 review, reported an up to 11% improvement in EF with ACE inhibitors/ARBs and β-blockers; most patients were receiving dual therapy. They reviewed results with CRT, reporting LVEFs that showed greatly divergent rates of improvement from 3.5% to 26%. This shows the difficulty in choosing the right patient for CRT application. Of course, it is well recognized that patients who respond to CRT more frequently have idiopathic (nonischemic) dilated cardiomyopathy [183].

In a review by Kramer et al. [184], five CRT studies were mentioned, totaling 1086 patients, with a decrease in ESV of 25.8 mL as compared with placebo. Obviously, these patients were on optimal pharmaceutical therapy. The difficulty in establishing practical criteria for the application of CRT is described in various working group reports.

Thus, in the American College of Cardiology/American Heart Association/Heart Rhythm Society (ACC/AHA/HRS) 2012 guidelines, a class I recommendation is given for patients with an EF ≤35%, a QRS duration longer than 150 ms, and a New York Heart Association (NYHA) class of II–IV [185, 186]. Similar indications are given by the ESC [186]. However, in patients with a previous MI, selection is obvious more difficult. Importantly, Sze and Daubert, who pioneered CRT, stress that LBBB may be "unsafe at any speed" (i.e., deleterious at any level of LVEF) [187].

Interestingly, in a very detailed study, Hessel et al. [188] stated that the etiology (ischemic versus nonischemic) was not a determining factor with regard to the response to CRT. Reverse REM was defined as a >10% decrease in the LVESV and was seen in 72% of patients by Yu et al. [189].

Here, the more recent CRT studies must be mentioned, because on the whole they recommend earlier application of the technique [190–196]. This is especially important because many authors of recent publications reiterate the importance of global noninvasive REM measurements to predict clinical outcomes. This was recently restated by Waring and Litwin [197]. Sekaran et al. [198] confirm the findings of review studies on the importance of both LV volumes and the left atrial EF (LAEF), but also stress the postulation of Gold et al. [196] that in patients with NYHA class I or II symptoms on optimal medical therapy, CRT is related to volumetric changes, and that at 6 months every 10% decrease in the LVESV reduces the adjusted risk ratio for mortality by 14%. This advocates not waiting for the patient with LBBB to develop HF, and possibly irreversible fibrosis, before deciding on CRT.

The Multicenter Automatic Defibrillator Implantation Trial with Cardiac Resynchronization Therapy (MADIT-CRT) trial [199] results further support these views. This trial included patients with NYHA class I–II symptoms, an EF ≤30%, and a QRS duration ≥130 ms; at 12 months, 40% of patients had complete left-sided reverse REM and lower rates of HF and death than patients with less reverse REM. According to the trial results, factors associated with complete left-sided reverse REM were female sex, absence of hypertension, better renal function, a QRS duration ≥150 ms, a smaller LA volume (LAV) index (<40 mL/m^2), and absence of previous MI. This last point poses many caveats, including the fact that in patients with IDCM and LBBB or a QRS duration ≥150 ms, one should not wait too long before applying CRT; however, patients with previous MI should not, in the author's view, be denied this benefit lightly. In such cases, refined application of echo and magnetic resonance imaging techniques should be further pursued.

These data bring into focus another consideration: whether in patients requiring permanent right ventricular (RV) pacing and with mild LV dysfunction (EF ≤50%, NYHA class I–II), biventricular pacing should be considered to avoid evolution toward REM and HF. In one trial, biventricular pacing was associated with better results at 24-month follow-up [200]. This report raises many questions regarding further approaches in this category of patients, encountered frequently in clinical practice.

A very interesting finding was reported some years ago by Vanderheyden et al. [201], who found that in the myocardium of patients not responding to CRT, β-MHC levels remained higher. The unfavorable functional characteristics of β-MHC have previously been reported [202].

Thus, the main message for applying CRT is to start as early as possible and, in cases of previous MI, to exhaust the eligibility criteria.

An "electrical" method that is not part of CRT is contractility modulation, which involves electrical signal application during the refractory period of the contractile cycle to modify contractility. It is followed by favorable protein modification and gene expression changes, and improvement in mitochondrial function, as reviewed by Liu et al. [203]. They reviewed four studies enrolling 723 participants. In comparison with the control arm, this modality did not affect all-cause mortality or hospitalization, although it improved the maximal oxygen uptake (VO_2 max) and 6-min walk test; arrhythmias decreased. Two studies showed opposite results with regard to HF outcomes. Thus, no concrete results or recommendations can be given regarding this modality.

13.2.4.2 Left Ventricular Assist Device Implantation

Goldfinger and Nair [182], in their aforementioned review, describe that LVAD support decreases fibrosis and CMC hypertrophy, and improves contractility. This technique is being used with increasing frequency, even as destination therapy, as will be further described.

Puehler et al. reported that pulsatile-flow LVADs allowed more frequent (threefold) weaning; surprisingly, they also found that continuous-flow devices permitted more reverse REM [204]. Imamura et al. [205] found more reverse REM with pulsatile-flow LVADs. It has also been reported that pulsatile flow is more likely to promote functional recovery [206].

13.3 Changes in Myocardial Characteristics

Many changes in CMC metabolism and apoptosis are seen, such as a decrease in tumor necrosis factor-α (TNF-α) [207].

Hall et al., from Sir Magdi Yacoub's group [208], studied six patients before and after LVAD insertion. They found 263 genes that were either up- or downregulated. On the whole, the following "signatures of recovery" were seen: upregulation of the integrin family and downregulation of exchange proteins directly activated by cAMP-2 (EPAC-2), which belongs to the cyclic adenosine monophosphate (cAMP) pathway. They reported change in various genes over many years [209, 210].

Blaxall et al. [209] found that the overall gene expression could significantly distinguish between pre- and post-LVAD status, especially concerning brain natriuretic peptide (BNP), collagen dystrophies, interleukin-8, metalloproteins, MMP, and TNF-α. Significantly, they also found β-MHC and skeletal α-actin downregulation, but only in nonischemic patients.

In patients with HF prior to and at 7 and 180 days post-LVAD placement, Mitchell et al. [210] found increases in the initially downregulated genes involved in cellular immune response antigen presentation and T-cell activation and survival, yet they remained significantly lower than in age- and sex-matched samples from healthy controls.

Ambardekar et al. [211] point out that the greatest regression in hypertrophy occurs in the subendocardium and the LV in comparison with the RV. They note alterations in the regulation of mitogen-activated protein kinases with regression of apoptosis, but also activation of IGF-1 and enhancement of transcription regulation of ribosomal biogenesis, which may counterbalance protein degradation pathways.

In an animal model, Topkara et al. [212] studied a huge number of genes, many overriding each other. In a Venn diagram they produced, >109 genes were normalized; 1845 new reverse REM genes were found, while 1538 genes were common between the two, representing persistently dysregulated HF genes. Interestingly, Jacobs et al. [213] found that partial support with low continuous flow produced less reverse REM than that achieved by a high-flow device.

Marinescu et al. [214] recently published a review on the association of reverse REM and the degree of myocardial recovery with which it is associated. They underlined in general that although most patients show a significant degree of reverse REM, very few exhibit sufficiently improved cardiac function to justify device explantation. They give an interesting historical perspective, highlighting the main strong early indications that a severely dilated heart could significantly improve from the use of LVADs. From these studies it can be summarized that reverse REM is seen in the majority of patients. They point out, however, that this improvement, which may achieve "reversal" as far as the phenotype is concerned, does not mean restitution to normal; in fact, it may be seen with other therapies [215, 216] and, according to de Groote et al. [217], HF may recur after β-blocker discontinuation. Also, they refer to the work of Givertz et al. [218], who reviewed the rate of spontaneous recovery in various forms of recent-onset dilated cardiomyopathy.

Marinescu et al. [214] propose use of the term "remission" instead of the term "recovery." They also propose, however, to reserve the term "recovered" for patients who remain normal, functionally and structurally, for an appreciably long time after LVAD removal. They also describe the various methods proposed for assessment and prediction of sustainability of recovery/remission. That description is beyond the scope of this chapter. However, it is important to highlight the factors that Marinescu et al. [214] enumerate as being associated with recovery/remission. They refer to a more recent report from the United Network for Organ Sharing database [219], describing 594 patients receiving a Heart Mate II and, as with an Heartware LVAD, support, for an average of 50 days in total. In a review by Drakos and Mehra [220], the incidence of recovery ranged from 9% to 63%. They underline that patients treated with intensive medical therapy and surveillance methods had higher recovery rates, as in the case of the very strong group of Sir Magdi Yacoub [54], who also use the β2-agonist clenbuterol as an inducer of physiological hypertrophy.

On the whole, patients with a higher probability of recovery are younger patients with a more recent onset of symptoms.

Moreover, Selzman et al. [221] also note that reverse REM is a multifactional process of returning the heart toward a normal phenotype. They present 13 studies with recovery rates, from 4.5% to 73%. They ascribe great importance to patient selection, stressing that pulsatile devices are associated with a greater reduction in BNP and greater LVEF improvement, and they describe various successful protocols.

A very simple element, present in all forms of REM and HF, should be taken into account: fibrosis. Kletz et al. [222] stress that in patients treated with an LVAD, intensive ACE inhibition therapy is crucial for regression of fibrosis. Apart from pharmacological approaches, various biological constructs and scaffold-free methods of advancing heart regeneration are also being used [223].

Also, manipulation of MMPs remains equally important as in the post-MI state [224].

Another aspect that has also been addressed is that fibrosis can predict the response to an LVAD [225], as evidenced by higher expression of collagens, fibronectin, MMPs, TIMPs, connective tissue growth factor, and TGF-β1.

Other factors [226] that should be addressed when evaluating and following up patients with an LVAD is the degree of persistent sympathetic activation, which seems to be higher with continuous-flow devices [226].

Persistent inflammatory activity and ways to combat it are important in every case of HF [227]. Continued upregulation of inflammatory markers has been shown to persist after LVAD use [228, 229].

Another important aspect is to prevent the emergence of atrophic REM, which may develop after prolonged LV unloading. The group of Taegtmeyer has worked consistently in this field [230, 231].

Use of drugs, including clenbuterol, and exercise are important, as already described.

All efforts, including cell and gene therapy, should continue. Moreover, the importance of the right ventricle is obvious [232].

13.4 Importance of Biomarkers

Ahmad et al. [233] studied plasma from 37 patients (median age 68 years) before LVAD implantation and afterward, at a median of 136 days (interquartile range 94–180 days). They found significant decreases in N-terminal (NT)-proBNP, interleukin 1 receptor-like 1 (ST2), galectin 3, growth/differentiation factor 15 (GDF15), high-sensitivity C-reactive protein ((hs)CRP), and copeptin, but not neutrophil gelatinase-associated lipocalin (NGAL). However, they noted that despite improvement, the absolute values of each biomarker remained extremely high.

MicroRNAs serve as predictors of recovery [234–236].

After reviewing the above data, two main questions remain today: what is the rate of myocardial recovery, and what is the survival rate with LVAD therapy?

In 2006, Topkara et al. [237] used multicenter data from the Interagency Registry for Mechanically Assisted Circulatory Support (INTERMACS) to study 13,454 adult patients. Device explantation rates with myocardial recovery were 0.9% at 1-year follow-up, 1.9% at 2 years, and 3.1% at 3 years. Independent predictors of device explantation with recovery were age <56 years, nonischemic etiology, time since initial diagnosis <2 years, suboptimal HF therapy before implantation, LVEDD <6.5 cm, pulmonary artery systolic pressure <50 mmHg, blood area nitrogen <30 mg/dL, and use of an axial-flow device. With regard to etiology, patients with myocarditis, postpartum cardiomyopathy, and Adriamycin (doxorubicin)–induced cardiomyopathy showed the highest rates of explantation. There was a significant overlap in explanted and not-explanted recovery.

Drakos et al. [238] reported the proceedings of a National Heart, Lung, and Blood Institute (NHLBI) working group, which included findings from 11 centers in patients receiving LVAD support for a duration of 3.5–11 months. The incidence rates of cardiac recovery ranged from 0% to 20% in patients with ischemic cardiomyopathy and from 13.5% to 73% in patients with nonischemic etiology. This shows the need for further work on this subject. The authors very pertinently pointed out that "Mechanical circulatory support (MCS) can be viewed as a research vehicle that could help advance the science of cardiac recovery"(Fig. 13.2).

The final, very practical question is: What is the survival rate with LVAD therapy?

Gustafson and Rogers [239] remind us that this therapy is currently being used both as a bridge to transplantation and also as a destination therapy. They mention current rates of survival of 80% at 1 year and 70% at 2 years. They stress that the results are better in stable patients that in those sliding on inotropes or in a desperate condition. Thus, they advise early referral and implantation.

Starling et al. [240] reported a 2-year survival rate of 70%. Heart Mate III gave very recently even better results [241].

In conclusion, an LVAD can significantly improve LV function and induce reverse REM. However, the actual "cure" rate in patients is still low. Earlier and more accurate selection, optimization of device characteristics, and continuous use of full pharmacological and other adjunctive therapies is essential for patients in

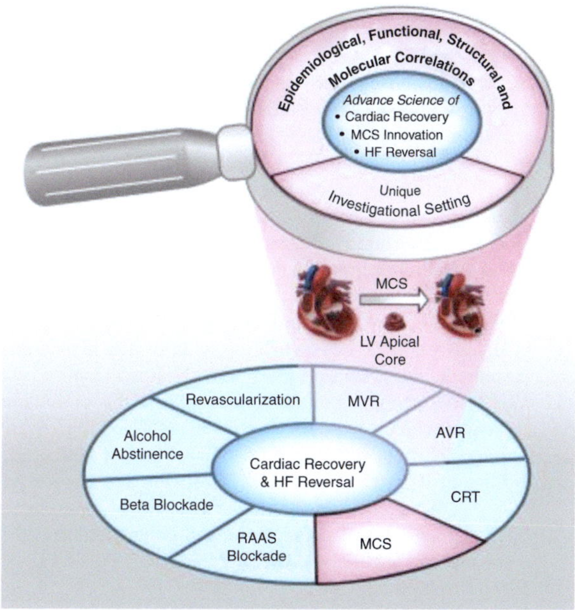

Fig. 13.2 Mechanical circulatory support (MCS) viewed as a "research vehicle" that could help advance the science of cardiac recovery. (Reproduced from Drakos et al. [238], with permission)

whom explantation is hoped for or in whom heart transplantation is contemplated. Finally, even if destination therapy is the only option, CMC regeneration either by cell or gene therapy still remains a hope; it may be aided by the improvement in LV function facilitated by LVAD therapy.

References

1. Yang XW, Hua W, Wang J, Liu ZM, Ding LG, Chen KP, et al. Regression of fragmented QRS complex: a marker of electrical reverse remodeling in cardiac resynchronization therapy. Ann Noninvasive Electrocardiol. 2015;20:18–27.
2. Poole JE, Singh JP, Birgersdotter-Green U. QRS duration or QRS morphology: what really matters in cardiac resynchronization therapy? J Am Coll Cardiol. 2016;67:1104–17.
3. Azevedo PS, Polegato BF, Minicucci MF, Paiva SA, Zornoff LA. Cardiac remodeling: concepts, clinical impact, pathophysiological mechanisms and pharmacologic treatment. Arq Bras Cardiol. 2016;106:62–9.
4. Bhatt AS, Ambrosy AP, Velazquez EJ. Adverse remodeling and reverse remodeling after myocardial infarction. Curr Cardiol Rep. 2017;19:71.
5. Migrino RQ, Young JB, Ellis SG, White HD, Lundergan CF, Miller DP, et al. End-systolic volume index at 90 to 180 minutes into reperfusion therapy for acute myocardial infarction is a strong predictor of early and late mortality. The Global Utilization of Streptokinase and t-PA for Occluded Coronary Arteries (GUSTO)-I Angiographic Investigators. Circulation. 1997;96:116–21.
6. White HD, Norris RM, Brown MA, Brandt PW, Whitlock RM, Wild CJ. Left ventricular end-systolic volume as the major determinant of survival after recovery from myocardial infarction. Circulation. 1987;76:44–51.

7. Kapetanakis S, Bhan A, Murgatroyd F, Kearney MT, Gall N, Zhang Q, et al. Real-time 3D echo in patient selection for cardiac resynchronization therapy. JACC Cardiovasc Imaging. 2011;4:16–26.
8. Lepper W, Kamp O, Vanoverschelde JL, Franke A, Sieswerda GT, Pasquet A, et al. Intravenous myocardial contrast echocardiography predicts left ventricular remodeling in patients with acute myocardial infarction. J Am Soc Echocardiogr. 2002;15:849–56.
9. Na HM, Cho GY, Lee JM, Cha MJ, Yoon YE, Lee SP, et al. Echocardiographic predictors for left ventricular remodeling after acute ST elevation myocardial infarction with low risk group: speckle tracking analysis. J Cardiovasc Ultrasound. 2016;24:128–34.
10. Gorcsan J, Kanzaki H, Bazaz R, Dohi K, Schwartzman D. Usefulness of echocardiographic tissue synchronization imaging to predict acute response to cardiac resynchronization therapy. Am J Cardiol. 2004;93:1178–81.
11. Mollema SA, Liem SS, Suffoletto MS, Bleeker GB, van der Hoeven BL, van de Veire NR, et al. Left ventricular dyssynchrony acutely after myocardial infarction predicts left ventricular remodeling. J Am Coll Cardiol. 2007;50:1532–40.
12. Yeh J Nihoyannopoulos P. Molecular imaging of inflammation using echocardiography. Advances with the use of microbubbles. Introduction to translational cardiovascular research. Springer 2015. p. 465–50.
13. Hoffmann R, von Bardeleben S, Kasprzak JD, Borges AC, ten Cate F, Firschke C, et al. Analysis of regional left ventricular function by cineventriculography, cardiac magnetic resonance imaging, and unenhanced and contrast-enhanced echocardiography: a multicenter comparison of methods. J Am Coll Cardiol. 2006;47:121–8.
14. Fieno DS, Kim RJ, Chen EL, Lomasney JW, Klocke FJ, Judd RM. Contrast-enhanced magnetic resonance imaging of myocardium at risk: distinction between reversible and irreversible injury throughout infarct healing. J Am Coll Cardiol. 2000;36:1985–91.
15. Tarantini G, Razzolini R, Cacciavillani L, Bilato C, Sarais C, Corbetti F, et al. Influence of transmurality, infarct size, and severe microvascular obstruction on left ventricular remodeling and function after primary coronary angioplasty. Am J Cardiol. 2006;98:1033–40.
16. Kim RJ, Fieno DS, Parrish TB, Harris K, Chen EL, Simonetti O, et al. Relationship of MRI delayed contrast enhancement to irreversible injury, infarct age, and contractile function. Circulation. 1999;100:1992–2002.
17. Bulluck H, Go YY, Crimi G, Ludman AJ, Rosmini S, Abdel-Gadir A, et al. Defining left ventricular remodeling following acute ST-segment elevation myocardial infarction using cardiovascular magnetic resonance. J Cardiovasc Magn Reson. 2017;19:26.
18. Bhat A, Gan GC, Tan TC, Hsu C, Denniss AR. Myocardial viability: from proof of concept to clinical practice. Cardiol Res Pract. 2016;2016:1020818. https://doi.org/10.1155/2016/1020818.
19. Thornhill RE, Prato FS, Wisenberg G. The assessment of myocardial viability: a review of current diagnostic imaging approaches. J Cardiovasc Magn Reson. 2002;4:381–410.
20. Anagnostopoulos CD, Cokkinos DV. Prediction of left ventricular remodelling by radionuclide imaging. Eur J Nucl Med Mol Imaging. 2011;38:1120–3.
21. Berti V, Sciagrà R, Acampa W, Ricci F, Cerisano G, Gallicchio R, et al. Relationship between infarct size and severity measured by gated SPECT and long-term left ventricular remodelling after acute myocardial infarction. Eur J Nucl Med Mol Imaging. 2011;38:1124–31.
22. Konstam MA, Kramer DG, Patel AR, Maron MS, Udelson JE. Left ventricular remodeling in heart failure: current concepts in clinical significance and assessment. JACC Cardiovasc Imaging. 2011;4:98–108.
23. Paschali A. Non invasive imaging modalities for cardiovascular translational research-technical considerations. Introduction to Translational Cardiovascular Research Springer 2015. p. 413–431.
24. Curley D, Lavin Plaza B, Shah AM, Botnar RM. Molecular imaging of cardiac remodelling after myocardial infarction. Basic Res Cardiol. 2018;113:10.
25. Kasama S, Toyama T, Sumino H, Nakazawa M, Matsumoto N, Sato Y, et al. Prognostic value of serial cardiac 123I-MIBG imaging in patients with stabilized chronic heart failure and reduced left ventricular ejection fraction. J Nucl Med. 2008;49:907–14.

26. Bengel FM. Imaging of post-infarct inflammation: moving forward toward clinical application. Circ Cardiovasc Imaging. 2016;9:e004713.
27. Fukushima K, Bravo PE, Higuchi T, Schuleri KH, Lin X, Abraham MR, et al. Molecular hybrid positron emission tomography/computed tomography imaging of cardiac angiotensin II type 1 receptors. J Am Coll Cardiol. 2012;60:2527–34.
28. Verjans JW, Lovhaug D, Narula N, Petrov AD, Indrevoll B, Bjurgert E, et al. Noninvasive imaging of angiotensin receptors after myocardial infarction. JACC Cardiovasc Imaging. 2008;1:354–62.
29. Jerosch-Herold M, Kwong R. Magnetic resonance imaging in the assessment of ventricular remodeling and viability. Curr Heart Fail Rep. 2008;5:5–10.
30. Vasan RS. Biomarkers of cardiovascular disease: molecular basis and practical considerations. Circulation. 2006;113:2335–62.
31. Biomarkers Definitions Working Group. Biomarkers and surrogate endpoints: preferred definitions and conceptual framework. Clin Pharmacol Ther. 2001;69:89–95.
32. Zannad F. What is measured by cardiac fibrosis biomarkers and imaging? Circ Heart Fail. 2014;7:239–42.
33. Ellims AH, Taylor AJ, Mariani JA, Ling LH, Iles LM, Maeder MT, et al. Evaluating the utility of circulating biomarkers of collagen synthesis in hypertrophic cardiomyopathy. Circ Heart Fail. 2014;7:271–8.
34. Azuaje F, Devaux Y, Wagner DR. Integrative pathway-centric modeling of ventricular dysfunction after myocardial infarction. PLoS One. 2010;5:e9661.
35. Yang J, Liu Y, Fan X, Li Z, Cheng Y. A pathway and network review on beta-adrenoceptor signaling and beta blockers in cardiac remodeling. Heart Fail Rev. 2014;19:799–814.
36. Funaro S, La Torre G, Madonna M, Galiuto L, Scarà A, Labbadia A, et al. Incidence, determinants, and prognostic value of reverse left ventricular remodelling after primary percutaneous coronary intervention: results of the Acute Myocardial Infarction Contrast Imaging (AMICI) multicenter study. Eur Heart J. 2009;30:566–75.
37. Rosenblatt-Velin N, Badoux S, Liaudet L. Pharmacological therapy in the heart as an alternative to cellular therapy: a place for the brain natriuretic peptide? Stem Cells Int. 2016;2016:5961342.
38. Ruvinov E, Harel-Adar T, Cohen S. Bioengineering the infarcted heart by applying bio-inspired materials. J Cardiovasc Transl Res. 2011;4:559–74.
39. Hausenloy DJ, Erik Bøtker H, Condorelli G, Ferdinandy P, Garcia-Dorado D, Heusch G, et al. Translating cardioprotection for patient benefit: position paper from the Working Group of Cellular Biology of the Heart of the European Society of Cardiology. Cardiovasc Res. 2013;98:7–27.
40. Hausenloy DJ, Garcia-Dorado D, Bøtker HE, Davidson SM, Downey J, Engel FB, et al. Novel targets and future strategies for acute cardioprotection: position paper of the European Society of Cardiology Working Group on Cellular Biology of the Heart. Cardiovasc Res. 2017;113:564–85.
41. Newton N, Croisille P, Gahide G, Rioufol G, Bonnefoy E, Sanchez I, et al. Effect of cyclosporine on left ventricular remodeling after reperfused myocardial infarction. J Am Coll Cardiol. 2010;55:1200–5.
42. Cung TT, Morel O, Cayla G, Rioufol G, Garcia-Dorado D, Angoulvant D, et al. Cyclosporine before PCI in patients with acute myocardial infarction. N Engl J Med. 2015;373:1021–31.
43. Ottani F, Latini R, Staszewsky L, La Vecchia L, Locuratolo N, Sicuro M, et al. Cyclosporine a in reperfused myocardial infarction: the multicenter, controlled, open-label CYCLE trial. J Am Coll Cardiol. 2016;67:365–74.
44. Monassier L, Ayme-Dietrich E, Aubertin-Kirch G, Pathak A. Targeting myocardial reperfusion injuries with cyclosporine in the CIRCUS trial—pharmacological reasons for failure. Fundam Clin Pharmacol. 2016;30:191–3.
45. Ishii H, Amano T, Matsubara T, Murohara T. Pharmacological intervention for prevention of left ventricular remodeling and improving prognosis in myocardial infarction. Circulation. 2008;118:2710–8.

46. Xie M, Burchfield JS, Hill JA. Pathological ventricular remodeling: therapies: part 2 of 2. Circulation. 2013;128:1021–30.
47. Cokkinos D. Le remodelage cardiaque après un infarctus: nouvelles données sur la prévention et le traintment. Bull Acad Natl Med 2015;199:1383–94.
48. Belogianneas C, Cokkinos DV. Left ventricular remodeling: a problem in search of solutions. European Cardiology Review 2016;11:29–35.
49. Tarone G, Balligand JL, Bauersachs J, Clerk A, De Windt L, Heymans S, et al. Targeting myocardial remodelling to develop novel therapies for heart failure: a position paper from the Working Group on Myocardial Function of the European Society of Cardiology. Eur J Heart Fail. 2014;16:494–508.
50. Miura T, Miki T. Limitation of myocardial infarct size in the clinical setting: current status and challenges in translating animal experiments into clinical therapy. Basic Res Cardiol. 2008;103:501–13.
51. Khattar RS. Effects of ACE-inhibitors and beta-blockers on left ventricular remodeling in chronic heart failure. Minerva Cardioangiol. 2003;51:143–54.
52. Lechat P, Packer M, Chalon S, Cucherat M, Arab T, Boissel JP. Clinical effects of beta-adrenergic blockade in chronic heart failure: a meta-analysis of double-blind, placebo-controlled, randomized trials. Circulation. 1998;98:1184–91.
53. Madamanchi A. Beta-adrenergic receptor signaling in cardiac function and heart failure. Mcgill J Med. 2007;10:99–104.
54. Birks EJ, Tansley PD, Hardy J, George RS, Bowles CT, Burke M, et al. Left ventricular assist device and drug therapy for the reversal of heart failure. N Engl J Med. 2006;355:1873–84.
55. Spanou D, Perimenis P, Mantzouratou P, Gomatos C, Cokkinos D, Mourouzis I, et al. Clenbuterol favorably remodels neonatal cardiac cells via activation of p38 MAPK signalling pathway. J Cardiovasc Surg. 2012;53:789–95.
56. Moens AL, Leyton-Mange JS, Niu X, Yang R, Cingolani O, Arkenbout EK, et al. Adverse ventricular remodeling and exacerbated NOS uncoupling from pressure-overload in mice lacking the beta3-adrenoreceptor. J Mol Cell Cardiol. 2009;47:576–85.
57. Kajstura J, Cigola E, Malhotra A, Li P, Cheng W, Meggs LG, et al. Angiotensin II induces apoptosis of adult ventricular myocytes in vitro. J Mol Cell Cardiol. 1997;29:859–70.
58. Jugdutt BI. Apoptosis after reperfused myocardial infarction: role of angiotensin II. Exp Clin Cardiol. 2004;9:219–28.
59. Albuquerque FN, Brandão AA, Silva DA, Mourilhe-Rocha R, Duque GS, Gondar AF, et al. Angiotensin-converting enzyme genetic polymorphism: its impact on cardiac remodeling. Arq Bras Cardiol. 2014;102:70–9.
60. Schieffer B, Wirger A, Meybrunn M, Seitz S, Holtz J, Riede UN, et al. Comparative effects of chronic angiotensin-converting enzyme inhibition and angiotensin II type 1 receptor blockade on cardiac remodeling after myocardial infarction in the rat. Circulation. 1994;89:2273–82.
61. McMurray JJ, Packer M, Desai AS, Gong J, Lefkowitz MP, Rizkala AR, et al. Angiotensin-neprilysin inhibition versus enalapril in heart failure. N Engl J Med. 2014;371:993–1004.
62. von Lueder TG, Wang BH, Kompa AR, Huang L, Webb R, Jordaan P, et al. Angiotensin receptor neprilysin inhibitor LCZ696 attenuates cardiac remodeling and dysfunction after myocardial infarction by reducing cardiac fibrosis and hypertrophy. Circ Heart Fail. 2015;8:71–8.
63. Pitt B, Remme W, Zannad F, Neaton J, Martinez F, Roniker B, et al. Eplerenone, a selective aldosterone blocker, in patients with left ventricular dysfunction after myocardial infarction. N Engl J Med. 2003;348:1309–21.
64. Iraqi W, Rossignol P, Angioi M, Fay R, Nuée J, Ketelslegers JM, et al. Extracellular cardiac matrix biomarkers in patients with acute myocardial infarction complicated by left ventricular dysfunction and heart failure: insights from the Eplerenone Post-acute Myocardial Infarction Heart Failure Efficacy and Survival Study (EPHESUS) study. Circulation. 2009;119:2471–9.
65. Kasama S, Toyama T, Kumakura H, Takayama Y, Ichikawa S, Suzuki T, et al. Effect of spironolactone on cardiac sympathetic nerve activity and left ventricular remodeling in patients with dilated cardiomyopathy. J Am Coll Cardiol. 2003;41:574–81.

66. Tsutamoto T, Wada A, Maeda K, Mabuchi N, Hayashi M, Tsutsui T, et al. Effect of spironolactone on plasma brain natriuretic peptide and left ventricular remodeling in patients with congestive heart failure. J Am Coll Cardiol. 2001;37:1228–33.
67. Hayashi M, Tsutamoto T, Wada A, Tsutsui T, Ishii C, Ohno K, et al. Immediate administration of mineralocorticoid receptor antagonist spironolactone prevents post-infarct left ventricular remodeling associated with suppression of a marker of myocardial collagen synthesis in patients with first anterior acute myocardial infarction. Circulation. 2003;107:2559–65.
68. Beygui F, Cayla G, Roule V, Roubille F, Delarche N, Silvain J, et al. Early aldosterone blockade in acute myocardial infarction: the ALBATROSS randomized clinical trial. J Am Coll Cardiol. 2016;67:1917–27.
69. Bell RM, Yellon DM. Atorvastatin, administered at the onset of reperfusion, and independent of lipid lowering, protects the myocardium by up-regulating a pro-survival pathway. J Am Coll Cardiol. 2003;41:508–15.
70. Kinlay S, Schwartz GG, Olsson AG, Rifai N, Leslie SJ, Sasiela WJ, et al. High-dose atorvastatin enhances the decline in inflammatory markers in patients with acute coronary syndromes in the MIRACL study. Circulation. 2003;108:1560–6.
71. Nahrendorf M, Sosnovik D, Chen JW, Panizzi P, Figueiredo JL, Aikawa E, et al. Activatable magnetic resonance imaging agent reports myeloperoxidase activity in healing infarcts and noninvasively detects the antiinflammatory effects of atorvastatin on ischemia–reperfusion injury. Circulation. 2008;117:1153–60.
72. Cheng CF, Juan SH, Chen JJ, Chao YC, Chen HH, Lian WS, et al. Pravastatin attenuates carboplatin-induced cardiotoxicity via inhibition of oxidative stress associated apoptosis. Apoptosis. 2008;13:883–94.
73. Lee TM, Lin MS, Tsai CH, Chang NC. Effects of pravastatin on ventricular remodeling by activation of myocardial KATP channels in infarcted rats: role of 70-kDa S6 kinase. Basic Res Cardiol. 2007;102:171–82.
74. Krum H, Ashton E, Reid C, Kalff V, Rogers J, Amarena J, et al. Double-blind, randomized, placebo-controlled study of high-dose HMG CoA reductase inhibitor therapy on ventricular remodeling, pro-inflammatory cytokines and neurohormonal parameters in patients with chronic systolic heart failure. J Card Fail. 2007;13:1–7.
75. Kjekshus J, Apetrei E, Barrios V, Böhm M, Cleland JG, Cornel JH, et al. Rosuvastatin in older patients with systolic heart failure. N Engl J Med. 2007;357:2248–61.
76. Tavazzi L, Maggioni AP, Marchioli R, Barlera S, Franzosi MG, Latini R, et al. Effect of rosuvastatin in patients with chronic heart failure (the GISSI-HF trial): a randomised, double-blind, placebo-controlled trial. Lancet. 2008;372:1231–9.
77. Kjekshus J. Are statins failing in heart failure? Eur Heart J. 2015;36:1502–4.
78. Preiss D, Campbell RT, Murray HM, Ford I, Packard CJ, Sattar N, et al. The effect of statin therapy on heart failure events: a collaborative meta-analysis of unpublished data from major randomized trials. Eur Heart J 2015;36:1536–1546.
79. Oerlemans MI, Liu J, Arslan F, den Ouden K, van Middelaar BJ, Doevendans PA, et al. Inhibition of RIP1-dependent necrosis prevents adverse cardiac remodeling after myocardial ischemia-reperfusion in vivo. Basic Res Cardiol. 2012;107:270. https://doi.org/10.1007/s00395-012-0270-8.
80. Luedde M, Lutz M, Carter N, Sosna J, Jacoby C, Vucur M, et al. RIP3, a kinase promoting necroptotic cell death, mediates adverse remodelling after myocardial infarction. Cardiovasc Res. 2014;103:206–16.
81. Letavernier E, Zafrani L, Perez J, Letavernier B, Haymann JP, Baud L. The role of calpains in myocardial remodelling and heart failure. Cardiovasc Res. 2012;96:38–45.
82. Portbury AL, Willis MS, Patterson C. Tearin' up my heart: proteolysis in the cardiac sarcomere. J Biol Chem. 2011;286:9929–34.
83. Spaeth CS, Boydston EA, Figard LR, Zuzek A, Bittner GD. A model for sealing plasmalemmal damage in neurons and other eukaryotic cells. J Neurosci. 2010;30:15790–800.
84. Eschenhagen T, Force T, Ewer MS, de Keulenaer GW, Suter TM, Anker SD, et al. Cardiovascular side effects of cancer therapies: a position statement from the Heart Failure Association of the European Society of Cardiology. Eur J Heart Fail. 2011;13:1–10.

85. Gao R, Zhang J, Cheng L, Wu X, Dong W, Yang X, et al. A phase II, randomized, double-blind, multicenter, based on standard therapy, placebo-controlled study of the efficacy and safety of recombinant human neuregulin-1 in patients with chronic heart failure. J Am Coll Cardiol. 2010;55:1907–14.
86. Jabbour A, Hayward CS, Keogh AM, Kotlyar E, McCrohon JA, England JF, et al. Parenteral administration of recombinant human neuregulin-1 to patients with stable chronic heart failure produces favourable acute and chronic haemodynamic responses. Eur J Heart Fail. 2011;13:83–92.
87. Fan GC, Kranias EG. Small heat shock protein 20 (HspB6) in cardiac hypertrophy and failure. J Mol Cell Cardiol. 2011;51:574–7.
88. De Acetis M, Notte A, Accornero F, Selvetella G, Brancaccio M, Vecchione C, et al. Cardiac overexpression of melusin protects from dilated cardiomyopathy due to long-standing pressure overload. Circ Res. 2005;96:1087–94.
89. Willis MS, Patterson C. Into the heart: the emerging role of the ubiquitin-proteasome system. J Mol Cell Cardiol. 2006;41:567–79.
90. Lee DI, Kass DA. Phosphodiesterases and cyclic GMP regulation in heart muscle. Physiology (Bethesda). 2012;27:248–58.
91. Guazzi M, Vicenzi M, Arena R, Guazzi MD. PDE5 inhibition with sildenafil improves left ventricular diastolic function, cardiac geometry, and clinical status in patients with stable systolic heart failure: results of a 1-year, prospective, randomized, placebo-controlled study. Circ Heart Fail. 2011;4:8–17.
92. Redfield MM, Chen HH, Borlaug BA, Semigran MJ, Lee KL, Lewis G, et al. Effect of phosphodiesterase-5 inhibition on exercise capacity and clinical status in heart failure with preserved ejection fraction: a randomized clinical trial. JAMA. 2013;309:1268–77.
93. Tocchetti CG, Stanley BA, Murray CI, Sivakumaran V, Donzelli S, Mancardi D, et al. Playing with cardiac “redox switches”: the “HNO way” to modulate cardiac function. Antioxid Redox Signal. 2011;14:1687–98.
94. Fraccarollo D, Widder JD, Galuppo P, Thum T, Tsikas D, Hoffmann M, et al. Improvement in left ventricular remodeling by the endothelial nitric oxide synthase enhancer AVE9488 after experimental myocardial infarction. Circulation. 2008;118:818–27.
95. Greenberg B, Butler J, Felker GM, Ponikowski P, Voors A, Desai AS, et al. Calcium upregulation by percutaneous administration of gene therapy in patients with cardiac disease (CUPID 2): a randomised, multinational, double-blind, placebo-controlled, phase 2b trial. Lancet. 2016;387:1178–86.
96. Jessup M, Greenberg B, Mancini D, Cappola T, Pauly DF, Jaski B, et al. Calcium Upregulation by Percutaneous Administration of Gene Therapy in Cardiac Disease (CUPID): a phase 2 trial of intracoronary gene therapy of sarcoplasmic reticulum Ca2+-ATPase in patients with advanced heart failure. Circulation. 2011;124:304–13.
97. Hajjar R. Resilient course of gene therapy in cardiovascular diseases. Lecture presented at the 1st Olympiad in Cardiovascular Medicine. International Symposium on Experimental & Clinical Cardiology, 17 May 2018, Athens.
98. Cleland JG, Teerlink JR, Senior R, Nifontov EM, Mc Murray JJ, Lang CC, et al. The effects of the cardiac myosin activator, omecamtiv mecarbil, on cardiac function in systolic heart failure: a double-blind, placebo-controlled, crossover, dose-ranging phase 2 trial. Lancet. 2011;378:676–83.
99. Teerlink JR, Clarke CP, Saikali KG, Lee JH, Chen MM, Escandon RD, et al. Dose-dependent augmentation of cardiac systolic function with the selective cardiac myosin activator, omecamtiv mecarbil: a first-in-man study. Lancet. 2011;378:667–75.
100. Teerlink JR, Felker GM, McMurray JJ, Solomon SD, Adams KF Jr, Cleland JG, et al. Chronic Oral Study of Myosin Activation to Increase Contractility in Heart Failure (COSMIC-HF): a phase 2, pharmacokinetic, randomised, placebo-controlled trial. Lancet. 2016;388:2895–903.
101. Gustafsson F, Guarracino F, Schwinger RHG. The inodilator levosimendan as a treatment for acute heart failure in various settings. Eur Heart J Suppl. 2017;19(Suppl C):C2–7.
102. Mavrogeni S, Giamouzis G, Papadopoulou E, Thomopoulou S, Dritsas A, Athanasopoulos G, et al. A 6-month follow-up of intermittent levosimendan administration effect on systolic

function, specific activity questionnaire, and arrhythmia in advanced heart failure. J Card Fail. 2007;13:556–9.
103. Silvetti S, Nieminen MS. Repeated or intermittent levosimendan treatment in advanced heart failure: an updated meta-analysis. Int J Cardiol. 2016;202:138–43.
104. Tarkia M, Stark C, Haavisto M, Kentala R, Vähäsilta T, Savunen T, et al. Effect of levosimendan therapy on myocardial infarct size and left ventricular function after acute coronary occlusion. Heart. 2016;102:465–71.
105. Louhelainen M, Vahtola E, Kaheinen P, Leskinen H, Merasto S, Kytö V, et al. Effects of levosimendan on cardiac remodeling and cardiomyocyte apoptosis in hypertensive Dahl/Rapp rats. Br J Pharmacol. 2007;150:851–61.
106. Tardif JC, O'Meara E, Komajda M, Böhm M, Borer JS, Ford I, et al. Effects of selective heart rate reduction with ivabradine on left ventricular remodelling and function: results from the SHIFT echocardiography substudy. Eur Heart J. 2011;32:2507–15.
107. Cittadini A, Napoli R, Monti MG, Rea D, Longobardi S, Netti PA, et al. Metformin prevents the development of chronic heart failure in the SHHF rat model. Diabetes. 2012;61:944–53.
108. Xiao H, Ma X, Feng W, Fu Y, Lu Z, Xu M, et al. Metformin attenuates cardiac fibrosis by inhibiting the TGFbeta1-Smad3 signalling pathway. Cardiovasc Res. 2010;87:504–13.
109. Zinman B, Wanner C, Lachin JM, Fitchett D, Bluhmki E, Hantel S, et al. Empagliflozin, cardiovascular outcomes, and mortality in type 2 diabetes. N Engl J Med. 2015;373:2117–28.
110. Byme NJ. Basic to translational science. JACC. 2017;2:347–54.
111. Verma S, Garg A, Yan AT, Gupta AK, Al-Omran M, Sabongui A, et al. Effect of empagliflozin on left ventricular mass and diastolic function in individuals with diabetes: an important clue to the EMPA-REG OUTCOME trial? Diabetes Care. 2016;39:e212–3.
112. Rastogi S, Sharov VG, Mishra S, Gupta RC, Blackburn B, Belardinelli L, et al. Ranolazine combined with enalapril or metoprolol prevents progressive LV dysfunction and remodeling in dogs with moderate heart failure. Am J Physiol Heart Circ Physiol. 2008;295:H2149–55.
113. Das S, Aiba T, Rosenberg M, Hessler K, Xiao C, Quintero PA, et al. Pathological role of serum- and glucocorticoid-regulated kinase 1 in adverse ventricular remodeling. Circulation. 2012;126:2208–19.
114. Wang S, Fan Y, Feng X, Sun C, Shi Z, Li T, et al. Nicorandil alleviates myocardial injury and post-infarction cardiac remodeling by inhibiting Mst1. Biochem Biophys Res Commun. 2018;495:292–9.
115. Lee TM, Lin MS, Chang NC. Inhibition of histone deacetylase on ventricular remodeling in infarcted rats. Am J Physiol Heart Circ Physiol. 2007;293:H968–77.
116. Kaludercic N, Carpi A, Menabò R, Di Lisa F, Paolocci N. Monoamine oxidases (MAO) in the pathogenesis of heart failure and ischemia/reperfusion injury. Biochim Biophys Acta. 1813;2011:1323–32.
117. Varela A, Mavroidis M, Katsimpoulas M, Sfiroera I, Kappa N, Mesa A, et al. The neuroprotective agent rasagiline mesylate attenuates cardiac remodeling after experimental myocardial infarction. ESC Heart Fail. 2017;4:331–40.
118. Hughes BG, Schulz R. Targeting MMP-2 to treat ischemic heart injury. Basic Res Cardiol. 2014;109:424.
119. Yabluchanskiy A, Li Y, Chilton RJ, Lindsey ML. Matrix metalloproteinases: drug targets for myocardial infarction. Curr Drug Targets. 2013;14:276–86.
120. Cerisano G, Buonamici P, Valenti R, Moschi G, Taddeucci E, Giurlani L, et al. Effects of a timely therapy with doxycycline on the left ventricular remodeling according to the pre-procedural TIMI flow grade in patients with ST-elevation acute myocardial infarction. Basic Res Cardiol. 2014;109:412.
121. Ago T, Sadoshima J. Thioredoxin and ventricular remodeling. J Mol Cell Cardiol. 2006;41:762–73.
122. Li HL, Liu C, de Couto G, Ouzounian M, Sun M, Wang AB, et al. Curcumin prevents and reverses murine cardiac hypertrophy. J Clin Invest. 2008;118:879–93.
123. Raj P, Aloud BM, Louis XL, Yu L, Zieroth S, Netticadan T. Resveratrol is equipotent to perindopril in attenuating post-infarct cardiac remodeling and contractile dysfunction in rats. J Nutr Biochem. 2016;28:155–63.

124. Ashrafian H, Czibik G, Bellahcene M, Aksentijević D, Smith AC, Mitchell SJ, et al. Fumarate is cardioprotective via activation of the Nrf2 antioxidant pathway. Cell Metab. 2012;15:361–71.
125. Nguyen B, Luong L, Naase H, Vives M, Jakaj G, Finch J, et al. Sulforaphane pretreatment prevents systemic inflammation and renal injury in response to cardiopulmonary bypass. J Thorac Cardiovasc Surg. 2014;148:690–697.e3.
126. Engberding N, Spiekermann S, Schaefer A, Heineke A, Wiencke A, Müller M, et al. Allopurinol attenuates left ventricular remodeling and dysfunction after experimental myocardial infarction: a new action for an old drug? Circulation. 2004;110:2175–9.
127. Xu X, Hu X, Lu Z, Zhang P, Zhao L, Wessale JL, et al. Xanthine oxidase inhibition with febuxostat attenuates systolic overload–induced left ventricular hypertrophy and dysfunction in mice. J Card Fail. 2008;14:746–53.
128. Gibson CM, Giugliano RP, Kloner RA, Bode C, Tendera M, Jánosi A, et al. EMBRACE STEMI study: a phase 2a trial to evaluate the safety, tolerability, and efficacy of intravenous MTP-131 on reperfusion injury in patients undergoing primary percutaneous coronary intervention. Eur Heart J. 2016;37:1296–303.
129. Atar D, Arheden H, Berdeaux A, Bonnet JL, Carlsson M, Clemmensen P, et al. Effect of intravenous TRO40303 as an adjunct to primary percutaneous coronary intervention for acute ST-elevation myocardial infarction: MITOCARE study results. Eur Heart J. 2015;36:112–9.
130. López B, González A, Hermida N, Valencia F, de Teresa E, Díez J. Role of lysyl oxidase in myocardial fibrosis: from basic science to clinical aspects. Am J Physiol Heart Circ Physiol. 2010;299:H1–9.
131. López B, Querejeta R, González A, Beaumont J, Larman M, Díez J. Impact of treatment on myocardial lysyl oxidase expression and collagen cross-linking in patients with heart failure. Hypertension. 2009;53:236–42.
132. TORAFIC Investigators Group. Effects of prolonged-release torasemide versus furosemide on myocardial fibrosis in hypertensive patients with chronic heart failure: a randomized, blinded-end point, active-controlled study. Clin Ther. 2011;33:1204–1213.e3.
133. Henry TD, Annex BH, McKendall GR, Azrin MA, Lopez JJ, Giordano FJ, et al. The VIVA trial: vascular endothelial growth factor in ischemia for vascular angiogenesis. Circulation. 2003;107:1359–65.
134. Rajagopalan S, Mohler E 3rd, Lederman RJ, Saucedo J, Mendelsohn FO, Olin J, et al. Regional angiogenesis with vascular endothelial growth factor (VEGF) in peripheral arterial disease: design of the RAVE trial. Am Heart J. 2003;145:1114–8.
135. Iwasaki H, Kawamoto A, Tjwa M, Horii M, Hayashi S, Oyamada A, et al. PLGF repairs myocardial ischemia through mechanisms of angiogenesis, cardioprotection and recruitment of myo-angiogenic competent marrow progenitors. PLoS One. 2011;6:e24872.
136. Talan MI, Ahmet I, Lakatta EG. Did clinical trials in which erythropoietin failed to reduce acute myocardial infarct size miss a narrow therapeutic window? PLoS One. 2012;7:e34819.
137. Brüel A, Christoffersen TE, Nyengaard JR. Growth hormone increases the proliferation of existing cardiac myocytes and the total number of cardiac myocytes in the rat heart. Cardiovasc Res. 2007;76:400–8.
138. Lee TM, Lin MS, Chou TF, Tsai CH, Chang NC. Adjunctive 17beta-estradiol administration reduces infarct size by altered expression of canine myocardial connexin43 protein. Cardiovasc Res. 2004;63:109–17.
139. Wang XF, Qu XQ, Zhang TT, Zhang JF. Testosterone suppresses ventricular remodeling and improves left ventricular function in rats following myocardial infarction. Exp Ther Med. 2015;9:1283–91.
140. Zaruba MM, Huber BC, Brunner S, Deindl E, David R, Fischer R, et al. Parathyroid hormone treatment after myocardial infarction promotes cardiac repair by enhanced neovascularization and cell survival. Cardiovasc Res. 2008;77:722–31.
141. Bodyak N, Ayus JC, Achinger S, Shivalingappa V, Ke Q, Chen YS, et al. Activated vitamin D attenuates left ventricular abnormalities induced by dietary sodium in Dahl salt-sensitive animals. Proc Natl Acad Sci U S A. 2007;104:16810–5.

142. Rafacho BP, Santos P, Assalin HB, Ardisson LP, Roscani MG, Polegato BF, et al. Role of vitamin D in the cardiac remodeling induced by tobacco smoke exposure. Int J Cardiol. 2012;155:472–3.
143. Park M, Sweeney G. Direct effects of adipokines on the heart: focus on adiponectin. Heart Fail Rev. 2013;18:631–44.
144. Soeki T, Kishimoto I, Schwenke DO, Tokudome T, Horio T, Yoshida M, et al. Ghrelin suppresses cardiac sympathetic activity and prevents early left ventricular remodeling in rats with myocardial infarction. Am J Physiol Heart Circ Physiol. 2008;294:H426–32.
145. Cokkinos DV, Chryssanthopoulos S. Thyroid hormones and cardiac remodeling. Heart Fail Rev. 2016;21:365–72.
146. Pantos C, Mourouzis I, Markakis K, Dimopoulos A, Xinaris C, Kokkinos AD, et al. Thyroid hormone attenuates cardiac remodeling and improves hemodynamics early after acute myocardial infarction in rats. Eur J Cardiothorac Surg. 2007;32:333–9.
147. Pantos C, Mourouzis I, Markakis K, Tsagoulis N, Panagiotou M, Cokkinos DV. Long-term thyroid hormone administration reshapes left ventricular chamber and improves cardiac function after myocardial infarction in rats. Basic Res Cardiol. 2008;103:308–18.
148. Pantos C, Mourouzis I, Tsagoulis N, Markakis K, Galanopoulos G, Roukounakis N et al. Thyroid hormone at supra-physiological dose optimizes cardiac geometry and improves cardiac function in rats with old myocardial infarction. J Physiol Pharmacol 2009;60:49–56.
149. Kalofoutis C, Mourouzis I, Galanopoulos G, Dimopoulos A, Perimenis P, Spanou D, et al. Thyroid hormone can favorably remodel the diabetic myocardium after acute myocardial infarction. Mol Cell Biochem. 2010;345:161–9.
150. Henderson KK, Danzi S, Paul JT, Leya G, Klein I, Samarel AM. Physiological replacement of T3 improves left ventricular function in an animal model of myocardial infarction–induced congestive heart failure. Circ Heart Fail. 2009;2:243–52.
151. Mahaffey KW, Raya TE, Pennock GD, Morkin E, Goldman S. Left ventricular performance and remodeling in rabbits after myocardial infarction. Effects of a thyroid hormone analogue. Circulation. 1995;91:794–801.
152. Chen YF, Weltman NY, Li X, Youmans S, Krause D, Gerdes AM. Improvement of left ventricular remodeling after myocardial infarction with eight weeks L-thyroxine treatment in rats. J Transl Med. 2013;11:40.
153. Chen YF, Pottala JV, Weltman NY, Ge X, Savinova OV, Gerdes AM. Regulation of gene expression with thyroid hormone in rats with myocardial infarction. PLoS One. 2012;7:e40161.
154. Chen YF, Kobayashi S, Chen J, Redetzke RA, Said S, Liang Q, et al. Short term triiodo-L-thyronine treatment inhibits cardiac myocyte apoptosis in border area after myocardial infarction in rats. J Mol Cell Cardiol. 2008;44:180–7.
155. Mourouzis I, Mantzouratou P, Galanopoulos G, Kostakou E, Roukounakis N, Kokkinos AD, et al. Dose-dependent effects of thyroid hormone on post-ischemic cardiac performance: potential involvement of Akt and ERK signalings. Mol Cell Biochem. 2012;363:235–43.
156. Fujio Y, Nguyen T, Wencker D, Kitsis RN, Walsh K. Akt promotes survival of cardiomyocytes in vitro and protects against ischemia–reperfusion injury in mouse heart. Circulation. 2000;101:660–7.
157. Matsui T, Tao J, del Monte F, Lee KH, Li L, Picard M, et al. Akt activation preserves cardiac function and prevents injury after transient cardiac ischemia in vivo. Circulation. 2001;104:330–5.
158. Matsui T, Li L, Wu JC, Cook SA, Nagoshi T, Picard MH, et al. Phenotypic spectrum caused by transgenic overexpression of activated Akt in the heart. J Biol Chem. 2002;277:22896–901.
159. Nagoshi T, Matsui T, Aoyama T, Leri A, Anversa P, Li L, et al. PI3K rescues the detrimental effects of chronic Akt activation in the heart during ischemia/reperfusion injury. J Clin Invest. 2005;115:2128–38.
160. Rajagopalan V, Gerdes AM. Role of thyroid hormones in ventricular remodeling. Curr Heart Fail Rep. 2015;12:141–9.
161. Goglia F, Moreno M, Lanni A. Action of thyroid hormones at the cellular level: the mitochondrial target. FEBS Lett. 1999;452:115–20.

162. Maity S, Kar D, De K, Chander V, Bandyopadhyay A. Hyperthyroidism causes cardiac dysfunction by mitochondrial impairment and energy depletion. J Endocrinol. 2013;217:215–28.
163. De Sibio MT, Luvizotto RA, Olimpio RM, Corrêa CR, Marino J, de Oliveira M, et al. A comparative genotoxicity study of a supraphysiological dose of triiodothyronine (T_3) in obese rats subjected to either calorie-restricted diet or hyperthyroidism. PLoS One. 2013;8(2):e56913.
164. Chen S, Shauer A, Zwas DR, Lotan C, Keren A, Gotsman I. The effect of thyroid function on clinical outcome in patients with heart failure. Eur J Heart Fail. 2014;16:217–26.
165. Lymvaios I, Mourouzis I, Cokkinos DV, Dimopoulos MA, Toumanidis ST, Pantos C. Thyroid hormone and recovery of cardiac function in patients with acute myocardial infarction: a strong association? Eur J Endocrinol. 2011;165:107–14.
166. Pingitore A, Nicolini G, Kusmic C, Iervasi G, Grigolini P, Forini F. Cardioprotection and thyroid hormones. Heart Fail Rev. 2016;21:391–9.
167. Iervasi G. THIRST. Thyroid hormone replacement therapy in ST elevation myocardial infarction (the PONTE study). Cambridge; January 31, 2012.
168. Pantos C, Mourouzis I. Translating thyroid hormone effects into clinical practice: the relevance of thyroid hormone receptor α1 in cardiac repair. Heart Fail Rev. 2015;20:273–82.
169. Pantos C, Mourouzis I, Paizis I, Malliopoulou V, Xinaris C, Moraitis P, et al. Pharmacological inhibition of TRalpha1 receptor potentiates the thyroxine effect on body weight reduction in rats: potential therapeutic implications in controlling body weight. Diabetes Obes Metab. 2007;9:136–8.
170. Kubin T, Pöling J, Kostin S, Gajawada P, Hein S, Rees W, et al. Oncostatin M is a major mediator of cardiomyocyte dedifferentiation and remodeling. Cell Stem Cell. 2011;9:420–32.
171. Garza MA, Wason EA, Zhang JQ. Cardiac remodeling and physical training post myocardial infarction. World J Cardiol. 2015;7:52–64.
172. Siu PM, Bryner RW, Martyn JK, Alway SE. Apoptotic adaptations from exercise training in skeletal and cardiac muscles. FASEB J. 2004;18:1150–2.
173. Linke A, Adams V, Schulze PC, Erbs S, Gielen S, Fiehn E, et al. Antioxidative effects of exercise training in patients with chronic heart failure: increase in radical scavenger enzyme activity in skeletal muscle. Circulation. 2005;111:1763–70.
174. Hammett CJ, Prapavessis H, Baldi JC, Varo N, Schoenbeck U, Ameratunga R, et al. Effects of exercise training on 5 inflammatory markers associated with cardiovascular risk. Am Heart J. 2006;151:367.e7–367.e16.
175. Giannuzzi P, Temporelli PL, Corrà U, Tavazzi L, ELVD-CHF Study Group. Antiremodeling effect of long-term exercise training in patients with stable chronic heart failure: results of the Exercise in Left Ventricular Dysfunction and Chronic Heart Failure (ELVD-CHF) trial. Circulation. 2003;108:554–9.
176. Dubach P, Myers J, Dziekan G, Goebbels U, Reinhart W, Vogt P, et al. Effect of exercise training on myocardial remodeling in patients with reduced left ventricular function after myocardial infarction: application of magnetic resonance imaging. Circulation. 1997;95:2060–7.
177. Haykowsky MJ, Liang Y, Pechter D, Jones LW, McAlister FA, Clark AM. A meta-analysis of the effect of exercise training on left ventricular remodeling in heart failure patients: the benefit depends on the type of training performed. J Am Coll Cardiol. 2007;49:2329–36.
178. Adamopoulos S, Gouziouta A, Mantzouratou P, Laoutaris ID, Dritsas A, Cokkinos DV, et al. Thyroid hormone signalling is altered in response to physical training in patients with end-stage heart failure and mechanical assist devices: potential physiological consequences? Interact Cardiovasc Thorac Surg. 2013;17:664–8.
179. Wei M, Xin P, Li S, Tao J, Li Y, Li J, et al. Repeated remote ischemic postconditioning protects against adverse left ventricular remodeling and improves survival in a rat model of myocardial infarction. Circ Res. 2011;108:1220–05.
180. Hausenloy D, Yellon D. Ischemic conditioning and reperfusion injury. Nat Rev Cardiol. 2016;13:193–209.
181. Clarke CL, Grunwald GK, Allen LA, Barón AE, Peterson PN, Brand DW, et al. Natural history of left ventricular ejection fraction in patients with heart failure. Circ Cardiovasc Qual Outcomes. 2013;6:680–6.

182. Goldfinger JZ, Nair AP. Myocardial recovery and the failing heart: medical, device and mechanical methods. Ann Glob Health. 2014;80:55–60.
183. Shah AM, Mann DL. In search of new therapeutic targets and strategies for heart failure: recent advances in basic science. Lancet. 2011;378:704–12.
184. Kramer DG, Trikalinos TA, Kent DM, Antonopoulos GV, Konstam MA, Udelson JE. Quantitative evaluation of drug or device effects on ventricular remodeling as predictors of therapeutic effects on mortality in patients with heart failure and reduced ejection fraction: a meta-analytic approach. J Am Coll Cardiol. 2010;56:392–406.
185. Tracy CM, Epstein AE, Darbar D, Dimarco JP, Dunbar SB, Estes NA 3rd, et al. ACCF/AHA/HRS focused update of the 2008 guidelines for device-based therapy of cardiac rhythm abnormalities: a report of the American College of Cardiology Foundation/American Heart Association Task Force on Practice Guidelines. J Am Coll Cardiol. 2012;60:1297–313.
186. European Society of Cardiology (ESC); European Heart Rhythm Association (EHRA), Brignole M, Auricchio A, Baron-Esquivias G, Bordachar P, Boriani G, et al. 2013 ESC guidelines on cardiac pacing and cardiac resynchronization therapy: the Task Force on Cardiac Pacing and Resynchronization Therapy of the European Society of Cardiology (ESC). Developed in collaboration with the European Heart Rhythm Association (EHRA). Europace. 2013;15:1070–118.
187. Sze E, Daubert JP. Left bundle branch block: is it "unsafe at any speed"? JACC Heart Fail. 2016;4:904–6.
188. Hessel MH, Bleeker GB, Bax JJ, Henneman MM, den Adel B, Klok M, et al. Reverse ventricular remodelling after cardiac resynchronization therapy is associated with a reduction in serum tenascin-C and plasma matrix metalloproteinase-9 levels. Eur J Heart Fail. 2007;9:1058–63.
189. Yu CM, Bleeker GB, Fung JW, Schalij MJ, Zhang Q, van der Wall EE, et al. Left ventricular reverse remodeling but not clinical improvement predicts long-term survival after cardiac resynchronization therapy. Circulation. 2005;112:1580–6.
190. St John Sutton MG, Plappert T, Abraham WT, Smith AL, Delurgio DB, Leon AR, et al. Effect of cardiac resynchronization therapy on left ventricular size and function in chronic heart failure. Circulation. 2003;107:1985–90.
191. Daubert C, Gold MR, Abraham WT, Ghio S, Hassager C, Goode G, et al. Prevention of disease progression by cardiac resynchronization therapy in patients with asymptomatic or mildly symptomatic left ventricular dysfunction: insights from the European cohort of the REVERSE (Resynchronization Reverses Remodeling in Systolic Left Ventricular Dysfunction) trial. J Am Coll Cardiol. 2009;54:1837–46.
192. Cleland JG, Daubert JC, Erdmann E, Freemantle N, Gras D, Kappenberger L, et al. The effect of cardiac resynchronization on morbidity and mortality in heart failure. N Engl J Med. 2005;352:1539–49.
193. Cleland JGF. Should we be trying to define responders to cardiac resynchronization therapy? J Am Coll Cardiol 2010;2010:04.003.
194. Solomon SD, Foster E, Bourgoun M, Shah A, Viloria E, Brown MW, et al. Effect of cardiac resynchronization therapy on reverse remodeling and relation to outcome: multicenter automatic defibrillator implantation trial: cardiac resynchronization therapy. Circulation. 2010;122:985–92.
195. St John Sutton M, Cerkvenik J, Borlaug BA, Daubert C, Gold MR, Ghio S, et al. Effects of cardiac resynchronization therapy on cardiac remodeling and contractile function: results from resynchronization reverses remodeling in systolic left ventricular dysfunction (REVERSE). J Am Heart Assoc. 2015;4:e002054.
196. Gold MR, Daubert C, Abraham WT, Ghio S, St John Sutton S, Hudnall JH, et al. The effect of reverse remodeling on long-term survival in mildly symptomatic patients with heart failure receiving cardiac resynchronization therapy: results of the REVERSE study. Heart Rhythm. 2015;12:524–30.
197. Waring AA, Litwin SE. Redefining reverse remodeling: can echocardiography refine our ability to assess response to heart failure treatments? J Am Coll Cardiol. 2016;68:1277–80.

198. Sekaran NK, Crowley AL, de Souza FR, Resende ES, Rao SV. The role for cardiovascular remodeling in cardiovascular outcomes. Curr Atheroscler Rep. 2017;19:23.
199. Mathias A, Moss AJ, McNitt S, Zareba W, Goldenberg I, Solomon SD, et al. Clinical implications of complete left-sided reverse remodeling with cardiac resynchronization therapy: a MADIT-CRT substudy. J Am Coll Cardiol. 2016;68:1268–76.
200. St John Sutton M, Plappert T, Adamson PB, Li P, Christman SA, Chung ES, et al. Left ventricular reverse remodeling with biventricular versus right ventricular pacing in patients with atrioventricular block and heart failure in the BLOCK HF trial. Circ Heart Fail. 2015;8:510–8.
201. Vanderheyden M, Mullens W, Delrue L, Goethals M, de Bruyne B, Wijns W, Geelen P, et al. Myocardial gene expression in heart failure patients treated with cardiac resynchronization therapy responders versus nonresponders. J Am Coll Cardiol. 2008;51:129–36.
202. Krenz M, Robbins J. Impact of beta-myosin heavy chain expression on cardiac function during stress. J Am Coll Cardiol. 2004;44:2390–7.
203. Liu X, Yang HJ, Ping HQ, Qiu S, Shi S, Yang B. The safety and efficacy of cardiac contractility modulation in heart failure: a meta-analysis of clinical trials. Herz. 2017; https://doi.org/10.1007/s00059-016-4514-5.
204. Puehler T, Ensminger S, Schoenbrodt M, Börgermann J, Rehn E, Hakim-Meibodi K, et al. Mechanical circulatory support devices as destination therapy—current evidence. Ann Cardiothorac Surg. 2014;3:513–24.
205. Imamura T, Kinugawa K, Nitta D, Hatano M, Kinoshita O, Nawata K, et al. Advantage of pulsatility in left ventricular reverse remodeling and aortic insufficiency prevention during left ventricular assist device treatment. Circ J. 2015;79:1994–9.
206. Krabatsch T, Schweiger M, Dandel M, Stepanenko A, Drews T, Potapov E, et al. Is bridge to recovery more likely with pulsatile left ventricular assist devices than with nonpulsatile-flow systems? Ann Thorac Surg. 2011;91:1335–40.
207. Torre-Amione G, Stetson SJ, Youker KA, Durand JB, Radovancevic B, Delgado RM, et al. Decreased expression of tumor necrosis factor-alpha in failing human myocardium after mechanical circulatory support: a potential mechanism for cardiac recovery. Circulation. 1999;100:1189–93.
208. Hall JL, Birks EJ, Grindle S, Cullen ME, Barton PJ, Rider JE, et al. Molecular signature of recovery following combination left ventricular assist device (LVAD) support and pharmacologic therapy. Eur Heart J. 2007;28:613–27.
209. Blaxall BC, Tschannen-Moran BM, Milano CA, Koch WJ. Differential gene expression and genomic patient stratification following left ventricular assist device support. J Am Coll Cardiol. 2003;41:1096–106.
210. Mitchell A, Guan W, Staggs R, Hamel A, Hozayen S, Adhikari N, et al. Identification of differentially expressed transcripts and pathways in blood one week and six months following implant of left ventricular assist devices. PLoS One. 2013;8:e77951.
211. Ambardekar AV, Buttrick PM. Reverse remodeling with left ventricular assist devices: a review of clinical, cellular, and molecular effects. Circ Heart Fail. 2011;4:224–33.
212. Topkara VK, Chambers KT, Yang KC, Tzeng HP, Evans S, Weinheimer C, et al. Functional significance of the discordance between transcriptional profile and left ventricular structure/function during reverse remodeling. JCI Insight. 2016;1:e86038.
213. Jacobs S, Geens J, Rega F, Burkhoff D, Meyns B. Continuous-flow left ventricular assist devices induce left ventricular reverse remodeling. J Heart Lung Transplant. 2013;32:466–8.
214. Marinescu KK, Uriel N, Mann DL, Burkhoff D. Left ventricular assist device-induced reverse remodeling: it's not just about myocardial recovery. Expert Rev Med Devices. 2017;14:15–26.
215. Basuray A, French B, Ky B, Vorovich E, Olt C, Sweitzer NK, et al. Heart failure with recovered ejection fraction: clinical description, biomarkers, and outcomes. Circulation. 2014;129:2380–7.
216. Basuray A, Fang JC. Management of patients with recovered systolic function. Prog Cardiovasc Dis. 2016;58:434–43.
217. de Groote P, Fertin M, Duva Pentiah A, Goéminne C, Lamblin N, Bauters C. Long-term functional and clinical follow-up of patients with heart failure with recovered left ventricular ejection fraction after β-blocker therapy. Circ Heart Fail. 2014;7:434–9.

218. Givertz MM, Mann DL. Epidemiology and natural history of recovery of left ventricular function in recent onset dilated cardiomyopathies. Curr Heart Fail Rep. 2013;10:321–30.
219. Pan S, Aksut B, Wever-Pinzon OE, Rao SD, Levin AP, Garan AR, et al. Incidence and predictors of myocardial recovery on long-term left ventricular assist device support: results from the United Network for Organ Sharing database. J Heart Lung Transplant. 2015;34:1624–9.
220. Drakos SG, Mehra MR. Clinical myocardial recovery during long-term mechanical support in advanced heart failure: insights into moving the field forward. J Heart Lung Transplant. 2016;35:413–20.
221. Selzman CH, Madden JL, Healy AH, McKellar SH, Koliopoulou A, Stehlik J, et al. Bridge to removal: a paradigm shift for left ventricular assist device therapy. Ann Thorac Surg. 2015;99:360–7.
222. Klotz S, Danser AH, Foronjy RF, Oz MC, Wang J, Mancini D, et al. The impact of angiotensin-converting enzyme inhibitor therapy on the extracellular collagen matrix during left ventricular assist device support in patients with end-stage heart failure. J Am Coll Cardiol. 2007;49:1166–74.
223. Soucy KG, Smith EF, Monreal G, Rokosh G, Keller BB, Yuan F, et al. Feasibility study of particulate extracellular matrix (P-ECM) and left ventricular assist device (HVAD) therapy in chronic ischemic heart failure bovine model. ASAIO J. 2015;61:161–9.
224. Zavadzkas JA, Stroud RE, Bouges S, Mukherjee R, Jones JR, Patel RK, et al. Targeted overexpression of tissue inhibitor of matrix metalloproteinase-4 modifies post-myocardial infarction remodeling in mice. Circ Res. 2014;114:1435–45.
225. Felkin LE, Lara-Pezzi E, George R, Yacoub MH, Birks EJ, Barton PJ. Expression of extracellular matrix genes during myocardial recovery from heart failure after left ventricular assist device support. J Heart Lung Transplant. 2009;28:117–22.
226. Markham DW, Fu Q, Palmer MD, Drazner MH, Meyer DM, Bethea BT, et al. Sympathetic neural and hemodynamic responses to upright tilt in patients with pulsatile and nonpulsatile left ventricular assist devices. Circ Heart Fail. 2013;6:293–9.
227. Westman PC, Lipinski MJ, Luger D, Waksman R, Bonow RO, Wu E, et al. Inflammation as a driver of adverse left ventricular remodeling after acute myocardial infarction. J Am Coll Cardiol. 2016;67:2050–60.
228. Grosman-Rimon L, Jacobs I, Tumiati LC, McDonald MA, Bar-Ziv SP, Fuks A, et al. Longitudinal assessment of inflammation in recipients of continuous-flow left ventricular assist devices. Can J Cardiol. 2015;31:348–56.
229. Grosman-Rimon L, McDonald MA, Jacobs I, Tumiati LC, Pollock Bar-Ziv S, Shogilev DJ, et al. Markers of inflammation in recipients of continuous-flow left ventricular assist devices. ASAIO J. 2014;60:657–63.
230. Baskin KK, Taegtmeyer H. Taking pressure off the heart: the ins and outs of atrophic remodelling. Cardiovasc Res. 2011;90:243–50.
231. Cao DJ, Jiang N, Blagg A, Johnstone JL, Gondalia R, Oh M, et al. Mechanical unloading activates FoxO3 to trigger Bnip3-dependent cardiomyocyte atrophy. J Am Heart Assoc. 2013;2:e000016.
232. Barbone A, Holmes JW, Heerdt PM, The' AH, Naka Y, Joshi N, et al. Comparison of right and left ventricular responses to left ventricular assist device support in patients with severe heart failure: a primary role of mechanical unloading underlying reverse remodeling. Circulation. 2001;104:670–5.
233. Ahmad T, Wang T, O'Brien EC, Samsky MD, Pura JA, Lokhnygina Y, et al. Effects of left ventricular assist device support on biomarkers of cardiovascular stress, fibrosis, fluid homeostasis, inflammation, and renal injury. JACC Heart Fail. 2015;3:30–9.
234. Matkovich SJ, Van Booven DJ, Youker KA, Torre-Amione G, Diwan A, Eschenbacher WH, et al. Reciprocal regulation of myocardial microRNAs and messenger RNA in human cardiomyopathy and reversal of the microRNA signature by biomechanical support. Circulation. 2009;119:1263–71.
235. Lok SI, de Jonge N, van Kuik J, van Geffen AJ, Huibers MM, van der Weide P, et al. MicroRNA expression in myocardial tissue and plasma of patients with end-stage heart

failure during LVAD support: comparison of continuous and pulsatile devices. PLoS One. 2015;10:e0136404.
236. Schipper ME, van Kuik J, de Jonge N, Dullens HF, de Weger RA. Changes in regulatory microRNA expression in myocardium of heart failure patients on left ventricular assist device support. J Heart Lung Transplant. 2008;27:1282–5.
237. Topkara VK, Garan AR, Fine B, Godier-Furnémont AF, Breskin A, Cagliostro B, et al. Myocardial recovery in patients receiving contemporary left ventricular assist devices: results from the Interagency Registry for Mechanically Assisted Circulatory Support (INTERMACS). Circ Heart Fail 2016;9. doi: 10.1161/CIRCHEARTFAILURE.116.003157.
238. Drakos SG, Pagani FD, Lundberg MS, Baldwin TJ. Advancing the science of myocardial recovery with mechanical circulatory support: a working group of the National Heart, Lung, and Blood Institute. J Thorac Cardiovasc Surg. 2017;154:165–70.
239. Gustafsson F, Rogers JG. Left ventricular assist device therapy in advanced heart failure: patient selection and outcomes. Eur J Heart Fail. 2017;19:595–602.
240. Starling RC, Estep JD, Horstmanshof DA, Milano CA, Stehlik J, Shah KB, et al. Risk assessment and comparative effectiveness of left ventricular assist device and medical management in ambulatory heart failure patients: the ROADMAP study 2-year results. JACC Heart Fail. 2017;5:518–27.
241. Mehra MR, Goldstein DJ, Uriel N, Cleveland JC, Yuzefpolskaya M, Salerno C, Walsh MN, Milano CA, Patel CB, Ewald GA, Itoh A, Dean D, Krishnamoorthy A, Cotts WG, Tatooles AJ, Jorde UP, Bruckner BA, Estep JD, Jeevanandam V, Sayer G, Horstmanshof D, Long JW, Gulati S, Skipper ER, O'Connell JB, Heatley G, Sood P, Naka Y. Two-Year Outcomes with a Magnetically Levitated Cardiac Pump in Heart Failure. N Eng J Med. 2018;378(15):1386–95.

Chapter 14
Conditioning of the Myocardium

Dennis V. Cokkinos

This term is used in its general meaning because pre-, peri-, and postconditioning and continuous conditioning have been described. This variety in time intervals has been recently very well described by Hausenloy and Yellon [1]. Over the years many protocols have emerged in the laboratory animal and in the human. Generally, smaller animals can be preconditioned with ischemia of shorter duration. Skyschally et al. [2] give a very detailed description of the various methods used. It represents a universal phenomenon, in humans, laboratory animals, and practically all organs and tissues and even isolated cells. It has even been documented in plants (saline environment, lack of water).

In essence, conditioning (C) signifies that the application of a noxious stimulus, low in intensity and for a limited time, can prevent the tissue to which it is applied against a subsequent stronger and longer application of the same type of stimulus which would otherwise be lethal. Obviously, this wide definition applies to preconditioning. In the other types (pre-, peri-, and postconditioning), protection against previous and ongoing injury is operative.

Ischemic C has been most widely studied. However, C can also be affected by exposure to hypoxia, thermal stress, cold stress, nerve and mechanical limb stimulation, stretch, immobilization, and bacterial toxins (lipopolysaccharide application).

The wide study of conditioning (C) was ushered by the seminal discovery of CE Murry [3] together with PB Jennings and KA Reimer.

In this case, as Louis Pasteur has quoted, "fortune aids the prepared mind." The researchers as stated in their article [3] were investigating why four repeated 10-min episodes of ischemia cause less damage and ATP depletion than one single period of 40 min [4]. In a canine model five cycles of intermittent occlusion of the left anterior descending artery produced a 75% reduction of myocardial infarct size [3].

D. V. Cokkinos (✉)
Heart and Vessel Department, Biomedical Research Foundation,
Academy of Athens - Gregory Skalkeas, Athens, Greece
e-mail: dcokkinos@bioacademy.gr

D. V. Cokkinos (ed.), *Myocardial Preservation*,
https://doi.org/10.1007/978-3-319-98186-4_14

14.1 Preconditioning-Mechanisms of Action

Many authors have described two phases of ischemic preconditioning of the myocardium (pre C): The first phase or "window" termed "classical" or "acute" starts immediately after the ischemic stimulus application and lasts for 2–3 h. This actually was the phenomenon described by Murry et al. [3].

After 12–24 h and lasting for 48–72 h, the second phase starts, termed the "late" or "delayed" pre C, representing the "second window" of cardioprotection. The mechanisms operative in the two phases seem to be different. The protection afforded by the second window is on the whole less robust than that of the first, according to Baines et al. [5].

It is didactically easier and simpler to describe the two phases separately:

Classical preconditioning. This will be subsequently described as pre C.

Trying to explain various reviews explaining the mechanisms of this phenomenon makes very interesting reading. Work in 1990–2000 pointed to opening K^+ATP channels as the final mediator of the protective effect [5–9].

It was soon realized that it is difficult to quantitate the degree of opening of the K^+ATP channels; Mocanu et al. [10], from Derek Yellon's group, studied K^+ATP membrane potential of either the cell (sarcolemmal) or the inner mitochondrial membrane.

Interestingly Lawrence et al. [11] had postulated that Na^+-activated K^+ current (K^+, Na^+) is present in guinea pig but not in rat ventricular myocytes.

An early finding which is still investigated today is the use of agents opening K^+ATP channels such as diazoxide, chromacalim, bimacalim, pinacidil, and importantly nicorandil, which has received wide clinical application [12–14], or closing them, such as the sulfonylurea glibenclamide [15] and 5-hydroxydecanoate [16].

Garlid [17] in an exhaustive review proposed that the main beneficial effect of the cardioprotective intervention is the maintenance of mitochondrial integrity and – up to a point – the upregulation of ROS production, which will be described later. Liu et al. [18] postulate that sarcolemmal K^+ATP channels are less potent than the mitochondrial (mito) ones.

Downey and Cohen [6] in a very detailed description of K^+ATP-sensitive K^+ channels stress that they open when ATP levels fall in the cell.

They further describe that sarcolemmal K^+ATP channels incorporate four pore-forming channel proteins, sulfonylurea-binding receptor proteins, which bind both ATP and sulfonylureas, which have already been described as abrogating pre C. The same authors discuss that the structure of the mitochondrial (mito) K^+ATP was not completely known at the time, but it was believed to incorporate elements of the two known inward rectifier ATP-sensitive K^+ channel proteins Kv6.1 and Kv6.2.

They also state that while cromakalim opens both channels, diazoxide is highly selective for mito channels and that mito K^+ATP opening is a trigger of pre C, and this is dependent on the production of ROS [19, 20].

Thus, Forbes et al. [19] have shown that the protective effect of diazoxide is blocked by antioxidants.

As Iliodromitis et al. [21] point out, it is realized that after pre C the myocardium is found to have a smaller adenine nucleotide pool, an excess of creatine phosphate and glucose, and a degree of cardiac dysfunction which is attributed to stunning [22, 23].

It is not clear whether this myocardial dysfunction is a requisite for the beneficial effect of pre C, as Garcia-Dorado et al. [24] pointed out quite early.

The authors postulate that inhibition of myofibrillar contractility, a result of uncontrolled calcium entry, could be a major protective mechanism. This question will also be addressed in postconditioning.

Also, pre C is accompanied by ischemic contracture. It is not known if contracture is a requisite for cardioprotection. Kolocassides et al. [25] tried three different protocols in isolated rat hearts subjected to normothermic global ischemia (35 min) and reperfusion (40 min), ischemic pre C, cardioplegia, and a combination of both. All three had similar post-ischemic contractile function; however, pre C accelerated, cardioplegia delayed, and the combination had little effect on contracture, thus creating questions as to its applicability as a predictor of protective efficacy.

Iliodromitis et al. [21] also point out that pre- and postconditioning which will be reviewed subsequently share some common pathways: adenosine, opioids, and bradykinins are important ligands [26].

pre C also involves activation of PI3K/Akt pathway and kinases of the MAPK family (MEK1/2 ERK1/2) which activate ROS production by the mitochondria, which activate pre C and subsequently open K^+ATP channels; these constitute the RISK (reperfusion injury salvage kinase) pathway. Importantly, K^+ATP opening produces closure of the mPTP [27, 28].

Another pathway, the SAFE (survival activating factor enhancement) which involves the TNFα receptor and STAT3 [29], is also operative in pre C.

Iliodromitis et al. [21] point out that contrary to adenosine, opioids and bradykinin activate K^+ATP channels directly. As regards bradykinin, it appears that B2 receptors are the ones operative in pre C [29].

Tyrosine kinase is also involved. Hattori et al. [30] tried a selective inhibitor of the Src tyrosine kinase family (PP1) in both pre- and post C. According to their results, they postulate that Src kinase activation triggers pre C either upstream of or parallel to the action of PKC-ε, i.e., it is a trigger but not a mediator.

Downey and Cohen [6] also discuss that while bradykinin and opioids trigger protection through mito K^+ATP opening, adenosine couples directly to PKC.

They also describe the trigger pathway for the muscarinic receptor which affects the mito K^+ATP in a complex way, finally activating PI3 which phosphorylates membrane phosphoinositide and finally activating Akt, which then phosphorylates eNOS [31].

Stokfisz et al. [32] give a recent detailed review, explaining the (classical) pre C; they suggest that even after 30 years of experience, it has not been clearly explained. They propose three main levels of signal transduction: triggers, intracellular mediator cascade, and effectors.

1. In the *triggers* they include:
   (a) Chemical stimuli, such as calcium ions, ROS, reactive nitrogen species, hydrogen sulfide
   (b) Autacoids, such as adenosine and bradykinin
   (c) Neurotransmitters and hormones such as acetylcholine and angiotensin
   (d) Cytokines, i.e., TNFα, interleukins b, and prostaglandins

Catecholamines act through the a-adrenergic receptors. Opioids act through receptors coupled to proteins and share part of their downstream signaling with adenosine and bradykinin.

2. *Intracellular mediator cascade* is effected by three pathways:
   (a) NO and NOS
   (b) RISK pathway (reperfusion injury salvage kinase)
   (c) SAFE pathway (survival activating factor enhancement)

The same authors [32] stress that the PKC activation in pre C remains controversial, since Vahlhaus et al. [33] showed in swine that its inhibitor staurosporine did not reduce infarct size, although this was seen in preconditioned rabbits [34].

3. *Effectors*. These are operative in the mitochondria where the crucial effectors finally meet, inhibiting the mPTP opening [35].

Stokfisz et al. [32] also describe other elements involved in pre C. Thus, they mention that inhibition of sarcolemmal connexin 43 prevents the spread of ischemic injury [36].

They also describe that protein nitrosation/nitrosylation is also involved [37].

14.2 Delayed or Second Window of Pre C

This observation came 7 years after pre C as described by Hausenloy and Yellon [38]; this phenomenon was discovered independently in 1993 by two research groups: Yellon's group, who termed it as the second window of cardioprotection (SWOP) [39], and Kuzuya et al. [40] who found a decrease of myocardial infarct size, either immediately or 24 h after a standard pre C application. The reviewers [38] point out that Szekeres et al. [41] had reported in the same year cardioprotection evidenced immediately and at 24 and 48 h after cardiac pacing.

Here, it must be reminded that ventricular pacing at the beginning of reperfusion can also induce postconditioning as described recently by Yang and Xi [42].

Its role against cardiac REM will be described in this chapter. Interestingly, Szekeres had described earlier (1983) pharmaceutical delayed preconditioning by prostacyclin [43].

The same author in 2000 [44] and Hausenloy and Yellon [38] describe that the following stimuli can also elicit delayed PC: ischemia, heat stress, pacing and exercise, as well as pharmacological agents.

In fact exercise can induce both early and delayed Pre C [45]. Also, remote preconditioning (RIPC) which will be described later, can cause both early and delayed Pre C [46].

The protocols using varying cycles of ischemia reperfusion are practically the same as in early pre C. Baxter et al. have shown that even a 5-min ischemic period can induce delayed Pre C [47].

Delayed preconditioning by heat stress was first described in 1988 [48]; the effects of ischemic early and delayed Pre C can be combined as described by Mullenheim et al. [49] and Stambaugh et al. [50].

Hausenloy and Yellon [38] remind that although many studies have assessed the benefits of delayed Pre C by measuring cell death, the degree of stunning has also been employed; delayed Pre C is also beneficial against endothelial dysfunction and platelet dysfunction which can produce microvascular obstruction [51].

The mechanisms underlying the protective effect of delayed Pre C have been described by many authors.

Hausenloy and Yellon [38] describe that in delayed Pre C, Akt, ERK1/2, PKC, and tyrosine kinase C activate many important transcription factors such as AP-1, HIF-1α, NFkB, Nrf2 (erythroid 2-related factor), and STAT 1/3.

These in turn induce the synthesis of COX-2, HSP-72, and iNOS. Adenosine is also involved, as in early pre C [52–54].

Bradykinin another autocoid besides adenosine has already been discussed in early pre C. Again, the B2 receptor is suggested as mediating the late response [55].

By the term autacoids, Heusch [56] describes substances that are released from cardiomyocytes, endothelium, and interstitial cells.

Importantly, Jaberansari et al. [57] have suggested that angiotensin-converting enzyme inhibitors can enhance subthreshold stimulus to an effective one toward eliciting delayed pre C.

Many other factors such as p38 MAPK, HSP27 [58], and MnSOD [59] are also involved in finally opening K^{+}ATP channels [60].

Opioids have also been implicated in delayed PC [61, 62]. However, it has already been discussed if these agents are pre- or post-conditioning mimetic or just cardioprotective [27]. As described by Hausenloy and Yellon [38], opioids act through the aforementioned signaling pathways [61, 62].

Apart from the already mentioned HSPs, expression of various proteins from the cell nucleus is also a hallmark of delayed pre C, according to Heusch [56] and Bolli et al. [63].

These proteins include PKC-ε [64], tyrosine kinases [65], and Janus kinases [66, 67].

Other important proteins are inducible (i)NOS [68], COX 2 [69], superoxide dismutase [70] aldose reductase [71], and heme oxygenase [72].

Heusch et al. [73] stress that delayed Pre C shares a protective phenotype with hibernating myocardium, including many of the already mentioned proteins [73].

In this context one may postulate if the diminished baseline and hyperemic coronary flow which characterizes hibernation play the role of repeated ischemic cycles causing delayed pre C.

Many factors, which include TNFα, IL-β, and IL-6, are generated in response to ischemia. As Hausenloy and Yellon [38] stress, they are not constitutively expressed in the heart. Dawn et al. [67] showed that IL-6$^{-/-}$ mice did not undergo delayed pre C and were characterized by attenuation of STAT1/3 activation and iNOS and COX-2 upregulation.

Apart from iNOS, eNOS also plays an important role in delayed pre C, by generating NO [74].

14.3 Hydrogen Sulfide

This factor, which is being recently widely discussed, has been proposed to signal delayed pre C [75, 76]. However, as Hausenloy and Yellon state [38] and Sivarajah et al. [77] in vivo showed, this molecule induced delayed pre C by endotoxin but not ischemia.

14.4 Reactive Oxygen Species (ROS)

These were already described in early pre C and are involved in late pre C as suggested by Sun et al. [78]. Their effects in delayed pre C can also be blocked by antioxidants and mimicked by exogenous ROS administration [70].

As in the case of early pre C, ROS generation opens K^+ATP channels [79].

After all these substances have been mentioned, Hausenloy and Yellon [38] classify them in: *Triggers,* which include adenosine, opioids, bradykinin, cytokines, ROS, NO and eNOS, and hydrogen sulfide.

Early mediators which include:

PKC, specifically PKC-ε [80]; tyrosine kinase, which was also mentioned in early pre C; and MAPKs [81], such as ERK 1/2 and JNK, activated upstream by the PKC-ε and also by opioids [82].

The PI3K- Akt pathway is also involved [83].

According to Hausenloy and Yellon [38], these early mediators produce their actions through the following transcription factors, many of which have already been mentioned: nuclear factor kB [84], activator protein-1, a stress sensor transcription factor [85], STAT1/3, and HIF-1α [86].

Hausenloy and Yellon [38] also classify as *distal mediators* MnSOD, HSPs, COX-2, aldose reductase [71], and heme oxygenase-1 [87].

However, the final effectors of all these mediators as Heusch stresses [56] are the mitochondria. They provide the amounts of ATP which are essential for cell integrity and function. Actually, transient mPTP opening is cardioprotective during preconditioning [88]. Their behavior characterizes the way of action of pre C; a little protects; a larger application damages. The inner mitochondrial K^+ATP channel [89] is already involved in the pre C effects, as already described.

The ubiquitous microRNAs (miRs) are also involved in delayed pre C, namely, 1, 21, and 24 [90, 91], found in the hearts of mice subjected to pre C [91].

Finally Hausenloy and Yellon [1] also point out that functional genomics may give further insights, as described by Varga et al. [92] and others [93].

In recapitulation of the above, Das and Malik [94] describe that classic pre C could be the result in the reprogramming of gene expression, translated into proteins during the late pre C. These already described genes are expressed by virtually any kind of stress (superoxide dismutase, glutathione peroxidase, heme oxygenase, HSPs). This process converts the “death signal” to the “survival signal.”

In this context very recently Gidlöf et al. [95] describe that pre C confers epigenetic repression of the mTOR gene and induction of autophagy. Hausenloy and Yellon [1], Stokfisz et al. [32], and Stenzel-Poore [96] have described the genetic involvement in late pre C.

14.5 Postconditioning

This very interesting mechanism was first described by Vinten-Johansen’s team in dogs [97] and was actually shown to be as robust in diminishing infarct size as pre C. The authors also found out that postconditioning (post C) was also associated with reduction of myocardial edema and reduction of polymorphonuclear (PMN) neutrophils in the infarct area and diminished PMN adherence in the endothelium mediated by downregulation of P-selectin. Additionally, lipid peroxidation was diminished. Buchholz et al. [98] reported similar results in rats but at a lower efficacy than preconditioning [97]. The same authors mention the work of Skyschally et al. [98], according to whom the effectiveness of post C as that of pre C depends on many factors, i.e., delay after reocclusion, duration, and number of occlusions and reperfusions. Obviously, as in all aspects of C, species similarities and differences between rodents and large animals have been shown. It is obvious that post C can have a greater clinical utility, since in humans it can be applied after the onset of an infarct and then before reperfusion. Many mechanisms have been proposed: In the initial study [97], oxidative stress, calcium overload, endothelial dysfunction improvement, and the reduction of inflammation were postulated. As further studies emerged, it was believed that post C shares many signaling pathways with pre C [99, 100], which according to Buchholz et al. [98] include G protein-coupled membrane receptors. They have shown that A1 adenosine receptors act as “triggers” [101].

The same authors [97, 98] also propose α1-adrenergic receptors as mediators, which may phosphorylate Akt which in turn would inhibit GSK-3b [102].

They also state that according to the group of Garcia Dorado [103], persistence of the acidotic state during reperfusion is essential for post C.

Interestingly and paradoxically, again in the sense of the yin and yang phenomenon, prolongation of acidosis can prevent activation of the pre-apoptotic calpains [103].

In this sense, intracellular acidosis is associated with the cardioprotection of post C by activating Akt and ERK [104] with prevention of mPTP opening as the final end point.

In fact activation of eNOS and the activation of P70S6K activate Akt downstream [105].

Post C also increases cGMP levels, the inhibition of which abolishes the protective effect of post C since guanylate cyclase blocks this effect, together with L-NAME, while NO donors enhance post C, pointing to this molecule as a mediator [105, 106].

Another player is activation of the PKG/c GMP pathway which according to Inserte et al. [107] may not be involved in the PI3/Akt cascade but may act through reduction of oxidative stress.

Skyschally et al. found that the RISK pathway mediates post C protection in rats [108] but not in pigs [109].

According to Gomez et al. [110], inhibition of GSK-3b by post C also acts by preventing the opening of mPTP independently of cyclophilin D.

According to Lim et al. from Yellon's group [111], both pre- and post C are involved in mPTP opening prevention. These authors showed in cyclophilin $D^{-/-}$ mice that no cardioprotective effect of these interventions was seen.

The role of cyclophilin D is described in the cell death chapter; Crisostomo et al. [112] point out that in comparison with the great deal of data available in pre C, post C remains less well explained than pre C. They mention that according to Kin et al. [113], in post C only adenosine 2 and 3 but not 1 receptors are involved.

They also point out that although both pre C and post C involve NO as a stimulus, in the former NO triggers formation of ROS, while in the latter it possibly acts through the NO-cGMP pathway.

Mewton et al. [114] discuss in a very focused review the elements of post C. They report the findings of Argaud et al. [115, 116] that mechanical post C and chemical post C with cyclosporine or NIM811 increase the Ca^{2+} load required for opening mPTP. The same authors also discuss the importance of mPTP and the role of cyclophilin D, which is considered an important component of mPTP. In the presence of high matrix Ca^{2+} concentration, it modifies the conformation of the inner mitochondrial membrane [117].

Cyclosporine inhibit mPTP opening by preventing the binding of CypD to the inner mitochondrial membrane.

In this context, Shanmuganathan et al. [118] have shown that the mPTP is a realistic target for cardioprotection in the human.

Argaud et al. [115] suggest that post C produces an enhanced resistance to Ca^{2+} overload.

Bice and Baxter [119] in 2015 reviewed the interspecies differences in post C effectiveness. They report that in the murine heart, a 30% reduction in infarct size is seen, while in larger animals, rabbits and dogs, a 50% reduction can be seen.

Here the interesting findings of Moriguchi et al. [120] should be described that inhibition of contractile activity during post C enhances cardioprotection, as discussed in pre C.

14.6 Time and Dosage of Post C Application

These are legions. However, before describing them, a very important fact should be considered, as described by Mewton et al. [114]: According to Argaud et al. [121], the mPTP remains closed during the whole period of ischemia, as discussed in the chapter on cell death. Thus, if post C was started 10 min after the onset of reperfusion, it was no longer protective. Similarly, Kin et al. [122] in rats and rabbits found that post C cycles were effective only when applied during the first minute of reperfusion. However, Roubille et al. [123] have shown in the mouse heart that post C can limit infarct size even after 30 min of reperfusion, a term described as delayed postconditioning. However, it is well known that as in pre C [124], times of application differ, being generally longer in larger animals. As regards application in humans, Skyschally et al. [109] describe that a delay of more than 1 min may be associated with a loss of protection. Here, another concept which may have an analogous action to post C must be described. The postulation of Hausenloy and Yellon [1] should be kept in mind that one can differentiate between early and delayed post C and gradual or gentle reperfusion which also has protective effects, analogous to those of post C [125, 126].

As Hausenloy and Yellon [38] describe, actually the term postconditioning was employed in 1996 by Na et al. [127] who showed that ventricular premature beats which would be expected to produce intermittent reperfusion prevented VF in cat hearts.

Yang and Xi [42] reported post C with intermittent ventricular pacing, as a potentially practical approach.

14.7 Other Effects of Post C

Apart from its effects on limiting infarct size post C in a way analogous to pre C, it exerts many other beneficial effects.

As Buchholz et al. [102] point out, besides reducing necrosis, post C may reduce apoptosis. Thus, Tian et al. [128] found a reduction in TUNEL-positive cells, through the already described Janus kinase 2/signal transducers, JAK-STAT3, and Bcl-2 pathways. Kin et al. [129] also found that it decreases caspase-3 activity through downregulation of NF-kB and TNFα.

Sun et al. [130] also found a decrease in cardiomyocyte loss with hypoxic post C; these authors also found [131] that apoptosis is decreased through inhibition of JNK and the p38 MAPK pathway.

As described in the chapter on cell death, this aspect is very important in the no-reflow phenomenon. It is associated with downregulation of NO synthesis [132] and increased neutrophil adhesion under the influence of P-selectin and increased ROS generation. Post C decreases all these unfavorable effects [38].

Actually Zhao et al. [133] described a decrease in the no-reflow phenomenon. The proposed action is an increase of neuronal and endothelial NO synthase. This effect is lost in hypercholesterolemia as will be further discussed.

A final important point is the effect on left ventricular function; Shinohara et al. [134] found that post C improved ventricular recovery in pigs.

Arrhythmias can also be diminished by post C:

Sasaki et al. [135] found this in rat heart; post C could terminate reperfusion arrhythmias.

Halkos et al. [136] also found a diminution in the incidence of ventricular fibrillation.

Similarly, Galagudza et al. [137] found that post C, started 15 min after reperfusion, converted ventricular fibrillation to sinus rhythm.

Reperfusion arrhythmias have in general been attributed to dysfunction of Ca^{2+} homeostasis.

14.8 Remote Conditioning (RIPC)

This extremely interesting phenomenon is being extensively studied for the reasons which will be described further. Maciel et al. [138] describe recently its mechanisms. They give the following reasons for its continuous and widening application: It is noninvasive, although it was first described by Przyklenk et al. [139] during an invasive procedure. Thus, the coronary arteries themselves are not directly involved, with avoidance of plaque rupture and distal embolization.

Subsequently application was extended to many other organs, such as the kidney, small intestine, and limbs [140, 141]. Conversely RIPC applied to other organs can protect the heart.

The most widely applied approach is intermittent occlusion of the arm.

As in locally applied pre C, the degree of protection afforded by RIPC depends on the number of cycle duration and effector organ mass. Johnsen et al. [142] recently described an algorithm based on these variables.

Thus, they found that four to six cycles afforded the greatest protection. Cycles lasting 2 min offered the same protection as 5 min, while cycles lasting 10 min inhibited protection. This brings into focus a point already discussed in pre C that too many cycles and too long duration may turn protection into injury [143–145].

As regards the operative mechanisms, many postulations have been offered. Heusch [56] and Hausenloy and Yellon [1] propose the following mechanisms:

14.8.1 Humoral Pathway

According to this concept humoral pathway reperfusion of the "remote" organ is necessary for RIPC, which implies that the factor generated by that organ must be transported to the heart [146, 147].

Also, Dickson et al. [148] showed that blood from a rabbit undergoing pre C reduced infarct size when transferred to a naive animal.

Shimizu et al. [149] also showed that transient limb ischemia can remotely protect through a humoral factor.

In a recent report by Gedik et al. [150], their results from 23 pts. undergoing RIPC were compared to 23 controls. They studied arterial plasma concentrations of 25 different cytokines; they found an increase of only interleukin-1α. They found, however, increased concentration of GDF-11, GHPH, IL-10, IL-6, IL-8, and IL-17, but did not attribute a preconditioning effect to these factors. They point out that IL-1α blockade has been found to induce IRI, but in isolated hearts its administration induces pre C [151] and also induces cardioprotection [152].

Maciel et al. [138] recently described that the coronary effluent from isolated rat hearts submitted to pre C was subjected to ultrafiltration in different molecular weight ranges. Only the <3.5–10 and <10 kDa fractions of hydrophobic eluate reduced IRI. Proteomic analysis identified 14 peptides; also PKC and K^+ATP channel activation was found in the 5–10 kDa fraction; the HSP70 protein was also identified by mass spectrometry.

Lim et al. [153] from Yellon's group postulated that RIPC requires both humoral and neural pathways.

Many other transferable factors are responsible for the effects of RIPC, i.e., adenosine [154], opioids [155], NO [156], and bradykinin [157], stromal-derived factor [158] and the calcitonin gene-related peptide [159] have been proposed according to Stokfisz et al. [32]. micro-RNA 144 has also been described as a circulating factor [160].

These factors are suggested to be thermolabile, hydrophobic, and < 15 kDa in size [149].

14.8.2 Neural Pathways

It is suggested that ischemia activates afferent neural pathways. Thus, renal nerve section abolished RIPC induced by renal artery occlusion [161].

Resection of the vagal nerve supply to the heart [162] also inhibits RIPC. Chemically, hexamethonium also inhibits RIPC [163].

Pickard et al. [164] in a report from the 8th Biennial Hatter Cardiovascular Institute Workshop discuss the actual pathway of the neural pathway. They report that the current paradigm postulates that autacoids – adenosine [165] and bradykinin – are produced in the remote tissue which stimulates local different sensory nerves [166].

14.9 Remote Ischemic Post C

As in the case of remote pre C, this technique is much less invasive and easy to perform. Accordingly, it is being implemented very frequently.

Indeed, as Kloner and Rezkalla point out [167], a theoretical concern is that multiple balloon inflations and deflations could cause microembolism. However, in the pioneering study of Laskey et al. [168], this complication was not seen in their patients.

As Bice and Baxter [119] describe, this also applies to interventions applied to organs distant from the heart. A detailed review was given by Schmidt et al. in 2015 [169], with the title "remote conditioning" since in the acute myocardial infarct setting, the borders between pre- and post C become less distinct. In fact, this technique is most frequently applied during the onset of reperfusion ([170, 171]). Actually, in the study of Loukogeorgakis et al. [171], the authors showed that remote post C can prevent local endothelial dysfunction.

McLeod et al. [172] have reviewed the efforts of remote ischemic "preconditioning" in acute myocardial infarction which will be discussed later in the "clinical results."

Repeated RIPC This concept is being advanced as a means toward decreasing left ventricular remodeling (REM) [173].

Wei et al. [174] applied repeated RIPC in post infarct rat hearts with a decrease in REM and improved survival.

Xu et al. [175] in a parallel effort found that hypoxia after an experimental myocardial infarction could reduce REM in rats. This would amount to chronic C [1].

14.10 Factors Affecting Pre C

This very powerful mechanism is affected by many factors: Ferdinandy et al. [176] give a very detailed review.

14.10.1 Left ventricular hypertrophy

Factors affecting LHV and its course from adaptive to maladaptive are discussed in the corresponding chapter. Very early studies by Moolman et al. [177] in spontaneous hypertensive rats (SHR) found that pre C is blunted. Here it must be reminded that SHR rats exhibit many myocardial abnormalities, developing heart failure quite early [178].

Speechly-Dick et al. [179] from Yellon's group found that in rat hearts rendered hypertrophic by DOCA administration pre C was preserved. Our group found the same results in LVH caused by abdominal aortic banding [180].

Rajesh et al. [181] reported exactly the same findings and added that this protective effect was abolished by glibenclamide or 5-HD, which signifies that $K^{+}ATP$ channels are involved.

Same results have been seen in Dahl salt-sensitive rats [182].

However, as will be subsequently discussed, when LV deteriorates toward HF, pre C is lost [183].

14.10.2 Age

Interestingly, Voucharas et al. [184] find that remote pre C is protective in hypertrophic but not in normal rat hearts.

Abete et al. [185] found that in 24-month-old rats, pre C was blunted. Tani et al. [186] reported similar results in middle-aged rats. Interestingly they found that exercise training restored the pre C effect [186].

However, Tomai et al. [187] did not find loss of pre C in elderly patients during PCI.

Abete et al. [188] give a detailed review on clinical application of pre C in the elderly.

They mention similar studies by Fenton et al. [189] and Bartling et al. [190].

The same authors also point out that the same effect is lost in diverse clinical situations [191–193]. Thus, pre-infarction angina does not protect elderly patients [194]; exercise pre C is also lost in the elderly hearts [195].

An opposite situation to an old age is the immature heart. Baker et al. [196] found that in rabbit hearts (age 7–10 days), protection against ischemia is preserved. The same researchers [197] found that these immature hearts are protected by pre C under normoxic but not hypoxic conditions [197].

Awad et al. [198] found that in isolated rat hearts, pre C develops within 7 days after birth. Iwaki et al. [199] found that in culture rat neonatal cardiomyocytes can produce HSP-70.

Ostádalová et al. [200] postulate that K^+ATP channels and NO protection in pre C may be ineffective in neonatal rat hearts.

The same group [201] recently reported a very interesting finding that chronic hypoxic exposure during early development may induce in utero a neonatal programming of various genes that can change the susceptibility of the adult heart to ischemic reperfusion in a gender-dependent manner.

14.10.3 Diabetes Mellitus

This is also a widely prevalent condition which affects cardiac structure and function in many ways. In earlier preclinical studies, Tosaki et al. [202] found that at the initial stages of diabetes induced in the rabbit, resistance to ischemia is increased, while it later decreases. Hadour et al. [203] found that diabetes represents a constantly preconditioned state.

Liu et al. [204] found that after streptozotocin administration, in the diabetic heart, the infarct size is reduced.

However, the additional protection of C may be blunted in diabetes and hyperglycemia [205] but is improved after insulin administration [206]. The same was found by Ebel et al. [207].

Kristiansen et al. [208] in rats also found the loss of pre C efficacy as Ravingerova et al. [209] found in the antiarrhythmic effect of pre C in rats. In a sheep model, pre C actually worsened the effect of IRI.

del Valle et al. [210] also found the loss of pre C protection in diabetic sheep.

Similarly, Lee and Chou [211] found diminution of the protective effects of pre C during angioplasty in diabetic patients.

Iliodromitis et al. suggest that in diabetic heart more intensive pre C is needed [21].

Also, Chang et al. [212] suggest that more pre C cycles are needed to diminish infarct size in the diabetic rat.

Ishihara et al. have [213] reported that pre-infarct angina was not protective in diabetic patients.

14.10.4 Hypercholesterolemia

Again not all studies report similar results. Szekeres et al. [214] found that pre C is diminished in hypercholesterolemia in rabbits.

Kremastinos et al. [215] however found that pre C is preserved, again in the rabbit.

Iliodromitis et al. [216] reported that past conditioning is ineffective in hypercholesterolemic rabbits [214].

Szilvassy et al. [217] found that pre C protection was lost in rabbits after 8 weeks of the hyperlipidemic diet. This was regained after a normal diet resumption; Ueda et al. [218] reported similar results, while Juhasz et al. [219] found that increasing PC cycles could even increase infarct size.

In the clinical setting, loss of pre C effectiveness was lost during PCI in hyperlipidemic patients [220, 221].

In studying late pre C in hyperlipidemic rabbits, Szekeres et al. [214] found that more ischemic cycles were needed to elicit protection.

Interestingly, statins although being cardioprotective in general and against IRI [222] have been shown to interfere with post C [223]. Possibly their overall protective effect may diminish the further beneficial effects of conditioning, in the concept that in the protected heart, conditioning has a smaller effect. Ferdinandy et al. [176] give an excellent overall review.

14.10.5 Thyroid Abnormalities

Our group has worked intensively by on this field. We have shown that pre C is more robust in hyperthyroid animals, while ischemic contracture is also intensified [224]. The question on the association of the degree of preconditioning-induced cardioprotection and intensity of contracture has already been discussed.

We have also shown that this protective effect is correlated to an increase in HSP-70 [225].

Interestingly, we found that although the hypothyroid heart shows increased tolerance to ischemia [226], it cannot be preconditioned [227].

14.10.6 Heart Failure

This aspect has not been adequately studied, yet its clinical importance is obvious, because protection by condition could be very important in the failing heart. Thus, Dekker et al. [228] found that in papillary muscles of rabbits with heart failure, ischemic pre C was not protective but actually injurious; probably this occurs because in the failing heart, any further ischemia even if light can be deleterious.

Ghosh et al. [229] also found that in chronic heart failure, pre C is inhibited.

Also, according to Miki et al. [230], pre C failed to protect the myocardium of remodeled rat hearts; this could be reversed with valsartan.

In this case, however, the question arises again if decreased contractility per se is cardioprotective, since as already reported contractility inhibition is protective in pre C but also in post C [120].

In this context, we have also shown that remodeling post MI rat hearts are protected against ischemia [231].

Masoud et al. [232] also found that remodeled mice hearts were more tolerant to ischemic injury.

Similarly Hu et al. [233] found that hibernating swine hearts show preservation of high-energy phosphate levels after simulated ischemia.

Yan et al. [234] also found that hibernation is associated with powerful cardioprotection which resembles pre C.

In the clinical context, Ishihara et al. [235] found that pre C effects of prodromal angina are lost in patients with a previous myocardial infarction.

These findings suggest a general behavior for the failing myocardium: Due to its decreased contractility, it is more protected, but cannot be further preconditioned.

14.10.7 Chronic Kidney Disease

Chronic kidney disease has been found to suppress Akt activation which plays a protective role in IRI and in pre C [236].

14.11 Comorbidities and Post C

As in pre C, many associated conditions can reduce its efficacy, a situation common in the human. Thus, in the presence of left ventricular hypertrophy (LVH), Penna et al. [237] showed that in rats which developed LVH by nandrolone treatment, its protective effect was abolished. As discussed in the case of pre C, not all models of LVH are similar or corresponding to the usual cause of LVH and hypertension. In this context, Fantinelli and Mosca [238] found that in LVH in SHR rats this beneficial effect is not abolished; the authors point out that specifically the PKC pathway is conserved.

Hypercholesterolemia may abolish the post C effect as already described by Iliodromitis et al. [216]. Kupai et al. found similar results [239].

Diabetes mellitus both type 1 and 2 may also decrease the post C effect in mice [240]; interestingly in the type 1 DM model, treatment re-established this protective effect. However, in another model type 2 DM, the post C beneficial action was reduced [241]. Other types of diabetes:

In the Zucker diabetic fatty rat model, Hjortbak et al. [242] found that the animals were endogenously protected and that conditioning reduced infarct size at 12 and 24 weeks. This actually involved pre C.

Zhu et al. [243] also showed that post C is ineffective in leptin-deficient obese ob/ob mice and type 2 diabetic mice.

14.12 Effects of remote preconditioning and comorbidities in other organs have also been intensively studied:

14.12.1 Kidney

A main effort has been against contrast medium-induced acute kidney injury. Er et al. have shown a positive effect in pts. with chronic kidney disease undergoing coronary interventions [244].

It has also been used in pts. undergoing aortocoronary bypass surgery [245].

Venugopal found the same in a secondary analysis of two small studies [246].

14.12.2 Brain

Here research is very intensive. Pre C has been seen to reduce infarct volume [247, 248].

Gidday gives a very detailed review in 2015 [249].

Another interesting aspect is cardiac resuscitation which is often associated with cerebral dysfunction. In this area, conditioning showed no benefit [250].

A type of conditioning which has and will be further discussed as regards the heart is “continuous C.” In this aspect, post TIA patients who were subjected to RIPC twice daily for 30 days had reduced MACE and improved cerebral perfusion [251].

14.12.3 Liver

Pre C showed improved survival and earlier organ function recovery [252]. Yin et al. [253] reported similar results. Koti et al. [254] have given an inclusive review.

Hardy et al. [255] reported somewhat more equivocal results in that they found that the prothrombin time was significantly improved; bilirubin, serum alkaline phosphatase, and alanine aminotransferase improved, but these did not reach significant improvement.

In the lung Soncul et al. found the benefit of pre C in lungs subjected to ischemia-reperfusion [256].

Also, the intestine can be protected by pre C [257].

Another area of pre C application is surgery of thoracoabdominal aneurysms where this technique has been applied to protect against spinal cord injury [258–261].

14.13 Paradigms of Conditioning in the Clinical Real-Life Setting

By discussing the instances where conditioning is present in various pathological conditions, the need of various applications as therapeutic interventions will emerge.

14.13.1 Effort Angina

The phenomenon of walk-through angina was described more than 200 years ago by Heberden [262].

The phenomenon of warm-up angina has a similar mechanism; in two consecutive efforts, either in everyday life or in exercise laboratory, pain occurs after greater exercise.

Mac Alpin and Kattus assessed this by electrocardiography [263].

Tomai [264] and Kelion et al. [265] gave pertinent description. Kelion et al. [265] found decreased ischemic myocardial dysfunction at the second exercise test.

Williams et al. found decreased lactic acid production with the two tests [266].

Okazaki and Kodama [267] also found a decrease in oxygen consumption. Both groups ascribe these effects to increased adenosine production.

In accordance to this postulation, Tomai et al. [268] found that glibenclamide, an inhibitor of K^+ATP opening, can inhibit exercise-induced pre C.

Maybaum et al. [269] found that in three consecutive treadmill exercise tests with the same work load, total ischemic time was markedly shortened in the last two tests.

Yellon's group shown that exercise can elicit delayed pre C [59]. Improvement in ischemic scintigraphic deficit after an exercise test has been found in conditions of early [270] and late [271] pre C.

Lalonde et al. [272] gave a very detailed meta-analysis in 2013.

14.13.2 Prodromal Angina

This has also been widely studied. It has been shown 20 years ago that it can limit infarct size [273, 274] and has shown that it can protect the myocardium for up to a week while according to Kloner et al. [275] for up to 2 days.

Also, in the TAMI [276], in TIMI-4 trials [277], and in the study by Ishihara et al. [213], an improvement was seen.

However, discrepant results have been reported, mostly in retrospective studies such as the TIMI II [278], the international tissue plasminogen activator/streptokinase mortality trial [279], and the GUSTO-1 trial [280].

The possible explanation can be advanced that in retrospective studies the time that has elapsed is difficult to accurately calculate and the protective effect of pre C can well have been lost. Further, multiple bouts of ischemia may have rendered the heart more vulnerable instead of being protected. The findings of the study of Abete et al. [194] that prodromal angina was much less protective in elderly pts. should not be forgotten.

14.13.3 Coronary Angioplasty (PCI)

Lesser ischemia hs been seen in the 2nd and 3rd inflation in older studies [281–283].

Masci et al. [284] found that in pts. with acute MI treated with primary PCI, those with prodromal angina have a higher myocardial salvage index and less microvascular damage.

Some pharmacological observations corroborate these findings. Thus, adenosine improves the stunning manifestations already seen by the first inflation [285]. On the contrary glibenclamide [286] and to a lesser degree glimepiride [287] blunt this response. Interestingly nitrates given 72 h before can induce protection during PCI [288]. The same can be seen with bradykinin [289].

14.14 Clinical Applications of Conditioning

Kloner and Rezkalla [167] describe the following circumstances in which conditioning can improve outcomes: cardiac surgery, myocardial infarction, PCI, cardiac transplantation, and cardiac resuscitation.

14.14.1 Cardiac Surgery:

A. Direct Pre C

Hausenloy and Yellon [1] remind the first successful application from Yellon's group [290]. They also mention a meta-analysis of 22 trials including 933 patients with positive results by Walsh et al. [291].

However, they comment on the difficulties of direct clamping, a frequently atherosclerotic aorta.

Sukkar [292] et al. recently give a systematic review and meta-analysis of the effect of ischemic conditioning in patients undergoing invasive procedures.

They identified 85 reports involving 13,800 patients; "central" C was investigated in 36% and RIPC in 64% of trials; in 65 trials anesthesia was used. Fifty-four percent of these volatile anesthetics were administered.

As regards outcomes, C did not affect all-cause mortality (RP 0.96), which was the primary outcome examined; C did not significantly reduce combined CV events or myocardial infarction. They postulate that it may reduce the risk of stroke (RP 0.72) but with very low quality evidence.

B. Remote Pre C

Pinaud et al. [293] found no effect on the heart or kidney protection of RIPC in pts undergoing aortic valve surgery.

Hausenloy and Yellon [1] report the results of major clinical studies of RIC (remote ischemic conditioning) in cardiac surgery. They mention eight positive studies (548 adults, 37 children) but also seven neutral studies (4663 pts).

Importantly, the last two very large trials by excellent groups yielded completely neutral results: the ERICA trial (1612 pts.) [294] and the RIPH heart study (1385 pts.) [295].

Zaugg and Lucchinetti [296] in an editorial postulate that RIPC in cardiac surgery is ineffective and may be risky; to support this argument they cite references of an increase of intracardiac expression of TNFα and myeloperoxidase activity.

14.14.2 Acute Myocardial Infarction

Mc Leod et al. [172] give a systematic review and meta-analysis of 11 articles involving 1220 patients in whom RIPC was assessed during acute myocardial infarction. Nowadays they involve PCI.

They found that the myocardial salvage index was higher and the infarct size was reduced, while the major cardiovascular events were lower. They do, however, stress the need for additional high-quality research.

Hausenloy et al. [1] also review seven completed studies of RIPC in STEMI (1521 patients) with a positive result. They point out in their conclusions that this setting offers the most promising data.

Blusztein et al. [297] performed a systematic review and meta-analysis evaluating ischemic C in PCI with and without MI.

During elective PCI, they found no decrease in mortality. In STEMI they found an improvement in myocardial salvage with RIP and diminution in infarct size in STEMI with local ischemic post C.

In this context Hausenloy and Yellon [1] mention six positive (393) and six neutral (129pts) trials with local post C in STEMI, excluding DANAMI 3.

In this very recent trial, local postconditioning in primary angioplasty in DANAMI 3 – a total of 1234 pts. – failed to show an effect with four repeated balloon occlusions [298].

As regards RIC in planned (elective) PCI, again Hausenloy and Yellon [1] mention six positive studies (1042 pts) and four neutral or negative studies (696 pts).

Concerning the neutral results in elective PCI and cardiac surgery, much discussion has been offered. The already described comorbidities may well play a role. Of course, elective PCI and surgery have currently very low morbidity and mortality and only low-grade IRI. Also, pre-existing medical therapy which continues during PCI and surgery offers protection which would not be easy to improve upon.

Van der Heide and Steenbergen [299] also discuss the pitfalls of applying laboratory C benefits to clinical practice. Apart from the reasons already given, they postulate that in animal studies thorough assessment of the effect on other organs is not carried out, while lesions in these organs may play an important role in the human. Heusch and Rassaf [300] in a review with the very provocative title "Time to Give Up on Cardioprotection" point out that adequate dose-finding phase II studies do not exist and that there exist only two phase II trials with RIPC in patients undergoing bypass surgery, both neutral. They conclude that it would be premature to give up cardioprotection. A pertinent point on RIPC is raised by many others in that sevoflurane volatile anesthetics offer cardioprotection on their own which can dampen the additional effect offered by C.

Propofol also confers cardioprotection although less than that of volatile anesthetics [301].

Thus, Li and Yuan [302] point out that compared with propofol, sevoflurane improved postoperative cardiac output, troponin I concentration, inotropic vasoconstrictor drug use, and atrial fibrillation incidence, but not ICU stay, post-op infarction, or mortality.

Yang et al. [303] also compared the effects of the 2 drugs in patients undergoing heart valve replacement surgery with cardiopulmonary bypass in 76 patients. They found lower TnI and CK-MB levels and the shorter ICU stay in the sevoflurane group.

Lucchinetti et al. [304] point out that with isoflurane pre C prevents activation of genomic remodeling program in rat hearts.

They again mention attenuation of RIPC by propofol [305] and isoflurane [306].

They also point out that the precise role of many comorbidities is an important factor. They conclude that the pursuit should continue with the quest for more effective protocols of C.

14.14.3 Cardiac Transplantation

Conditioning has been proposed since 20 years but apparently is not being used widely [307, 308].

14.14.4 Cardiopulmonary Resuscitation

Obviously, pre- and post C is difficult to apply in this setting. Ovize et al. [309] are currently studying cyclosporine in this setting. Thyroid hormones have given promising experimental results in preserving the donor heart before it is transplanted [310, 311] and are used clinically.

Bartos et al. [312] also give a detailed review in post C in this crucial situation.

14.14.5 TAVR

Recent studies have been reported with RIPC in transfemoral transcatheter aortic valve implantation.

Kahlert et al. [313] reported no protection of the heart, kidneys, and brain and no differences in mortality and MACE.

Repeated RIPC to Prevent Cardiac Remodeling As Hausenloy and Yellon describe [1] and Thijssen et al. [173] report in a very pertinent review on RIPC, there are two clinical trials in the UK and Canada, according to the experimental work of Wei et al. [174] and more recently of Yamaguchi et al. [314].

Conditioning is mentioned as an adjunct of cardioprotection by a group of experts in 2013 [315].

The same group in 2017 again remarked on various drugs and PIPC but again without more concrete recommendations [316].

The place of C in cardioprotection is well presented by G. Heusch [317].

Finally, Ovize's group very prominent in this field [309] give a very detailed and thoughtful review in 2013. They focus mainly on postconditioning.

In the area of STEMI treatment, they point out that although management of the culprit vessel is near optimal, treatment of the injured myocardium has not been as successful. As regards post C, they point out that for phase III trials, major adverse cardiovascular events reported are death, heart failure, reinfarction, unstable angina, stroke, and need for revascularization at the various time points. They stress that LV remodeling and arrhythmias should also be used, but also that too great a combination of end points presents the risk of lowering the statistical power of the study. They also discuss the optional time window for applying post C and discuss the efficacy of pharmacological versus ischemic post C.

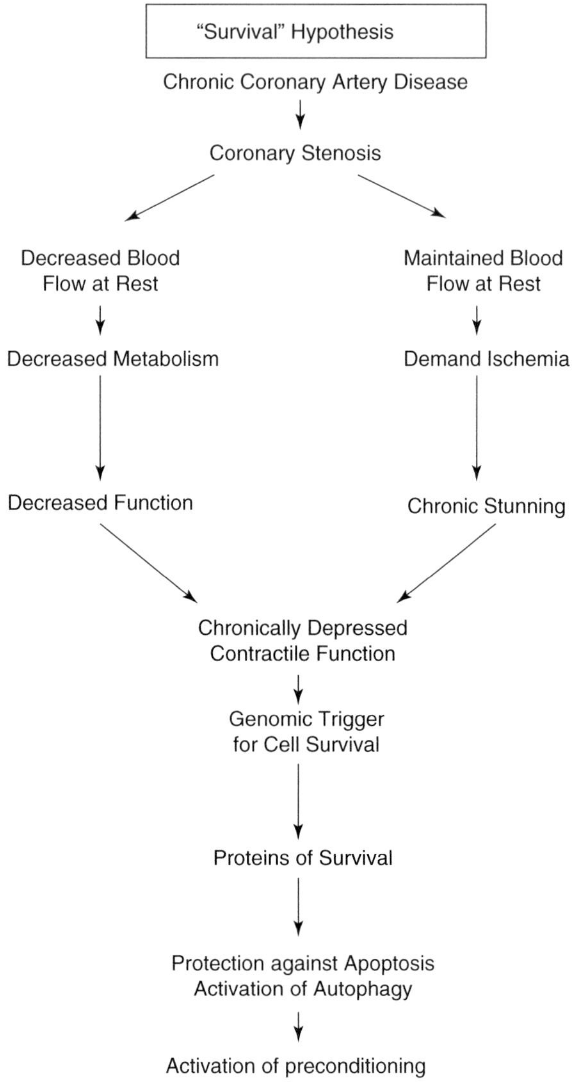

Fig. 14.1 Cell survival hypothesis for chronically ischemic myocardium. The figure illustrates the mechanisms of myocardial hibernation, comparing the "smart heart" hypothesis (left) and the "repetitive stunning" hypothesis (right), and shows how an adaptation of gene and protein expression and the regulation of intracellular processes (inhibition of apoptosis and activation of autophagy) lead to the maintained viability of the ischemic tissue. (Reproduced with permission from Depré and Stephen [318])

They discuss RIPC and point out the need to be removed from phase II to clinical outcomes trials.

Hausenloy and Yellon [1] reiterate in their very recent review that conditioning can be pre-, (classical and delayed), per-, post-, and delayed post- or continuous, thus covering all phases of cardioprotection and supporting cardiac preservation.

Depré and Vatner [318] place preconditioning in the survival hypothesis in pts. with chronic artery disease (Fig. 14.1).

In conclusion, after just more than 30 years since its discovery, conditioning in all its aspects remains a subject of intensive research which constantly brings new information. However, the clinical application is still being discussed and tried. It is obvious that combination of pre- and post C, local and remote together with exercise and pharmaceutical therapy, epigenetic interventions, and cell and gene therapy, must be implemented. As will be repeatedly stressed in other chapters of this book, no single therapy is to be considered any longer but as many interventions as possible must be employed in concerted efforts.

References

1. Hausenloy DJ, Yellon DM. Ischaemic conditioning and reperfusion injury. Nat Rev Cardiol. 2016;13:193–209.
2. Skyschally A, van Caster P, Iliodromitis EK, Schulz R, Kremastinos DT, Heusch G. Ischemic postconditioning: experimental models and protocol algorithms. Basic Res Cardiol. 2009;104:469–83.
3. Murry CE, Jennings RB, Reimer KA. Preconditioning with ischemia: a delay of lethal cell injury in ischemic myocardium. Circulation. 1986;74:1124–36.
4. Reimer KA, Murry CE, Yamasawa I, Hill ML, Jennings RB. Four brief periods of myocardial ischemia cause no cumulative ATP loss or necrosis. Am J Phys. 1986;251:H1306–15.
5. Baines CP, Pass JM, Ping P. Protein kinases and kinase-modulated effectors in the late phase of ischemic preconditioning. Basic Res Cardiol. 2001;96:207–18.
6. Downey JM, Cohen MV. Do mitochondrial K(ATP) channels serve as triggers rather than end-effectors of ischemic preconditioning's protection. Basic Res Cardiol. 2000:95272–4.
7. Gross GJ, Auchampach JA. Blockade of ATP-sensitive potassium channels prevents myocardial preconditioning in dogs. Circ Res. 1992:70223–33.
8. Downey JM, Cohen MV. Ischemic precondition. In: Cokkinos DV, Pantos C, Heusch G, Taegtmeyer H, editors. Myocardial ischemia: New York Springer; 2006. p. 99–112.
9. Baines CP, Cohen MV, Downey JM. Signal transduction in ischemic preconditioning: the role of kinases and mitochondrial K(ATP) channels. J Cardiovasc Electrophysiol. 1999;10:741–54.
10. Mocanu MM, Maddock HL, Baxter GF, Lawrence CL, Standen NB, Yellon DM. Glimepiride, a novel sulfonylurea, does not abolish myocardial protection afforded by either ischemic preconditioning or diazoxide. Circulation. 2001;103:3111–6.
11. Lawrence C, Rodrigo GC. A Na+–activated K+ current (IK, Na) is present in Guinea-pig but not rat ventricular myocytes. Pflugers Arch. 1999;437:831–8.
12. Garlid KD, Paucek P, Yarov-Yarovoy V, Murray HN, Darbenzio RB, D'Alonzo AJ, et al. Cardioprotective effect of diazoxide and its interaction with mitochondrial ATP-sensitive K^+ channels. Possible mechanism of cardioprotection. Circ Res. 1997;81:1072–82.
13. Grover GJ, Newburger J, Sleph PG, Dzwonczyk S, Taylor SC, Ahmed SZ, et al. Cardioprotective effects of the potassium channel opener cromakalim: stereoselectivity and effects on myocardial adenine nucleotides. J Pharmacol Exp Ther. 1991;257:156–62.
14. Grover GJ. Garlid KD.ATP-sensitive potassium channels: a review of their cardioprotective pharmacology. J Mol Cell Cardiol. 2000;32:677–95.
15. Geisen K, Végh A, Krause E, Papp JG. Cardiovascular effects of conventional sulfonylureas and glimepiride. Horm Metab Res. 1996;28:496–507.
16. Sato T, O'Rourke B, Marbán E. Modulation of mitochondrial ATP-dependent K+ channels by protein kinase C. Circ Res. 1998;83:110–4.
17. Garlid KD. Opening mitochondrial K(ATP) in the heart--what happens, and what does not happen. Basic Res Cardiol. 2000;95:275–9.
18. Liu Y, Sato T, O'Rourke B, Marban E. Mitochondrial ATP-dependent potassium channels: novel effectors of cardioprotection? Circulation. 1998;97:2463–9.
19. Forbes RA, Steenbergen C, Murphy E. Diazoxide-induced cardioprotection requires signaling through a redox-sensitive mechanism. Circ Res. 2001;88:802–9.

20. Pain T, Yang XM, Critz SD, Yue Y, Nakano A, Liu GS, et al. Opening of mitochondrial K (ATP) channels triggers the preconditioned state by generating free radicals. Circ Res. 2000;87:460–6.
21. Iliodromitis EK, Andreadou I, Dagres N, Kremastinos DT. Pre- Peri- Post-Conditioning the ischemic myocardium: Challenges, Confounders and Expectations. Introduction to Translational Cardiovascular Research Cokkinos DV, editor. Cham Springer, 2015. p. 541–52.
22. Murry CE, Richard VJ, Jennings RB, Reimer KA. Myocardial protection is lost before contractile function recovers from ischemic preconditioning. Am J Phys. 1991;260:H796–804.
23. Jennings RB, Sebbag L, Schwartz LM, Crago MS, Reimer KA. Metabolism of preconditioned myocardium: effect of loss and reinstatement of cardioprotection. J Mol Cell Cardiol. 2001;33:1571–88.
24. Garcia-Dorado D, Théroux P, Duran JM, Solares J, Alonso J, Sanz E, et al. Selective inhibition of the contractile apparatus. A new approach to modification of infarct size, infarct composition, and infarct geometry during coronary artery occlusion and reperfusion. Circulation. 1992;85:1160–74.
25. Kolocassides KG, Galiñanes M, Hearse DJ. Dichotomy of ischemic preconditioning: improved postischemic contractile function despite intensification of ischemic contracture. Circulation. 1996;93:1725–33.
26. Xin W, Yang X, Rich TC, Krieg T, Barrington R, Cohen MV, et al. All preconditioning-related G protein-coupled receptors can be demonstrated in the rabbit cardiomyocyte. J Cardiovasc Pharmacol Ther. 2012;17:190–8.
27. Hausenloy DJ, Tsang A, Mocanu MM, Yellon DM. Ischemic preconditioning protects by activating prosurvival kinases at reperfusion. Am J Physiol Heart Circ Physiol. 2005;288:H971–6.
28. Schulz R, Cohen MV, Behrends M, Downey JM, Heusch G. Signal transduction of ischemic preconditioning. Cardiovasc Res. 2001;52:181–98.
29. Yang XP, Liu YH, Scicli GM, Webb CR, Carretero OA. Role of kinins in the cardioprotective effect of preconditioning: study of myocardial ischemia/reperfusion injury in B2 kinin receptor knockout mice and kininogen-deficient rats. Hypertension. 1997;30:735–40.
30. Hattori R, Otani H, Uchiyama T, Imamura H, Cui J, Maulik N, et al. Src tyrosine kinase is the trigger but not the mediator of ischemic preconditioning. Am J Physiol Heart Circ Physiol. 2001;281:H1066–74.
31. Krieg T, Qin Q, Philipp S, Alexeyev MF, Cohen MV, Downey JM. Acetylcholine and bradykinin trigger preconditioning in the heart through a pathway that includes Akt and NOS. Am J Physiol Heart Circ Physiol. 2004;287:H2606–11.
32. Stokfisz K, Ledakowicz-Polak A, Zagorski M, Zielinska M. Ischaemic preconditioning - current knowledge and potential future applications after 30 years of experience. Adv Med Sci. 2017;62:307–16.
33. Vahlhaus C, Schulz R, Post H, Onallah R, Heusch G. No prevention of ischemic preconditioning by the protein kinase C inhibitor staurosporine in swine. Circ Res. 1996;79:407–14.
34. Ytrehus K, Liu Y, Downey JM. Preconditioning protects ischemic rabbit heart by protein kinase C activation. Am J Phys. 1994;266:H1145–52.
35. Hausenloy DJ, Maddock HL, Baxter GF, Yellon DM. Inhibiting mitochondrial permeability transition pore opening: a new paradigm for myocardial preconditioning? Cardiovasc Res. 2002;55:534–43.
36. Garcia-Dorado D, Inserte J, Ruiz-Meana M, González MA, Solares J, Juliá M, et al. Gap junction uncoupler heptanol prevents cell-to-cell progression of hypercontracture and limits necrosis during myocardial reperfusion. Circulation. 1997;96:3579–86.
37. Sun J. Protein S-nitrosylation: a role of nitric oxide signaling in cardiac ischemic preconditioning. Sheng Li Xue Bao. 2007;59:544–52.
38. Hausenloy DJ, Yellon DM. The second window of preconditioning (SWOP) where are we now? Cardiovasc Drugs Ther. 2010;24:235–54.

39. Marber MS, Latchman DS, Walker JM, Yellon DM. Cardiac stress protein elevation 24 hours after brief ischemia or heat stress is associated with resistance to myocardial infarction. Circulation. 1993;88:1264–72.
40. Kuzuya T, Hoshida S, Yamashita N, Fuji H, Oe H, Hori M, et al. Delayed effects of sublethal ischemia on the acquisition of tolerance to ischemia. Circ Res. 1993;72:1293–9.
41. Szekeres L, Papp JG, Szilvássy Z, Udvary E, Vegh A. Moderate stress by cardiac pacing may induce both short term and long term cardioprotection. Cardiovasc Res. 1993;27:593–6.
42. Yang F, Xi L. Postconditioning of ischemic heart by intermittent ventricular pacing at the beginning of reperfusion: novel mechanisms and potential utilities in interventional cardiology settings. Am J Physiol Heart Circ Physiol. 2016;310:H1–3.
43. Szekeres L. Drug-induced delayed cardiac protection against the effects of myocardial ischemia. Pharmacol Ther. 2005;108:269–80.
44. Szekeres L Exp Clin Cardiol 2000;5:116–21 underlines that late pre-C produced by stronger stressors. No archives available mentioned in Ref.
45. Domenech R, Macho P, Schwarze H, Sánchez G. Exercise induces early and late myocardial preconditioning in dogs. Cardiovasc Res. 2002;55:561–6.
46. Loukogeorgakis SP, Panagiotidou AT, Broadhead MW, Donald A, Deanfield JE, MacAllister RJ. Remote ischemic preconditioning provides early and late protection against endothelial ischemia-reperfusion injury in humans: role of the autonomic nervous system. J Am Coll Cardiol. 2005;46:450–6.
47. Baxter GF, Goma FM, Yellon DM. Characterisation of the infarct-limiting effect of delayed preconditioning: timecourse and dose-dependency studies in rabbit myocardium. Basic Res Cardiol. 1997;92:159–67.
48. Currie RW, Karmazyn M, Kloc M, Mailer K. Heat-shock response is associated with enhanced postischemic ventricular recovery. Circ Res. 1988;63:543–9.
49. Müllenheim J, Schlack W, Frässdorf J, Heinen A, Preckel B, Thämer V. Additive protective effects of late and early ischaemic preconditioning are mediated by the opening of KATP channels in vivo. Pflugers Arch. 2001;442:178–87.
50. Stambaugh K, Elliott GT, Jacobson KA, Liang BT. Additive effects of late preconditioning produced by monophosphoryl lipid a and the early preconditioning mediated by adenosine receptors and KATP channel. Circulation. 1999;99:3300–7.
51. Kaeffer N, Richard V, Thuillez C. Delayed coronary endothelial protection 24 hours after preconditioning: role of free radicals. Circulation. 1997;96:2311–6.
52. Guo Y, Stein AB, Wu WJ, Zhu X, Tan W, Li Q, Bolli R. Late preconditioning induced by NO donors, adenosine A1 receptor agonists, and delta1-opioid receptor agonists is mediated by iNOS. Am J Physiol Heart Circ Physiol. 2005;289:H2251–7.
53. Baxter GF, Marber MS, Patel VC, Yellon DM. Adenosine receptor involvement in a delayed phase of myocardial protection 24 hours after ischemic preconditioning. Circulation. 1994;90:2993–3000.
54. Dana A, Baxter GF, Walker JM, Yellon DM. Prolonging the delayed phase of myocardial protection: repetitive adenosine A1 receptor activation maintains rabbit myocardium in a preconditioned state. J Am Coll Cardiol. 1998;31:1142–9.
55. Kositprapa C, Ockaili RA, Kukreja RC. Bradykinin B2 receptor is involved in the late phase of preconditioning in rabbit heart. J Mol Cell Cardiol. 2001;33:1355–62.
56. Heusch G. Molecular basis of cardioprotection: signal transduction in ischemic pre-, post-, and remote conditioning. Circ Res. 2015;116:674–99.
57. Jaberansari MT, Baxter GF, Muller CA, Latouf SE, Röth E, Opie LH, et al. Angiotensin-converting enzyme inhibition enhances a subthreshold stimulus to elicit delayed preconditioning in pig myocardium. J Am Coll Cardiol. 2001;37:1996–2001.
58. Dana A, Skarli M, Papakrivopoulou J, Yellon DM. Adenosine a(1) receptor induced delayed preconditioning in rabbits: induction of p38 mitogen-activated protein kinase activation and Hsp27 phosphorylation via a tyrosine kinase- and protein kinase C-dependent mechanism. Circ Res. 2000;86:989–97.

59. Dana A, Jonassen AK, Yamashita N, Yellon DM. Adenosine a (1) receptor activation induces delayed preconditioning in rats mediated by manganese superoxide dismutase. Circulation. 2000;101:2841–8.
60. Bernardo NL, Okubo S, Maaieh MM, Wood MA, Kukreja RC. Delayed preconditioning with adenosine is mediated by opening of ATP-sensitive K(+) channels in rabbit heart. Am J Phys. 1999;277(1 Pt 2):H128–35.
61. Gross ER, Peart JN, Hsu AK, Auchampach JA, Gross GJ. Extending the cardioprotective window using a novel delta-opioid agonist fentanyl isothiocyanate via the PI3-kinase pathway. Am J Physiol Heart Circ Physiol. 2005;288:H2744–9.
62. Yu CK, Li YH, Wong GT, Wong TM, Irwin MG. Remifentanil preconditioning confers delayed cardioprotection in the rat. Br J Anaesth. 2007;99:632–8.
63. Bolli R, Li QH, Tang XL, Guo Y, Xuan YT, Rokosh G, et al. The late phase of preconditioning and its natural clinical application--gene therapy. Heart Fail Rev. 2007;12:189–99.
64. Qiu Y, Ping P, Tang XL, Manchikalapudi S, Rizvi A, Zhang J, et al. Direct evidence that protein kinase C plays an essential role in the development of late preconditioning against myocardial stunning in conscious rabbits and that epsilon is the isoform involved. J Clin Invest. 1998;101:2182–98.
65. Vahlhaus C, Schulz R, Post H, Rose J, Heusch G. Prevention of ischemic preconditioning only by combined inhibition of protein kinase C and protein tyrosine kinase in pigs. J Mol Cell Cardiol. 1998;30:197–209.
66. Xuan YT, Guo Y, Han H, Zhu Y, Bolli R. An essential role of the JAK-STAT pathway in ischemic preconditioning. Proc Natl Acad Sci U S A. 2001;98:9050–5.
67. Dawn B, Xuan YT, Guo Y, Rezazadeh A, Stein AB, Hunt G, et al. IL-6 plays an obligatory role in late preconditioning via JAK-STAT signaling and upregulation of iNOS and COX-2. Cardiovasc Res. 2004;64:61–71.
68. Bolli R, Manchikalapudi S, Tang XL, Takano H, Qiu Y, Guo Y, et al. The protective effect of late preconditioning against myocardial stunning in conscious rabbits is mediated by nitric oxide synthase. Evidence that nitric oxide acts both as a trigger and as a mediator of the late phase of ischemic preconditioning. Circ Res. 1997;81:1094–107.
69. Guo Y, Bao W, Wu WJ, Shinmura K, Tang XL, Bolli R. Evidence for an essential role of cyclooxygenase-2 as a mediator of the late phase of ischemic preconditioning in mice. Basic Res Cardiol. 2000;95:479–84.
70. Zhou X, Zhai X, Ashraf M. Direct evidence that initial oxidative stress triggered by preconditioning contributes to second window of protection by endogenous antioxidant enzyme in myocytes. Circulation. 1996;93:1177–784.
71. Shinmura K, Bolli R, Liu SQ, Tang XL, Kodani E, Xuan YT, et al. Aldose reductase is an obligatory mediator of the late phase of ischemic preconditioning. Circ Res. 2002;91:240–6.
72. Brooks AC, Guo Y, Singh M, McCracken J, Xuan YT, Srivastava S, et al. Endoplasmic reticulum stress-dependent activation of ATF3 mediates the late phase of ischemic preconditioning. J Mol Cell Cardiol. 2014;76:138–47.
73. Heusch G, Schulz R, Rahimtoola SH. Myocardial hibernation: a delicate balance. Am J Physiol Heart Circ Physiol. 2005;288:H984–99.
74. Takano H, Manchikalapudi S, Tang XL, Qiu Y, Rizvi A, Jadoon AK, et al. Nitric oxide synthase is the mediator of late preconditioning against myocardial infarction in conscious rabbits. Circulation. 1998;98:441–9.
75. Hu LF, Pan TT, Neo KL, Yong QC, Bian JS. Cyclooxygenase-2 mediates the delayed cardioprotection induced by hydrogen sulfide preconditioning in isolated rat cardiomyocytes. Pflugers Arch. 2008;455:971–8.
76. Calvert JW, Jha S, Gundewar S, Elrod JW, Ramachandran A, Pattillo CB, et al. Hydrogen sulfide mediates cardioprotection through Nrf2 signaling. Circ Res. 2009;105:365–74.
77. Sivarajah A, McDonald MC, Thiemermann C. The production of hydrogen sulfide limits myocardial ischemia and reperfusion injury and contributes to the cardioprotective effects of preconditioning with endotoxin, but not ischemia in the rat. Shock. 2006;26:154–61.

78. Sun JZ, Tang XL, Park SW, Qiu Y, Turrens JF, Bolli R. Evidence for an essential role of reactive oxygen species in the genesis of late preconditioning against myocardial stunning in conscious pigs. J Clin Invest. 1996;97:562–76.
79. Gross ER, Peart JN, Hsu AK, Grover GJ, Gross GJ. K(ATP) opener-induced delayed cardioprotection: involvement of sarcolemmal and mitochondrial K(ATP) channels, free radicals and MEK1/2. J Mol Cell Cardiol. 2003;35:985–92.
80. Xuan YT, Guo Y, Zhu Y, Wang OL, Rokosh G, Messing RO, et al. Role of the protein kinase C-epsilon-Raf-1-MEK-1/2-p44/42 MAPK signaling cascade in the activation of signal transducers and activators of transcription 1 and 3 and induction of cyclooxygenase-2 after ischemic preconditioning. Circulation. 2005;112:1971–8.
81. Maulik N, Watanabe M, Zu YL, Huang CK, Cordis GA, Schley JA, et al. Ischemic preconditioning triggers the activation of MAP kinases and MAPKAP kinase 2 in rat hearts. FEBS Lett. 1996;396:233–7.
82. Fryer RM, Hsu AK, Gross GJ. ERK and p38 MAP kinase activation are components of opioid-induced delayed cardioprotection. Basic Res Cardiol. 2001;96:136–42.
83. Kis A, Yellon DM, Baxter GF. Second window of protection following myocardial preconditioning: an essential role for PI3 kinase and p70S6 kinase. J Mol Cell Cardiol. 2003;35:1063–71.
84. Xuan YT, Tang XL, Banerjee S, Takano H, Li RC, Han H, et al. Nuclear factor-kappaB plays an essential role in the late phase of ischemic preconditioning in conscious rabbits. Circ Res. 1999;84:1095–109.
85. Li RC, Ping P, Zhang J, Wead WB, Cao X, Gao J, et al. PKCepsilon modulates NF-kappaB and AP-1 via mitogen-activated protein kinases in adult rabbit cardiomyocytes. Am J Physiol Heart Circ Physiol. 2000;279:H1679–89.
86. Cai Z, Manalo DJ, Wei G, Rodriguez ER, Fox-Talbot K, et al. Hearts from rodents exposed to intermittent hypoxia or erythropoietin are protected against ischemia-reperfusion injury. Circulation. 2003;108:79–85.
87. Jancsó G, Cserepes B, Gasz B, Benkó L, Borsiczky B, Ferenc A, et al. Expression and protective role of heme oxygenase-1 in delayed myocardial preconditioning. Ann N Y Acad Sci. 2007;1095:251–61.
88. Hausenloy D, Wynne A, Duchen M, Yellon D. Transient mitochondrial permeability transition pore opening mediates preconditioning-induced protection. Circulation. 2004;109:1714–7.
89. Ardehali H, O'Rourke B. Mitochondrial K(ATP) channels in cell survival and death. J Mol Cell Cardiol. 2005;39:7–16.
90. Yin C, Wang X, Kukreja RC. Endogenous microRNAs induced by heat-shock reduce myocardial infarction following ischemia-reperfusion in mice. FEBS Lett. 2008;582:4137–42.
91. Yin C, Salloum FN, Kukreja RC. A novel role of microRNA in late preconditioning: upregulation of endothelial nitric oxide synthase and heat shock protein 70. Circ Res. 2009;104:572–5.
92. Varga ZV, Giricz Z, Bencsik P, Madonna R, Gyongyosi M, Schulz R, et al. Functional genomics of cardioprotection by ischemic conditioning and the influence of comorbid conditions: implications in target identification. Curr Drug Targets. 2015;16:904–11.
93. Onody A, Zvara A, Hackler L Jr, Vígh L, Ferdinandy P, Puskás LG. Effect of classic preconditioning on the gene expression pattern of rat hearts: a DNA microarray study. FEBS Lett. 2003;536:35–40.
94. Das DK, Maulik N. Cardiac genomic response following preconditioning stimulus. Cardiovasc Res. 2006;70:254–63.
95. Gidlöf O, Johnstone AL, Bader K, Khomtchouk BB, O'Reilly JJ, Celik S, et al. Ischemic preconditioning confers epigenetic repression of mTOR and induction of autophagy through G9a-dependent H3K9 dimethylation. J Am Heart Assoc. 2016;5
96. Stenzel-Poore MP, Stevens SL, Simon RP. Genomics of preconditioning. Stroke. 2004;35:2683–6.
97. Zhao ZQ, Corvera JS, Halkos ME, Kerendi F, Wang NP, Guyton RA, et al. Inhibition of myocardial injury by ischemic postconditioning during reperfusion: comparison with isch-

emic preconditioning. This is very interesting mechanism. Am J Physiol Heart Circ Physiol. 2003;285:H579–88.
98. Buchholz B, Donato M, D'Annunzio V, Gelpi RJ. Ischemic postconditioning: mechanisms, comorbidities, and clinical application. Mol Cell Biochem. 2014;392:1–12.
99. Bell RM, Yellon DM. Conditioning the whole heart--not just the cardiomyocyte. J Mol Cell Cardiol. 2012;53:24–32.
100. Ovize M, Baxter GF, Di Lisa F, Ferdinandy P, Garcia-Dorado D, Hausenloy DJ, et al. Postconditioning and protection from reperfusion injury: where do we stand? Position paper from the working Group of Cellular Biology of the heart of the European society of cardiology. Cardiovasc Res. 2010;87:406–23.
101. Donato M, D'Annunzio V, Berg G, Gonzalez G, Schreier L, Morales C, et al. Ischemic postconditioning reduces infarct size by activation of A1 receptors and K+(ATP) channels in both normal and hypercholesterolemic rabbits. J Cardiovasc Pharmacol. 2007;49:287–92.
102. Buchholz B, D Annunzio V, Giani JF, Siachoque N, Dominici FP, Turyn D, et al. Ischemic postconditioning reduces infarct size through the α1-adrenergic receptor pathway. J Cardiovasc Pharmacol. 2014;63:504–11.
103. Inserte J, Barba I, Hernando V, Garcia-Dorado D. Delayed recovery of intracellular acidosis during reperfusion prevents calpain activation and determines protection in postconditioned myocardium. Cardiovasc Res. 2009;81:116–22.
104. Fujita M, Asanuma H, Hirata A, Wakeno M, Takahama H, Sasaki H, et al. Prolonged transient acidosis during early reperfusion contributes to the cardioprotective effects of postconditioning. Am J Physiol Heart Circ Physiol. 2007;292:H2004–8.
105. Yang XM, Proctor JB, Cui L, Krieg T, Downey JM, Cohen MV. Multiple, brief coronary occlusions during early reperfusion protect rabbit hearts by targeting cell signaling pathways. J Am Coll Cardiol. 2004;44:1103–10.
106. Penna C, Cappello S, Mancardi D, Raimondo S, Rastaldo R, Gattullo D, et al. Postconditioning reduces infarct size in the isolated rat heart: role of coronary flow and pressure and the nitric oxide/cGMP pathway. Basic Res Cardiol. 2006;101:168–79.
107. Inserte J, Hernando V, Vilardosa Ú, Abad E, Poncelas-Nozal M, Garcia-Dorado D. Activation of cGMP/protein kinase G pathway in postconditioned myocardium depends on reduced oxidative stress and preserved endothelial nitric oxide synthase coupling. J Am Heart Assoc. 2013;2:e005975.
108. Skyschally A, Gent S, Amanakis G, Schulte C, Kleinbongard P, Heusch G. Across-species transfer of protection by remote ischemic preconditioning with species-specific myocardial signal transduction by reperfusion injury salvage kinase and survival activating factor enhancement pathways. Circ Res. 2015;117:279–88.
109. Skyschally A, van Caster P, Boengler K, Gres P, Musiolik J, Schilawa D, et al. Ischemic postconditioning in pigs: no causal role for RISK activation. Circ Res. 2009;104:15–18. However, according to the same group activation showed that the phosphorylation of the RISK pathway does not reduce infarct size (113).
110. Gomez L, Paillard M, Thibault H, Derumeaux G, Ovize M. Inhibition of GSK3beta by postconditioning is required to prevent opening of the mitochondrial permeability transition pore during reperfusion. Circulation. 2008;117:2761–18.
111. Lim SY, Davidson SM, Hausenloy DJ, Yellon DM. Preconditioning and postconditioning: the essential role of the mitochondrial permeability transition pore. Cardiovasc Res. 2007;75:530–5.
112. Crisostomo PR, Wairiuko GM, Wang M, Tsai BM, Morrell ED, Meldrum DR. Preconditioning versus postconditioning: mechanisms and therapeutic potentials. J Am Coll Surg. 2006;202:797–812.
113. Kin H, Zatta AJ, Lofye MT, Amerson BS, Halkos ME, Kerendi F, et al. Postconditioning reduces infarct size via adenosine receptor activation by endogenous adenosine. Cardiovasc Res. 2005;67:124–33.

114. Mewton N, Ivanès F, Cour M, Ovize M. Postconditioning: from experimental proof to clinical concept. Dis Model Mech. 2010;3:39–44.
115. Argaud L, Gateau-Roesch O, Raisky O, Loufouat J, Robert D, Ovize M. Postconditioning inhibits mitochondrial permeability transition. Circulation. 2005;111:194–7.
116. Argaud L, Gomez L, Gateau-Roesch O, Couture-Lepetit E, Loufouat J, Robert D, et al. Trimetazidine inhibits mitochondrial permeability transition pore opening and prevents lethal ischemia-reperfusion injury. J Mol Cell Cardiol. 2005;39:893–9.
117. Baines CP, Kaiser RA, Purcell NH, Blair NS, Osinska H, Hambleton MA, et al. Loss of cyclophilin D reveals a critical role for mitochondrial permeability transition in cell death. Nature. 2005;434:658–62.
118. Shanmuganathan S, Hausenloy DJ, Duchen MR, Yellon DM. Mitochondrial permeability transition pore as a target for cardioprotection in the human heart. Am J Physiol Heart Circ Physiol. 2005;28:H237–42.
119. Bice JS, Baxter GF. Postconditioning signalling in the heart: mechanisms and translatability. Br J Pharmacol. 2015;172:1933–46.
120. Moriguchi A, Otani H, Yoshioka K, Shimazu T, Fujita M, Okazaki T, et al. Inhibition of contractile activity during postconditioning enhances cardioprotection by restoring sarcolemmal dystrophin through phosphatidylinositol 3-kinase. Circ J. 2010;74:2393–402.
121. Argaud L, Loufouat J, Gateau-Roesch O, Gomez L, Robert D, Ovize M. Persistent inhibition of mitochondrial permeability transition by preconditioning during the first hours of reperfusion. Shock. 2008;30:552–6.
122. Kin H, Zhao ZQ, Sun HY, Wang NP, Corvera JS, Halkos ME, et al. Postconditioning attenuates myocardial ischemia-reperfusion injury by inhibiting events in the early minutes of reperfusion. Cardiovasc Res. 2004;62:74–85.
123. Roubille F, Franck-Miclo A, Covinhes A, Lafont C, Cransac F, Combes S, et al. Delayed postconditioning in the mouse heart in vivo. Circulation. 2011;124:1330–1336. Staat et al (128) applied 4 cycles of 1-minute ischemia.
124. Staat P, Rioufol G, Piot C, Cottin Y, Cung TT, L'Huillier I, et al. Postconditioning the human heart. Circulation. 2005;112:2143–8.
125. Sato H, Jordan JE, Zhao ZQ, Sarvotham SS, Vinten-Johansen J. Gradual reperfusion reduces infarct size and endothelial injury but augments neutrophil accumulation. Ann Thorac Surg. 1997;64:1099–107.
126. Okamoto F, Allen BS, Buckberg GD, Bugyi H, Leaf J. Reperfusion conditions: importance of ensuring gentle versus sudden reperfusion during relief of coronary occlusion. J Thorac Cardiovasc Surg. 1986;92:613–20.
127. Na HS, Kim YI, Yoon YW, Han HC, Nahm SH, Hong SK. Ventricular premature beat-driven intermittent restoration of coronary blood flow reduces the incidence of reperfusion-induced ventricular fibrillation in a cat model of regional ischemia. Am Heart J. 1996;132:78–83.
128. Tian Y, Zhang W, Xia D, Modi P, Liang D, Wei M. Postconditioning inhibits myocardial apoptosis during prolonged reperfusion via a JAK2-STAT3-Bcl-2 pathway. J Biomed Sci. 2011;18:53.
129. Kin H, Wang NP, Mykytenko J, Reeves J, Deneve J, Jiang R, et al. Inhibition of myocardial apoptosis by postconditioning is associated with attenuation of oxidative stress-mediated nuclear factor-kappa B translocation and TNF alpha release. Shock. 2008;29:761–8.
130. Sun HY, Wang NP, Kerendi F, Halkos M, Kin H, Guyton RA, et al. Hypoxic postconditioning reduces cardiomyocyte loss by inhibiting ROS generation and intracellular Ca2+ overload. Am J Physiol Heart Circ Physiol. 2005;288:H1900–98.
131. Sun HY, Wang NP, Halkos M, Kerendi F, Kin H, Guyton RA, et al. Postconditioning attenuates cardiomyocyte apoptosis via inhibition of JNK and p38 mitogen-activated protein kinase signaling pathways. Apoptosis. 2006;11:1583–93.

132. Engelman DT, Watanabe M, Engelman RM, Rousou JA, Flack JE 3rd, Deaton DW, et al. Constitutive nitric oxide release is impaired after ischemia and reperfusion. J Thorac Cardiovasc Surg. 1995;110:1047–53.
133. Zhao JL, Yang YJ, You SJ, Cui CJ, Gao RL. Different effects of postconditioning on myocardial no-reflow in the normal and hypercholesterolemic mini-swines. Microvasc Res. 2007;73:137–42.
134. Shinohara G, Morita K, Nagahori R, Koh Y, Kinouchi K, Abe T, et al. Ischemic postconditioning promotes left ventricular functional recovery after cardioplegic arrest in an in vivo piglet model of global ischemia reperfusion injury on cardiopulmonary bypass. J Thorac Cardiovasc Surg. 2011;142:926–32.
135. Sasaki H, Shimizu M, Ogawa K, Okazaki F, Taniguchi M, Taniguchi I, et al. Brief ischemia-reperfusion performed after prolonged ischemia (ischemic postconditioning) can terminate reperfusion arrhythmias with no reduction of cardiac function in rats. Int Heart J. 2007;48:205–13.
136. Halkos ME, Kerendi F, Corvera JS, Wang NP, Kin H, Payne CS, et al. Myocardial protection with postconditioning is not enhanced by ischemic preconditioning. Ann Thorac Surg. 2004;78:961–9. discussion 969.
137. Galagudza M, Kurapeev D, Minasian S, Valen G, Vaage J. Ischemic postconditioning: brief ischemia during reperfusion converts persistent ventricular fibrillation into regular rhythm. Eur J Cardiothorac Surg. 2004;25:1006–10.
138. Maciel L, de Oliveira DF, Verissimo Da Costa GC, Bisch PM, Jhm N. Cardioprotection by the transfer of coronary effluent from ischaemic preconditioned rat hearts: identification of cardioprotective humoral factors. Basic Res Cardiol. 2017;112:152.
139. Przyklenk K, Bauer B, Ovize M, Kloner RA, Whittaker P. Regional ischemic 'preconditioning' protects remote virgin myocardium from subsequent sustained coronary occlusion. Circulation. 1993;87:893–9.
140. Birnbaum Y, Hale SL, Kloner RA. Ischemic preconditioning at a distance: reduction of myocardial infarct size by partial reduction of blood supply combined with rapid stimulation of the gastrocnemius muscle in the rabbit. Circulation. 1997;96:1641–6.
141. Kharbanda RK, Mortensen UM, White PA, Kristiansen SB, Schmidt MR, Hoschtitzky JA, et al. Transient limb ischemia induces remote ischemic preconditioning in vivo. Circulation. 2002;106:2881–3.
142. Johnsen J, Pryds K, Salman R, Løfgren B, Kristiansen SB, Bøtker HE. The remote ischemic preconditioning algorithm: effect of number of cycles, cycle duration and effector organ mass on efficacy of protection. Basic Res Cardiol. 2016;111:10.
143. Li GC, Vasquez JA, Gallagher KP, Lucchesi BR. Myocardial protection with preconditioning. Circulation. 1990;82:609–19.
144. Cohen MV, Yang XM, Downey JM. Conscious rabbits become tolerant to multiple episodes of ischemic preconditioning. Circ Res. 1994;74:998–1004.
145. Iliodromitis EK, Kremastinos DT, Katritsis DG, Papadopoulos CC, Hearse DJ. Multiple cycles of preconditioning cause loss of protection in open-chest rabbits. J Mol Cell Cardiol. 1997;29:915–20.
146. Serejo FC, Rodrigues LF Jr, da Silva Tavares KC, de Carvalho AC, Nascimento JH. Cardioprotective properties of humoral factors released from rat hearts subject to ischemic preconditioning. J Cardiovasc Pharmacol. 2007;49:214–20.
147. Gho BC, Schoemaker RG, van den Doel MA, Duncker DJ, Verdouw PD. Myocardial protection by brief ischemia in noncardiac tissue. Circulation. 1996;94:2193–200.
148. Dickson EW, Reinhardt CP, Renzi FP, Becker RC, Porcaro WA, Heard SO. Ischemic preconditioning may be transferable via whole blood transfusion: preliminary evidence. J Thromb Thrombolysis. 1999;8:123–9.
149. Shimizu M, Tropak M, Diaz RJ, Suto F, Surendra H, Kuzmin E, et al. Transient limb ischaemia remotely preconditions through a humoral mechanism acting directly on the myocardium: evidence suggesting cross-species protection. Clin Sci (Lond). 2009;117:191–200.

150. Gedik N, Kottenberg E, Thielmann M, Frey UH, Jakob H, Peters J, et al. Potential humoral mediators of remote ischemic preconditioning in patients undergoing surgical coronary revascularization. Sci Rep. 2017;7:12660.
151. Maulik N, Engelman RM, Wei Z, Lu D, Rousou JA, Das DK. Interleukin-1 alpha preconditioning reduces myocardial ischemia reperfusion injury. Circulation. 1993;88:II387–94.
152. Nogae C, Makino N, Hata T, Nogae I, Takahashi S, Suzuki K, et al. Interleukin 1 alpha-induced expression of manganous superoxide dismutase reduces myocardial reperfusion injury in the rat. J Mol Cell Cardiol. 1995;27:2091–9.
153. Lim SY, Yellon DM, Hausenloy DJ. The neural and humoral pathways in remote limb ischemic preconditioning. Basic Res Cardiol. 2010;105:651–5.
154. Leung CH, Wang L, Nielsen JM, Tropak MB, Fu YY, Kato H, et al. Remote cardioprotection by transfer of coronary effluent from ischemic preconditioned rabbit heart preserves mitochondrial integrity and function via adenosine receptor activation. Cardiovasc Drugs Ther. 2014;28:7–17.
155. Dickson EW, Blehar DJ, Carraway RE, Heard SO, Steinberg G, Przyklenk K. Naloxone blocks transferred preconditioning in isolated rabbit hearts. J Mol Cell Cardiol. 2001;33:1751–6.
156. Rassaf T, Totzeck M, Hendgen-Cotta UB, Shiva S, Heusch G, Kelm M. Circulating nitrite contributes to cardioprotection by remote ischemic preconditioning. Circ Res. 2014;114:1601–10.
157. Schoemaker RG, van Heijningen CL. Bradykinin mediates cardiac preconditioning at a distance. Am J Physiol Heart Circ Physiol. 2000;278:H1571–6.
158. Davidson SM, Selvaraj P, He D, Boi-Doku C, Yellon RL, Vicencio JM, et al. Remote ischaemic preconditioning involves signalling through the SDF-1α/CXCR4 signalling axis. Basic Res Cardiol. 2013;108:377.
159. Brzozowski T, Konturek PC, Konturek SJ, Pajdo R, Kwiecien S, Pawlik M, et al. Ischemic preconditioning of remote organs attenuates gastric ischemia-reperfusion injury through involvement of prostaglandins and sensory nerves Eur J Pharmacol. 2004 Sep 19;499:201–213. Among the ubiquitous miRs, microRNA-144 has also been recently described (165).
160. Li J, Rohailla S, Gelber N, Rutka J, Sabah N, Gladstone RA, et al. MicroRNA-144 is a circulating effector of remote ischemic preconditioning. Basic Res Cardiol. 2014;109:423.
161. Ding YF, Zhang MM, He RR. Role of renal nerve in cardioprotection provided by renal ischemic preconditioning in anesthetized rabbits. Sheng Li Xue Bao. 2001;53:7–12.
162. Dong JH, Liu YX, Zhao J, Ma HJ, Guo SM, He RR. High-frequency electrical stimulation of femoral nerve reduces infarct size following myocardial ischemia-reperfusion in rats. Sheng Li Xue Bao. 2004;56:620–4.
163. Donato M, Buchholz B, Rodríguez M, Pérez V, Inserte J, García-Dorado D, et al. Role of the parasympathetic nervous system in cardioprotection by remote hindlimb ischaemic preconditioning. Exp Physiol. 2013;98:425–34.
164. Pickard JM, Bøtker HE, Crimi G, Davidson B, Davidson SM, Dutka D, et al. Remote ischemic conditioning: from experimental observation to clinical application: report from the 8th biennial hatter cardiovascular institute workshop. Basic Res Cardiol. 2015;110:453.
165. Liem DA, Verdouw PD, Ploeg H, Kazim S, Duncker DJ. Sites of action of adenosine in interorgan preconditioning of the heart. Am J Physiol Heart Circ Physiol. 2002;283:H29–37.
166. Wolfrum S, Schneider K, Heidbreder M, Nienstedt J, Dominiak P, Dendorfer A. Remote preconditioning protects the heart by activating myocardial PKCepsilon-isoform. Cardiovasc Res. 2002;55:583–9.
167. Kloner RA, Rezkalla SH. Preconditioning, postconditioning and their application to clinical cardiology. Cardiovasc Res. 2006;70:297–307.
168. Laskey WK. Brief repetitive balloon occlusions enhance reperfusion during percutaneous coronary intervention for acute myocardial infarction: a pilot study. Catheter Cardiovasc Interv. 2005;65:361–7.
169. Schmidt MR, Redington A, Bøtker HE. Remote conditioning the heart overview: translatability and mechanism. Br J Pharmacol. 2015;172:1947–60.

170. Kharbanda RK, Peters M, Walton B, Kattenhorn M, Mullen M, Klein N, et al. Ischemic preconditioning prevents endothelial injury and systemic neutrophil activation during ischemia-reperfusion in humans in vivo. Circulation. 2001;103:1624–30.
171. Loukogeorgakis SP, Panagiotidou AT, Yellon DM, Deanfield JE, MacAllister RJ. Postconditioning protects against endothelial ischemia-reperfusion injury in the human forearm. Circulation. 2006;113:1015–9.
172. McLeod SL, Iansavichene A, Cheskes S. Remote ischemic perconditioning to reduce reperfusion injury during acute ST-segment-elevation myocardial infarction: a systematic review and meta-analysis. J Am Heart Assoc. 2017;6
173. Thijssen D, Maxwell J, Green DJ, Cable NT, Jones H. Repeated ischaemic preconditioning: a novel therapeutic intervention and potential underlying mechanisms. Exp Physiol. 2016;101:677–92.
174. Wei M, Xin P, Li S, Tao J, Li Y, Li J, et al. Repeated remote ischemic postconditioning protects against adverse left ventricular remodeling and improves survival in a rat model of myocardial infarction. Circ Res. 2011;108:1220–5.
175. Xu WQ, Yu Z, Xie Y, Huang GQ, Shu XH, Zhu Y, et al. Therapeutic effect of intermittent hypobaric hypoxia on myocardial infarction in rats. Basic Res Cardiol. 2011;106:329–42.
176. Ferdinandy P, Schulz R, Baxter GF. Interaction of cardiovascular risk factors with myocardial ischemia/reperfusion injury, preconditioning, and postconditioning. Pharmacol Rev. 2007;59:418–58.
177. Moolman JA, Genade S, Tromp E, Opie LH, Lochner A. Ischaemic preconditioning does not protect hypertrophied myocardium against ischaemia. S Afr Med J. 1997;87(Suppl 3):C151–6.
178. Brooks WW, Shen SS, Conrad CH, Goldstein RH, Bing OH. Transition from compensated hypertrophy to systolic heart failure in the spontaneously hypertensive rat: structure, function, and transcript analysis. Genomics. 2010;95:84–92.
179. Speechly-Dick ME, Baxter GF, Yellon DM. Ischaemic preconditioning protects hypertrophied myocardium. Cardiovasc Res. 1994;28:1025–9.
180. Pantos CI, Davos CH, Carageorgiou HC, Varonos DV, Cokkinos DV. Ischaemic preconditioning protects against myocardial dysfunction caused by ischaemia in isolated hypertrophied rat hearts. Basic Res Cardiol. 1996;91:444–9.
181. Rajesh KG, Sasaguri S, Suzuki R, Xing Y, Maeda H. Ischemic preconditioning prevents reperfusion heart injury in cardiac hypertrophy by activation of mitochondrial KATP channels. Int J Cardiol. 2004;96:41–9.
182. Butler KL, Huang AH, Gwathmey JK. AT1-receptor blockade enhances ischemic preconditioning in hypertrophied rat myocardium. Am J Phys. 1999;277:H2482–7.
183. Behr TM, Nerurkar SS, Nelson AH, Coatney RW, Woods TN, Sulpizio A, et al. Hypertensive end-organ damage and premature mortality are p38 mitogen-activated protein kinase-dependent in a rat model of cardiac hypertrophy and dysfunction. Circulation. 2001;104:1292–8.
184. Voucharas C, Lazou A, Triposkiadis F, Tsilimingas N. Remote preconditioning in normal and hypertrophic rat hearts. J Cardiothorac Surg. 2011;6:34.
185. Abete P, Ferrara N, Cioppa A, Ferrara P, Bianco S, Calabrese C, et al. Preconditioning does not prevent postischemic dysfunction in aging heart. J Am Coll Cardiol. 1996;27:1777–86.
186. Tani M, Honma Y, Hasegawa H, Tamaki K. Direct activation of mitochondrial K(ATP) channels mimics preconditioning but protein kinase C activation is less effective in middle-aged rat hearts. Cardiovasc Res. 2001;49:56–68.
187. Tomai F, Crea F, Ghini AS, Proietti I, Gaspardone A, Versaci F, et al. Ischemic preconditioning during coronary angioplasty is preserved in elderly patients. Ital Heart J. 2000;1:562–8.
188. Abete P, Cacciatore F, Testa G, Della-Morte D, Galizia G, Ferrara N, et al. Clinical application of ischemic preconditioning in the elderly. Dose Response. 2009;8:34–40.
189. Fenton RA, Dickson EW, Meyer TE, Dobson JG Jr. Aging reduces the cardioprotective effect of ischemic preconditioning in the rat heart. J Mol Cell Cardiol. 2000;32:1371–15.

190. Bartling B, Friedrich I, Silber RE, Simm A. Ischemic preconditioning is not cardioprotective in senescent human myocardium. Ann Thorac Surg. 2003;76:105–11.
191. Longobardi G, Abete P, Ferrara N, Papa A, Rosiello R, Furgi G, et al. "Warm-up" phenomenon in adult and elderly patients with coronary artery disease: further evidence of the loss of "ischemic preconditioning" in the aging heart. J Gerontol A Biol Sci Med Sci. 2000;55:M124–9.
192. Wu ZK, Pehkonen E, Laurikka J, Kaukinen L, Honkonen EL, Kaukinen S, et al. The protective effects of preconditioning decline in aged patients undergoing coronary artery bypass grafting. J Thorac Cardiovasc Surg. 2001;122:972–8.
193. Ebrahim Z, Yellon DM, Baxter GF. Ischemic preconditioning is lost in aging hypertensive rat heart: independent effects of aging and longstanding hypertension. Exp Gerontol. 2007;42:807–14.
194. Abete P, Ferrara N, Cacciatore F, Madrid A, Bianco S, Calabrese C, et al. Angina-induced protection against myocardial infarction in adult and elderly patients: a loss of preconditioning mechanism in the aging heart? J Am Coll Cardiol. 1997;30:947–54.
195. Ye JX, Chen DZ. Novel cardioprotective strategy combining three different preconditioning methods to prevent ischemia/reperfusion injury in aged hearts in an improved rabbit model. Exp Ther Med. 2015;10:1339–47.
196. Baker JE, Holman P, Gross GJ. Preconditioning in immature rabbit hearts: role of KATP channels. Circulation. 1999;99:1249–54.
197. Baker EJ, Boerboom LE, Olinger GN, Baker JE. Tolerance of the developing heart to ischemia: impact of hypoxemia from birth. Am J Phys. 1995;268:H1165–73.
198. Awad WI, Shattock MJ, Chambers DJ. Ischemic preconditioning in immature myocardium. Circulation. 1998;98:II206–13.
199. Iwaki K, Chi SH, Dillmann WH, Mestril R. Induction of HSP70 in cultured rat neonatal cardiomyocytes by hypoxia and metabolic stress. Circulation. 1993;87:2023–32.
200. Ostádalová I, Ostádal B, Jarkovská D, Kolár F. Ischemic preconditioning in chronically hypoxic neonatal rat heart. Pediatr Res. 2002;52:561–7.
201. Ostadalova B, Ostadalova I, Kolar F, Sedmera D. Developmental determinants of cardiac sensitivity to hypoxia. Can J Physiol Pharmacol. 2014;92:566–74.
202. Tosaki A, Engelman DT, Engelman RM, Das DK. The evolution of diabetic response to ischemia/reperfusion and preconditioning in isolated working rat hearts. Cardiovasc Res. 1996;31:526–36.
203. Hadour G, Ferrera R, Sebbag L, Forrat R, Delaye J, de Lorgeril M. Improved myocardial tolerance to ischaemia in the diabetic rabbit. J Mol Cell Cardiol. 1998;30:1869–75.
204. Liu Y, Thornton JD, Cohen MV, Downey JM, Schaffer SW. Streptozotocin-induced non-insulin-dependent diabetes protects the heart from infarction. Circulation. 1993;88:1273–8.
205. Kersten JR, Montgomery MW, Ghassemi T, Gross ER, Toller WG, Pagel PS, et al. Diabetes and hyperglycemia impair activation of mitochondrial K(ATP) channels. Am J Physiol Heart Circ Physiol. 2001;280:H1744–50.
206. Kersten JR, Toller WG, Gross ER, Pagel PS, Warltier DC. Diabetes abolishes ischemic preconditioning: role of glucose, insulin, and osmolality. Am J Physiol Heart Circ Physiol. 2000;278:H1218–24.
207. Ebel D, Müllenheim J, Frässdorf J, Heinen A, Huhn R, Bohlen T, et al. Effect of acute hyperglycaemia and diabetes mellitus with and without short-term insulin treatment on myocardial ischaemic late preconditioning in the rabbit heart in vivo. Pflugers Arch. 2003;446:175–82.
208. Kristiansen SB, Løfgren B, Støttrup NB, Khatir D, Nielsen-Kudsk JE, Nielsen TT, et al. Ischaemic preconditioning does not protect the heart in obese and lean animal models of type 2 diabetes. Diabetologia. 2004;47:1716–21.
209. Ravingerová T, Stetka R, Pancza D, Ulicná O, Ziegelhöffer A, Styk J. Susceptibility to ischemia-induced arrhythmias and the effect of preconditioning in the diabetic rat heart. Physiol Res. 2000;49:607–16.

210. del Valle HF, Lascano EC, Negroni JA, Crottogini AJ. Absence of ischemic preconditioning protection in diabetic sheep hearts: role of sarcolemmal KATP channel dysfunction. Mol Cell Biochem. 2003;249:21–30.
211. Lee TM, Chou TF. Impairment of myocardial protection in type 2 diabetic patients. J Clin Endocrinol Metab. 2003;88:531–7.
212. Tsang A, Hausenloy DJ, Mocanu MM, Carr RD, Yellon DM. Preconditioning the diabetic heart - the importance of Akt phosphorylation. Diabetes. 2005;54:2360–4.
213. Ishihara M, Sato H, Tateishi H, Kawagoe T, Shimatani Y, Kurisu S, et al. Implications of prodromal angina pectoris in anterior wall acute myocardial infarction: acute angiographic findings and long-term prognosis. J Am Coll Cardiol. 1997;30:970–5.
214. Szekeres L, Szilvássy Z, Ferdinandy P, Nagy I, Karcsu S, Csáti S. Delayed cardiac protection against harmful consequences of stress can be induced in experimental atherosclerosis in rabbits. J Mol Cell Cardiol. 1997;29:1977–83.
215. Kremastinos DT, Bofilis E, Karavolias GK, Papalois A, Kaklamanis L, Iliodromitis EK. Preconditioning limits myocardial infarct size in hypercholesterolemic rabbits. Atherosclerosis. 2000;150:81–9.
216. Iliodromitis EK, Zoga A, Vrettou A, Andreadou I, Paraskevaidis IA, Kaklamanis L, et al. The effectiveness of postconditioning and preconditioning on infarct size in hypercholesterolemic and normal anesthetized rabbits. Atherosclerosis. 2006;188:356–62.
217. Szilvassy Z, Ferdinandy P, Szilvassy J, Nagy I, Karcsu S, Lonovics J, et al. The loss of pacing-induced preconditioning in atherosclerotic rabbits: role of hypercholesterolaemia. J Mol Cell Cardiol. 1995;27:2559–69.
218. Ueda Y, Kitakaze M, Komamura K, Minamino T, Asanuma H, Sato H, et al. Pravastatin restored the infarct size-limiting effect of ischemic preconditioning blunted by hypercholesterolemia in the rabbit model of myocardial infarction. J Am Coll Cardiol. 1999;34:2120–05.
219. Juhasz B, Der P, Turoczi T, Bacskay I, Varga E, Tosaki A. Preconditioning in intact and previously diseased myocardium: laboratory or clinical dilemma? Antioxid Redox Signal. 2004;6:325–33.
220. Kyriakides ZS, Psychari S, Iliodromitis EK, Kolettis TM, Sbarouni E, Kremastinos DT. Hyperlipidemia prevents the expected reduction of myocardial ischemia on repeated balloon inflations during angioplasty. Chest. 2002;121:1211–5.
221. Ungi I, Ungi T, Ruzsa Z, Nagy E, Zimmermann Z, Csont T, et al. Hypercholesterolemia attenuates the anti-ischemic effect of preconditioning during coronary angioplasty. Chest. 2005;128:1623–8.
222. Di Napoli P, Antonio Taccardi A, Grilli A, Spina R, Felaco M, Barsotti A, et al. Simvastatin reduces reperfusion injury by modulating nitric oxide synthase expression: an ex vivo study in isolated working rat hearts. Cardiovasc Res. 2001;51:283–93.
223. Fan Y, Yang S, Cao Y, Huang Y. Effects of acute and chronic atorvastatin on cardioprotection of ischemic postconditioning in isolated rat hearts. Cardiovasc Ther. 2013;31:187–92.
224. Pantos C, Cokkinos DD, Tzeis SM, Malliopoulou V, Mourouzis IS, Carageorgiou HC, et al. Hyperthyroidism is associated with preserved preconditioning capacity but intensified and accelerated ischaemic contracture in rat heart. Basic Res Cardiol. 1999;94:254–60.
225. Pantos C, Malliopoulou V, Mourouzis I, Thempeyioti A, Paizis I, Dimopoulos A, et al. Hyperthyroid hearts display a phenotype of cardioprotection against ischemic stress: a possible involvement of heat shock protein 70. Horm Metab Res. 2006;38:308–13.
226. Pantos C, Malliopoulou V, Mourouzis I, Sfakianoudis K, Tzeis S, Doumba P, et al. Propylthiouracil-induced hypothyroidism is associated with increased tolerance of the isolated rat heart to ischaemia-reperfusion. J Endocrinol. 2003;178:427–35.
227. Mourouzis I, Dimopoulos A, Saranteas T, Tsinarakis N, Livadarou E, Spanou D, et al. Ischemic preconditioning fails to confer additional protection against ischemia-reperfusion injury in the hypothyroid rat heart. Physiol Res. 2009;58:29–38.
228. Dekker LR, Rademaker H, Vermeulen JT, Opthof T, Coronel R, Spaan JA, et al. Cellular uncoupling during ischemia in hypertrophied and failing rabbit ventricular myocardium: effects of preconditioning. Circulation. 1998;97:1724–30.

229. Ghosh S, Standen NB, Galiñianes M. Failure to precondition pathological human myocardium. J Am Coll Cardiol. 2001;37:711–8.
230. Miki T, Miura T, Tsuchida A, Nakano A, Hasegawa T, Fukuma T, et al. Cardioprotective mechanism of ischemic preconditioning is impaired by postinfarct ventricular remodeling through angiotensin II type 1 receptor activation. Circulation. 2000;102:458–63.
231. Pantos C, Mourouzis I, Dimopoulos A, Markakis K, Panagiotou M, Xinaris C, et al. Enhanced tolerance of the rat myocardium to ischemia and reperfusion injury early after acute myocardial infarction. Basic Res Cardiol. 2007;102:327–33.
232. Masoud WG, Abo Al-Rob O, Yang Y, Lopaschuk GD, Clanachan AS. Tolerance to ischaemic injury in remodelled mouse hearts: less ischaemic glycogenolysis and preserved metabolic efficiency. Cardiovasc Res. 2015;107:499–508.
233. Hu Q, Suzuki G, Young RF, Page BJ, Fallavollita JA, Canty JM Jr. Reductions in mitochondrial O(2) consumption and preservation of high-energy phosphate levels after simulated ischemia in chronic hibernating myocardium. Am J Physiol Heart Circ Physiol. 2009;297:H223–32.
234. Yan L, Kudej RK, Vatner DE, Vatner SF. Myocardial ischemic protection in natural mammalian hibernation. Basic Res Cardiol. 2015;110:9.
235. Ishihara M, Inoue I, Kawagoe T, Shimatani Y, Kurisu S, Hata T, et al. Ischaemic preconditioning effect of prodromal angina pectoris is lost in patients with prior myocardial infarction. Heart. 2006;92:973–4.
236. Nishizawa K, Yano T, Tanno M, Miki T, Kuno A, Tobisawa T, et al. Chronic treatment with an erythropoietin receptor ligand prevents chronic kidney disease-induced enlargement of myocardial infarct size. Hypertension. 2016;68:697–706.
237. Penna C, Rastaldo R, Mancardi D, Raimondo S, Cappello S, Gattullo D, et al. Post-conditioning induced cardioprotection requires signaling through a redox-sensitive mechanism, mitochondrial ATP-sensitive K+ channel and protein kinase C activation. Basic Res Cardiol. 2006;101:180–9.
238. Fantinelli JC, Mosca SM. Comparative effects of ischemic pre and postconditioning on ischemia-reperfusion injury in spontaneously hypertensive rats (SHR). Mol Cell Biochem. 2007;296:45–51.
239. Kupai K, Csonka C, Fekete V, Odendaal L, van Rooyen J, Marais DW, et al. Cholesterol diet-induced hyperlipidemia impairs the cardioprotective effect of postconditioning: role of peroxynitrite. Am J Physiol Heart Circ Physiol. 2009;297:H1729–35.
240. Przyklenk K, Maynard M, Greiner DL, Whittaker P. Cardioprotection with postconditioning: loss of efficacy in murine models of type-2 and type-1 diabetes. Antioxid Redox Signal. 2011;14:781–90.
241. Oosterlinck W, Dresselaers T, Geldhof V, Nevelsteen I, Janssens S, Himmelreich U, et al. Diabetes mellitus and the metabolic syndrome do not abolish, but might reduce, the cardioprotective effect of ischemic postconditioning. J Thorac Cardiovasc Surg. 2013;145:1595–602.
242. Hjortbak MV, Hjort J, Povlsen JA, Jensen VR, Støttrup NB, Laursen MR, et al. Influence of diabetes mellitus duration on the efficacy of ischemic preconditioning in a Zucker diabetic fatty rat model. PLoS One. 2018;13:e0192981. Published online 2018 Feb 23. https://doi.org/10.1371/journal.pone.0192981.
243. Zhu SG, Xi L, Kukreja RC. Type 2 diabetic obese db/db mice are refractory to myocardial ischaemic post-conditioning in vivo: potential role for Hsp20, F1-ATPase δ and Echs1. J Cell Mol Med. 2012;16:950–8.
244. Er F, Nia AM, Dopp H, Hellmich M, Dahlem KM, Caglayan E, et al. Ischemic preconditioning for prevention of contrast medium-induced nephropathy: randomized pilot RenPro trial (renal protection trial). Circulation. 2012;126:296–303.
245. Zimmerman RF, Ezeanuna PU, Kane JC, Cleland CD, Kempananjappa TJ, Lucas FL, et al. Ischemic preconditioning at a remote site prevents acute kidney injury in patients following cardiac surgery. Kidney Int. 2011;80:861–7.
246. Venugopal V, Laing CM, Ludman A, Yellon DM, Hausenloy D. Effect of remote ischemic preconditioning on acute kidney injury in nondiabetic patients undergoing coronary artery

bypass graft surgery: a secondary analysis of 2 small randomized trials. Am J Kidney Dis. 2010;56:1043–9.
247. Mergenthaler P, Dirnagl U. Protective conditioning of the brain: expressway or roadblock? J Physiol. 2011;589:4147–55.
248. Hess DC, Hoda MN, Bhatia K. Remote limb perconditioning [corrected] and postconditioning: will it translate into a promising treatment for acute stroke? Stroke. 2013;44:1191–7.
249. Gidday J. Cerebrovascular ischemic protection by pre- and post-conditioning. Brain Circ. 2015;1:97–103.
250. Xu J, Sun S, Lu X, Hu X, Yang M, Tang W. Remote ischemic pre- and postconditioning improve postresuscitation myocardial and cerebral function in a rat model of cardiac arrest and resuscitation. Crit Care Med. 2015;43:e12–8.
251. Meng R, Asmaro K, Meng L, Liu Y, Ma C, Xi C, et al. Upper limb ischemic preconditioning prevents recurrent stroke in intracranial arterial stenosis. Neurology. 2012;79:1853–61.
252. Lloris-Carsí JM, Cejalvo D, Toledo-Pereyra LH, Calvo MA, Suzuki S. Preconditioning: effect upon lesion modulation in warm liver ischemia. Transplant Proc. 1993;25:3303–4.
253. Yin DP, Sankary HN, Chong AS, Ma LL, Shen J, Foster P, Williams JW. Protective effect of ischemic preconditioning on liver preservation-reperfusion injury in rats. Transplantation. 1998;66:152–7.
254. Koti RS, Seifalian AM, Davidson BR. Protection of the liver by ischemic preconditioning: a review of mechanisms and clinical applications. Dig Surg. 2003;20:383–96.
255. Hardy KJ, McClure DN, Subwongcharoen S. Ischaemic preconditioning of the liver: a preliminary study. Aust N Z J Surg. 1996;6:707–10.
256. Soncul H, Oz E, Kalaycioglu S. Role of ischemic preconditioning on ischemia-reperfusion injury of the lung. Chest. 1999;115:1672–7.
257. Erling Junior N, Montero EF, Sannomiya P, Poli-De-Figueiredo LF. Local and remote ischemic preconditioning protect against intestinal ischemic/reperfusion injury after supraceliac aortic clamping. Clinics (Sao Paulo). 2013;68:1548–54.
258. Selimoglu O, Ugurlucan M, Basaran M, Gungor F, Banach M, Cucu O, et al. Efficacy of remote ischaemic preconditioning for spinal cord protection against ischaemic injury: association with heat shock protein expression. Folia Neuropathol. 2008;46:204–12.
259. Dong HL, Zhang Y, Su BX, Zhu ZH, Gu QH, Sang HF, et al. Limb remote ischemic preconditioning protects the spinal cord from ischemia-reperfusion injury: a newly identified nonneuronal but reactive oxygen species-dependent pathway. Anesthesiology. 2010;112:881–91.
260. Toumpoulis IK, Papakostas JC, Matsagas MI, Malamou-Mitsi VD, Pappa LS, Drossos GE, et al. Superiority of early relative to late ischemic preconditioning in spinal cord protection after descending thoracic aortic occlusion. J Thorac Cardiovasc Surg. 2004;128:724–30.
261. Etz CD, Weigang E, Hartert M, Lonn L, Mestres CA, Di Bartolomeo R, et al. Contemporary spinal cord protection during thoracic and thoracoabdominal aortic surgery and endovascular aortic repair: a position paper of the vascular domain of the European Association for Cardio-Thoracic Surgery†. Eur J Cardiothorac Surg. 2015;47:943–57.
262. Heberden W A letter to Dr. Heberden concerning the angina pectoris: and an account of the dissection of the one who had been troubled by that disorder. Read at the college, Nov.17, 1772. Medical Transactions published by the College of Physicians in London 1785;3:1–11.
263. MacAlpin RN, Kattus AA. Adaptation to exercise in angina pectoris. The electrocardiogram during treadmill walking and coronary angiographic findings. Circulation. 1966;33:183–201.
264. Tomai F. Warm up phenomenon and preconditioning in clinical practice. Heart. 2002;87:99–100.
265. Kelion AD, Webb TP, Gardner MA, Ormerod OJ, Banning AP. The warm-up effect protects against ischemic left ventricular dysfunction in patients with angina. J Am Coll Cardiol. 2001;37:705–10.
266. Williams DO, Bass TA, Gewirtz H, Most AS. Adaptation to the stress of tachycardia in patients with coronary artery disease: insight into the mechanism of the warm-up phenomenon. Circulation. 1985;71:687–92.

267. Okazaki Y, Kodama K, Sato H, Kitakaze M, Hirayama A, Mishima M, et al. Attenuation of increased regional myocardial oxygen consumption during exercise as a major cause of warm-up phenomenon. J Am Coll Cardiol. 1993;21:1597–604.
268. Tomai F, Crea F, Danesi A, Perino M, Gaspardone A, Ghini AS, et al. Mechanisms of the warm-up phenomenon. Eur Heart J. 1996;17:1022–7.
269. Maybaum S, Ilan M, Mogilevsky J, Tzivoni D. Improvement in ischemic parameters during repeated exercise testing: a possible model for myocardial preconditioning. Am J Cardiol. 1996;78:1087–91.
270. Koutelou M, Katsikis A, Theodorakos A, Tsapaki V, Kouzoumi A, Dritsas A, et al. Stress test with dual isotope studies for the documentation of classical ischemic preconditioning. Atherosclerosis. 2010;210:445–51.
271. Iliodromitis EK, Koutelou M, Paraskevaidis IA, Theodorakos A, Farmakis D, Tsoutsanis J, et al. Treadmill exercise test with dual isotope scintigraphy documents the second window of preconditioning in humans. Atherosclerosis. 2008;198:122–8.
272. Lalonde F, Poirier P, Sylvestre MP, Arvisais D, Curnier D. Exercise-induced ischemic preconditioning detected by sequential exercise stress tests: a meta-analysis. Eur J Prev Cardiol. 2015;22:100–12.
273. Ottani F, Galvani M, Ferrini D, Sorbello F, Limonetti P, Pantoli D, et al. Prodromal angina limits infarct size. A role for ischemic preconditioning. Circulation. 1995;91:291–7.
274. Nakagawa Y, Ito H, Kitakaze M, Kusuoka H, Hori M, Kuzuya T, et al. Effect of angina pectoris on myocardial protection in patients with reperfused anterior wall myocardial infarction: retrospective clinical evidence of "preconditioning". J Am Coll Cardiol. 1995;25:1076–83.
275. Kloner RA, Shook T, Antman EM, Cannon CP, Przyklenk K, McCabe CH, et al. TIMI 9 investigators [abst]. Circulation. 1996;94:I–611.
276. Muller DW, Topol EJ, Califf RM, Sigmon KN, Gorman L, George BS, et al. Relationship between antecedent angina pectoris and short-term prognosis after thrombolytic therapy for acute myocardial infarction. Thrombolysis and angioplasty in myocardial infarction (TAMI) study group. Am Heart J. 1990;119:224–31.
277. Kloner RA, Shook T, Przyklenk K, Davis VG, Junio L, Matthews RVM, et al. Previous angina alters in-hospital outcome in TIMI 4. A clinical correlate to preconditioning? Circulation. 1995;91:37–45.
278. Ruocco NA Jr, Bergelson BA, Jacobs AK, Frederick MM, Faxon DP, Ryan TJ. Invasive versus conservative strategy after thrombolytic therapy for acute myocardial infarction in patients with antecedent angina. A report from thrombolysis in myocardial infarction phase II (TIMI II). J Am Coll Cardiol. 1992;20:1445–51.
279. Barbash G, White HD, Modan M, Van de Werf F. Antecedent angina pectoris predicts worse outcome after myocardial infarction in patients receiving thrombolytic therapy: experience gleaned from the international tissue plasminogen activator/streptokinase mortality trial. J Am Coll Cardiol. 1992;20:36–41.
280. Migrino RQ, Moliterno DJ, Topol EJ. Preinfarction angina. Letter. N Engl J Med. 1996;335:59.
281. Deutsch E, Berger M, Kussmaul WG, Hirshfeld JW Jr, Herrmann HC, Laskey WK. Adaptation to ischemia during percutaneous transluminal coronary angioplasty. Clinical, hemodynamic, and metabolic features. Circulation. 1990;82:2044–51.
282. Cribier A, Korsatz L, Koning R, Rath P, Gamra H, Stix G, et al. Improved myocardial ischemic response and enhanced collateral circulation with long repetitive coronary occlusion during angioplasty: a prospective study. J Am Coll Cardiol. 1992;20:578–86.
283. Matsubara T, Minatoguchi S, Matsuo H, Hayakawa K, Segawa T, Matsuno Y, et al. Three minute, but not one minute, ischemia and nicorandil have a preconditioning effect in patients with coronary artery disease. J Am Coll Cardiol. 2000;35:345–51.
284. Masci PG, Andreini D, Francone M, Bertella E, De Luca L, Coceani M, et al. Prodromal angina is associated with myocardial salvage in acute ST-segment elevation myocardial infarction. Eur Heart J Cardiovasc Imaging. 2013;14:1041–8.

285. Leesar MA, Stoddard M, Ahmed M, Broadbent J, Bolli R. Preconditioning of human myocardium with adenosine during coronary angioplasty. Circulation. 1997;95:2500–7.
286. Tomai F, Crea F, Gaspardone A, Versaci F, De Paulis R, Penta De Peppo A, et al. Ischemic preconditioning during coronary angioplasty is prevented by glibenclamide, a selective ATP-sensitive K+ channel blocker. Circulation. 1994;90:700–5.
287. Klepzig H, Kober G, Matter C, Luus H, Schneider H, Boedeker KH, et al. Sulfonylureas and ischaemic preconditioning; a double-blind, placebo-controlled evaluation of glimepiride and glibenclamide. Eur Heart J. 1999;20:439–46.
288. Leesar MA, Stoddard MF, Dawn B, Jasti VG, Masden R, Bolli R. Delayed preconditioning-mimetic action of nitroglycerin in patients undergoing coronary angioplasty. Circulation. 2001;103:2935–41.
289. Leesar MA, Stoddard MF, Manchikalapudi S, Bolli R. Bradykinin-induced preconditioning in patients undergoing coronary angioplasty. J Am Coll Cardiol. 1999;34:639–50.
290. Yellon DM, Alkhulaifi AM, Pugsley WB. Preconditioning the human myocardium. Lancet. 1993;342:276–7.
291. Walsh SR, Tang TY, Kullar P, Jenkins DP, Dutka DP, Gaunt ME. Ischaemic preconditioning during cardiac surgery: systematic review and meta-analysis of perioperative outcomes in randomised clinical trials. Eur J Cardiothorac Surg. 2008;34:985–94.
292. Sukkar L, Hong D, Wong MG, Badve SV, Rogers K, Perkovic V, et al. Effects of ischaemic conditioning on major clinical outcomes in people undergoing invasive procedures: systematic review and meta-analysis. BMJ. 2016;355:i5599.
293. Pinaud F, Corbeau JJ, Baufreton C, Binuani JP, De Brux JL, Fouquet O, et al. Remote ischemic preconditioning in aortic valve surgery: results of a randomized controlled study. J Cardiol. 2016;67:36–41.
294. Hausenloy DJ, Candilio L, Evans R, Ariti C, Jenkins DP, Kolvekar S, et al. Remote ischemic preconditioning and outcomes of cardiac surgery. N Engl J Med. 2015;373:1408–17.
295. Meybohm P, Bein B, Brosteanu O, Cremer J, Gruenewald M, Stoppe C, et al. A multicenter trial of remote ischemic preconditioning for heart surgery. N Engl J Med. 2015;373:1397–407.
296. Zaugg M, Lucchinetti E. Remote ischemic preconditioning in cardiac surgery--ineffective and risky? N Engl J Med. 2015;373:1470–2.
297. Blusztein DI, Brooks MJ, Andrews DT. A systematic review and meta-analysis evaluating ischemic conditioning during percutaneous coronary intervention. Futur Cardiol. 2017;13:579–92.
298. Engstrøm T, Kelbæk H, Helqvist S, Høfsten DE, Kløvgaard L, Clemmensen P, et al. Effect of ischemic postconditioning during primary percutaneous coronary intervention for patients with ST-segment elevation myocardial infarction: a randomized clinical trial. JAMA Cardiol. 2017;2:490–7.
299. Vander Heide RS, Steenbergen C. Cardioprotection and myocardial reperfusion: pitfalls to clinical application. Circ Res. 2013;113:464–77.
300. Heusch G, Rassaf T. Time to give up on cardioprotection? A critical appraisal of clinical studies on ischemic pre-, post-, and remote conditioning. Circ Res. 2016;119:676–95.
301. Lin E, Symons JA. Volatile anaesthetic myocardial protection: a review of the current literature. HSR Proc Intensive Care Cardiovasc Anesth. 2010;2:105–9.
302. Li F, Yuan Y. Meta-analysis of the cardioprotective effect of sevoflurane versus propofol during cardiac surgery. BMC Anesthesiol. 2015;15:128.
303. Yang XL, Wang D, Zhang GY, Guo XL. Comparison of the myocardial protective effect of sevoflurane versus propofol in patients undergoing heart valve replacement surgery with cardiopulmonary bypass. BMC Anesthesiol. 2017;17:37.
304. Lucchinetti E, da Silva R, Pasch T, Schaub MC, Zaugg M. Anaesthetic preconditioning but not postconditioning prevents early activation of the deleterious cardiac remodelling programme: evidence of opposing genomic responses in cardioprotection by pre- and postconditioning. Br J Anaesth. 2005;95:140–52.

305. Bautin AE, Galagudza MM, Datsenko SV, Tashkhanov DM, Marichev AO, Bakanov AI, et al. Effects of remote ischemic preconditioning on perioperative period in elective aortic valve replacement. Anesteziol Reanimatol. 2014:11–7.
306. Zhou C, Liu Y, Yao Y, Zhou S, Fang N, Wang W, et al. β-Blockers and volatile anesthetics may attenuate cardioprotection by remote preconditioning in adult cardiac surgery: a meta-analysis of 15 randomized trials. J Cardiothorac Vasc Anesth. 2013;27:305–11.
307. Landymore RW, Bayes AJ, Murphy JT, Fris JH. Preconditioning prevents myocardial stunning after cardiac transplantation. Ann Thorac Surg. 1998;66:1953–7.
308. Cope JT, Mauney MC, Banks D, Binns OA, Moore CL, Rentz JJ, et al. Intravenous phenylephrine preconditioning of cardiac grafts from non-heart-beating donors. Ann Thorac Surg. 1997;63:1664–8.
309. Ovize M, Thibault H, Przyklenk K. Myocardial conditioning: opportunities for clinical translation. Circ Res. 2013;113:439–50.
310. Salim A, Vassiliu P, Velmahos GC, Sava J, Murray JA, Belzberg H, et al. The role of thyroid hormone administration in potential organ donors. Arch Surg. 2001;136:1377–80.
311. Cooper LB, Milano CA, Williams M, Swafford W, Croezen D, Van Bakel AB, et al. Thyroid hormone use during cardiac transplant organ procurement. Clin Transpl. 2016;30:1578–83.
312. Bartos JA, Debaty G, Matsuura T, Yannopoulos D. Post-conditioning to improve cardiopulmonary resuscitation. Curr Opin Crit Care. 2014;20:242–9.
313. Kahlert P, Hildebrandt HA, Patsalis PC, Al-Rashid F, Jánosi RA, Nensa F, et al. No protection of heart, kidneys and brain by remote ischemic preconditioning before transfemoral transcatheter aortic valve implantation: interim-analysis of a randomized single-blinded, placebo-controlled, single-center trial. Int J Cardiol. 2017;231:248–54.
314. Yamaguchi T, Izumi Y, Nakamura Y, Yamazaki T, Shiota M, Sano S, et al. Repeated remote ischemic conditioning attenuates left ventricular remodeling via exosome-mediated intercellular communication on chronic heart failure after myocardial infarction. Int J Cardiol. 2015;178:239–46.
315. Hausenloy DJ, Erik Bøtker H, Condorelli G, Ferdinandy P, Garcia-Dorado D, Heusch G, et al. Translating cardioprotection for patient benefit: position paper from the working Group of Cellular Biology of the heart of the European Society of Cardiology. Cardiovasc Res. 2013;98:7–27.
316. Hausenloy DJ, Garcia-Dorado D, Bøtker HE, Davidson SM, Downey J, Engel FB, et al. Novel targets and future strategies for acute cardioprotection: position paper of the European Society of Cardiology Working Group on cellular biology of the heart. Cardiovasc Res. 2017;113:564–85.
317. Heusch G. Cardioprotection: changes and challenges of its translation to the clinic. Lancet. 2013;381:166–75.
318. Depré C, Vatner SF. Cardioprotection in stunned and hibernating myocardium. Heart Fail Rev. 2007;12:307–17.

Chapter 15
Fibrosis–Inflammation of the Cardiovascular System

Evangelos Oikonomou and Dimitris Tousoulis

15.1 Introduction

The roles of inflammation and activation of the innate immune system in cardiovascular diseases have been well described, since the nineteenth century, in autopsy studies, in vitro data, in vivo preclinical experiments, and even clinical research. Activation of the immune system—macrophage accumulation, cytokine generation and secretion, and adhesion molecule production—may therefore be considered a common pathophysiological background shared by atherosclerosis, heart failure, ischemic heart disease, dilated cardiomyopathy, other cardiomyopathies, myocarditis, and even thoracic aortic diseases (Fig. 15.1) [1–6]. Importantly, the recently conducted Canakinumab Anti-inflammatory Thrombosis Outcomes Study (CANTOS) [7] not only showed that targeting inflammation may be a clinical meaningful approach but also stands out as a proof of concept for the central role of inflammation in the genesis and progression of atheromatosis.

Recently, attention has been focused on the roles of fibrosis, extracellular matrix (ECM) adaptations, and remodeling, especially concerning heart failure and cardiomyopathies, but also the ECM scaffold of the arterial wall. Fibrosis may be considered a reparative mechanism when the tissue architecture is damaged, aimed at preserving the integrity of the structure [8]. However, fibroblasts and the ECM lack functional properties and progressive scarring causes latter-stage impairment of function and organ damage. Cumulative evidence suggests fibrosis is the common pathobiological lesion in patients with heart failure caused by different etiologies and insults [9–11]. Biomarkers of fibrosis are considered an adverse prognostic sign in patients with heart failure, and extensive fibrosis in the cardiovascular system, assessed by various imaging modalities, has been associated with an adverse prognosis [9–12].

E. Oikonomou · D. Tousoulis (✉)
1st Cardiology Department, Hippokration Hospital, Athens University Medical School, Athens, Greece

D. V. Cokkinos (ed.), *Myocardial Preservation*,
https://doi.org/10.1007/978-3-319-98186-4_15

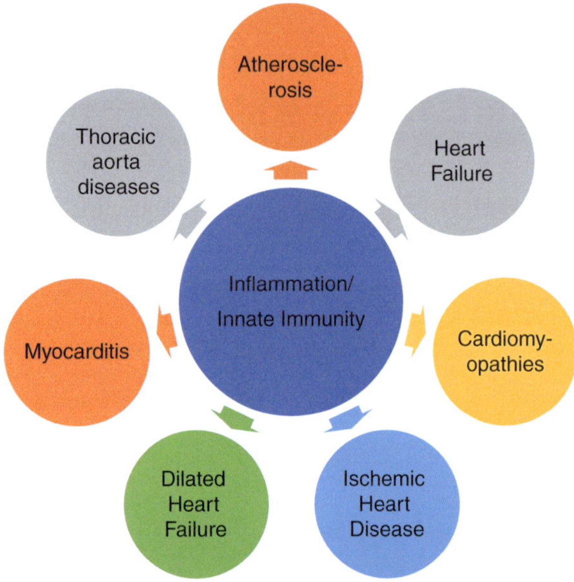

Fig. 15.1 Cardiovascular entities directly or indirectly associated with inflammation

Interestingly, the interrelationship between fibrosis and inflammation makes even more fascinating the combined study of the roles of these processes in the health and disease of the cardiovascular system.

15.2 The Extracellular Matrix

The ECM consists mainly of inactive components (noncellular). Water, proteins, polysaccharides, proteoglycans, and fibrous proteins (elastins, collagens, laminins, and fibronectins) are the main constituents of the ECM [13–15]. Despite the inactive composition of the ECM, this is unique to each tissue and organ as a dynamic interpolation between several cell types responsible for synthesis and regeneration of fibrous tissue (e.g., epithelial tissue, macrophages, fibroblasts, adipocytes, and endothelial elements).

Two systems are responsible for proteolysis and degradation of the ECM: (i) the fibrinolytic (plasminogen/plasmin) system; and (ii) mainly the matrix metalloproteinase (MMP) system. MMPs consist of a whole group of different zinc-dependent endopeptidases capable of degrading most ECM components [16]. MMPs are differentiated into gelatinases, stromelysins, collagenases, and membrane-type MMPs (MT-MMPs) [17].

Disproportionate activity of MMPs and their tissue inhibitors (TIMPs) may contribute to the generation and physical course of cardiovascular diseases such as atherosclerosis, vascular remodeling, and progression of heart failure (Fig. 15.2) [18, 19].

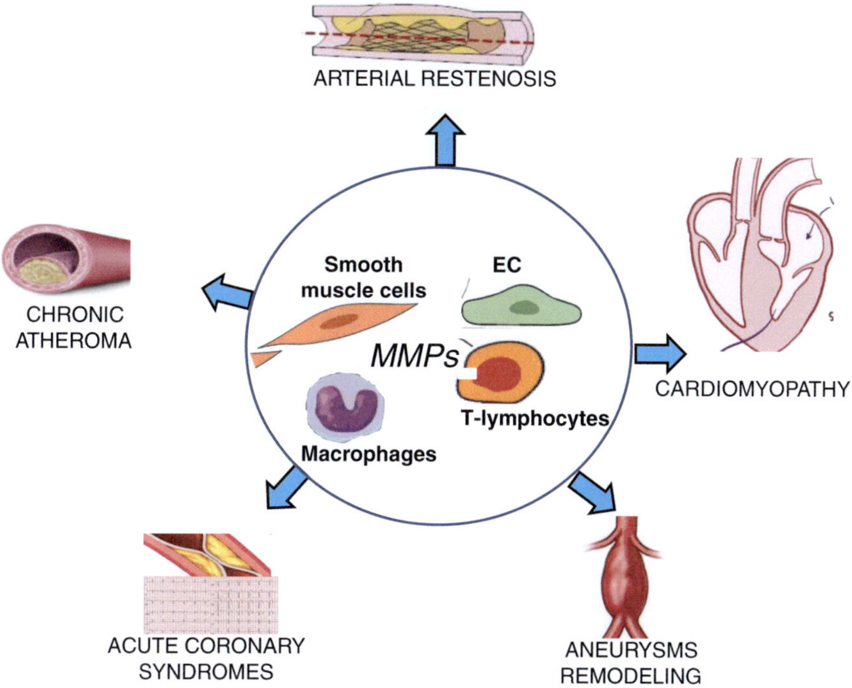

Fig. 15.2 Cell types involved in extracellular matrix production and degradation

15.3 Inflammation and the Extracellular Matrix Modulation System

Inflammation, oxidative stress, tissue injury, shear stress, and wall stress are significant determinants of vascular and myocardial remodeling and may activate or cease MMP activity [20] (Table 15.1). Macrophages and, to a lesser degree, other inflammatory cells produce MMPs [22].

The first step in MMP regulation is considered a gene transcription process [32] mediated by cyclic adenosine monophosphate (cAMP) and prostaglandin (PG) E2 [21].

At the second step, driven by inflammatory molecules and cytokines [i.e., tumor necrosis factor (TNF)-α, interleukin (IL)-6, and IL-1], there is increased secretion of MMPs into the target tissue [22]. Growth factors [vascular endothelial growth factor (VEGF), epidermal growth factor (EGF), platelet-derived growth factor (PDGF), stromal cell–derived factor (SDF)-1, basic fibroblast growth factor (bFGF), and insulin] also contribute to the modulation of macrophages and stromal cells (i.e., epithelial cells and fibroblasts) and to a secretory switch toward MMP production and secretion [22, 23]. In the opposite direction, anti-inflammatory stimuli (e.g., IL-4) downregulate MMP gene transcription [24].

Table 15.1 Molecules involved in matrix metalloproteinase (MMP) expression

Molecules	Target levels/cells/actions	Effects on ECM degradation
cAMP, PGE2 [21]	Activate mRNA gene transcription of MMPs	↑
TNF-α, IL-6, IL-1 [22]	Activate secretion from fibroblasts, macrophages, stromal cells, etc.	↑
VEGF, EGF, PDGF, bFGF, insulin [23]	Modulate macrophages and stromal cells (i.e., epithelial cells and fibroblasts) to secrete MMPs	↑
IL-4 [24]	Downregulates mRNA gene transcription of MMPs	↓
TGF-β1 [25, 26]	Stimulates MMP-2 and MMP-9 expression in monocytes Inhibits MMP-1, MMP-3, and MMP-12 synthesis in circulating macrophages	↑↓
SDF-1 [26, 27]	Reduces MMP-9 expression in monocytes Increases MMP-9 expression in megakaryocytes	↑↓
Oxidized LDL [28]	Increases MMP-9 mRNA transcription in monocytes and macrophages Inhibits TIMP-1 expression	↑
MicroRNA-29b [29]	Increases MMP-9 expression	↑
$ONOO^-$ [30]	Induces MMP-1, MMP-8, and MMP-9 secretion	↑
NO [31]	Downregulates MMP-9 and MMP-2 expression in SMCs	↓

bFGF basic fibroblast growth factor, *cAMP* cyclic adenosine monophosphate, *ECM* extracellular matrix, *EGF* epidermal growth factor, *IL* interleukin, *LDL* low-density lipoprotein, *mRNA* messenger RNA, *NO* nitric oxide, *$ONOO^-$* peroxynitrite, *PDGF* platelet-derived growth factor, *PGE2* prostaglandin E2, *SDF* stromal cell–derived factor, *SMC* smooth muscle cell, *TGF* transforming growth factor, *TIMP* tissue inhibitor of metalloproteinase, *TNF* tumor necrosis factor, *VEGF* vascular endothelial growth factor

However, we should note that the same stimuli may act differently concerning up- or downregulation of different MMPs and different cell types. Transforming growth factor (TGF)-β1, when acting on monocytes, stimulates expression of MMP-2 and MMP-9 but, when acting on human peripheral blood macrophages, inhibits MMP-1, MMP-3, and MMP-12 synthesis [25, 26]. SDF-1 in monocytes of patients with acute coronary syndromes reduces MMP-9 expression, while in megakaryocytes it causes release of MMP-9 [26, 27].

Oxidative stress may also act as an activation factor for MMP activity. Hypoxia causes MMP-2 messenger RNA (mRNA) upregulation. Conversely, reoxygenation also upregulates mRNA expression specific for MT1-MMP [33]. Oxidized low-density lipoprotein (LDL) in monocytes and tissue macrophages increases transcription of MMP-9 mRNA, with a parallel decrease in TIMP-1 expression [28]. Data from preclinical studies also confirm the impact of oxidized LDL on MMP-2 and MMP-9 activity through epigenetic modifications caused by microRNA-29b [29].

Peroxynitrite ($ONOO^-$) also induces secretion of MMP-1, MMP-8, and MMP-9 [30]. Interestingly, the smooth muscle cell (SMC) gene, purified with endothelial nitric oxide synthase (eNOS), downregulates expression of MMP-9 and MMP-2. Nevertheless, the actions of NO on SMCs are also mediated by reactive oxygen products cause by neighboring inflammatory cells [31]. Interestingly, NO in diseased vessels exacerbates inequality between MMPs and TIMPs in the direction of ECM degradation, while in healthy vascular tissue it has a favorable outcome [34].

Wall stress also has an active role in the regulation of MMP expression. Accordingly, MMP-2 expression in the arterial wall may be considered flow dependent and changes in hemodynamic status may alter ECM synthesis more actively than vascular injury itself [35]. Confirmatory data come from murine models where cessation of carotid artery flow causes uptitration of MMP-9 and forced remodeling [36]. Increased arterial wall pressure in an ex vivo model confirms the uptitration of MMP-9 and MMP-2, highlighting the role of ECM remodeling in arterial hypertension–associated vascular remodeling [37].

15.4 Cardiovascular Risk Factors and Extracellular Matrix Synthesis

Well established atherosclerotic and coronary artery disease risk factors are positively associated with extracellular protease levels. Both MMP-9 and TIMP-1 are consistently found to be elevated in smokers [38–41]. In rabbit models with hypercholesterolemia or hypertension, elastin levels were uptitrated. From epidemiological studies and especially the Framingham Heart Study, the associations of MMP-9 and TIMP-1 levels with hypertension and LDL cholesterol levels were documented [38, 40, 42, 43]. Interestingly, diabetes mellitus was associated with low TIMP-1 levels and increased MMP-9 [40, 44], although the latter finding was not confirmed by subsequent studies [45].

15.5 Roles of the Extracellular Matrix and Fibrosis in Cardiac Remodeling

All types of injury in the heart may activate ECM synthesis and cause cardiac remodeling. Fibrosis is characterized by expansion of the extracellular-inactive component of the myocardium. Following myocardial infarction and myocyte cell death, animal studies have documented the activation of several classes of proteases (MMP-1, MMP-2, MMP-3, and MMP-9) during the remodeling process [46–50]. Several cell types contribute to ECM modulation and myocardial fibrosis following myocardial infarction (i.e., inflammatory cells, fibroblast-like cells, and cardiomyocytes). All cell types in an oxidative and inflammatory environment are activated to produce MMPs, which are found to be elevated as early as 24 h following the initial event [46–50], highlighting the active roles of ECM degradation and

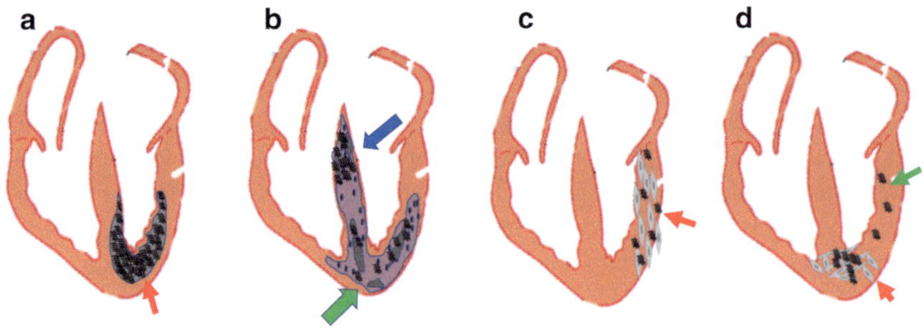

Fig. 15.3 Schematic representation of four different patterns of myocardial fibrosis. (**a**) Infarct zone with replacement fibrosis (*red arrow*). (**b**) Myocarditis with edema, regions of myocyte cell death, replacement fibrosis, and interstitial fibrosis (*red arrow:* zone of myocarditis with edema; *green arrow:* interstitial fibrosis; *blue arrow:* necrotic zones with replacement fibrosis). (**c**) Hypertensive cardiomyopathy with myocardial hypertrophy and interstitial fibrosis (*red arrow*). (**d**) Hypertrophic cardiomyopathy with myocardial cell disarray, replacement fibrosis, and interstitial fibrosis (*red arrow:* zone of hypertrophy with myocardial cell disarray and replacement fibrosis; *green arrow:* interstitial fibrosis)

synthesis in the healing process. As was shown in animal models, activation of MMP-9 has a central role in wound healing following myocardial infarction. Lack of MMP-9 activity in mice ameliorates degradation of the necrotic infarct zone and protects against rupture or aneurysm formation [51]. Inactivation of MMP-9 also protects against left ventricular (LV) cavity enlargement and outward remodeling accompanied by lower inflammatory infiltration and decreased collagen in the infarct territory [19, 52].

Fibrosis is also a common feature of several cardiomyopathies. In patients with dilated cardiomyopathy, the activity of several MMPs is increased [53–56]. Tachycardia-induced cardiomyopathy may be associated with degradation of the natural ECM and domination of fibrosis since inactivation of MMPs experimentally ameliorates LV dilatation caused by rapid pacing in pigs [57, 58] (Fig. 15.3).

15.5.1 Myocardial Infarction

Myocardial infarction occurs following obstruction of an epicardial coronary artery, causing necrosis of myocardial cells. As there is no blood flow in the infarct area (at least during the first hours of infarction), circulating immune cells cannot accumulate and myofibroblasts may take over the role of macrophages, degrading dead cells [59]. At the second step, neutrophils, monocytes, and tissue macrophages are accumulated [60]. Toll-like receptors (TLRs) have a central role in the perturbation of inflammation, causing expression of monocyte chemoattractant protein (MCP)-1, TNF-α, and IL-6 [61–63]; activation of inflammatory cells; and degradation of the ECM. All of these processes are followed by a proliferative phase with macrophage secretion of growth factors and cytokines to activate mesenchymal cells to deposit the ECM. Several studies have documented the role of galectin-3 (a profibrotic and proinflammatory protein) in postinfarction remodeling and in close association with the development of heart failure, systolic impairment, and diastolic impairment [64]. TGF-β is another potent player, stimulating hypertrophy of the cardiomyocytes and promoting ECM deposition (collagen and fibronectin production) [65]. Interestingly, while in the infarct zone there is replacement fibrosis, the surrounding noninfarct ischemic or jeopardized zone presents perivascular and interstitial fibrosis [66]. Of note, fibrosis preserves the structural integrity of the heart and maintains its function as a pump. Balanced activation of macrophages and fibroblasts, ECM degradation, and recovery of fibrin proteins protects against adverse remodeling, heart failure, aneurysm formation, and rupture of the LV.

15.5.2 Myocarditis and Myocarditis-Associated Cardiomyopathies

By definition, inflammation and the innate and adaptive immune system play central roles in the progression of this entity. Cardiac specific viruses adhere and ender cardiomyocytes, replicate and damage the integrity of the cardiomyocytes and leading to uncoupling of the ECM and cardiomyocytes. In addition, apoptosis and necrosis of cardiomyocytes is repaired with fibrotic tissue [67, 68]. At the following step, the subacute stage, natural killer cells attack infected cells and macrophages contribute to degradation of apoptotic cells. Activation of the innate adaptive system is followed by a cascade of inflammatory cytokines. In the following phase the central role in the depletion of destroyed and infected cells is undertaken by adaptive immunity and especially by cytotoxic T cells. Myocardial cell loss is replaced by scar formation with TGF-β as the main profibrotic factor [69, 70]. However, perturbation of inflammation may cause a chronic condition with further myocardial loss and fibrosis, especially interstitially, which causes dilated cardiomyopathy [68].

15.5.3 Heart Failure

The so-called cytokine hypothesis emphasizes that heart failure is caused at least in part by the damaging action of inflammatory cytokines. Inflammatory cytokines exert significant effects on the process of ventricular remodeling. The most important role is mediated by IL-1 and TNF-α. In experimental models knocked out for IL-1β and IL-18, attenuation of ventricular dilation is observed following myocardial infarction [71]. Conversely, adverse LV remodeling with dilation and changes in collagen composition are observed in models overexpressing TNF-α [72]. The anti-inflammatory cytokine IL-10, when administered in animal models of heart failure, causes attenuation of immune activation with parallel beneficial effects in remodeling of the LV after myocardial infarction [73]. Similarly, blockade of nuclear factor-κB attenuates remodeling after myocardial infarction, favorably affecting fibroblast activation and myocardial fibrosis [74].

15.5.4 Hypertrophic Cardiomyopathy

The main finding in hypertrophic cardiomyopathy is increased LV wall thickness. Additionally, it is characterized by myocardial fibrosis, which is inherent in the phenotype of the disease. Cardiac magnetic resonance imaging can reveal the extent of fibrosis in hypertrophic cardiomyopathy [75]. Late gadolinium enhancement coincides with the regions of hypertrophy and presents a midwall patchy pattern. Additionally, cardiac magnetic resonance imaging can identify expansion of the interstitial volume [76, 77].

Importantly, late gadolinium enhancement is associated with LV stiffness, cardiac remodeling, and diastolic and systolic dysfunction. Moreover, the extent of late gadolinium enhancement may provide additional data on the prognosis and the risk of malignant ventricular arrhythmias [78].

Interestingly, in sarcomere mutation carriers without the phenotype of the disease, levels of serum C-terminal propeptide of type I procollagen were significantly higher, which denoted that a profibrotic state may precede the development of LV hypertrophy [79].

15.5.5 Hypertension–Hypertensive Cardiomyopathy

Neurohormonal activation plays a key role in hypertension. Increased shear stress in hypertension not only impairs endothelial cells but also may be associated with perivascular fibrosis with collagen deposition in arterial adventitia. These structural changes impair arterial wall elasticity, causing a further increment in blood pressure and a vicious circle, further damaging arterial wall properties. Similar changes are also observed in the microcirculation, causing microvascular remodeling and rarefaction [80]. Hypertension combined with decreased arterial elasticity increases cardiac afterload, leading finally to ECM changes and interstitial fibrosis in the heart, not directly associated with myocardial loss but probably as a reparative mechanism to compensate for wall stress [81]. Perturbation of hypertension may cause myocardial hypertrophy and myocardial loss, which may be associated with systolic dysfunction [82]. In hypertensive heart failure there is also mobilization of the inflammatory pathway and angiotensin II overexpression may be associated with IL-6 and TGF-β exacerbations [83].

15.5.6 *Atrial Fibrillation and Fibrosis*

Impulse conduction heterogeneity caused by fibrosis of the atria is considered one of the main mechanisms of the genesis and perpetuation of fibrillate waves in the atria. Moreover, when atrial fibrosis is advanced there are more frequent episodes of atrial fibrillation and the arrhythmia tends to progress to a permanent state. Interestingly, when there is expansion of the extracellular volume in the atria as a result of interstitial fibrosis, rhythm control is difficult to achieve in patients with atrial fibrillation. A few profibrotic signals have been identified in patients with atrial fibrillation, such as TGF-β, angiotensin II, and PDGF [84]. Interestingly, atrial fibrillation may be initiated in patients with systemic infections and especially when there is inflammatory pericarditis. Additionally, biomarkers of inflammation contribute to an adverse prognosis in patients with atrial fibrillation [85].

15.6 Roles of the Extracellular Matrix and Fibrosis in Aortic Diseases

In MMP-9-deficient mice, increased arterial wall pressure is associated with an increase in the pressure–diameter relationship [86]. In specimens from abdominal aortic aneurysms, levels of MMP-2 and MMP-9 were found to be uptitrated [87, 88]. SMCs isolated from aortic aneurysms also produce increased levels of MMP-2 and MMP-9 [89], and may be associated with increased MMP-9 expression and a tendency toward aortic aneurysm formation [90]. Conversely, mice incapable of MMP-9 production resist aneurysm formation following aortic injury [91].

Marfan syndrome is an inherited connective tissue disorder which, among other consequences, causes dilation of the ascending aorta and is caused mainly by mutations in genes encoding fibrillin. In the progression of the disease the role of TGF-β is significant, and inhibition of this growth factor by targeting angiotensin II type 1 receptors can attenuate the progression of the disease [92].

Additionally, positron emission tomography studies in patients with repaired coarctation of the aorta have not only shown disseminated inflammation of the aortic wall but also identified an association of TGF-β with aortic and arterial stiffening in this population [3, 93].

15.7 Roles of Fibrosis–Inflammation in Atherosclerosis

As previously mentioned, SMCs are normally found in the medial layer of the arterial wall. A few SMCs can be observed in the intima early in life. However, as atheromatous plaque evolves beyond recruitment of macrophages and changes in endothelial cell function, SMCs are recruited from the media to the intima.

SMCs in the intima are less differentiated, exhibiting an embryonic phenotype with an embryonic myosin isoform and a rough endoplasmic reticulum. Concerning replication of SMCs, although this appears infrequent in stable atherosclerotic plaques, in vulnerable plaques it may be exacerbated, contributing to aggravation of atherosclerotic plaques.

Interestingly, inflammatory cytokines and immune cells found in the intima may potentiate programmed SMC death. Indeed, a balance between SMC migration, proliferation, and apoptosis regulates the numbers of these cells in evolving atheromatic plaques, diverting the functional futures of the plaques to either a vulnerable or a stable phenotype [94].

The volume of an atherosclerotic plaque is highly dependent on the ECM, which mainly consists of collagen fibers (types I and III), elastin, and proteoglycans. These molecules are produced by SMCs under the stimulus of chemokines such as PDGF and TGF-β.

Of note, the composition of the ECM components depends on a balance between MMPs, which catabolize components of this extracellular network, and their inhibitors—TIMPs.

MMPs and TIMPs play major roles not only in ECM degradation but also in mediating cell migration and proliferation, and tissue remodeling. SMC migration through a dense layer of extracellular components depends on this balance between MMPs and TIMPs.

The incidence of acute coronary events is not associated with the degree of stenosis or the plaque volume, and a significant proportion of acute coronary events happens in atherosclerotic plaques causing less than 50% stenosis [95, 96].

Plaque characteristics that predispose to vulnerability have been identified based on pathological studies and are described by the general term "thin-cap fibroatheroma." The characteristics of such a vulnerable plaque include—among others—a thin fibrous cap, outward remodeling and infiltration of the plaque with inflammatory cells [97–99].

15.8 Fibrosis Evaluation

Since fibrosis of the cardiovascular system has a central pathogenetic role in several cardiovascular entities, identification, quantification, and long-term monitoring of ECM components is of importance. However, since imaging and examination modalities have difficulty in characterizing tissue characteristics, we have limited options. Of course, autopsy studies may provide important information, but from a clinical perspective they are not of importance, while myocardial biopsies are a high-risk invasive strategy, which is not indicated in humans.

Another approach is to use—as a surrogate for fibrosis—specific circulating biomarkers. The most relevant are galectin-3, ST-2, procollagen 3, N-terminal peptide, carboxyterminal propeptide of type I procollagen, and syndecan-4, which are also associated with the prognosis and clinical course of heart failure [1]. However, this strategy also has significant limitations since, of the biomarkers in use, some are not an absolute signal of fibrosis but may also be associated with inflammation. Moreover, they lack cardiac specificity and may be found to be elevated in other fibrosis-associated diseases.

The most applied imaging modality in heart failure (echocardiography) can provide only indirect information such as the level and progression of diastolic dysfunction. Until now the most useful modality to evaluate cardiac fibrosis has been cardiac magnetic resonance. Late gadolinium enhancement may characterize the region of myocardial infarction and extensive areas of myocardial damage caused by myocarditis. However, interstitial fibrosis is difficult to determine (only increments in extracellular volumes can be defined) with T1 mapping and is not tissue specific; nor may it be accurately quantified in the whole myocardial mass [100].

15.9 Treatment of Extracellular Matrix Remodeling and Fibrosis

Cardiovascular drugs have been examined for their ability to modulate ECM synthesis and fibrosis. Amlodipine and diltiazem, when applied to cultured vascular endothelial cells, increase the activity of MMP-1 and MMP-2, with parallel increases in IL-6 mRNA transcription and TIMP-1 [101]. Angiotensin II has been found to uptitrate levels of MMP-1 [102], while losartan, when acting on SMCs, increases the activity of MMP-2. In macrophages, nitroglycerin may cause activation of MMP-2, MMP-7, and MMP-9, with a corresponding decrease in TIMP-1 expression [103].

Hydroxy-methyl-glutaryl coenzyme (HMG-CoA) reductase inhibitors, or statins, are another potent type of medicine, with pleiotropic effects in the cardiovascular system and especially in the modulation of atherosclerosis [104, 105]. Human endothelial cells incubated with fluvastatin and lovastatin present reduced MMP-1 activity [106]. Similarly, macrophages exposed to statins show downregulated MMP-9 activity [107]. Immunocytochemistry in carotid arteries has also shown that pravastatin and simvastatin cause inhibition of MMP-9 and MMP-2 and secretion of TIMP-1 associated with carotid plaques [108, 109].

In patients with ischemic heart failure, spironolactone decreases MMP-9, TIMP-1, and the MMP-9 to TIMP-1 ratio, with a parallel beneficial impact on cardiac remodeling [110]. Accordingly, in patients with LV systolic dysfunction but without heart failure, eplerenone significantly decreased MMP-2 and increased MMP-9 over 24 weeks relative to placebo [111].

Omega-3 polyunsaturated fatty acids may lower levels of MMP-2, MMP-9, and their tissue inhibitors in plasma, indicating a possible favorable effect in vascular remodeling [112]. Recently, we have shown that in patients with heart failure, omega-3 polyunsaturated fatty acids may improve the LV end-diastolic volume and diastolic function [113].

Beta-adrenergic blockers may modulate MMP levels in subjects with heart failure; however, there are no data on the role of this class of drugs in atherosclerotic plaque remodeling [114].

However, we should note that at the moment there are no specific treatments targeting fibrosis, since there are a lot of unanswered questions. Following myocardial infarction, attenuation of fibrosis may be of importance; however, when this happen in the proliferative phase (i.e., when treatment with cortisone is applied in the first days after myocardial infarction) it may cause cardiac rupture or aneurysm formation and heart failure [115]. Similarly, anti-inflammatory and immunosuppressive treatments have not proved useful in chronic myocarditis [116]. In addition, the quality of the ECM may affect the final impact of myocardial remodeling and fibrosis. Crosslinked collagen fibers may be especially responsible for diastolic dysfunction and heart failure following pressure overload. Expression of osteopontin is able to induce the crosslinking enzyme lysyl oxidase when cardiac fibroblasts express syndecam-4, and may be a target of future treatment [117].

In conclusion, in recent years, inflammation has been revealed as an underlying mechanism implicated in most, if not all, cardiovascular diseases. Extracellular matrix remodeling and pathological fibrous formation (quantitative and qualitative) have been recognized as maladaptive tissue responses to most cardiovascular complications. Ample data give insights into the strong regulatory roles of regional and systemic inflammation in the modulation of extracellular matrix degradation and regeneration in a balanced bidirectional connection. Undoubtedly, left ventricular fibrosis and adverse remodeling in cardiomyopathies, in heart failure, and following myocardial infarction will continue to be the focus of research interest in the coming years, not only to improve our understanding of the fundamental mechanisms of extracellular matrix composition and synthesis but also to achieve beneficial modification of extracellular remodeling.

References

1. Oikonomou E, Vogiatzi G, Tsalamandris S, et al. Non-natriuretic peptide biomarkers in heart failure with preserved and reduced ejection fraction. Biomark Med. 2018;12:783–97.
2. Oikonomou E, Tousoulis D. Inflammation: a pathogenetic mechanism or a mediator, linking risk factors and cardiovascular disease? Int J Cardiol. 2018;264:170–1.
3. Brili S, Oikonomou E, Antonopoulos AS, et al. 18F-Fluorodeoxyglucose positron emission tomography/computed tomographic imaging detects aortic wall inflammation in patients with repaired coarctation of aorta. Circ Cardiovasc Imaging. 2018;11:e007002.
4. Antonopoulos AS, Papanikolaou E, Vogiatzi G, Oikonomou E, Tousoulis D. Anti-inflammatory agents in peripheral arterial disease. Curr Opin Pharmacol. 2017;39:1–8.
5. Tousoulis D, Oikonomou E, Economou EK, Crea F, Kaski JC. Inflammatory cytokines in atherosclerosis: current therapeutic approaches. Eur Heart J. 2016;37:1723–32.
6. Oikonomou E, Tousoulis D, Siasos G, Zaromitidou M, Papavassiliou AG, Stefanadis C. The role of inflammation in heart failure: new therapeutic approaches. Hell J Cardiol. 2011;52:30–40.

7. Ridker PM, Everett BM, Thuren T, et al. Antiinflammatory therapy with canakinumab for atherosclerotic disease. N Engl J Med. 2017;377:1119–31.
8. Suthahar N, Meijers WC, Sillje HHW, de Boer RA. From inflammation to fibrosis—molecular and cellular mechanisms of myocardial tissue remodelling and perspectives on differential treatment opportunities. Curr Heart Fail Rep. 2017;14:235–50.
9. Gawor M, Spiewak M, Kubik A, et al. Circulating biomarkers of hypertrophy and fibrosis in patients with hypertrophic cardiomyopathy assessed by cardiac magnetic resonance. Biomarkers. 2018:1–7. https://doi.org/10.1080/1354750X.2018.1474261.
10. Pedretti S, Vargiu S, Baroni M, et al. Complexity of scar and ventricular arrhythmias in dilated cardiomyopathy of any etiology: long-term data from the SCARFEAR (Cardiovascular Magnetic Resonance Predictors of Appropriate Implantable Cardioverter–Defibrillator Therapy Delivery) registry. Clin Cardiol. 2018;41:494–501.
11. Siasos G, Tousoulis D, Kioufis S, et al. Inflammatory mechanisms in atherosclerosis: the impact of matrix metalloproteinases. Curr Top Med Chem. 2012;12:1132–48.
12. Siebermair J, Kholmovski EG, Marrouche N. Assessment of left atrial fibrosis by late gadolinium enhancement magnetic resonance imaging: methodology and clinical implications. JACC Clin Electrophysiol. 2017;3:791–802.
13. Frantz C, Stewart KM, Weaver VM. The extracellular matrix at a glance. J Cell Sci. 2010;123:4195–200.
14. Schaefer L, Schaefer RM. Proteoglycans: from structural compounds to signaling molecules. Cell Tissue Res. 2010;339:237–46.
15. Jarvelainen H, Sainio A, Koulu M, Wight TN, Penttinen R. Extracellular matrix molecules: potential targets in pharmacotherapy. Pharmacol Rev. 2009;61:198–223.
16. McCawley LJ, Matrisian LM. Matrix metalloproteinases: they're not just for matrix anymore! Curr Opin Cell Biol. 2001;13:534–40.
17. Garcia-Touchard A, Henry TD, Sangiorgi G, et al. Extracellular proteases in atherosclerosis and restenosis. Arterioscler Thromb Vasc Biol. 2005;25:1119–27.
18. Plutzky J. The vascular biology of atherosclerosis. Am J Med. 2003;115(Suppl 8A):55S–61S.
19. Creemers EE, Cleutjens JP, Smits JF, Daemen MJ. Matrix metalloproteinase inhibition after myocardial infarction: a new approach to prevent heart failure? Circ Res. 2001;89:201–10.
20. Galis ZS, Khatri JJ. Matrix metalloproteinases in vascular remodeling and atherogenesis: the good, the bad, and the ugly. Circ Res. 2002;90:251–62.
21. Corcoran ML, Stetler-Stevenson WG, DeWitt DL, Wahl LM. Effect of cholera toxin and pertussis toxin on prostaglandin H synthase-2, prostaglandin E2, and matrix metalloproteinase production by human monocytes. Arch Biochem Biophys. 1994;310:481–8.
22. Galis ZS, Sukhova GK, Lark MW, Libby P. Increased expression of matrix metalloproteinases and matrix degrading activity in vulnerable regions of human atherosclerotic plaques. J Clin Invest. 1994;94:2493–503.
23. Libby P, Galis ZS. Cytokines regulate genes involved in atherogenesis. Ann N Y Acad Sci. 1995;748:158–68. discussion 168–170.
24. Wassenaar A, Verschoor T, Kievits F, et al. CD40 engagement modulates the production of matrix metalloproteinases by gingival fibroblasts. Clin Exp Immunol. 1999;115:161–7.
25. Feinberg MW, Jain MK, Werner F, et al. Transforming growth factor-beta 1 inhibits cytokine-mediated induction of human metalloelastase in macrophages. J Biol Chem. 2000;275:25766–73.
26. Li YY, McTiernan CF, Feldman AM. Interplay of matrix metalloproteinases, tissue inhibitors of metalloproteinases and their regulators in cardiac matrix remodeling. Cardiovasc Res. 2000;46:214–24.
27. Lane WJ, Dias S, Hattori K, et al. Stromal-derived factor 1–induced megakaryocyte migration and platelet production is dependent on matrix metalloproteinases. Blood. 2000;96:4152–9.
28. Xu XP, Meisel SR, Ong JM, et al. Oxidized low-density lipoprotein regulates matrix metalloproteinase-9 and its tissue inhibitor in human monocyte–derived macrophages. Circulation. 1999;99:993–8.

29. Chen KC, Wang YS, Hu CY, et al. OxLDL up-regulates microRNA-29b, leading to epigenetic modifications of MMP-2/MMP-9 genes: a novel mechanism for cardiovascular diseases. FASEB J. 2011;25:1718–28.
30. Okamoto T, Akaike T, Nagano T, et al. Activation of human neutrophil procollagenase by nitrogen dioxide and peroxynitrite: a novel mechanism for procollagenase activation involving nitric oxide. Arch Biochem Biophys. 1997;342:261–74.
31. Cai H, Harrison DG. Endothelial dysfunction in cardiovascular diseases: the role of oxidant stress. Circ Res. 2000;87:840–4.
32. Ye S. Polymorphism in matrix metalloproteinase gene promoters: implication in regulation of gene expression and susceptibility of various diseases. Matrix Biol. 2000;19:623–9.
33. Ben-Yosef Y, Lahat N, Shapiro S, Bitterman H, Miller A. Regulation of endothelial matrix metalloproteinase-2 by hypoxia/reoxygenation. Circ Res. 2002;90:784–91.
34. Rajagopalan S, Meng XP, Ramasamy S, Harrison DG, Galis ZS. Reactive oxygen species produced by macrophage-derived foam cells regulate the activity of vascular matrix metalloproteinases in vitro: implications for atherosclerotic plaque stability. J Clin Invest. 1996;98:2572–9.
35. Bassiouny HS, Song RH, Hong XF, Singh A, Kocharyan H, Glagov S. Flow regulation of 72-kD collagenase IV (MMP-2) after experimental arterial injury. Circulation. 1998;98:157–63.
36. Godin D, Ivan E, Johnson C, Magid R, Galis ZS. Remodeling of carotid artery is associated with increased expression of matrix metalloproteinases in mouse blood flow cessation model. Circulation. 2000;102:2861–6.
37. Chesler NC, Ku DN, Galis ZS. Transmural pressure induces matrix-degrading activity in porcine arteries ex vivo. Am J Phys. 1999;277:H2002–9.
38. Sundstrom J, Evans JC, Benjamin EJ, et al. Relations of plasma matrix metalloproteinase-9 to clinical cardiovascular risk factors and echocardiographic left ventricular measures: the Framingham Heart Study. Circulation. 2004;109:2850–6.
39. Abboud RT, Fera T, Johal S, Richter A, Gibson N. Effect of smoking on plasma neutrophil elastase levels. J Lab Clin Med. 1986;108:294–300.
40. Sundstrom J, Evans JC, Benjamin EJ, et al. Relations of plasma total TIMP-1 levels to cardiovascular risk factors and echocardiographic measures: the Framingham Heart Study. Eur Heart J. 2004;25:1509–16.
41. Nakamura T, Ebihara I, Shimada N, Koide H. Effect of cigarette smoking on plasma metalloproteinase-9 concentration. Clin Chim Acta. 1998;276:173–7.
42. Koh KK, Ahn JY, Kang MH, et al. Effects of hormone replacement therapy on plaque stability, inflammation, and fibrinolysis in hypertensive or overweight postmenopausal women. Am J Cardiol. 2001;88:1423–6. A8
43. Kalela A, Ponnio M, Koivu TA, et al. Association of serum sialic acid and MMP-9 with lipids and inflammatory markers. Eur J Clin Investig. 2000;30:99–104.
44. Marx N, Froehlich J, Siam L, et al. Antidiabetic PPAR gamma-activator rosiglitazone reduces MMP-9 serum levels in type 2 diabetic patients with coronary artery disease. Arterioscler Thromb Vasc Biol. 2003;23:283–8.
45. Papazafiropoulou A, Perrea D, Moyssakis I, Kokkinos A, Katsilambros N, Tentolouris N. Plasma levels of MMP-2, MMP-9 and TIMP-1 are not associated with arterial stiffness in subjects with type 2 diabetes mellitus. J Diabetes Complications. 2010;24:20–7.
46. Carlyle WC, Jacobson AW, Judd DL, et al. Delayed reperfusion alters matrix metalloproteinase activity and fibronectin mRNA expression in the infarct zone of the ligated rat heart. J Mol Cell Cardiol. 1997;29:2451–63.
47. Cleutjens JP, Kandala JC, Guarda E, Guntaka RV, Weber KT. Regulation of collagen degradation in the rat myocardium after infarction. J Mol Cell Cardiol. 1995;27:1281–92.
48. Tyagi SC, Kumar SG, Haas SJ, et al. Post-transcriptional regulation of extracellular matrix metalloproteinase in human heart end-stage failure secondary to ischemic cardiomyopathy. J Mol Cell Cardiol. 1996;28:1415–28.

49. Sato S, Ashraf M, Millard RW, Fujiwara H, Schwartz A. Connective tissue changes in early ischemia of porcine myocardium: an ultrastructural study. J Mol Cell Cardiol. 1983;15:261–75.
50. Danielsen CC, Wiggers H, Andersen HR. Increased amounts of collagenase and gelatinase in porcine myocardium following ischemia and reperfusion. J Mol Cell Cardiol. 1998;30:1431–42.
51. Heymans S, Luttun A, Nuyens D, et al. Inhibition of plasminogen activators or matrix metalloproteinases prevents cardiac rupture but impairs therapeutic angiogenesis and causes cardiac failure. Nat Med. 1999;5:1135–42.
52. Ducharme A, Frantz S, Aikawa M, et al. Targeted deletion of matrix metalloproteinase-9 attenuates left ventricular enlargement and collagen accumulation after experimental myocardial infarction. J Clin Invest. 2000;106:55–62.
53. Thomas CV, Coker ML, Zellner JL, Handy JR, Crumbley AJ 3rd, Spinale FG. Increased matrix metalloproteinase activity and selective upregulation in LV myocardium from patients with end-stage dilated cardiomyopathy. Circulation. 1998;97:1708–15.
54. Tyagi SC, Kumar S, Voelker DJ, Reddy HK, Janicki JS, Curtis JJ. Differential gene expression of extracellular matrix components in dilated cardiomyopathy. J Cell Biochem. 1996;63:185–98.
55. Spinale FG, Coker ML, Thomas CV, Walker JD, Mukherjee R, Hebbar L. Time-dependent changes in matrix metalloproteinase activity and expression during the progression of congestive heart failure: relation to ventricular and myocyte function. Circ Res. 1998;82:482–95.
56. Li YY, Feldman AM, Sun Y, McTiernan CF. Differential expression of tissue inhibitors of metalloproteinases in the failing human heart. Circulation. 1998;98:1728–34.
57. Coker ML, Thomas CV, Clair MJ, et al. Myocardial matrix metalloproteinase activity and abundance with congestive heart failure. Am J Phys 1998; 274:H1516–HH1523.
58. Spinale FG, Coker ML, Krombach SR, et al. Matrix metalloproteinase inhibition during the development of congestive heart failure: effects on left ventricular dimensions and function. Circ Res. 1999;85:364–76.
59. Nakaya M, Watari K, Tajima M, et al. Cardiac myofibroblast engulfment of dead cells facilitates recovery after myocardial infarction. J Clin Invest. 2017;127:383–401.
60. Frangogiannis NG. The inflammatory response in myocardial injury, repair, and remodelling. Nat Rev Cardiol. 2014;11:255–65.
61. Hohensinner PJ, Kaun C, Rychli K, et al. Monocyte chemoattractant protein (MCP-1) is expressed in human cardiac cells and is differentially regulated by inflammatory mediators and hypoxia. FEBS Lett. 2006;580:3532–8.
62. Gabriel AS, Martinsson A, Wretlind B, Ahnve S. IL-6 levels in acute and post myocardial infarction: their relation to CRP levels, infarction size, left ventricular systolic function, and heart failure. Eur J Intern Med. 2004;15:523–8.
63. Nah DY, Rhee MY. The inflammatory response and cardiac repair after myocardial infarction. Korean Circ J. 2009;39:393–8.
64. Meijers WC, van der Velde AR, Pascual-Figal DA, de Boer RA. Galectin-3 and post-myocardial infarction cardiac remodeling. Eur J Pharmacol. 2015;763:115–21.
65. Bujak M, Frangogiannis NG. The role of TGF-beta signaling in myocardial infarction and cardiac remodeling. Cardiovasc Res. 2007;74:184–95.
66. Talman V, Ruskoaho H. Cardiac fibrosis in myocardial infarction—from repair and remodeling to regeneration. Cell Tissue Res. 2016;365:563–81.
67. Wang Q, Wehrens XH. Connecting enterovirus infection to dystrophin dysfunction in dilated cardiomyopathy. Ann Transl Med. 2016;4:S23.
68. Corsten MF, Schroen B, Heymans S. Inflammation in viral myocarditis: friend or foe? Trends Mol Med. 2012;18:426–37.
69. Schwimmbeck PL, Rohn G, Wrusch A, et al. Enteroviral and immune mediated myocarditis in SCID mice. Herz. 2000;25:240–4.

70. Li K, Xu W, Guo Q, et al. Differential macrophage polarization in male and female BALB/c mice infected with coxsackievirus B3 defines susceptibility to viral myocarditis. Circ Res. 2009;105:353–64.
71. Frantz S, Ducharme A, Sawyer D, et al. Targeted deletion of caspase-1 reduces early mortality and left ventricular dilatation following myocardial infarction. J Mol Cell Cardiol. 2003;35:685–94.
72. Diwan A, Dibbs Z, Nemoto S, et al. Targeted overexpression of noncleavable and secreted forms of tumor necrosis factor provokes disparate cardiac phenotypes. Circulation. 2004;109:262–8.
73. Krishnamurthy P, Rajasingh J, Lambers E, Qin G, Losordo DW, Kishore R. IL-10 inhibits inflammation and attenuates left ventricular remodeling after myocardial infarction via activation of STAT3 and suppression of HuR. Circ Res. 2009;104:e9–18.
74. Frantz S, Hu K, Bayer B, et al. Absence of NF-kappaB subunit p50 improves heart failure after myocardial infarction. FASEB J. 2006;20:1918–20.
75. Authors/Task Force Members, Elliott PM, Anastasakis A, et al. 2014 ESC guidelines on diagnosis and management of hypertrophic cardiomyopathy: the Task Force for the Diagnosis and Management of Hypertrophic Cardiomyopathy of the European Society of Cardiology (ESC). Eur Heart J. 2014;35:2733–79.
76. Rudolph A, Abdel-Aty H, Bohl S, et al. Noninvasive detection of fibrosis applying contrast-enhanced cardiac magnetic resonance in different forms of left ventricular hypertrophy relation to remodeling. J Am Coll Cardiol. 2009;53:284–91.
77. Moon JC, Reed E, Sheppard MN, et al. The histologic basis of late gadolinium enhancement cardiovascular magnetic resonance in hypertrophic cardiomyopathy. J Am Coll Cardiol. 2004;43:2260–4.
78. O'Hanlon R, Grasso A, Roughton M, et al. Prognostic significance of myocardial fibrosis in hypertrophic cardiomyopathy. J Am Coll Cardiol. 2010;56:867–74.
79. Ho CY, Lopez B, Coelho-Filho OR, et al. Myocardial fibrosis as an early manifestation of hypertrophic cardiomyopathy. N Engl J Med. 2010;363:552–63.
80. Harvey A, Montezano AC, Lopes RA, Rios F, Touyz RM. Vascular fibrosis in aging and hypertension: molecular mechanisms and clinical implications. Can J Cardiol. 2016;32:659–68.
81. Bleakley C, Hamilton PK, Pumb R, Harbinson M, McVeigh GE. Endothelial function in hypertension: victim or culprit? J Clin Hypertens (Greenwich). 2015;17:651–4.
82. Diez J. Mechanisms of cardiac fibrosis in hypertension. J Clin Hypertens (Greenwich). 2007;9:546–50.
83. Gonzalez GE, Rhaleb NE, D'Ambrosio MA, et al. Deletion of interleukin-6 prevents cardiac inflammation, fibrosis and dysfunction without affecting blood pressure in angiotensin II–high salt-induced hypertension. J Hypertens. 2015;33:144–52.
84. Burstein B, Nattel S. Atrial fibrosis: mechanisms and clinical relevance in atrial fibrillation. J Am Coll Cardiol. 2008;51:802–9.
85. Mazaris S, Siasos G, Oikonomou E, et al. Atrial fibrillation: biomarkers determining prognosis. Curr Med Chem. Epub 2017 Jul 27. https://doi.org/10.2174/092986732466617072711564 2.
86. Lehoux S, Lemarie CA, Esposito B, Lijnen HR, Tedgui A. Pressure-induced matrix metalloproteinase-9 contributes to early hypertensive remodeling. Circulation. 2004;109:1041–7.
87. Thompson RW, Parks WC. Role of matrix metalloproteinases in abdominal aortic aneurysms. Ann N Y Acad Sci. 1996;800:157–74.
88. Boden N, Cheng Y, Knowles PF. Equilibrium and non-equilibrium conformations of peptides in lipid bilayers. Biophys Chem. 1997;65:205–10.
89. Patel MI, Melrose J, Ghosh P, Appleberg M. Increased synthesis of matrix metalloproteinases by aortic smooth muscle cells is implicated in the etiopathogenesis of abdominal aortic aneurysms. J Vasc Surg. 1996;24:82–92.

90. McMillan WD, Tamarina NA, Cipollone M, Johnson DA, Parker MA, Pearce WH. Size matters: the relationship between MMP-9 expression and aortic diameter. Circulation. 1997;96:2228–32.
91. Pyo R, Lee JK, Shipley JM, et al. Targeted gene disruption of matrix metalloproteinase-9 (gelatinase B) suppresses development of experimental abdominal aortic aneurysms. J Clin Invest. 2000;105:1641–9.
92. Habashi JP, Judge DP, Holm TM, et al. Losartan, an AT1 antagonist, prevents aortic aneurysm in a mouse model of Marfan syndrome. Science. 2006;312:117–21.
93. Brili S, Antonopoulos AS, Oikonomou E, et al. Impairment of arterial elastic properties and elevated circulating levels of transforming growth factor-beta in subjects with repaired coarctation of aorta. Int J Cardiol. 2016;207:282–3.
94. Bentzon JF, Weile C, Sondergaard CS, Hindkjaer J, Kassem M, Falk E. Smooth muscle cells in atherosclerosis originate from the local vessel wall and not circulating progenitor cells in ApoE knockout mice. Arterioscler Thromb Vasc Biol. 2006;26:2696–702.
95. Falk E, Shah PK, Fuster V. Coronary plaque disruption. Circulation. 1995;92:657–71.
96. Motoyama S, Ito H, Sarai M, et al. Plaque characterization by coronary computed tomography angiography and the likelihood of acute coronary events in mid-term follow-up. J Am Coll Cardiol. 2015;66:337–46.
97. Schaar JA, Muller JE, Falk E, et al. Terminology for high-risk and vulnerable coronary artery plaques. Report of a meeting on the vulnerable plaque, June 17 and 18, 2003, Santorini, Greece. Eur Heart J. 2004;25:1077–82.
98. Varnava AM, Mills PG, Davies MJ. Relationship between coronary artery remodeling and plaque vulnerability. Circulation. 2002;105:939–43.
99. Arbustini E, Dal Bello B, Morbini P, et al. Plaque erosion is a major substrate for coronary thrombosis in acute myocardial infarction. Heart. 1999;82:269–72.
100. Masci PG, Doulaptsis C, Bertella E, et al. Incremental prognostic value of myocardial fibrosis in patients with non-ischemic cardiomyopathy without congestive heart failure. Circ Heart Fail. 2014;7:448–56.
101. Eickelberg O, Roth M, Mussmann R, et al. Calcium channel blockers activate the interleukin-6 gene via the transcription factors NF-IL6 and NF-kappaB in primary human vascular smooth muscle cells. Circulation. 1999;99:2276–82.
102. Funck RC, Wilke A, Rupp H, Brilla CG. Regulation and role of myocardial collagen matrix remodeling in hypertensive heart disease. Adv Exp Med Biol. 1997;432:35–44.
103. Death AK, Nakhla S, McGrath KC, et al. Nitroglycerin upregulates matrix metalloproteinase expression by human macrophages. J Am Coll Cardiol. 2002;39:1943–50.
104. Tousoulis D, Antoniades C, Vasiliadou C, et al. Effects of atorvastatin and vitamin C on forearm hyperaemic blood flow, asymmetrical dimethylarginine levels and the inflammatory process in patients with type 2 diabetes mellitus. Heart. 2007;93:244–6.
105. Tousoulis D, Charakida M, Stefanadi E, Siasos G, Latsios G, Stefanadis C. Statins in heart failure: beyond the lipid lowering effect. Int J Cardiol. 2007;115:144–50.
106. Ikeda U, Shimpo M, Ohki R, et al. Fluvastatin inhibits matrix metalloproteinase-1 expression in human vascular endothelial cells. Hypertension. 2000;36:325–9.
107. Bellosta S, Via D, Canavesi M, et al. HMG-CoA reductase inhibitors reduce MMP-9 secretion by macrophages. Arterioscler Thromb Vasc Biol. 1998;18:1671–8.
108. Crisby M, Nordin-Fredriksson G, Shah PK, Yano J, Zhu J, Nilsson J. Pravastatin treatment increases collagen content and decreases lipid content, inflammation, metalloproteinases, and cell death in human carotid plaques: implications for plaque stabilization. Circulation. 2001;103:926–33.
109. Cipollone F, Fazia M, Iezzi A, et al. Suppression of the functionally coupled cyclooxygenase-2/prostaglandin E synthase as a basis of simvastatin-dependent plaque stabilization in humans. Circulation. 2003;107:1479–85.
110. Li MJ, Huang CX, Okello E, Yanhong T, Mohamed S. Treatment with spironolactone for 24 weeks decreases the level of matrix metalloproteinases and improves cardiac function in patients with chronic heart failure of ischemic etiology. Can J Cardiol. 2009;25:523–6.

111. Weir RA, Mark PB, Petrie CJ, et al. Left ventricular remodeling after acute myocardial infarction: does eplerenone have an effect? Am Heart J. 2009;157:1088–96.
112. Derosa G, Maffioli P, D'Angelo A, et al. Effects of long chain omega-3 fatty acids on metalloproteinases and their inhibitors in combined dyslipidemia patients. Expert Opin Pharmacother. 2009;10:1239–47.
113. Oikonomou E, Vogiatzi G, Karlis D, et al. Effects of omega-3 polyunsaturated fatty acids on fibrosis, endothelial function and myocardial performance, in ischemic heart failure patients. Clin Nutr. Epub 2018 May 3. https://doi.org/10.1016/j.clnu.2018.04.017.
114. Wu TC, Chen YH, Leu HB, et al. Carvedilol, a pharmacological antioxidant, inhibits neointimal matrix metalloproteinase-2 and -9 in experimental atherosclerosis. Free Radic Biol Med. 2007;43:1508–22.
115. Gonzalez GE, Cassaglia P, Noli Truant S, et al. Galectin-3 is essential for early wound healing and ventricular remodeling after myocardial infarction in mice. Int J Cardiol. 2014;176:1423–5.
116. Mason JW, O'Connell JB, Herskowitz A, et al. A clinical trial of immunosuppressive therapy for myocarditis. The Myocarditis Treatment Trial Investigators. N Engl J Med. 1995;333:269–75.
117. Herum KM, Lunde IG, Skrbic B, et al. Syndecan-4 is a key determinant of collagen cross-linking and passive myocardial stiffness in the pressure-overloaded heart. Cardiovasc Res. 2015;106:217–26.

Chapter 16
Endogenous Regeneration of the Mammalian Heart

Konstantinos Malliaras

16.1 Introduction

The mammalian heart was traditionally viewed as a static organ, containing terminally differentiated postmitotic myocytes, devoid of any regenerative capacity. This belief, adopted by the majority of the scientific community for over a century, should not come as a surprise. After all, it is well established that myocardial injury resulting in myocyte death heals by replacement fibrosis, without any readily detectable regeneration at the macroscopic level. In addition, the incidence of primary cardiac tumors derived from myocytes (i.e., rhabdomyomas/rhabdomyosarcomas) is extremely low [1]. However, during the last decade, the concept of the mammalian heart as a regenerative organ has gained significant traction. It is now firmly established that traceable endogenous cardiomyocyte replenishment occurs throughout life both in rodents and in humans [2–4]. While this regenerative capacity is limited (and clearly insufficient to remuscularize the heart in pathologic conditions characterized by substantial myocyte losses), it certainly carries immense appeal from a therapeutic standpoint; exogenous stimulation of innate regenerative mechanisms would most likely lead to development of more effective therapeutic strategies for a wide spectrum of cardiac diseases. In this chapter, we will discuss:

(a) The rates of myocyte turnover in the mammalian heart during normal aging and after cardiac injury
(b) The cellular sources of myocyte replenishment (proliferation of resident myocytes versus cardiomyogenic differentiation endogenous progenitors)
(c) The roles of the nervous system and the immune system in cardiac regeneration
(d) Therapeutic strategies to stimulate endogenous cardiac regeneration

---

K. Malliaras (✉)
Department of Cardiology, Laikon Hospital, Athens, Greece

D. V. Cokkinos (ed.), *Myocardial Preservation*,
https://doi.org/10.1007/978-3-319-98186-4_16

16.2 Rates of Myocyte Turnover in the Mammalian Heart

The most convincing evidence demonstrating that myocyte turnover does indeed occur in the human heart during normal aging was provided by the Frisen group [5, 6]. These researchers recognized that the aboveground nuclear weapon testing that occurred in the late 1950s resulted in a worldwide ^{14}C pulse, which could be used to retrospectively measure myocyte turnover. They used accelerator mass spectrometry to perform radiocarbon dating of myocyte DNA obtained from 12 (age range: 19–73 years) [5] and 51 (age range: 8–75 years) [6] explanted hearts. Using mathematical modeling, they calculated that myocyte turnover reaches its peak in early childhood and then decreases exponentially with age. More specifically, *myocyte turnover* occurs at an annual rate of ~3–4% during the first decade of life and then gradually decreases at ~2%/year at age 10, ~1%/year at age 20, and at ~0.4%/year at age 75; thus, ~50% of myocytes are replenished during an average lifespan. Similar rates of human myocyte turnover were reported by Mollova et al., who performed immunostaining for proteins associated with cell cycle progression and cytokinesis in 36 explanted hearts (age range 0–59 years) [7]. They found that human myocyte cycling was highest in infants and then decreased gradually to an estimated annual turnover rate of ~1.9% at 20 years of age and to 0.04% at >40 years of age. A nearly identical temporal pattern of changes in myocyte turnover has also been reported in mice. More specifically, in the healthy mouse heart, myocyte turnover is highest during the early postnatal period [8–10] and then decreases exponentially with age (to an annual turnover rate of 0.7–1.3% in adult mice) [8, 11, 12].

What happens after myocardial injury? The neonatal mouse heart has an impressive ability for near-complete regeneration in response to a wide range of injurious stimuli, including apical resection ([13], but cf. [14]), myocardial infarction [15, 16], and cryoinjury [17]. More specifically, Porello et al. demonstrated that apical resection performed in the hearts of 1-day-old mice triggers robust cardiomyocyte proliferation and angiogenesis at the injury site, resulting in complete regeneration of the resected myocardium over 21 days, with minimal fibrosis ([13], but cf. [14]). A similar regenerative response was observed by the same research group after induction of myocardial infarction in the hearts of 1-day-old mice [15]. However, this capacity for robust endogenous cardiac regeneration (which resembles the regenerative potential possessed by lower vertebrates such as newts [18] and zebrafish [19]) was lost by postnatal day 7 [15]. Whether a similar transient capacity for robust regeneration exists in large mammals (including humans) remains unknown; however, anecdotal evidence suggests that the neonatal human heart may also possess substantial regenerative capacity. To that end, a case series reported minimal long-term scarring and functional recovery of left ventricular function in 14 pediatric patients with surgically corrected anomalous left coronary artery from the pulmonary artery, despite evidence of scarring and compromised cardiac function prior to surgery [20]. In addition, Haubner et al. described a case of a newborn child who, on postnatal day 1, suffered a large anteroseptal myocardial infarction requiring inotropic therapy and mechanical circulatory support with an extracorporeal membrane oxygenation device. Intriguingly, despite the large ischemic insult and the late administration of thrombolysis (28 h post myocardial infarction), the pediatric patient displayed complete normalization of cardiac function over a period of 6 weeks [21].

Contrary to the neonatal heart, the injured adult mammalian heart harbors very limited regenerative potential, which is clearly insufficient to replace lost myocytes at a clinically relevant degree following injury. However, multiple lines of evidence suggest that a detectable increase in new myocyte formation occurs after cardiac injury. Specifically, Beltrami et al. reported a 70-fold increase in the rate of myocyte proliferation (based on the detection of mitotic figures in myocyte nuclei) in the border zone of infarcted human hearts compared to healthy control hearts [22]. Kajstura et al. reported a 10-fold increase in the rate of myocyte proliferation (based on the detection of mitotic figures) in failing human hearts compared to healthy control hearts [23]. In addition, several independent research groups have demonstrated a ~10- to 20-fold increase in myocyte regeneration (or in myocyte cycling) in the border zone of infarcted adult mouse hearts, compared to healthy control hearts [8, 11, 12].

In conclusion, it has been now convincingly demonstrated that the healthy mammalian heart undergoes continuous cardiomyocyte replenishment throughout life. The rate of myocyte turnover seems to be highest during infancy/childhood and then to decrease exponentially with age. In addition, myocardial injury appears to trigger a robust regenerative response in neonatal hearts, but only a small (but traceable) increase in myocyte replenishment in adult hearts. In the next section, we will discuss the cellular sources of the postnatally generated myocytes, which have been at the epicenter of intense debate.

16.3 Cellular Sources of Myocyte Replenishment

Whether newly formed myocytes arise from proliferation of resident myocytes, from myogenic differentiation of endogenous cardiac progenitors, or from both processes at the same time has been the focus of intensive research.

Genetic fate-mapping experiments have demonstrated that proliferation of preexisting cardiomyocytes appears to be the dominant mechanism of myocyte replenishment after cardiac injury in the *neonatal* mouse heart [13, 15]. With regard to the *adult* mouse heart, studies from two independent laboratories which combined genetic fate mapping with *pulse-chase* approaches have shown that myocyte replenishment during normal aging occurs almost exclusively via proliferation of preexisting myocytes (and not via myogenic differentiation of endogenous progenitors) [8, 12]. These proliferating myocytes are smaller in size and mononucleated [12, 24] and – based on the findings of Kimura et al. – express hypoxia-inducible factor 1a (consistent with a hypoxic phenotype) [24]. This hypoxic phenotype may render cycling cardiomyocytes resistant to oxidative DNA damage; the latter purportedly induces cell cycle arrest as myocytes transition from the hypoxic intrauterine environment to the oxygen-rich postnatal environment [25].

Induction of myocardial infarction in adult mouse hearts results (as mentioned earlier in this review) in a 10–20-fold increase in resident *myocyte proliferation* in the infarct border zone [8, 11, 12]. While the increased proliferation of resident adult myocytes post myocardial infarction is accepted by the majority of the research community [26], controversy surrounds the potential role of *progenitor cells* in cardiomyogenesis following cardiac injury. The first study that provided convincing evidence suggesting that endogenous progenitors contribute significantly to myocyte replenishment in the infarcted mouse heart was performed by Hsieh et al. [27]. These researchers used bitransgenic αMHC-MerCreMer/ZEG mice, in which induction of Cre recombinase activity (via tamoxifen administration) results in genetic labeling of ~80% of resident myocytes with green fluorescent protein (GFP). Since endogenous progenitors are presumably not labeled by GFP, any progenitor cell-mediated cardiomyocyte replacement would result in dilution of the GFP+ pool by GFP- cardiomyocytes. Hsieh et al. reported that during normal aging, the percentage of GFP+ myocytes remained unchanged, suggesting that in the normal adult mouse heart, no detectable progenitor cell-mediated cardiomyocyte replenishment occurs. However, following induction of myocardial infarction, the percentage of GFP+ myocytes decreased significantly, suggesting that substantial myogenic differentiation of (unlabeled) endogenous progenitors occurs following cardiac injury [27]. These findings were reproduced by several independent groups using similar methodology [12, 28, 29].

In an effort to better document the activation of these committed progenitors post-injury, Malliaras et al. used the bitransgenic αMHC-MerCreMer/ZEG mice described above but induced the activity of Cre recombinase following (and not prior to) myocardial infarction [30]. In this way, the researchers achieved genetic labeling of the endogenous progenitors, as they became activated (i.e., switched on the αMHC promoter). These endogenous progenitors were rare in normal hearts (comprising ~0.2% of non-myocyte cardiac cells). Importantly, cardiac injury stimulated the robust activation of the said progenitors (which comprised ~1.5% of the non-myocyte pool after myocardial injury). These activated progenitors could spontaneously contract ex vivo (after isolation) and expressed cardiac transcription factors, sarcomeric proteins, and cycling proteins. They neither arose from differentiation of bone marrow cells nor from dedifferentiation of mature myocytes. In addition, they could form mature myocytes, structurally integrated in host myocardium, after delivery into recipient hearts. While the genetic approach employed by Malliaras et al. enables characterization of the activated, partially differentiated cardiac progenitors, it cannot elucidate the identity/properties of the uncommitted, undifferentiated parent stem cell.

What is the identity of the said parent stem cells? During the past 18 years, several populations of putative adult cardiac stem cells have been proposed, including c-kit+ cells (CD117) [31], sca-1+ (stem cell antigen-1+) cells [32], cardiac side-population cells [33], SSEA-1+ cells (stage-specific embryonic antigen-1) [34], epicardium-derived cardiac progenitor cells [35], and cardiosphere-derived cells

(CDCs) [36, 37]. All the above cell types can differentiate into all three major cardiac lineages (cardiomyocytes, vascular smooth muscle cells, and endothelial cells) in vitro and possibly in vivo after exogenous administration. However, their physiologic role (if any) in the naturally occurring myocyte turnover remains controversial. In the study by Malliaras et al. (described above) [30], the activated progenitors were negative for c-kit, SSEA-1, PDGFRα (platelet-derived growth factor receptor alpha), and CD34; 50% of the activated progenitors were positive for Sca-1, and 10% were positive for nestin. However, the optimal way to identify a potential contribution of the aforementioned purported cardiac progenitor cells to postnatal cardiomyogenesis is via prospective (forward) fate-mapping studies. Multiple such studies have recently been published. Reviewing the published data in their totality, the main findings can be summarized as follows:

(a) The role of cardiac *c-kit+ cells* in postnatal cardiomyogenesis has been the subject of intense debate. A fate-mapping study by Ellison et al. reported that, following isoproterenol-mediated myocardial injury (a disease model that mimics stress-mediated cardiomyopathy), c-kit+ cells give rise to a substantial number of newly formed myocytes (replenishing ~4–7% of the myocyte pool over a period of 4 weeks) [28]. However, several subsequent fate-mapping studies from independent laboratories demonstrated that the contributions of c-kit+ cells to the myocyte pool (both in the healthy and in the infarcted heart) are negligible [38–40]. Perhaps these inconsistent results can be explained by the different fate-mapping approaches employed in these studies. Ellison et al. used in situ genetic labeling c-kit+ cells by infecting the hearts of reporter mice with a lentiviral vector expressing Cre recombinase under the control of the c-kit promoter [28]. On the other hand, the other studies used knock-in transgenic mice [38–40]. Even though critiques have arisen regarding both approaches [41–44], currently the consensus is that c-kit+ cells do not give rise to myocytes at a clinically meaningful degree [26].

(b) Forward fate-mapping studies have also investigated the potential roles of Sca-1+ cells [45], Bmi1+ cells [46], neural crest-derived cells [47], and epicardium-derived cells in innate cardiac regeneration [48]. Specifically, Uchida et al. reported that Sca-1+ cells (which have been isolated from mouse but not from human hearts) give rise to a traceable but physiologically irrelevant number of myocytes during normal aging, after myocardial infarction, or after pressure overload [45]. Valiente-Alandi et al. reported that Bm1+ progenitor cells annually replenish 7% of myocytes in the adult mouse heart [46]. Tamura et al. reported that while neural crest-derived cells (which express nestin) minimally contribute to postnatal cardiomyogenesis during normal aging, they regenerate a substantial portion of myocytes after myocardial infarction (~3% of myocytes in the infarct border zone) [47]. Finally, the ability of epicardium-derived cells to form myocytes in the healthy or injured heart has been the subject of intense debate. The consensus is that the contribution of epicardium-derived cells to postnatal cardiomyogenesis is negligible [48]; however, the cardiomyogenic capacity of epicardium-derived cells may be amplified by priming the epicardium with exogenous factors [49, 50].

In conclusion, the *neonatal* mammalian heart appears to replenish lost myocytes through robust proliferation of preexisting myocytes, similarly to the regenerative response observed in newts [18] and zebrafish [19]. Likewise, myocyte turnover in the adult mammalian heart during normal aging appears to occur predominantly via proliferation of preexisting (small, mononucleated, and possibly hypoxic) myocytes [8, 12, 24, 51], without any significant contributions by endogenous progenitors [8, 12, 27]. Myocardial injury in the adult heart results in upregulation of resident myocyte proliferation, primarily in the infarct border zone [8, 11, 12]. In addition, it may stimulate activation and cardiomyogenic differentiation of endogenous progenitors, resulting in traceable progenitor cell-derived contributions to the myocyte pool of the injured heart [12, 27–29, 30, 47, 52]. However, the identity of the said endogenous progenitors has not yet been elucidated.

16.4 Neonatal Cardiac Regeneration: The Roles of the Nervous and Immune Systems

The transient robust regenerative potential of the neonatal mouse heart has enabled researchers to gain insight into some of the mechanisms governing mammalian cardiac regeneration. To that end, recent studies have highlighted the role of peripheral nerves and the role of inflammation in the regenerative response observed after injury in the neonatal mouse heart.

The nervous system plays a critical role in orchestrating tissue regeneration in many species (including newts [53], zebrafish [54], and mammals [55]). To that end, recent evidence suggests that nerves are required for the regeneration of the neonatal mouse heart [56, 57]. Specifically, Mahmoud et al. demonstrated that parasympathetic denervation of the neonatal mouse heart (achieved through mechanical disruption of the vagus nerve or through systemic administration of atropine) attenuates myocyte proliferation and impairs cardiac regeneration following injury [56]. Interestingly, gene expression analysis revealed that parasympathetic denervation resulted in blunted expression of inflammatory genes post-injury; specifically, significant downregulation of genes involved in inflammation, would healing, and chemotaxis was observed in denervated hearts. Importantly from a therapeutic standpoint, the negative effects of parasympathetic denervation on cardiac regeneration could partially be rescued by the administration of neuregulin 1 and nerve growth factor recombinant proteins. White et al. investigated the effect of sympathetic nerves on neonatal hear regeneration [57]. They demonstrated (using a fate-mapping approach) that resection of the ventricular apex in neonatal hearts triggers neurogenesis, as sympathetic nerves regrow into the regenerating apical myocardium. Interestingly, chemical sympathetic denervation (achieved through administration of 6-hydroxydopamine hydrobromide) of the neonatal mouse heart inhibited both sympathetic regrowth and myocardial regeneration following apical resection. The results of these studies suggest that autonomic nerves, perhaps both through release of trophic factors and through modulation of the immune response, are required for the robust regenerative response observed in the injured neonatal mouse heart.

The type of inflammatory response that develops following injury plays a central role in promoting or constraining tissue regeneration in many species like, newts [58] and frogs [59]. Recent studies have highlighted the role of the immune system in regulating the regenerative capacity of the neonatal mouse heart. Aurora et al. demonstrated that neonatal macrophages are required for the robust cardiomyogenesis and vasculogenesis observed following myocardial injury; depletion of macrophages resulted in attenuation of the regenerative response and in fibrotic scar formation [60]. Interestingly, depletion of neonatal macrophages did not appear to directly affect the proliferative capacity of cardiomyocytes; however, it significantly impaired angiogenesis in the injured area. Importantly, the researchers performed a comparison between "regenerative" macrophages (obtained from infarcted P1 mice with robust regenerative potential) and "non-regenerative" macrophages (obtained from infarcted P14 mice, which have lost the capacity for complete regeneration following injury). They found that "regenerative" macrophages have a unique phenotype (distinct from M1 and M2), characterized by increased expression of several genes involved in immune modulation, angiogenesis, response to oxidative stress, and production of soluble factors. The important role of the inflammatory immune response in the regenerative response of the injured neonatal heart was also highlighted in a study by Han et al. [61]. These researchers demonstrated that systemic immunosuppression with corticosteroids in neonatal mice prevented the regenerative response that is normally observed after apical resection; instead, immunosuppressed injured neonatal hearts healed by fibrotic scarring. In addition, they showed that IL-6 signaling was necessary for neonatal cardiomyocyte proliferation. Taken together, these studies implicate the inflammatory immune response in cardiac regeneration. In addition, macrophages appear to play a crucial role in the regenerative process, acting presumably through secretion of paracrine factors that promote angiogenesis and regeneration of the neonatal mouse heart after injury.

16.5 Exogenous Stimulation of Endogenous Cardiac Regeneration

Exogenous amplification of endogenous regenerative processes carries an obvious therapeutic appeal; while current treatment strategies in cardiology focus on cardioprotection (e.g., prompt coronary reperfusion) and attenuation of disease progression (e.g., anti-remodeling drugs), stimulation of endogenous cardiac regeneration would offer patients a truly regenerative approach. Thus, the research efforts devoted toward this aim have been immense. Here, we will briefly review therapeutic strategies that have been shown to presumably stimulate endogenous regeneration in vivo (i.e., in experimental animals). Some of these strategies are depicted schematically in Fig. 16.1.

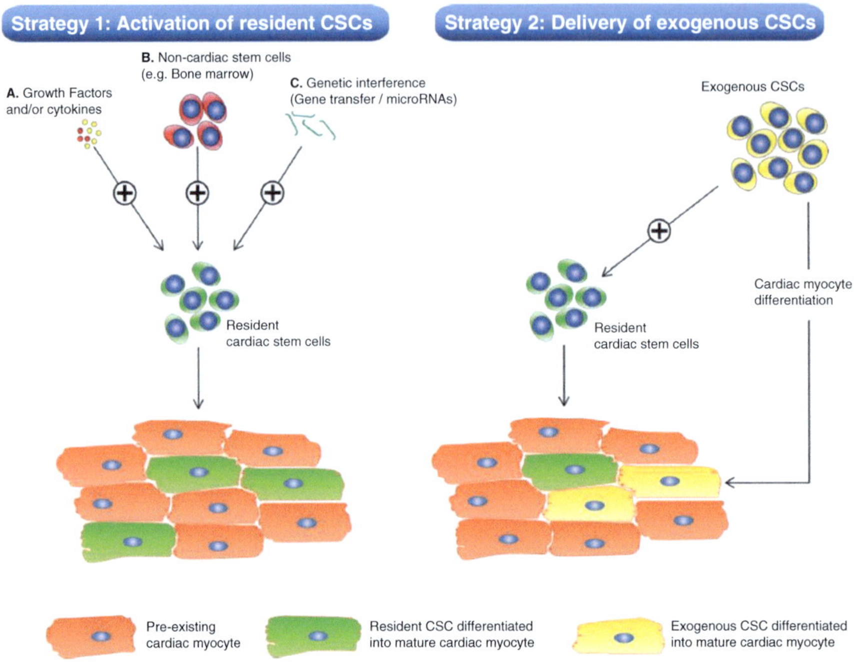

Fig. 16.1 Strategies for therapeutic cardiac regeneration. The first approach (depicted on the left) focuses on exogenous stimulation of endogenous cardiac regeneration, via administration of microRNAs, genes that manipulate the cell cycle, mitogenic factors, growth factors, and progenitor cells. The other approach (depicted on the right) focuses on delivery of progenitor cells (mainly embryonic stem cells or induced pluripotent stem cells), which – through direct differentiation into mature cardiac cells – could form new myocardium. (Obtained from Koudstaal et al. [99] by permission from Stem Cells Transl Med 2013;432:43)

Most mammalian cardiomyocytes withdraw from the cell cycle and become quiescent soon after birth. Therefore, one attempt to amplify division of resident cardiomyocytes has been through genetic manipulation of the cell cycle. Overexpression of cell cycle activators (e.g., *cyclin D2* [62], *cyclin A2* [63, 64], or a combination of *cyclin-dependent kinase 1* [CDK1], *CDK4*, *cyclin B1*, and *cyclin D1* [65]) in cardiomyocytes has been shown to increase myocyte proliferation and confer functional benefits in infarcted mouse hearts. Conversely, suppression of cell cycle inhibitors (e.g., genetic deletion of *retinoblastoma* and *p130* proteins [66]) may also result in increased myocyte proliferation (albeit at the expense of decreased myocyte contractility). In addition, genetic deletion of *Meis1* (a transcription factor that appears to govern myocytes' cell cycle arrest through activation of the CDK inhibitors p15, p16, and p21) has also been shown to upregulate myocyte proliferation, without any negative impact on cardiac function [67].

Mitogenic stimulation of adult myocytes has also been attempted through genetic manipulation of the *Hippo pathway* [68], an evolutionary conserved pathway that controls organ size and participates in cardiac organogenesis [69]. Healen et al.

demonstrated that the Hippo signaling pathway, when active, inhibits cardiomyocyte proliferation both in the developing [70] and in the adult [71] mouse heart. Importantly from a therapeutic perspective, genetic disruption of the Hippo pathway (achieved through genetic inactivation of either Salvador scaffold protein or the large tumor suppressor homolog kinases 1 and 2) stimulated myocyte proliferation in the normal and infarcted mouse heart [71]. Likewise, genetic activation of *Yes-associated protein* (YAP protein, which promotes cellular proliferation and is normally restrained by the Hippo pathway) results in increased myocyte proliferation and enhances cardiac regeneration in infarcted adult mouse hearts [72, 73]. In addition, genetic overexpression of paired-like homeodomain transcription factor 2 (Pitx2, a transcription factor which interacts with YAP and has been found to be upregulated in Hippo-deficient mice) stimulates myocyte proliferation and bestows substantial regenerative capacity in infarcted hearts of adult mice [74]. These results indicate that repression of the Hippo pathway may constitute a valid therapeutic target that could promote endogenous regeneration in the injured mammalian heart.

Stimulation of myocyte proliferation has also been attempted through genetic manipulation of *microRNA* (miRNA) expression. To that end, (a) overexpression of miR-199a [75], miR-590 [75], miR-17-92 [76], and miR-302-367 [77] or (b) suppression of expression of the miR-15 family [15], the miR-99/100 family, and the let-7a/c miRNA family [78] in infarcted adult mouse hearts has been shown to increase myocyte proliferation and promote regeneration. Interestingly, regarding miR-302-367, Tian et al. demonstrated that its sustained overexpression resulted in myocyte dedifferentiation and development of heart failure, while its transient overexpression (using miRNA mimics) conferred regenerative effects without any deleterious consequences [77]. This suggests that the temporal pattern of exogenous stimulation of endogenous regeneration may be of critical importance, as prolonged stimulation could lead to adverse outcomes (e.g., development of heart failure or tumorigenesis).

Another approach for upregulation of adult myocyte proliferation may be through exogenous delivery of mitogenic factors like periostin [79, 80], neuregulin [81], fibroblast growth factor 1 [82], and follistatin-like 1 [83]. These factors have been shown to stimulate myocyte division and promote regeneration in infarcted mouse [79, 81–83] and pig hearts [80, 83]. Neuregulin signaling in particular has attracted significant attention, as transient genetic activation of neuregulin's receptor *ERBB2* (without concurrent administration of exogenous neuregulin) has also been shown to promote myocyte proliferation and regeneration in infarcted hearts of adult mice [84]. Nevertheless, the mitogenic effects of periostin [85] and neuregulin [86] on adult cardiac myocytes have been called into question by some research groups.

Finally, mitogenic stimulation of adult cardiomyocytes has been attempted through induction of systemic hypoxemia. Nakada et al. demonstrated that exposure of infarcted adult mice to hypoxia (FiO2 7%) for 2 weeks stimulated myocyte proliferation and conferred regenerative effects [87]. The researchers suggest that the exposure to a hypoxic environment (which mimics the intrauterine environment) inhibits oxidative metabolism, reduces formation of reactive oxygen species, and ultimately decreases oxidative DNA damage in myocytes. Since oxidative DNA damage may be responsible for the cell cycle arrest observed in mammalian myocytes soon after birth [25], its decrease via exposure to systemic hypoxemia may force myocytes to reenter the cell cycle and proliferate.

Apart from upregulation of adult myocyte proliferation, research efforts have also focused on stimulation of progenitor cell-mediated innate regeneration. In bitransgenic αMHC-MerCreMer/reporter mice (similar to the ones used by Hsieh et al.), administration of either *secreted frizzled related protein 2* (Sfrp2, a canonical Wnt inhibitor) [88] or prostaglandin E2 [52] resulted in amplification of endogenous progenitor cell-mediated cardiac regeneration in infarcted hearts, as evidenced by dilution of the GFP+ myocyte pool by GFP- myocytes. Interestingly, in both studies progenitor cell-mediated regeneration appeared to occur through activation and cardiomyogenic differentiation of Sca-1+ cells. Furthermore, Zangi et al., using a growth factor-based approach, demonstrated that transient local cardiac delivery of vascular endothelial growth factor-A (achieved through intramyocardial injections of synthetic modified RNA) activates epicardial-derived endogenous progenitors and promotes cardiac regeneration in infarcted hearts of adult mice [49]. While only a small minority of epicardial-derived progenitors underwent cardiomyogenic differentiation, a substantial proportion differentiated into endothelial and vascular smooth muscle cells and contributed to angiogenesis. This limited capacity of epicardial-derived progenitors for cardiomyogenic differentiation could possibly be enhanced through cardiac priming with thymosin beta-1, as reported by Smart et al. [50].

All the aforementioned experimental strategies to bolster endogenous cardiac regeneration have been tested (almost exclusively) in small animals. Thus, clinical translation appears distant for the time being. On the contrary, three readily translatable therapeutic approaches (already implemented in patients) that may stimulate endogenous regeneration are exercise, cell therapy, and mechanical unloading with left ventricular assist devices. These approaches are considered individually below. First, regarding exercise, Vujic et al. demonstrated that running exercise stimulated myocyte proliferation in infarcted hearts of adult mice [89]. The mitogenic effects of exercise were abolished after inhibition of miR-222, which is known to increase with exercise in both mice and humans [90, 91]. Second, mounting evidence suggests that cell therapy with adult progenitor cells may indirectly promote endogenous regenerative processes. To that end, cell therapy with cardiosphere-derived cells appears to amplify both resident myocyte proliferation [12, 92–94] and activation of endogenous progenitors after myocardial infarction [30, 93]. Similar effects have been also reported after cell therapy with mesenchymal stromal cells [94] and c-kit cells (derived either from the heart [95] or the bone marrow [29]). Finally, chronic mechanical circulatory support with left ventricular assist devices [96] may also stimulate myocyte proliferation [97]; this finding is in concordance with pathologic studies reporting an increase in diploid cardiomyocytes (consistent with formation of newly generated myocytes) after mechanical unloading [98].

In conclusion, during the past decade, a remarkable shift in our view of the mammalian heart has taken place; once viewed as a postmitotic organ, the adult mammalian heart is now considered a regenerative organ. The human heart's innate capacity for myocyte replenishment appears to peak during childhood and to decrease exponentially with age. In addition, studies in neonatal mice suggest that a limited time window exists immediately after birth, during which the neonatal heart possesses remarkable regenerative potential and is capable of near-complete regeneration post-injury. While the regenerative potential of the adult mammalian heart is clearly limited and irrelevant from a clinical standpoint, the study of the cellular sources of innate regeneration and the molecular pathways that govern it is certainly merited; elucidation of the endogenous regenerative mechanisms of the mammalian heart could enable their therapeutic exploitation. With regard to the cellular sources of myocyte turnover, cardiomyocyte proliferation has emerged as the dominant mechanism of myocyte replenishment in the injured neonatal heart and in the healthy adult heart during normal aging. Following myocardial injury of the adult heart, myocyte proliferation increases. Endogenous progenitors may also contribute to cardiomyogenesis in the injured mammalian heart, although this is not universally accepted and remains a subject of intense debate. Regarding therapeutic ways to stimulate cardiac regeneration, several strategies have yielded promising results in animal testing, including genetic manipulation of the cell cycle, regulation of miRNA expression, modulation of the Hippo and neuregulin/ERBB signaling pathways, administration of mitogenic factors, exposure to hypoxia, exercise, cell therapy, and mechanical unloading with left ventricular assist devices. Clinical translation of such therapeutic strategies is of utmost importance, as safe and reliable exogenous stimulation of endogenous regenerative processes will undoubtedly enable development of more effective treatments for a wide spectrum of cardiac diseases.

References

1. Castillo JG, Silvay G. Characterization and management of cardiac tumors. Semin Cardiothorac Vasc Anesth. 2010;14(1):6–20.
2. Laflamme MA, Murry CE. Heart regeneration. Nature. 2011;473(7347):326–35.
3. Malliaras K, Terrovitis J. Cardiomyocyte proliferation vs progenitor cells in myocardial regeneration: the debate continues. Glob Cardiol Sci Pract. 2013;2013(3):303–15.
4. Malliaras K, Vakrou S, Kapelios CJ, Nanas JN. Innate heart regeneration: endogenous cellular sources and exogenous therapeutic amplification. Expert Opin Biol Ther. 2016;16(11):1341–52.
5. Bergmann O, Bhardwaj RD, Bernard S, et al. Evidence for cardiomyocyte renewal in humans. Science. 2009;324(5923):98–102.
6. Bergmann O, Zdunek S, Felker A, et al. Dynamics of cell generation and turnover in the human heart. Cell. 2015;161(7):1566–75.
7. Mollova M, Bersell K, Walsh S, et al. Cardiomyocyte proliferation contributes to heart growth in young humans. Proc Natl Acad Sci USA. 2013;110(4):1446–51.

8. Senyo SE, Steinhauser ML, Pizzimenti CL, et al. Mammalian heart renewal by pre-existing cardiomyocytes. Nature. 2013;493(7432):433–6.
9. Alkass K, Panula J, Westman M, et al. No evidence for cardiomyocyte number expansion in preadolescent mice. Cell. 2015;163(4):1026–36.
10. Soonpaa MH, Zebrowski DC, Platt C, et al. Cardiomyocyte cell-cycle activity during preadolescence. Cell. 2015;163(4):781–2.
11. Soonpaa MH, Field LJ. Assessment of cardiomyocyte DNA synthesis in normal and injured adult mouse hearts. Am J Physiol. 1997;272(1 Pt 2):H220–6.
12. Malliaras K, Zhang Y, Seinfeld J, et al. Cardiomyocyte proliferation and progenitor cell recruitment underlie therapeutic regeneration after myocardial infarction in the adult mouse heart. EMBO Mol Med. 2013;5(2):191–209.
13. Porrello ER, Mahmoud AI, Simpson E, et al. Transient regenerative potential of the neonatal mouse heart. Science. 2011;331(6020):1078–1080.
14. Andersen DC, Ganesalingam S, Jensen CH, Sheikh SP. Do neonatal mouse hearts regenerate following heart apex resection?. Stem Cell Rep. 2014;2:406–13.
15. Porrello ER, Mahmoud AI, Simpson E, et al. Regulation of neonatal and adult mammalian heart regeneration by the miR-15 family. Proc Natl Acad Sci USA. 2013;110(1): 187–192.
16. Haubner BJ, Adamowicz-Brice M, Khadayate S, Tiefenthaler V, Metzler B, Aitman T, Penninger JM. Complete cardiac regeneration in a mouse model of myocardial infarction. Aging (Albany NY). 2012;4:966–977.
17. Jesty SA, Steffey MA, Lee FK, et al. c-kit+ precursors support postinfarction myogenesis in the neonatal, but not adult, heart. Proc Natl Acad Sci USA. 2012;109(33):13380–5.
18. Oberpriller JO, Oberpriller JC. Response of the adult newt ventricle to injury. J Exp Zool. 1974;187(2):249–53.
19. Poss KD, Wilson LG, Keating MT. Heart regeneration in zebrafish. Science. 2002;298(5601):2188–90.
20. Fratz S, Hager A, Schreiber C, Schwaiger M, Hess J, Stern HC. Long-term myocardial scarring after operation for anomalous left coronary artery from the pulmonary artery. Ann Thorac Surg. 2011;92:1761–5.
21. Haubner BJ, Schneider J, Schweigmann U, Schuetz T, Dichtl W, Velik-Salchner C, Stein JI, Penninger JM. Functional recovery of a human neonatal heart after severe myocardial infarction. Circ Res. 2016;118(2):216–21.
22. Beltrami AP, Urbanek K, Kajstura J, et al. Evidence that human cardiac myocytes divide after myocardial infarction. N Engl J Med. 2001;334(23):1750–7.
23. Kajstura J, Leri A, Finato N, et al. Myocyte proliferation in end-stage cardiac failure in humans. Proc Natl Acad Sci USA. 1998;95(15):8801–5.
24. Kimura W, Xiao F, Canseco DC, et al. Hypoxia fate mapping identifies cycling cardiomyocytes in the adult heart. Nature. 2015;523(7559):226–30.
25. Puente BN, Kimura W, Muralidhar SA, et al. The oxygen-rich postnatal environment induces cardiomyocyte cell-cycle arrest through DNA damage response. Cell. 2014;157(3):565–79. https://doi.org/10.1016/j.cell.2014.03.032.
26. Eschenhagen T, Bolli R, Braun T, Field LJ, et al. Cardiomyocyte regeneration: a consensus statement. Circulation. 2017;136(7):680–86.
27. Hsieh PC, Segers VF, Davis ME, et al. Evidence from a genetic fate-mapping study that stem cells refresh adult mammalian cardiomyocytes after injury. Nat Med. 2007;13(8):970–74.
28. Ellison GM, Vicinanza C, Smith AJ, et al. Adult c-kit(pos) cardiac stem cells are necessary and sufficient for functional cardiac regeneration and repair. Cell. 2013;154(4):827–42.
29. Loffredo FS, Steinhauser ML, Gannon J, Lee RT. Bone marrow-derived cell therapy stimulates endogenous cardiomyocyte progenitors and promotes cardiac repair. Cell Stem Cell. 2011;8(4):389–98.
30. Malliaras K, Ibrahim A, Tseliou E, et al. Stimulation of endogenous cardioblasts by exogenous cell therapy after myocardial infarction. EMBO Mol Med. 2014;6(6):760–77.

31. Beltrami AP, Barlucchi L, Torella D, Baker M, Limana F, Chimenti S, et al. Adult cardiac stem cells are pluripotent and support myocardial regeneration. Cell. 2003;114:763–6.
32. Oh H, Bradfute SB, Gallardo TD, Nakamura T, Gaussin V, Mishina Y, et al. Cardiac progenitor cells from adult myocardium: homing, differentiation, and fusion after infarction. Proc Natl Acad Sci U S A. 2003;100:12313–8.
33. Martin CM, Meeson AP, Robertson SM, Hawke TJ, Richardson JA, Bates S, et al. Persistent expression of the ATP-binding cassette transporter, Abcg2, identifies cardiac SP cells in the developing and adult heart. Dev Biol. 2004;265:262–75.
34. Ott HC, Matthiesen TS, Brechtken J, Grindle S, Goh SK, Nelson W, et al. The adult human heart as a source for stem cells: repair strategies with embryonic-like progenitor cells. Nat Clin Pract Cardiovasc Med. 2007;4(Suppl 1):S27–39.
35. Zhou B, Ma Q, Rajagopal S, Wu SM, Domian I, Rivera-Feliciano J, et al. Epicardial progenitors contribute to the cardiomyocyte lineage in the developing heart. Nature. 2008;454:109–13.
36. Messina E, De Angelis L, Frati G, Morrone S, Chimenti S, Fiordaliso F, et al. Isolation and expansion of adult cardiac stem cells from human and murine heart. Circ Res. 2004;95:911–21.
37. Smith RR, Barile L, Cho HC, Leppo MK, Hare JM, Messina E, et al. Regenerative potential of cardiosphere-derived cells expanded from percutaneous endomyocardial biopsy specimens. Circulation. 2007;115:896–908.
38. van Berlo JH, Kanisicak O, Maillet M, et al. c-kit+ cells minimally contribute cardiomyocytes to the heart. Nature. 2014;509(7500):337–41.
39. Liu Q, Yang R, Huang X, et al. Genetic lineage tracing identifies in situ Kit-expressing cardiomyocytes. Cell Res. 2016;26(1):119–30.
40. Sultana N, Zhang L, Yan J, et al. Resident c-kit(+) cells in the heart are not cardiac stem cells. Nat Commun. 2015;6:8701.
41. Molkentin JD, Houser SR. Are resident c-Kit+ cardiac stem cells really all that are needed to mend a broken heart? Circ Res. 2013;113(9):1037–9.
42. Nadal-Ginard B, Ellison GM, Torella D. Absence of evidence is not evidence of absence: pitfalls of cre knock-ins in the c-Kit locus. Circ Res. 2014;115(4):415–8.
43. Vicinanza C, Aquila I, Cianflone E, et al. Kit^{cre} knock-in mice fail to fate-map cardiac stem cells. Nature. 2018;555(7697):E1–E5.
44. van Berlo JH, Kanisicak O, Maillet M, Vagnozzi RJ, Karch J, Lin SJ, Middleton RC, Marbán E, Molkentin JD. van Berlo et al. reply. Nature. 2018;555(7697):E18.
45. Uchida S, De Gaspari P, Kostin S, et al. Sca1-derived cells are a source of myocardial renewal in the murine adult heart. Stem Cell Rep. 2013;1(5):397–410.
46. Valiente-Alandi I, Albo-Castellanos C, Herrero D, et al. Cardiac Bmi1(+) cells contribute to myocardial renewal in the murine adult heart. Stem Cell Res Ther. 2015;6:205.
47. Tamura Y, Matsumura K, Sano M, et al. Neural crest-derived stem cells migrate and differentiate into cardiomyocytes after myocardial infarction. Arterioscler Thromb Vasc Biol. 2011;31(3):582–9.
48. Smits AM, Dronkers E, Goumans MJ. The epicardium as a source of multipotent adult cardiac progenitor cells: their origin, role and fate. Pharmacol Res. 2018;127:129–40.
49. Zangi L, Lui KO, von Gise A, et al. Modified mRNA directs the fate of heart progenitor cells and induces vascular regeneration after myocardial infarction. Nat Biotechnol. 2013;31(10):898–907.
50. Smart N, Bollini S, Dubé KN, et al. De novo cardiomyocytes from within the activated adult heart after injury. Nature. 2011;474(7353):640–4.
51. Ali SR, Hippenmeyer S, Saadat LV, et al. Existing cardiomyocytes generate cardiomyocytes at a low rate after birth in mice. Proc Natl Acad Sci U S A. 2014;111(24):8850–5.
52. Hsueh YC, Wu JM, Yu CK, et al. Prostaglandin E2 promotes post-infarction cardiomyocyte replenishment by endogenous stem cells. EMBO Mol Med. 2014;6(4):496–503.
53. Kumar A, Godwin JW, Gates PB, Garza-Garcia AA, Brockes JP. Molecular basis for the nerve dependence of limb regeneration in an adult vertebrate. Science. 2007;318:772–7.

54. Rojas-Muñoz A, Rajadhyksha S, Gilmour D, van Bebber F, Antos C, Rodríguez Esteban C, Nüsslein-Volhard C, Izpisúa Belmonte JC. ErbB2 and ErbB3 regulate amputation-induced proliferation and migration during vertebrate regeneration. Dev Biol. 2009;327:177–90.
55. Lucas D, Scheiermann C, Chow A, Kunisaki Y, Bruns I, Barrick C, Tessarollo L, Frenette PS. Chemotherapy-induced bone marrow nerve injury impairs hematopoietic regeneration. Nat Med. 2013;19, 695–703.
56. Mahmoud AI, O'Meara CC, Gemberling M, Zhao L, Bryant DM, Zheng R, Gannon JB, Cai L, Choi W-Y, Egnaczyk GF, et al. Nerves regulate cardiomyocyte proliferation and heart regeneration. Dev Cell. 2015;34:387–99.
57. White IA, Gordon J, Balkan W, Hare JM. Sympathetic reinnervation is required for mammalian cardiac regeneration. Circ Res. 2015;117:990–4.
58. Godwin JW, Pinto AR, Rosenthal NA. Macrophages are required for adult salamander limb regeneration. Proc Natl Acad Sci USA. 2013;110:9415–20.
59. Grow M, Neff AW, Mescher AL, King MW. Global analysis of gene expression in Xenopus hindlimbs during stage-dependent complete and incomplete regeneration. Dev Dyn. 2006;235:2667–85.
60. Aurora AB, Porrello ER, Tan W, Mahmoud AI, Hill JA, Bassel-Duby R, Sadek HA, Olson EN. Macrophages are required for neonatal heart regeneration. J Clin Invest. 2014;124: 1382–92.
61. Han C, Nie Y, Lian H, Liu R, He F, Huang H, Hu S. Acute inflammation stimulates a regenerative response in the neonatal mouse heart. Cell Res. 2015;25(10):1137–51.
62. Pasumarthi KB, Nakajima H, Nakajima HO, et al. Targeted expression of cyclin D2 results in cardiomyocyte DNA synthesis and infarct regression in transgenic mice. Circ Res. 2005;96(1):110–8,
63. Woo YJ, Panlilio CM, Cheng RK, et al. Therapeutic delivery of cyclin A2 induces myocardial regeneration and enhances cardiac function in ischemic heart failure. Circulation. 2006;114(1 Suppl):I206–13.
64. Shapiro SD, Ranjan AK, Kawase Y, et al. Cyclin A2 induces cardiac regeneration after myocardial infarction through cytokinesis of adult cardiomyocytes. Sci Transl Med. 2014;6(224):224ra27.
65. Mohamed TMA, Ang YS, Radzinsky E, Zhou P, Huang Y, Elfenbein A, Foley A, Magnitsky S, Srivastava D. Regulation of Cell cycle to stimulate adult cardiomyocyte proliferation and cardiac regeneration. Cell. 2018;173(1):104–116.e12.
66. Sdek P, Zhao P, Wang Y, et al. Rb and p130 control cell cycle gene silencing to maintain the postmitotic phenotype in cardiac myocytes. J Cell Biol. 2011;194(3):407–23.
67. Mahmoud AI, Kocabas F, Muralidhar SA, et al. Meis1 regulates postnatal cardiomyocyte cell cycle arrest. Nature. 2013;497(7448):249–53.
68. Zhou Q, Li L, Zhao B, Guan K-L. The hippo pathway in heart development, regeneration, and diseases. Circ Res. 2015;116:1431–47.
69. Miesfeld JB, Link BA. Establishment of transgenic lines to monitor and manipulate Yap/Taz-Tead activity in zebrafish reveals both evolutionarily conserved and divergent functions of the Hippo pathway. Mech Dev. 2014;133:177–88.
70. Heallen T. Hippo pathway inhibits Wnt signaling to restrain cardiomyocyte proliferation and heart size. Science. 2011;332:458–61.
71. Heallen T, Morikawa Y, Leach J, Tao G, Willerson JT, Johnson RL, Martin JF. Hippo signaling impedes adult heart regeneration. Development. 2013;140:4683–90.
72. Xin M, Kim Y, Sutherland LB, et al. Hippo pathway effector Yap promotes cardiac regeneration. Proc Natl Acad Sci U S A. 2013;110(34):13839–44.
73. Lin Z, von Gise A, Zhou P, et al. Cardiac specific YAP activation improves cardiac function and survival inan experimental murine MI model. Circ Res. 2014;115(3):354–63.
74. Tao G, Kahr PC, Morikawa Y, Zhang M, Rahmani M, Heallen TR, Li L, Sun Z, Olson EN, Amendt BA, Martin JF. Pitx2 promotes heart repair by activating the antioxidant response after cardiac injury. Nature. 2016;534:119–123.

75. Eulalio A, Mano M, Dal Ferro M, et al. Functional screening identifies miRNAs inducing cardiac regeneration. Nature. 2012;492(7429):376–81.
76. Chen J, Huang ZP, Seok HY, et al. mir-17-92 cluster is required for and sufficient to induce cardiomyocyte proliferation in postnatal and adult hearts. Circ Res. 2013;112(12): 1557–66.
77. Tian Y, Liu Y, Wang T, et al. A microRNA-Hippo pathway that promotes cardiomyocyte proliferation and cardiac regeneration in mice. Sci Transl Med. 2015;7(279):279ra38.
78. Aguirre A, In vivo activation of a conserved microRNA program induces mammalian heart regeneration. Cell Stem Cell. 2014;15:589–604. https://doi.org/10.1016/j.stem.2014.10.003.
79. Kuhn B, del Monte F, Hajjar RJ, et al. Periostin induces proliferation of differentiated cardiomyocytes and promotes cardiac repair. Nat Med. 2007;13(8):962–9.
80. Polizzotti BD, Arab S, Kühn B. Intrapericardial delivery of gelfoam enables the targeted delivery of Periostin peptide after myocardial infarction by inducing fibrin clot formation. PLoS One. 2012;7(5):e36788.
81. Bersell K, Arab S, Haring B, Kuhn B. Neuregulin1/ErbB4 signaling induces cardiomyocyte proliferation and repair of heart injury. Cell. 2009;138(2):257–70.
82. Engel FB, Hsieh PC, Lee RT, Keating MT. FGF1/p38 MAP kinase inhibitor therapy induces cardiomyocyte mitosis, reduces scarring, and rescues function after myocardial infarction. Proc Natl Acad Sci U S A. 2006;103(42):15546–51.
83. Wei K, et al. Epicardial FSTL1 reconstitution regenerates the adult mammalian heart. Nature. 2015;525:479–85. https://doi.org/10.1038/nature15372.
84. D'Uva G, Aharonov A, Lauriola M, et al. ERBB2 triggers mammalian heart regeneration by promoting cardiomyocyte dedifferentiation and proliferation. Nat Cell Biol. 2015;17(5): 627–38.
85. Lorts A, Schwanekamp JA, Elrod JW, et al. Genetic manipulation of periostin expression in the heart does not affect myocyte content, cell cycle activity, or cardiac repair. Circ Res. 2009;104(1):e1–7.
86. Reuter S, Soonpaa MH, Firulli AB, et al. Recombinant neuregulin 1 does not activate cardiomyocyte DNA synthesis in normal or infarcted adult mice. PLoS ONE 2014;9(12):e115871.
87. Nakada Y, Canseco DC, Thet S, et al. Hypoxia induces heart regeneration in adult mice. Nature. 2017;541(7636):222–7.
88. Schmeckpeper J, Verma A, Yin L, et al. Inhibition of Wnt6 by Sfrp2 regulates adult cardiac progenitor cell differentiation by differential modulation of Wnt pathways. J Mol Cell Cardiol. 2015;85:215–25.
89. Vujic A, Lerchenmüller C, Wu TD, Guillermier C, Rabolli CP, Gonzalez E, Senyo SE, Liu X, Guerquin-Kern JL, Steinhauser ML, Lee RT, Rosenzweig A. Exercise induces new cardiomyocyte generation in the adult mammalian heart. Nat Commun. 2018;9(1):1659.
90. Liu X, Xiao J, Zhu H, et al. miR-222 is necessary for exercise-induced cardiac growth and protects against pathological cardiac remodeling. Cell Metab. 2015;21(4):584–95.
91. Baggish AL, et al. Dynamic regulation of circulating microRNA during acute exhaustive exercise and sustained aerobic exercise training. J. Physiol. 2011;589:3983–94.
92. Malliaras K, Li TS, Luthringer D, et al. Safety and efficacy of allogeneic cell therapy in infarcted rats transplanted with mismatched cardiosphere-derived cells. Circulation. 2012;125:100–12.
93. Malliaras K, Smith RR, Kanazawa H, et al. Validation of contrast-enhanced magnetic resonance imaging to monitor regenerative efficacy after cell therapy in a porcine model of convalescent myocardial infarction. Circulation. 2013;128:2764–75.
94. Weil BR, Suzuki G, Leiker MM, Fallavollita JA, Canty JM. Comparative Efficacy of Intracoronary Allogeneic Mesenchymal Stem Cells and Cardiosphere-Derived Cells in Swine with Hibernating Myocardium. Circ Res. 2015;117:634–44.
95. Tang XL, Li Q, Rokosh G, et al. Long-Term Outcome of Administration of c-kitPOS Cardiac Progenitor Cells After Acute Myocardial Infarction: Transplanted Cells Do not Become Cardiomyocytes, but Structural and Functional Improvement and Proliferation of Endogenous Cells Persist for at Least One Year. Circ Res. 2016;118(7):1091–105.

96. Malliaras KG, Terrovitis JV, Drakos SG, Nanas JN. Reverse cardiac remodeling enabled by mechanical unloading of the left ventricle. J Cardiovasc Transl Res. 2009;2(1):114–25.
97. Canseco DC, Kimura W, Garg S, et al. Human ventricular unloading induces cardiomyocyte proliferation. J Am Coll Cardiol. 2015;65(9):892–900.
98. Wohlschlaeger, B. Levkau, G. Brockhoff, et al. Hemodynamic support by left ventricular assist devices reduces cardiomyocyte DNA content in the failing human heart. Circulation. 2010;121(8) :989–96.
99. Koudstaal S, Jansen Of Lorkeers SJ, Gaetani R, Gho JM, van Slochteren FJ, Sluijter JP, Doevendans PA, Ellison GM, Chamuleau SA. Concise review: heart regeneration and the role of cardiac stem cells. Stem Cells Transl Med. 2013;2(6):434–43.

Chapter 17
Cell Therapy for Heart Disease: Ready for Prime Time or Lost in Translation?

Konstantinos Malliaras and Dennis V. Cokkinos

When for various reasons a certain number of cardiomyocytes die, replacement fibrosis, cardiac remodeling, and heart failure ensue. Ideally, the injured cells must either be protected, regenerated (from endogenous sources), or replaced (by exogenous cells). Cell therapy is being tested clinically for all the aforementioned purposes since 2000. The amount of basic, clinical, and translational research carried out in this field has been vast, as the effective replacement of lost cardiomyocytes carries an obvious therapeutic appeal. Moreover, it has opened new exciting paths for research of cell life and the various molecular players which govern it. However, many unanswered questions must be pointed out.

17.1 Cell Types Used

The different cell types that have been used for cardiac repair are legion and are depicted schematically in Fig. 17.1. Here, only those with an appreciable number of preclinical studies and those that have undergone clinical testing will be described. The desirable attributes of the ideal cell type for heart repair, as outlined by Malliaras et al. [1, 2], should be reminded. Specifically, the ideal progenitor cell for heart repair must have the following properties:

1. Be safe (not creating tumors or promoting generation of arrhythmias).
2. Produce clinically meaningful improvement in cardiac function.

K. Malliaras (✉)
Department of Cardiology, Laikon Hospital, Athens, Greece

D. V. Cokkinos
Heart and Vessel Department, Biomedical Research Foundation, Academy of Athens - Gregory Skalkeas, Athens, Greece

D. V. Cokkinos (ed.), *Myocardial Preservation*,
https://doi.org/10.1007/978-3-319-98186-4_17

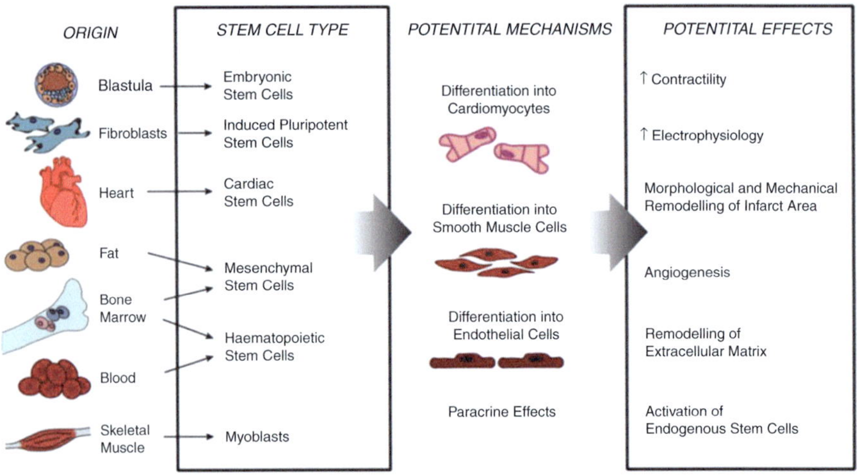

Fig. 17.1 Sources of adult progenitor cells for heart repair and proposed mechanisms of action. The most widely used cell types in clinical trials have been bone marrow-derived mononuclear cells, mesenchymal stromal cells (derived either from the bone marrow or from adipose tissue), skeletal myoblasts, and heart-derived cells (c-kit+ cells and cardiosphere-derived cells). (Figure obtained from Ref. [138]) reproduced by permission from Duelen R, Sampaolesi M. EBioMedicine 2017;16:30–40

3. Create healthy muscle and vessels which will be incorporated and function in the host tissue. The failure to achieve this prerequisite (at least to a clinically relevant degree) remains a major problem with all cell types utilized to date.
4. Be easily harvested, grown in large numbers and practically delivered, without eliciting a significant immune response.
5. Not raise ethical concerns.

The same authors stress that as of now the ideal stem cell has not been found [1, 2].

17.1.1 Embryonic Stem Cells

Considered as the prototypical stem cells, *embryonic stem cells* are derived from the inner mass of the developing embryo at the blastocyst stage. They are pluripotent (can differentiate into every cell type) and can be self-renewed and clonally expanded [3]. Experimentally, they can form a substantial amount of newly generated myocardial tissue, structurally and functionally integrated in the host issue [4]. However, they have tumorigenic potential [5], are by default allogeneic and therefore immunogenic (and thus require immunosuppression of the host), may promote arrhythmogenesis [4], and raise obvious ethical issues, all of which have precluded their widespread use in clinical trials. Currently only in the ESCORT trial are such cells being tested clinically [6].

An alternative approach is the in vitro creation of embryonic-like pluripotent stem cells (*induced pluripotent stem cells*, *iPSCs*) from adult somatic cells, such as fibroblasts, through nuclear reprogramming by exogenously delivered transcription factors (Oct4, Sox2, c-Myc, Klf4, Nanog, Lin2) [7, 8]. Patient-specific iPSCs are particularly attractive for cellular cardiomyoplasty, as their autologous nature would theoretically obviate the need for chronic immunosuppression of the host. Still, they do present many problems including tumorigenicity, arrhythmogenicity [9], and possibly immunogenicity (despite their autologous origin) [10]. They are also costly and do not presently appear to be close to clinical testing.

17.1.2 Clinically-Used Progenitor Cells

17.1.2.1 Skeletal Myoblasts

Skeletal myoblasts were the first cell type that was administered in clinical trials of cell therapy for heart disease (first application in humans in 2000) [11]. Their further use has been hampered by the finding that they may promote generation of reentrant ventricular arrhythmias; in recipient myocardium, skeletal myoblasts differentiate into multinucleated myofibers [12] that lack expression of gap junctions, thus forming areas of conduction block that facilitate reentry [13]. The concern for increased arrhythmogenicity raised by preclinical studies was confirmed at the clinical level in the MAGIC [14] and MARVEL-1 [15] trials, but not in the SEISMIC trial [16]. Additionally, even though skeletal myoblasts demonstrate a contractile phenotype, it has not been proven that they can effectively differentiate into cardiomyocytes [12]. Their use has declined, and new trials are not forthcoming.

17.1.2.2 Bone Marrow-Derived Cells

The bone marrow contains a large variety of cells, including hematopoietic stem cells (at various stages of maturation) [17], mesenchymal stromal cells [18], and endothelial progenitor cells [19]. Bone marrow-derived cells were the second cellular product that was tested in humans (for the first time in 2001) [20], shortly after the publication of the first proof-of-concept studies in small animals [21]. The rapid clinical translation was achieved by capitalizing on the pre-existing experience of bone marrow transplantation for hematopoietic disorders. In the clinical field of cardiac cell therapy, bone marrow-derived cells have been (for the most part) delivered in the following two forms: (a) autologous *bone marrow mononuclear cells* (BMMNCs) either unfractionated or after purification for a progenitor cell surface marker and (b) *mesenchymal stromal cells* (either autologous or allogeneic). These cellular products are considered individually below.

Bone Marrow-Derived Mononuclear Cells

Autologous BMMNCs, isolated by density centrifugation of bone marrow aspirates, comprise the most widely used cellular product in clinical trials of cell therapy for heart disease to date. Autologous BMMNCs have been primarily used in the setting of acute or recent myocardial infarction and are typically delivered intracoronarily (into the infarct-related artery) using standard angiography catheters. So far, intracoronary infusion of autologous BMMNCs has been shown to be feasible and safe. However, its efficacy remains in doubt, as results of randomized controlled trials have ranged from positive (REPAIR-AMI, FINCELL) [22, 23] to resoundingly negative (ASTAMI, HEBE, SCAMI, TIME, LateTIME, SWISS-AMI) [24–29]. The definitive answer regarding the potential therapeutic efficacy of autologous BMMNCs in acute myocardial infarction will be provided by the BAMI trial, a large phase 3 trial currently underway in Europe with its time from randomization to all-cause death as the primary endpoint [30]. BAMI will enroll ~3000 pts. with reperfused acute myocardial infarction and left ventricular dysfunction across 11 European countries; it is powered to detect a 25% decrease in all case mortality [30].

Since the unprocessed bone marrow in reality contains few genuine stem cells (<4% of cells in the bone marrow aspirate are true progenitor cells) [31], this population can be enriched by magnetic activated cell-sorting techniques for progenitor cell surface markers such as CD34+ [32, 33]. Higher counts of cells with these markers may yield increased functional benefits.

Bone Marrow-Derived Mesenchymal Stromal Cells

They are mesoderm-derived stromal cells, isolated by preferential adherence to plastic in tissue culture. They can readily undergo osteogenic, chondrogenic, and adipogenic differentiation [18] and under special conditions may transdifferentiate into cardiac muscle (at least in vitro) [34]. In the clinical setting, they have been primarily administered in patients with chronic ischemic cardiomyopathy or heart failure, via catheter-guided transendocardial injections. In a head-to-head comparison of autologous bone marrow-derived mesenchymal stromal cells versus autologous BMMNCs in patients with chronic ischemic cardiomyopathy (TAC-HFT study), mesenchymal stromal cells appeared to be superior in terms of scar shrinkage and improvement in regional contractility [35].

The beneficial effects of autologous mesenchymal stromal cell therapy may be enhanced by exposure of the cultured cells in vitro to a cocktail of cytokines and growth factors that promotes "cardiopoiesis," i.e., the adoption of a cardiac phenotype by the bone marrow-derived cells [36]. Such an approach, developed by Terzic et al., has yielded mixed results in the clinical setting; while transendocardial injection of "cardiopoietic" mesenchymal stromal cells in patients with chronic ischemic cardiomyopathy yielded impressive efficacy signals in the early phase C-CURE trial (in terms of cardiac function improvement and reversal of adverse cardiac remodeling) [37], these signals were not reproduced in the subsequent larger phase 3 CHART-1 trial [38]. The potential efficacy of autologous "cardiopoietic" bone marrow-derived mesenchymal stromal cells in patients with chronic ischemic cardiomyopathy is currently being tested in the phase 3 CHART-2 trial (NCT02317458).

Importantly from a translational perspective, mesenchymal stromal cells appear to be hypoimmunogenic in vivo [39]. The low immunogenicity of mesenchymal stromal cells may be attributed both to the lack of surface expression of MHC II antigens or co-stimulatory molecules and to the secretion of plethora of immunosuppressive and immunomodulatory factors. This hypoimmunogenic profile has rendered allogeneic applications exceptionally attractive. The POSEIDON [40] and POSEIDON-DCM [41] trials performed a head-to-head comparison between allogeneic and autologous bone marrow-derived mesenchymal stromal cells in patients with ischemic and nonischemic cardiomyopathy, respectively. Both trials demonstrated safety of allogeneic cells and equal potency between allogeneic and autologous cellular products. In addition, transendocardial injection of allogeneic mesenchymal precursor cells (a variant of mesenchymal stromal cells after purification for the surface markers STRO-1 and STRO-3 [42]) in patients with heart failure did not raise safety concerns, in terms of recipient alloimmunization [43]. Nowadays, a substantial portion of clinical trials of mesenchymal stromal cells for heart repair are conducted using cells grown from allogeneic sources (e.g., the phase 3 DREAM-HF1 trial [NCT02032004]).

17.1.2.3 Heart-Derived Progenitor Cells

The adult human heart is now considered as a self-regenerative organ capable of limited (but traceable) endogenous cardiomyocyte replenishment [44]. Whether the endogenous regeneration of cardiomyocytes occurs via proliferation of pre-existing resident cardiomyocytes or via differentiation of cardiac stem cells remains the subject of intense debate [45–47]. Nevertheless, during the past 15 years, several populations of putative adult cardiac stem cells have been proposed, including *c-kit+* (CD 117+) cells [48], *sca-1+* (stem cell antigen-1+) cells [49], cardiac *side-population cells* [50], *SSEA-1+* (stage-specific embryonic antigen-1+) cells [51], *epicardium-derived cardiac progenitor cells* [52], and *cardiosphere-derived cells* (CDCs) [53, 54]. While all aforementioned cell types have the capacity to differentiate into all three major cardiac cell types (cardiomyocytes, vascular smooth muscle cells, and endothelial cells) in vitro, their physiologic role (if any) in the naturally occurring endogenous cardiomyocyte replenishment remains controversial. In this review, we will focus on c-kit+ cells and CDCs, as they are the only heart-derived cellular products that have been tested clinically. Both cellular products were delivered in humans for the first time in 2009.

In humans c-kit+ cells were studied in the SCIPIO study [55, 56]. SCIPIO aimed to assess the feasibility, safety, and potential efficacy of intracoronary infusion of autologous c-kit+ cells in surgically revascularized patients with ischemic heart failure. C-kit+ cells were isolated by immunomagnetic selection from the right atrial appendage, harvested during coronary bypass surgery. Following isolation, c-kit+ cells were expanded in vitro and were subsequently administered by intracoronary infusion 4 months after the initial operation. An interim analysis of SCIPIO reported that intracoronary infusion of c-kit+ cells resulted in impressive improvement in ejection fraction (measured by echocardiography) that was not observed in controls [55]. MRI (performed only in a subset of treated patients but not in controls) demonstrated scar shrinkage and an increase in viable myocardium after therapy with c-kit+ cells [56]. Currently, the potential efficacy of autologous c-kit+ cells (delivered alone or in combination with autologous mesenchymal stromal cells) in ischemic heart failure is being tested in the phase 2 CONCERT-HF trial (NCT02501811). In addition, the potential efficacy of allogeneic c-kit+ cells in acute myocardial infarction is currently being tested in the phase 1/2 CAREMI study [57].

CDCs are CD105+/CD45- heart-derived cells, generated from multicellular spheroid microtissues, termed *cardiospheres* [53, 54]. CDCs can be expanded to clinically relevant numbers from a limited amount of starting cardiac tissue (e.g., percutaneous endomyocardial biopsy specimens) [54]. In the CADUCEUS study, intracoronary infusion of autologous CDCs (grown from endomyocardial biopsies) in patients with convalescent myocardial infarction resulted in decreased scar size, increased viable myocardium, and improved regional (but not global) cardiac function compared to usual care [58, 59]. In addition, autologous CDCs have demonstrated intriguing efficacy signals in early phase trials enrolling pediatric patients with hypoplastic left heart syndrome [60, 61] or single-ventricle physiology [62]. Importantly, CDCs – similar to mesenchymal stromal cells – are hypoimmunogenic and thus attractive for allogeneic applications [63–65]. Preclinical studies have demonstrated equal potency of allogeneic and autologous CDCs [63, 66], while early phase clinical trials have shown safety and possibly efficacy of allogeneic CDCs in heart failure [67] and dystrophic cardiomyopathy [68]. Currently, the potential efficacy of allogeneic CDCs in patients with prior myocardial infarction is being tested in the phase 2 ALLSTAR trial [69].

17.1.2.4 Adipose-Derived Mesenchymal Stromal Cells

Mesenchymal stromal cells can also be derived from the adipose tissue (besides the bone marrow, as described earlier). A major advantage of adipose-derived over bone marrow-derived mesenchymal stromal cells is that the former can be easily procured in clinically relevant numbers (without the need for in vitro expansion) by liposuction. This allows the application of autologous adipose-derived stromal cells in the acute setting. In the clinical setting, delivery of adipose-derived mesenchymal stromal cells in patients with acute myocardial infarction (APOLLO trial) [70] or with chronic ischemic cardiomyopathy (PRECISE trial) [71] proved to be safe and possibly effective. In addition, delivery of culture-expanded, adipose-derived mesenchymal stromal cells stimulated by VEGF-a in patients with refractory angina proved to be safe but not effective in increasing exercise capacity in the MyStromalCell Trial [72].

17.2 Real Life Results

A vast number of clinical trials has been reported or is currently underway. Overall, while cell therapy in general has established an excellent safety profile, results regarding its potential efficacy have been conflicting and perhaps (given the overwhelmingly positive results of animal studies) somewhat disappointing. A recently published trial sequential analysis of two Cochrane Reviews examined the effect of bone marrow-derived cells (mainly mononuclear cells or mesenchymal stromal cells) [73] on mortality, heart failure hospitalizations, and left ventricular ejection fraction (LVEF) in patients with either acute myocardial infarction or chronic heart failure.

With regard to acute myocardial infarction, the analysis included 41 randomized clinical trials (2739 participants). No effect of bone marrow-derived cell therapy was observed on mortality or hospitalization for heart failure. In addition, cell therapy with bone marrow-derived cells did not result in improvement in LVEF, as measured by MRI. Since an improvement in LVEF was the main and initial target of cell therapy in acute myocardial infarction, these findings are disappointing.

With regard to heart failure, the analysis included 24 randomized clinical trials (1094 participants). Bone marrow-derived cell therapy resulted in a significant reduction in cardiac mortality (15.9% in controls vs 5.6% in cell-treated patients, RR: 0.42, $p < 0.0001$). However, it should be noted that a substantial portion of this difference in mortality stems from a study [74], which found a 38.9% mortality in 54 controls (an extremely high figure), vs 10.9% in 55 pts. receiving cell therapy at 1 year of follow-up. If this study is not included, the results of mortality are 4.88% (for cell-treated patients) vs 11.11% (for control patients) at 1 year. Bone marrow-derived cell therapy was also associated with a decrease in the incidence of rehospitalization for HF (22.5% vs 6.4%). Somewhat paradoxically, no effect on LVEF was observed, even though the authors of the analysis stress that it was significantly well-powered to detect such a difference. To a clinician this discrepancy between cardiac function and mortality is difficult to reconcile, unless a reduction in arrhythmic cell death can be subsequently detected.

What can we learn from these results? It appears that patients with heart failure may represent a more fertile target for cell therapy clinical testing compared to patients with acute MI [75]. This may be rationalized by the fact that nowadays, prompt reperfusion in the setting of acute myocardial infarction combined with state-of-the-art drug therapy post-myocardial infarction usually results in preservation of systolic function of infarcted hearts. Therefore, patients with acute myocardial infarction may not be sick enough to derive any meaningful benefit from cell therapy. In contrast, multiple lines of evidence suggest that the sicker patients are the ones who are benefited the most by the administered cells [75]. This finding has major implications for the design of future studies; clinical testing of cell therapy should perhaps focus on sicker patients with substantial room for improvement. To that end, patients with advanced heart failure may represent a more fertile target for cell therapy.

17.3 Other Paradigms of Cell Therapy for Cardiac Diseases

As described earlier, most of the clinical trials of cell therapy to date have focused on the setting of acute/convalescent myocardial infarction or chronic ischemic cardiomyopathy/heart failure. However, the potential efficacy of cell therapy has also been explored in other forms of cardiac diseases, including:

17.3.1 Refractory Angina Pectoris

BMMNCs and granulocyte colony-stimulating factor (GCSF)-mobilized *CD34+ cells* (isolated from the peripheral blood via leukapheresis) have been used in the setting of refractory angina. Several early phase randomized controlled studies have been performed, and efficacy has been evaluated based on imaging of myocardial perfusion or measurement of exercise capacity or assessment of angina frequency. So far, results from these early phase trials have not raised significant safety concerns. However, with regard to efficacy, results have been conflicting, ranging from negative (i.e., no significant effect of cell therapy) [76, 77] to positive (increased myocardial perfusion or decreased angina frequency or improved exercise tolerance) [32, 78, 79]. CD34+ cells for refractory angina pectoris were recently tested in the phase 3 RENEW trial; the trial was stopped prematurely (after enrollment of 112 of planned 444 patients) by the sponsor due to "strategic considerations" [80]. Despite the premature termination, some encouraging efficacy signals were observed, as cell-treated patients exhibited a trend toward improved exercise capacity compared to controls. Thus, a definitive phase 3 trial, adequately powered to assess efficacy, is still warranted.

17.3.2 Nonischemic Cardiomyopathy

Cell therapy has not been tested systematically in the setting of nonischemic cardiomyopathy. In a large study that enrolled 110 patients with nonischemic dilated cardiomyopathy, intracoronary administration of GCSF-mobilized autologous CD34+ cells resulted in improved cardiac function and increased 6 min walking distance compared to standard therapy at 5 years post cell delivery [33]. In addition, intriguing hints of efficacy were observed after intracoronary allogeneic CDC delivery in young patients with Duchenne muscular dystrophy and cardiomyopathy. Intriguingly, CDC therapy not only conferred cardiac improvements (decreased scarring and improved regional function) but also improved the function of the skeletal muscles of the upper extremities [68]. In animal models, cell therapy has also been tested in the setting of anthracycline-induced cardiomyopathy [81] and acute myocarditis [82].

17.3.3 *Mechanical Circulatory Support*

Tseng et al., in a comprehensive review, propose that the heart unloaded by a left ventricular assist device (LVAD) may provide a less hostile milieu to regenerative therapy than the recently infarcted heart [83]. So far, the effect of a combinatory therapeutic approach comprising cell therapy in conjunction with mechanical circulatory support (with a LVAD) has been investigated in only one randomized trial [84]. Thirty patients with end-stage heart failure were randomized to undergo LVAD implantation combined with intramyocardial injection of allogeneic mesenchymal stromal cells or LVAD implantation alone. Delivery of allogeneic cells did not raise significant safety concerns, and a trend toward increased rate of successful temporary LVAD weaning in cell-treated patients compared to controls was observed. Currently, a larger follow-up trial enrolling 159 patients is underway (NCT02362646).

17.4 Proposed Mechanisms of Action

The major finding of the last decade in cell therapy for heart disease is the elucidation of its mechanism of action. The administration of adult stem cells was originally based on the assumption that they would differentiate into organized, normally contracting and conducting cardiac tissue which would replace lost myocardium (cardiogenesis), vasculature (angiogenesis), or both. However, after 17 years of efforts, it is no longer believed that this occurs, at least to a clinically meaningful degree. It is now well recognized that the great majority of exogenously delivered progenitor cells survive in the myocardium for not more than a week [85]. Although differentiation of progenitor cells into all types of cardiac cells, including cardiomyocytes, vascular smooth muscle cells, and endothelial cells may sporadically occur, the generation of fully functional, structurally integrated tissue, either myocardial or vascular, remains elusive.

Nowadays, a purely indirect mechanism of action is being advanced [86]: through paracrine mechanisms, progenitor cells exert a cardioprotective effect by attenuating cell death, fibrosis, and inflammation. In addition, exogenously delivered progenitor cells may stimulate endogenous regenerative mechanisms, by promoting differentiation and recruitment of resident cardiac stem or by enhancing resident cardiomyocyte proliferation (Fig. 17.1). It is important to note, as stressed by Dzau's group [86], that the paracrine factors released by progenitor cells have pleiotropic actions and that act at multiple time points. The paracrinic effects of the administered progenitor cells are further described below.

17.4.1 *Cardioprotection*

Adult stem cells secrete various factors that may confer a cardioprotective effect to acutely injured cardiomyocytes. This acute cardioprotective effect (termed "cellular postconditioning" by the Marbán group [87]) is distinct from the cell therapy-induced regenerative effect. Obviously, for this cardioprotective effect to materialize, exogenous cells need to be administered early after the ischemic insult, as the majority of myocytes die within hours following the onset of ischemia. Potential cardioprotective factors secreted by the administered cells include (but are not limited to) VEGF, FGF-2, HGF, IGF-I, TB4 [88], and secreted frizzled-related protein 2 (sfrp2) which antagonizes caspase-3 and HASF (hypoxia-induced Akt-regulated stem cell factor) [89].

17.4.2 Immune Modulation of Inflammation

Delivery of exogenous adult stem cells has been shown to modify the inflammatory milieu in the setting of myocardial injury. Specifically, progenitor cells can down-regulate the pro-inflammatory factors TNFa, IL-1, IL-6, and MCP-1 while simultaneously upregulating the expression of anti-inflammatory cytokines, like IL-10 [86]. While the underlying mechanisms have not been fully elucidated, a cell therapy-induced polarization of resident macrophages from the pro-inflammatory M1 to the anti-inflammatory M2 phenotype has been proposed [90–92].

17.4.3 Stimulation of Endogenous Regeneration

Preclinical mechanistic studies have suggested that adult stem cells may stimulate endogenous regenerative pathways. More specifically, bone marrow-derived mesenchymal stromal cells [93] and CDCs [94] have been shown to upregulate proliferation of resident cardiomyocytes, possibly through both contact-dependent mechanisms [95] and secretion of exosomes [96], rich in microRNAs. With regard to the latter, exosomes (i.e., extracellular vesicles secreted by the administered cells) have recently attracted significant interest and are now considered as key mediators of cell-cell communication, immune modulation, cell proliferation, cell senescence, and differentiation [97–99, 121, 122]. In addition, several different cell types (including bone marrow c-kit+ cells and CDCs) have been shown to stimulate the recruitment and differentiation of endogenous progenitors [100, 101], partially through secretion of SDF-1a by the administered cells [101].

17.4.4 Cardiac Remodeling

Adult stem cells may also exert antifibrotic effects, by decreasing collagen deposition, increasing collagen degradation, and enhancing the expression of extracellular matrix metalloproteinases [102]. The underlying mechanisms may involve inhibition of Tgf-β1/smad signaling [103] or secretion of antifibrotic factors by the administered cells, like tissue inhibitors of matrix metalloproteinases [104, 105] or the already-mentioned sfrp2 [89].

17.4.5 Metabolism and Contractility

Stem cell injection may also preserve the normal metabolic processes in the surviving myocardium following injury [106]. In addition, adult stem cells may secrete factors that directly improve myocyte contractility; such factors include IGF-1 [107] and IL-6 [108].

17.4.6 Neoangiogenesis

Various proangiogenic factors have been identified in the secretome of adult stem cells. These factors include (but are not limited to) VEGF, bFGF, IGF-1, thrombopoietin, and HGF [109]. They are produced by mesenchymal stromal cells [105, 110], endothelial progenitor cells [111], and CDCs [112].

17.5 Lessons from the Preclinical and Clinical Studies of Cell Therapy for Heart Disease

A vast number of preclinical and clinical studies of cell therapy for heart disease have been performed to date. While results have been somewhat conflicting and perhaps disappointing, a few take-home messages (described in detail elsewhere [1, 2]) must be highlighted:

1. The administered cells do not differentiate into myocardium (at least to a clinically relevant degree) but only exert a paracrine antiapoptotic, trophic, and perhaps regenerative effect.
2. Efficacy, as assessed by LVEF, is modest at best. However, LVEF is load-dependent and only provides a crude assessment of cardiac function. More sophisticated methods, like MRI assessment of regional function and fibrosis, need to be employed in future studies.
3. So far, cell therapy clinical trials have focused on relatively "healthy" patients with acute myocardial infarction undergoing prompt reperfusion. Such patients have a baseline LVEF of ~50%, with little room for improvement. Targeting sicker patients (e.g., patients with advanced heart failure) may maximize the chance to demonstrate efficacy of cell therapy [75].
4. Acute retention of administered cells is low and long-term survival is miniscule. The search for efficient ways to boost cardiac cell retention and long-term survival is certainly warranted (more on this later).

5. Two dominant routes of cell delivery have emerged: the intracoronary and the transendocardial route. Each one is associated with a distinct set of advantages and disadvantages. Specifically, intracoronary cell administration is technically straightforward (thus facilitating broad clinical application) and achieves widespread and homogeneous myocardial coverage [113, 114]. However, administration of high cell doses (especially when it comes to relative large cells like heart-derived cells or mesenchymal stromal cells) is hampered by microvascular occlusion [115], and overall cardiac retention is low [116]. On the other hand, transendocardial injection of cells results in higher cell retention [116] and can enable administration of very high cells doses [37]. However, transendocardial injection is technically demanding and results in highly-localized delivery (with cells clustered near the injection sites) [113].
6. The use of *allogeneic cells* is gaining traction. Important advantages of allogeneic cell therapy include (a) the circumvention of several technical, financial, and logistic hurdles associated with the culture of autologous cells and (b) the ability to generate highly standardized "off-the-shelf" cellular products, which can be stored and delivered in the acute setting. Obviously, the use of allogeneic cells is associated with the risk of recipient allosensitization; however, the clinical results obtained so far suggest that the incidence of allosensitization is low, and when such allosensitization occurs, it is transient and resolves after a few months [40, 41, 43, 67].

17.6 Strategies to Boost Cell Retention and Survival

In brief, such strategies can be broadly divided into two approaches: (a) increasing survival of administered cells by combating the hostile milieu of the recipient myocardium through pretreatment of recipient tissue or preconditioning of administered cells and (b) enhancing retention of administered cells through development of effective carrier materials/tissue engineering. These approaches are considered individually below.

17.6.1 Combating the Hostile Milieu

Abdelwahid et al. [117] point out that several approaches can be helpful to reverse the hostile environment of the damaged myocardium (which is acidic, hypoxic, glucose-deprived, and inflammatory) or to increase the administered cells' resistance to it. A vast number of approaches have been investigated in preclinical and clinical studies, including:

- Inhibition of apoptotic cell signaling in administered cells, through overexpression of genes that promote cell survival. Examples of pro-survival genes that, once overexpressed in administered cells, may block apoptotic cell death include Akt [118], Pim-1 kinase [119], and heme oxygenase-1 [120].

- Hypoxic preconditioning of administered cells [121], which has been shown to upregulate expression of pro-survival, angiogenic, and migratory genes, such as Akt, VEGF, and CXCR-4 [122–124].
- Pharmacologic preconditioning of cells, by culturing cells in a cocktail of growth factors (containing activin A, IGF1, FGF-2, TGF-β1, BMP-4, retinoic acid, α-thrombin, and IL-6) to promote "cardiopoiesis," i.e., acquisition of a cardiac phenotype (lineage specification) in bone marrow-derived cells [36]. This approach was tested clinically in the C-CURE [37] and CHART-1 [38] clinical trials, as described earlier.
- Priming of myocardium by extracorporeal application of shockwaves (which purportedly increases tissue expression of chemoattractants like SDF-1 and VEGF) [125] or by local intramyocardial delivery of SDF-1 [126].
- Increasing cardiac homing of administered cells through ultrasound-mediated microbubble destruction [127, 128] through magnetic attraction of iron-loaded cells [129] or through use of biospecific antibodies that bind cells to cardiac-specific antigens only expressed in injured myocardium [130].
- Repeated injections of STEM is being proposed.

17.6.1.1 Tissue Engineering

As Alferai et al. [131] point out, emphasis recently is given on tissue engineering methods that mimic biological and biomechanical components of the natural myocardial tissue to maintain cell integrity.

Biomimetic Scaffolds

These are made of polymers such as collagen, fibrin, alginate, matrigel, chitosan, and hyaluronic acid, similar to the natural extracellular matrix. Synthetic polymers (e.g., polyethylene glycol) can also be used, with the caveat of eliciting inflammatory responses once transplanted in host myocardium. When used together with cells, the scaffolds support and protect the cells. Electrical stimulation can be employed as a supplemental process to promote ex vivo maturation of immature cardiomyocytes embedded in scaffolds [132].

Scaffold-Free Constructs

They are in effect flexible cell sheets produced by specialized cell culture conditions. Miyugawa et al. transplanted 3D sheets of stacked monolayers of neonatal rat cardiomyocytes after experimental MI [133]. The sheets attached to the native myocardium, expressed connexin-43, and displayed angiogenesis. Recently, the same researchers reported the transplantation of an autologous cell sheet containing skeletal myoblasts in 15 ischemic and 12 delated cardiomyopathy patients, with encouraging efficacy signals [134]. However, no data are available with regard to the fate of the transplanted cells.

Engineering Bioartificial Hearts

The general concept is to decellularize hearts by intracoronary perfusion with detergents, preserve the natural extracellular matrix, and then use progenitor cells to repopulate the intact decellularized matrix. While promising preliminary results have been reported using animal hearts [135], this approach still remains far from clinical translation.

17.7 Translational Conclusions

As a conclusion the position paper European Society of Cardiology Working Group Cellular Biology of the Heart should be reviewed [136]. This group included many experts in the field of STEM therapy and cardioprotection. Their main proposals and conclusions can be summarized as follows:

- They underline that successful preclinical studies are not accompanied by clinical efficacy.
- They advocate the further improvement of cell tracking systems to evaluate the fate of transplanted cells.
- They advocate the correct monitoring of the use of controls, reproducibility, standardization, and data quality.
- They attach great importance to correct clinical trial design.
- They advocate recording and evaluation of clinically relevant delivery routes, cell dose, and timing of delivery. They describe ways to assess the clinical benefit of cell therapy, including follow-up.
- They summarize their final recommendations as follows:
  - Future preclinical studies should be designed to examine modes of delivery and mechanisms of efficacy rather than safety and efficacy endpoints only.
  - Careful selection of cell source is deemed essential. Therefore, clinical studies comparing the efficacy of different cell types or their combinations are warranted.
  - Future clinical studies should focus on careful characterization of the administered cellular product, including assessment of cell number and viability.
  - Given that cell retention is low, strategies to enhance cell retention (including development of effective carrier materials, tissue engineering approaches, or pretreatment strategies) should be developed.

- The usage of hard, clinically meaningful endpoints is mandatory to clarify whether functional improvement translates into increased survival.

17.7.1 Last Comments

Lader et al. [137] summarize the current state of cell therapy for heart disease as follows: promising but not ready for prime time. They conclude that a tremendous need remains for cell-based therapies and that much work remains to be done, but the future looks bright.

References

1. Malliaras K, Marbán E. Cardiac cell therapy: where we've been, where we are, and where we should be headed. Br Med Bull. 2011;98:161–85.
2. Malliaras K, Kreke M, Marbán E. The stuttering progress of cell therapy for heart disease. Clin Pharmacol Ther. 2011;90:532–41.
3. Murry CE, Keller G. Differentiation of embryonic stem cells to clinically relevant populations: lessons from embryonic development. Cell. 2008;132:661–80.
4. Chong JJ, et al. Human embryonic-stem-cell-derived cardiomyocytes regenerate non-human primate hearts. Nature. 2014;510:273–7.
5. Nussbaum J, Minami E, Laflamme MA, et al. Transplantation of undifferentiated murine embryonic stem cells in the heart: teratoma formation and immune response. FASEB J. 2007;21:1345–57.
6. Menasche P, et al. Human embryonic stem cell-derived cardiac progenitors for severe heart failure treatment: first clinical case report. Eur Heart J. 2015;36:2011–7.
7. Nazaraki G, Uosaki H, Teranishi M, et al. Directed and systematic differentiation of cardiovascular cells from mouse induced pluripotent stem cells. Circulation. 2008;118:498–506.
8. Nelson TJ, Martinez-Fernandez A, Yamada S, et al. Repair of acute myocardial infarction by human stemness factors induced pluripotent stem cells. Circulation. 2009;120:408–16.
9. Shiba Y, et al. Allogeneic transplantation of iPS cell-derived cardiomyocytes regenerates primate hearts. Nature. 2016;538:388–91.
10. Zhao T, Zhang ZN, Rong Z, Xu Y. Immunogenicity of induced pluripotent stem cells. Nature. 2011;474:212–5.
11. Menasché P, Hagège A, Scorsin M, Pouzet B, Desnos M, Duboc D, Schwartz K, Vilquin JT, Marolleau JP. Autologous skeletal myoblast transplantation for cardiac insufficiency. First clinical case. Arch Mal Coeur Vaiss. 2001;94(3):180–2.
12. Reinecke H, Poppa V, Murry CE. Skeletal muscle stem cells do not transdifferentiate into cardiomyocytes after cardiac grafting. J Mol Cell Cardiol. 2002;34:241–9.
13. Abraham MR, Henrikson CA, Tung L, et al. Antiarrhythmic engineering of skeletal myoblasts for cardiac transplantation. Circ Res. 2005;97:159–67.
14. Menasché P, Alfieri O, Janssens S, McKenna W, Reichenspurner H, Trinquart L, et al. The myoblast autologous grafting in ischemic cardiomyopathy (MAGIC) trial: first randomized placebo-controlled study of myoblast transplantation. Circulation. 2008;117:1189–200.
15. Povsic TJ, O'Connor CM, Henry T, et al. A double-blind, randomized, controlled, multicenter study to assess the safety and cardiovascular effects of skeletal myoblast implantation by cath-

eter delivery in patients with chronic heart failure after myocardial infarction. Am Heart J. 2011;162:654–62.
16. Duckers HJ, Houtgraaf J, Hehrlein C, Schofer J, Waltenberger J, Gershlick A, et al. Final results of a phase IIa, randomised, open-label trial to evaluate the percutaneous intramyocardial transplantation of autologous skeletal myoblasts in congestive heart failure patients: the SEISMIC trial. EuroIntervention. 2011;6:805–12.
17. Civin CI, Gore SD. Antigenic analysis of hematopoiesis: a review. J Hematother. 1993;2:137–44.
18. Dominici M, Le Blanc K, Mueller I, et al. Minimal criteria for defining multipotent mesenchymal stromal cells. The International Society for Cellular Therapy position statement. Cytotherapy. 2006;8:315–7.
19. Crosby JR, Kaminski WE, Schatteman G, et al. Endothelial cells of hematopoietic origin make a significant contribution to adult blood vessel formation. Circ Res. 2000;87:728–30.
20. Strauer BE, Brehm M, Zeus T, et al. Intracoronary, human autologous stem cell transplantation for myocardial regeneration following myocardial infarction. Dtsch Med Wochenschr. 2001;126:932–8.
21. Orlic D, Kajstura J, Chimenti S, et al. Bone marrow cells regenerate infarcted myocardium. Nature. 2001;410:701–5.
22. Schächinger V, Erbs S, Elsässer A, et al. Intracoronary bone marrow-derived progenitor cells in acute myocardial infarction. N Engl J Med. 2006;355:1210–21.
23. Huikuri HV, Kervinen K, Niemelä M, et al. Effects of intracoronary injection of mononuclear bone marrow cells on left ventricular function, arrhythmia risk profile, and restenosis after thrombolytic therapy of acute myocardial infarction. Eur Heart J. 2008;29:2723–32.
24. Lunde K, Solheim S, Aakhus S, et al. Intracoronary injection of mononuclear bone marrow cells in acute myocardial infarction. N Engl J Med. 2006;355:1199–209.
25. Hirsch A, Nijveldt R, van der Vleuten PA, et al. Intracoronary infusion of mononuclear cells from bone marrow or peripheral blood compared with standard therapy in patients after acute myocardial infarction treated by primary percutaneous coronary intervention: results of the randomized controlled HEBE trial. Eur Heart J. 2010;32:1736–47. https://doi.org/10.1093/eurheartj/ehq449.
26. Wöhrle J, Merkle N, Mailänder V, et al. Results of intracoronary stem cell therapy after acute myocardial infarction. Am J Cardiol. 2010;105:804–12.
27. Traverse JH, Henry TD, Pepine CJ, Willerson JT, Chugh A, Yang PC, Zhao DXM, Ellis SG, Forder JR, Perin EC, Penn MS, Hatzopoulos AK, Chambers JC, Baran KW, Raveendran G, Gee AP, Taylor DA, Moyé L, Ebert RF, Simari RD. TIME trial: effect of timing of stem cell delivery following ST-elevation myocardial infarction on the recovery of global and regional left ventricular function: final 2-year analysis. Circ Res. 2018;122(3):479–88.
28. Traverse JH, Henry TD, Ellis SG, Pepine CJ, Willerson JT, et al. Effect of intracoronary delivery of autologous bone marrow mononuclear cells 2 to 3 weeks following acute myocardial infarction on left ventricular function: the LateTIME randomized trial. JAMA. 2011;306(19):2110–9.
29. Sürder D, Manka R, Lo Cicero V, et al. Intracoronary injection of bone marrow-derived mononuclear cells early or late after acute myocardial infarction: effects on global left ventricular function. Circulation. 2013;127(19):1968–79.
30. Mathur A, Arnold R, Assmus B, Bartunek J, et al. The effect of intracoronary infusion of bone marrow-derived mononuclear cells on all-cause mortality in acute myocardial infarction: rationale and design of the BAMI trial. Eur J Heart Fail. 2017;19(11):1545–50.
31. Dimmeler S, Zeiher AM. Cell therapy of acute myocardial infarction: open questions. Cardiology. 2009;113:155–60.
32. Losordo DW, Henry TD, Davidson C, Sup Lee J, Costa MA, Bass T, et al. Intramyocardial, autologous CD34+ cell therapy for refractory angina. Circ Res. 2011;109:428–36.

33. Vrtovec B, Poglajen G, Lezaic L, Sever M, Domanovic D, Cernelc P, et al. Effects of intracoronary CD34+ stem cell transplantation in nonischemic dilated cardiomyopathy patients: 5-year follow-up. Circ Res. 2013;112:165–73.
34. Pijnappels DA, Schalij MJ, Ramkisoensing AA, van Tuyn J, de Vries AA, van der Laarse A, et al. Forced alignment of mesenchymal stem cells undergoing cardiomyogenic differentiation affects functional integration with cardiomyocyte cultures. Circ Res. 2008;103:167–76.
35. Heldman AW, Difede DL, Fishman JE, Zambrano JP, Trachtenberg BH, et al. Transendocardial mesenchymal stem cells and mononuclear bone marrow cells for ischemic cardiomyopathy: the TAC-HFT randomized trial. JAMA. 2013;311:62–73. https://doi.org/10.1001/jama.2013.282909.
36. Behfar A, Yamada S, Crespo-Diaz R, Nesbitt JJ, Rowe LA, Perez-Terzic C, et al. Guided cardiopoiesis enhances therapeutic benefit of bone marrow human mesenchymal stem cells in chronic myocardial infarction. J Am Coll Cardiol. 2010;56:721–34.
37. Bartunek J, Behfar A, Dolatabadi D, Vanderheyden M, Ostojic M, Dens J, et al. Cardiopoietic stem cell therapy in heart failure: the C-CURE (Cardiopoietic stem cell therapy in heart failURE) multicenter randomized trial with lineage-specified biologics. J Am Coll Cardiol. 2013;61:2329–38.
38. Bartunek J, Terzic A, Davison BA, et al. Cardiopoietic cell therapy for advanced ischaemic heart failure: results at 39 weeks of the prospective, randomized, double blind, sham-controlled CHART-1 clinical trial. Eur Heart J. 2017;38(9):648–60.
39. Ankrum JA, Ong JF, Karp JM. Mesenchymal stem cells: immune evasive, not immune privileged. Nat Biotechnol. 2014;32(3):252–60.
40. Hare JM, Fishman JE, Gerstenblith G, DiFede Velazquez DL, Zambrano JP, Suncion VY, et al. Comparison of allogeneic vs autologous bone marrow-derived mesenchymal stem cells delivered by transendocardial injection in patients with ischemic cardiomyopathy: the POSEIDON randomized trial. JAMA. 2012;308:2369–79.
41. Hare JM, Difede DL, Rieger AC, Florea V, Landin AM, El-Khorazaty J, et al. Randomized comparison of allogeneic versus autologous mesenchymal stem cells for nonischemic dilated cardiomyopathy: POSEIDON-DCM trial. J Am Coll Cardiol. 2017;69(5):526–37.
42. Psaltis PJ, et al. Enrichment for STRO-1 expression enhances the cardiovascular paracrine activity of human bone marrow-derived mesenchymal cell populations. J Cell Physiol. 2010;223:530–40.
43. Perin EC, et al. A phase II dose-escalation study of allogeneic mesenchymal precursor cells in patients with ischemic or nonischemic heart failure. Circ Res. 2015;117:576–84.
44. Bergmann O, Bhardwaj RD, Bernard S, Zdunek S, Barnabé-Heider F, Walsh S, Zupicich J, Alkass K, Buchholz BA, Druid H, Jovinge S, Frisén J. Evidence for cardiomyocyte renewal in humans. Science. 2009;324(5923):98–102.
45. Laflamme MA, Murry CE. Heart regeneration. Nature. 2011;473(7347):326–35.
46. Malliaras K, Terrovitis J. Cardiomyocyte proliferation vs progenitor cells in myocardial regeneration: the debate continues. Glob Cardiol Sci Pract. 2013;2013(3):303–15.
47. Malliaras K, Vakrou S, Kapelios CJ, Nanas JN. Innate heart regeneration: endogenous cellular sources and exogenous therapeutic amplification. Expert Opin Biol Ther. 2016;16(11):1341–52.
48. Beltrami AP, Barlucchi L, Torella D, Baker M, Limana F, Chimenti S, et al. Adult cardiac stem cells are pluripotent and support myocardial regeneration. Cell. 2003;114:763–6.
49. Oh H, Bradfute SB, Gallardo TD, Nakamura T, Gaussin V, Mishina Y, et al. Cardiac progenitor cells from adult myocardium: homing, differentiation, and fusion after infarction. Proc Natl Acad Sci U S A. 2003;100:12313–8.
50. Martin CM, Meeson AP, Robertson SM, Hawke TJ, Richardson JA, Bates S, et al. Persistent expression of the ATP-binding cassette transporter, Abcg2, identifies cardiac SP cells in the developing and adult heart. Dev Biol. 2004;265:262–75.

51. Ott HC, Matthiesen TS, Brechtken J, Grindle S, Goh SK, Nelson W, et al. The adult human heart as a source for stem cells: repair strategies with embryonic-like progenitor cells. Nat Clin Pract Cardiovasc Med. 2007;4(Suppl 1):S27–39.
52. Zhou B, Ma Q, Rajagopal S, Wu SM, Domian I, Rivera-Feliciano J, et al. Epicardial progenitors contribute to the cardiomyocyte lineage in the developing heart. Nature. 2008;454:109–13.
53. Messina E, De Angelis L, Frati G, Morrone S, Chimenti S, Fiordaliso F, et al. Isolation and expansion of adult cardiac stem cells from human and murine heart. Circ Res. 2004;95:911–21.
54. Smith RR, Barile L, Cho HC, Leppo MK, Hare JM, Messina E, et al. Regenerative potential of cardiosphere-derived cells expanded from percutaneous endomyocardial biopsy specimens. Circulation. 2007;115:896–908.
55. Bolli R, Chugh AR, D'Amario D, Loughran JH, Stoddard MF, Ikram S, et al. Cardiac stem cells in patients with ischaemic cardiomyopathy (SCIPIO): initial results of a randomised phase 1 trial. Lancet. 2011;378:1847–57.
56. Chugh AR, Beache GM, Loughran JH, Mewton N, Elmore B, Kajstura J, et al. Administration of cardiac stem cells in patients with ischemic cardiomyopathy: the SCIPIO trial: surgical aspects and interim analysis of myocardial function and viability by magnetic resonance. Circulation. 2012;126(11 Suppl 1):554–64.
57. Sanz-Ruiz R, Casado Plasencia A, Borlado LR, et al. Rationale and design of a clinical trial to evaluate the safety and efficacy of intracoronary infusion of allogeneic human cardiac stem cells in patients with acute myocardial infarction and left ventricular dysfunction: the randomized multicenter double-blind controlled CAREMI trial (cardiac stem cells in patients with acute myocardial infarction). Circ Res. 2017;121:71–80.
58. Makkar RR, Smith RR, Cheng K, Malliaras K, Thomson LE, Berman D, et al. Intracoronary cardiosphere-derived cells for heart regeneration after myocardial infarction (CADUCEUS): a prospective, randomised phase 1 trial. Lancet. 2012;379:895–904.
59. Malliaras K, Makkar RR, Smith RR, Cheng K, Wu E, Bonow RO, et al. Intracoronary cardiosphere-derived cells after myocardial infarction: evidence for therapeutic regeneration in the final 1-year results of the CADUCEUS trial. J Am Coll Cardiol. 2014;63:110–22.
60. Ishigami S, Ohtsuki S, Tarui S, et al. Intracoronary autologous cardiac progenitor cell transfer in patients with hypoplastic left heart syndrome: the TICAP prospective phase 1 controlled trial. Circ Res. 2017;116:653–64.
61. Tarui S, Ishigami S, Ousaka D, Kasahara S, Ohtsuki S, Sano S, Oh H. Transcoronary infusion of cardiac progenitor cells in hypoplastic left heart syndrome: three-year follow-up of the Transcoronary Infusion of Cardiac Progenitor Cells in Patients With Single-Ventricle Physiology (TICAP) trial. J Thorac Cardiovasc Surg. 2015;150:1198–1207, 1208.e1. https://doi.org/10.1016/j.jtcvs.2015.06.076.
62. Ishigami S, Ohtsuki S, Eitoku T, et al. Intracoronary cardiac progenitor cells in single ventricle physiology: the PERSEUS (cardiac progenitor cell infusion to treat Univentricular heart disease) randomized phase 2 trial. Circ Res. 2017;120:1162–73.
63. Malliaras K, Li TS, Luthringer D, et al. Safety and efficacy of allogeneic cell therapy in infarcted rats transplanted with mismatched cardiosphere-derived cells. Circulation. 2012;125:100–12.
64. Lauden L, Boukouaci W, Borlado LR, et al. Allogenicity of human cardiac stem/progenitor cells orchestrated by programmed death ligand 1. Circ Res. 2013;112:451–64.
65. Kapelios CJ, Nanas JN, Malliaras K. Allogeneic cardiosphere-derived cells for myocardial regeneration: current progress and recent results. Futur Cardiol. 2016;12(1):87–100.
66. Malliaras K, Smith RR, Kanazawa H, et al. Validation of contrast-enhanced magnetic resonance imaging to monitor regenerative efficacy after cell therapy in a porcine model of convalescent myocardial infarction. Circulation. 2013;128:2764–75.
67. Chakravarty T, Makkar R, Henry T, et al. TCT-820 multivessel intracoronary infusion of allogeneic cardiosphere derived cells in dilated cardiomyopathy: long term outcomes of the

Dilated Cardiomyopathy Intervention with Allogeneic Myocardially-Regenerative Cells (DYNAMIC Trial). J Am Coll Cardiol. 2016;68:B332 (abstract).
68. http://www.abstractsonline.com/pp8/#!/4412/presentation/52588.
69. Chakravarty T, Makkar RR, Ascheim DD, Traverse JH, Schatz R, Demaria A, Francis GS, Povsic TJ, Smith RR, Lima JA, Pogoda JM, Marbán L, Henry TD. ALLogeneic heart STem cells to achieve myocardial regeneration (ALLSTAR) trial: rationale and design. Cell Transplant. 2017;26(2):205–14.
70. Houtgraaf JH, den Dekker WK, van Dalen BM, Springeling T, de Jong R, van Geuns RJ, et al. First experience in humans using adipose tissue-derived regenerative cells in the treatment of patients with ST-segment elevation myocardial infarction. J Am Coll Cardiol. 2012;59:539–40.
71. Perin EC, Sanz-Ruiz R, Sánchez PL, Lasso J, Pérez-Cano R, Alonso-Farto JC, et al. Adipose-derived regenerative cells in patients with ischemic cardiomyopathy: the PRECISE Trial. Am Heart J. 2014; 168:88–95.e2.
72. Qayyum AA, Mathiasen AB, Mygind ND, Kühl JT, Jørgensen E, Helqvist S, Elberg JJ, Kofoed KF, Vejlstrup NG, Fischer-Nielsen A, Haack-Sørensen M, Ekblond A, Kastrup J. Adipose-derived stromal cells for treatment of patients with chronic ischemic heart disease (MyStromalCell trial): a randomized placebo-controlled study. Stem Cells Int. 2017;2017:5237063.
73. Fisher SA, Doree C, Taggart DP, Mathur A, Martin-Rendon E. Cell therapy for heart disease: trial sequential analyses of two Cochrane reviews. Clin Pharmacol Ther. 2016;100:88–101.
74. Pokushalov E, Romanov A, Chernyavsky A, Larionov P, Terekhov I, Artyomenko S, Poveshenko O, Kliver E, Shirokova N, Karaskov A, Dib N. Efficiency of intramyocardial injections of autologous bone marrow mononuclear cells in patients with ischemic heart failure: a randomized study. J Cardiovasc Transl Res. 2010;3(2):160–8.
75. Malliaras K, Marbán E. Moving beyond surrogate endpoints in cell therapy trials for heart disease. Stem Cells Transl Med. 2014;3(1):2–6.
76. Losordo DW, Schatz RA, White CJ, Udelson JA, Veereshwarayya V, Durgin M, et al. Intramyocardial transplantation of autologous CD34+ stem cells for intractable angina. A phase I/IIa double-blind, randomized Controlled Trial. Circulation. 2007;115:3165–72.
77. Tse HF, Thambar S, Kwong YL, Rowlings P, Bellamy G, McCrohon J, et al. Prospective randomized trial of direct endomyocardial implantation of bone marrow cells for treatment of severe coronary diseases (PROTECT-CAD trial). Eur Heart J. 2007;28:2998–3005.
78. van Ramshorst J, Bax JJ, Beeres SL, Dibbets-Schneider P, Roes SD, Stokkel MP, et al. Intramyocardial bone marrow cell injection for chronic myocardial ischemia: a randomized controlled trial. JAMA. 2009;301:1997–2004.
79. Wang S, Cui J, Peng W, Lu M. Intracoronary autologous CD34+ stem cell therapy for intractable angina. Cardiology. 2010;117:140–7.
80. Povsic TJ, Henry TD, Traverse JH, et al. The RENEW trial: efficacy and safety of Intramyocardial autologous CD34(+) cell Administration in Patients with Refractory Angina. JACC Cardiovasc Interv. 2016;9(15):1576–85.
81. De Angelis A, Piegari E, Cappetta D, Marino L, Filippelli A, Berrino L, et al. Anthracycline cardiomyopathy is mediated by depletion of the cardiac stem cell pool and is rescued by restoration of progenitor cell function. Circulation. 2010;121:276–92.
82. Van Linthout S, Savvatis K, Miteva K, Peng J, Ringe J, Warstat K, et al. Mesenchymal stem cells improve murine acute coxsackievirus B3-induced myocarditis. Eur Heart J. 2011;32:2168–78.
83. Tseng CC, Ramjankhan FZ, de Jonge N, Chamuleau SA. Advanced strategies for end-stage heart failure: combining regenerative approaches with LVAD, a new horizon? Front Surg. 2015;2:10.
84. Ascheim DD, Gelijns AC, Goldstein D, et al. Mesenchymal precursor cells as adjunctive therapy in recipients of contemporary left ventricular assist devices. Circulation.

2014;129(22):2287–96. https://doi.org/10.1161/CIRCULATIONAHA.113.007412. Epub 2014 Mar 28.

85. Terrovitis JV, Smith RR, Marbán E. Assessment and optimization of cell engraftment after transplantation into the heart. Circ Res. 2010;106(3):479–94. https://doi.org/10.1161/CIRCRESAHA.109.208991.
86. Hodgkinson CP, Bareja A, Gomez JA, Dzau VJ. Emerging concepts in paracrine mechanisms in regenerative cardiovascular medicine and biology. Circ Res. 2016;118:95–107.
87. Kanazawa H, Tseliou E, Malliaras K, et al. Cellular postconditioning: allogeneic cardiosphere-derived cells reduce infarct size and attenuate microvascular obstruction when administered after reperfusion in pigs with acute myocardial infarction. Circ Heart Fail. 2015;8(2):322–32.
88. Gnecchi M, He H, Noiseux N, Liang OD, Zhang L, Morello F, Mu H, Melo LG, Pratt RE, Ingwall JS, Dzau VJ. Evidence supporting paracrine hypothesis for Akt-modified mesenchymal stem cell-mediated cardiac protection and functional improvement. FASEB J. 2006;20:661–9.
89. Mirotsou M, Zhang Z, Deb A, Zhang L, Gnecchi M, Noiseux N, et al. Secreted frizzled related protein 2 (Sfrp2) is the key Akt-mesenchymal stem cell-released paracrine factor mediating myocardial survival and repair. Proc Natl Acad Sci U S A. 2007;104:1643–8.
90. Zhang QZ, Su WR, Shi SH, Wilder-Smith P, Xiang AP, Wong A, Nguyen AL, Kwon CW, Le AD. Human gingiva-derived mesenchymal stem cells elicit polarization of m2 macrophages and enhance cutaneous wound healing. Stem Cells. 2010;28:1856–68.
91. Kim J, Hematti P. Mesenchymal stem cell-educated macrophages: a novel type of alternatively activated macrophages. Exp Hematol. 2009;37:1445–53.
92. Dayan V, Yannarelli G, Billia F, Filomeno P, Wang XH, Davies JE, Keating A. Mesenchymal stromal cells mediate a switch to alternatively activated monocytes/macrophages after acute myocardial infarction. Basic Res Cardiol. 2011;106:1299–310.
93. Weil BR, Suzuki G, Leiker MM, Fallavollita JA, Canty JM. Comparative efficacy of intracoronary allogeneic mesenchymal stem cells and Cardiosphere-derived cells in swine with hibernating myocardium. Circ Res. 2015;117:634–44.
94. Malliaras K, Zhang Y, Seinfeld J, Galang G, Tseliou E, Cheng K, et al. Cardiomyocyte proliferation and progenitor cell recruitment underlie therapeutic regeneration after myocardial infarction in the adult mouse heart. EMBO Mol Med. 2013;5:191–209.
95. Xie Y, Ibrahim A, Cheng K, Wu Z, Liang W, Malliaras K, Sun B, Liu W, Shen D, Cheol Cho H, Li T, Lu L, Lu G, Marbán E. Importance of cell-cell contact in the therapeutic benefits of cardiosphere-derived cells. Stem Cells. 2014;32(9):2397–406.
96. Ibrahim AG, Cheng K, Marban E. Exosomes as critical agents of cardiac regeneration triggered by cell therapy. Stem Cell Rep. 2014;2:606–19.
97. Ibrahim A, Marban E. Exosomes: fundamental biology and roles in cardiovascular physiology. Annu Rev Physiol. 2016;78:67–83.
98. De Jong OG, Van Balkom BW, Schiffelers RM, Bouten CV, Verhaar MC. Extracellular vesicles: potential roles in regenerative medicine. Front Immunol. 2014;5:608.
99. Rani S, Ryan AE, Griffin MD, Ritter T. Mesenchymal stem cell-derived extracellular vesicles: toward cell-free therapeutic applications. Mol Ther. 2015;23:812–23.
100. Loffredo FS, Steinhauser ML, Gannon J, Lee RT. Bone marrow-derived cell therapy stimulates endogenous cardiomyocyte progenitors and promotes cardiac repair. Cell Stem Cell. 2011;8(4):389–98. https://doi.org/10.1016/j.stem.2011.02.002.
101. Malliaras K, Ibrahim A, Tseliou E, et al. Stimulation of endogenous cardioblasts by exogenous cell therapy after myocardial infarction. EMBO Mol Med. 2014;6:760–77.
102. Tseliou E, de Couto G, Terrovitis J, Sun B, Weixin L, Marbán L, Marbán E. Angiogenesis, cardiomyocyte proliferation and anti-fibrotic effects underlie structural preservation post-infarction by intramyocardially-injected cardiospheres. PLoS One. 2014;9(2):e88590.
103. Tseliou E, Reich H, de Couto G, Terrovitis J, Sun B, Liu W, Marbán E. Cardiospheres reverse adverse remodeling in chronic rat myocardial infarction: roles of soluble endoglin and Tgf-β signaling. Basic Res Cardiol. 2014;109(6):443.

104. Xu X, Xu Z, Xu Y, Cui G. Effects of mesenchymal stem cell transplantation on extracellular matrix after myocardial infarction in rats. Coron Artery Dis. 2005;16:245–55.
105. Nguyen BK, Maltais S, Perrault LP, et al. Improved function and myocardial repair of infarcted heart by intracoronary injection of mesenchymal stem cell-derived growth factors. J Cardiovasc Transl Res. 2010;3:547–58.
106. Gnecchi M, He H, Melo LG, Noiseaux N, Morello F, de Boer RA, et al. Early beneficial effects of bone marrow-derived mesenchymal stem cells overexpressing Akt on cardiac metabolism after myocardial infarction. Stem Cells. 2009;27:971–9.
107. Freestone NS, Ribaric S, Mason WT. The effect of insulin-like growth factor-1 on adult rat cardiac contractility. Mol Cell Biochem. 1996;163–164:223–229.
108. Maxeiner H1, Mufti S, Krehbiehl N, Dülfer F, Helmig S, Schneider J, Böning A, Matejec R, Weigand MA, Schlüter KD, Wenzel S. Interleukin-6 contributes to the paracrine effects of cardiospheres cultured from human, murine and rat hearts. J Cell Physiol. 2014;229(11):1681–9. doi: https://doi.org/10.1002/jcp.24613.
109. Wu R, Hu X, Wang J. Concise review: optimized strategies for stem cell-based therapy in myocardial repair: clinical translatability and potential limitation. Stem Cells. 2018;36(4):482–500. https://doi.org/10.1002/stem.2778. Epub 2018 Jan 26.
110. Danieli P, Malpasso G, Ciuffreda MC, et al. Conditioned medium from human amniotic mesenchymal stromal cells limits infarct size and enhances angiogenesis. Stem Cells Transl Med. 2015;4:448–58.
111. Hynes B, Kumar AH, O'sullivan J, et al. Potent endothelial progenitor cell conditioned media-related anti-apoptotic, cardiotrophic, and pro-angiogenic effects post-myocardial infarction are mediated by insulin-like growth factor-1. Eur Heart J. 2013;34:782–9.
112. Chimenti I, Smith RR, Li TS, Gerstenblith G, Messina E, Giacomello A, et al. Relative roles of direct regeneration versus paracrine effects of human cardiosphere-derived cells transplanted into infarcted mice. Circ Res. 2010;106:971–80.
113. Li Q, Guo Y, Ou Q, et al. Intracoronary administration of cardiac stem cells in mice: a new, improved technique for cell therapy in murine models. Basic Res Cardiol. 2011;106:849–64.
114. Tseliou E, Kanazawa H, Dawkins J, et al. Widespread myocardial delivery of heart-derived stem cells by nonocclusive triple-vessel intracoronary infusion in porcine ischemic cardiomyopathy: superior attenuation of adverse remodeling documented by magnetic resonance imaging and histology. PLoS One. 2016;11:e0144523.
115. Johnston PV, Sasano T, Mills K, Evers R, Lee ST, Smith RR, et al. Engraftment, differentiation, and functional benefits of autologous cardiosphere-derived cells in porcine ischemic cardiomyopathy. Circulation. 2009;120:1075–83.
116. Freyman T, Polin G, Osman H, et al. A quantitative, randomized study evaluating three methods of mesenchymal stem cell delivery following myocardial infarction. Eur Heart J. 2006;27:1114–22.
117. Abdelwahid E, Kalvelyte A, Stulpinas A, de Carvalho KA, Guarita-Souza LC, Foldes G. Stem cell death and survival in heart regeneration and repair. Apoptosis. 2016;21:252–68.
118. Mangi AA, Noiseux N, Kong D, He H, Rezvani M, Ingwall JS, et al. Mesenchymal stem cells modified with Akt prevent remodeling and restore performance of infarcted hearts. Nat Med. 2003;9:1195–201.
119. Siddiqi S, Sussman MA. Cell and gene therapy for severe heart failure patients: the time and place for Pim-1 kinase. Expert Rev Cardiovasc Ther. 2013;11:949–57.
120. Improved graft mesenchymal stem cell survival in ischemic heart with a hypoxia-regulated heme oxygenase-1 vector. J Am Coll Cardiol. 2005;46:1339–1350.
121. Yu SP, Wei Z, Wei L. Preconditioning strategy in stem cell transplantation therapy. Transl Stroke Res. 2013;4(1):76–88.
122. Hypoxic preconditioning enhances the benefit of cardiac progenitor cell therapy for treatment of myocardial infarction by inducing CXCR4 expression. Circ Res. 2009;104:1209–1216.
123. Hypoxic preconditioning augments efficacy of human endothelial progenitor cells for therapeutic neovascularization. Lab Invest. 2003;83:65–73.

124. Hypoxic preconditioning results in increased motility and improved therapeutic potential of human mesenchymal stem cells. Stem Cells. 2008;26:2173–2182.
125. Assmus B, Walter DH, Seeger FH, Leistner DM, Steiner J, Ziegler I, Lutz A, Khaled W, Klotsche J, Tonn T, Dimmeler S, Zeiher AM. Effect of shock wave-facilitated intracoronary cell therapy on LVEF in patients with chronic heart failure: the CELLWAVE randomized clinical trial. JAMA. 2013;309(15):1622–31.
126. Yamaguchi J, Kusano KF, Masuo O, Kawamoto A, Silver M, Murasawa S, Bosch-Marce M, Masuda H, Losordo DW, Isner JM, Asahara T. Stromal cell-derived factor-1 effects on ex vivo expanded endothelial progenitor cell recruitment for ischemic neovascularization. Circulation. 2003;107(9):1322–8.
127. Zen K, Okigaki M, Hosokawa Y, Adachi Y, Nozawa Y, Takamiya M, Tatsumi T, Urao N, Tateishi K, Takahashi T, Matsubara H. Myocardium-targeted delivery of endothelial progenitor cells by ultrasound-mediated microbubble destruction improves cardiac function via an angiogenic response. J Mol Cell Cardiol. 2006;40(6):799–809. Epub 2006 May 5
128. Ghanem A, Steingen C, Brenig F, Funcke F, Bai ZY, Hall C, Chin CT, Nickenig G, Bloch W, Tiemann K. Focused ultrasound-induced stimulation of microbubbles augments site-targeted engraftment of mesenchymal stem cells after acute myocardial infarction. J Mol Cell Cardiol. 2009;47(3):411–8.
129. Cheng K, Malliaras K, Li TS, Sun B, Houde C, Galang G, et al. Magnetic enhancement of cell retention, engraftment, and functional benefit after intracoronary delivery of cardiac-derived stem cells in a rat model of ischemia/reperfusion. Cell Transplant. 2012;21:1121–35.
130. Zhao TC, Tseng A, Yano N, Tseng Y, Davol PA, Lee RJ, Lum LG, Padbury JF. Targeting human CD34+ hematopoietic stem cells with anti-CD45 x anti-myosin light-chain bispecific antibody preserves cardiac function in myocardial infarction. J Appl Physiol (1985). 2008;104(6):1793–800. https://doi.org/10.1152/japplphysiol.01109.2007. Epub 2008 Feb 21.
131. Alrefai MT, Murali D, Paul A, Ridwan KM, Connell JM, Shum-Tim D. Cardiac tissue engineering and regeneration using cell-based therapy. Stem Cells Cloning. 2015;8:81–101.
132. Radisic M, Park H, Shing H, Consi T, Schoen FJ, Langer R, et al. Functional assembly of engineered myocardium by electrical stimulation of cardiac myocytes cultured on scaffolds. Proc Natl Acad Sci U S A. 2004;101:18129–34.
133. Miyagawa S, Sawa Y, Sakakida S, Taketani S, Kondoh H, Memon IA, et al. Tissue cardiomyoplasty using bioengineered contractile cardiomyocyte sheets to repair damaged myocardium: their integration with recipient myocardium. Transplantation. 2005;80:1586–95.
134. Miyagawa S, Domae K, Yoshikawa Y, Fukushima S, Nakamura T, Saito A, et al. Phase I clinical trial of autologous stem cell—sheet transplantation therapy for treating cardiomyopathy. J Am Heart Assoc. 2017;6:e003918.
135. Ott HC, Matthiesen TS, Goh SK, Black LD, Kren SM, Netoff TI, et al. Perfusion-decellularized matrix: using nature's platform to engineer a bioartificial heart. Nat Med. 2008;14:213–21.
136. Madonna R, Van Laake LW, Davidson SM, Engel FB, Hausenloy DJ, Lecour S, et al. Position paper of the European Society of Cardiology Working Group Cellular Biology of the heart: cell-based therapies for myocardial repair and regeneration in ischemic heart disease and heart failure. Eur Heart J. 2016;37:1789–98.
137. Lader J, Stachel M, Bu L. Cardiac stem cells for myocardial regeneration: promising but not ready for prime time. Curr Opin Biotechnol. 2017;47:30–5.
138. Duelen R, Sampaolesi M. Stem cell Technology in Cardiac Regeneration: a pluripotent stem cell promise. EBioMedicine. 2017;16:30–40. https://doi.org/10.1016/j.ebiom.2017.01.029. Epub 2017 Jan 27

Chapter 18
Gene Therapy in Cardiac Disease

Styliani Vakrou and Konstantinos Malliaras

18.1 Introduction

Gene therapy emerged as a potentially viable therapeutic approach for inherited and acquired diseases approximately 45 years ago [1, 2], following the demonstration of successful exogenous genetic modification of mammalian cells [3, 4]. In principle, gene therapy can induce sustained production of missing or dysfunctional endogenous proteins, after possibly only a single application; thus, gene therapy carries extraordinary therapeutic potential, as it can not only attenuate disease progression and provide symptomatic relief but also theoretically alter the disease's natural history. Clinical translation of gene therapy was first achieved in 1990 [5]. However, initial clinical applications not only failed to demonstrate efficacy but also raised significant safety concerns, including the widely publicized death of Jesse Gelsinger in 1999 [6]. These disappointing results prompted the NIH to recommend a return from "bedside to bench," highlighting the need to focus more on the basic aspects of somatic gene therapy in order to improve gene delivery and achieve sustained and high-level expression of transferred genes [7]. Over the past 20 years, remarkable advances in vector technology have enabled effective and sustained genetic modification of target tissues [1]. In addition, intensive basic research efforts have enabled better understanding of the pathophysiology of several diseases, enabling identification of key "molecular players" which can serve as potential therapeutic targets for gene therapy.

Heart disease is the number one killer in the world [8]. Thus, it has naturally become a prime target for gene therapy. In this chapter, we focus on gene therapy for heart failure and – to a lesser extent – coronary artery disease. We first touch upon the basic principles of gene transfer for cardiac disease, including discussion of different vectors and delivery methods. We then review gene-based therapeutic

S. Vakrou · K. Malliaras (✉)
Department of Cardiology, Laikon Hospital, Athens, Greece

D. V. Cokkinos (ed.), *Myocardial Preservation*,
https://doi.org/10.1007/978-3-319-98186-4_18

interventions that have been tested clinically in patients, primarily focusing on randomized, placebo-controlled clinical trials. Discussion of gene-based therapeutic interventions that have only been investigated in animal models is intentionally cursory; the reader is referred elsewhere for excellent reviews on this topic [9].

18.2 Vectors and Delivery Methods

The efficient transfer of exogenous genetic material to the target tissue is a prerequisite for successful gene therapy. There are two main categories of vehicles used for gene delivery, nonviral and viral vectors. Here we will focus on the vectors used in cardiovascular gene therapy, which are depicted schematically in Table 18.1.

Table 18.1 Vectors used in cardiovascular applications of gene therapy

Vector	Nonviral	Adenoviral	AAV	Lentiviral
Diameter	N/A	60–90 nm	20–25 nm	100 nm
Genome	DNA	dsDNA	ssDNA	ssRNA
Insert capacity, kb	>50 kb	7–36 kb	4.8 kb	7–10 kb
Integration	No	No	No	Pseudorandom
Cell type	Dividing/ nondividing	Dividing/nondividing	Dividing/ nondividing	Dividing/ nondividing
Peak cardiac expression	2–4 days	1–4 days	2–4 weeks	4–6 days
Pattern of transgene expression	Low – transient	High – transient	Moderate – long term	Moderate – long term
Tissue tropism	No	Liver, neuronal, striated muscles, respiratory	Heart for cardiotropic AAVs	$CD4^+$ cells
Pathogenicity	No	Common cold	No	HIV-related virus
Neutralizing antibodies	None	Present	Present in 2–80 % of population	Maybe
Immune response	Low inflammatory	Robust, cytotoxic and immunogenic	Minimal and transient	Minimal
Risk of insertional mutagenesis	None	Low	Rare	Present
Production	Easy	Easy	Moderate	Difficult
Genetic manipulation	Easy	Moderate	Difficult	Moderate
Clinical trial approved	Yes	Yes	Yes	No

AAV adeno-associated viruses, *CAR* coxsackie-adenovirus receptor, *HSPG* heparan sulfate proteoglycan, *EGFR* epidermal growth factor receptor

Obtained from [85] Naim C, Yerevanian A, Hajjar RJ by permission from Curr Cardiol Rep 2013;15:333

Two types of *nonviral vectors* have been used: transfection with naked *plasmid* DNA and – more recently – transfection with mRNAs with modified nucleotides (*modified mRNAs [modRNAs]*) [10]. Transfection with naked plasmid DNA allows transgenes of any size to be used (no size limit). In addition, plasmids can be readily manufactured at a large scale and are associated with limited immunogenicity. The latter allows repeat administrations, which is important from a therapeutic standpoint considering the short-term expression of the transgene. However, the low transfection efficiency is a significant disadvantage of this vector. Transfection with naked plasmid DNA has been employed clinically in the STOP-HF [11] and RETRO-HF [12] clinical trials of gene therapy for heart failure and in the VIVA [13], Euroinject One [14], and NORTHERN trials [15] of gene therapy for coronary artery disease (discussed later).

Recently, gene transfer using modRNAs was developed [16]. ModRNAs are single-stranded mRNA molecules that have undergone chemical modification to increase their stability. Given that they act as mRNAs, nuclear translocation is not required; thus, potential insertional mutagenesis or promoter dependency is obviated. In addition, the ability of modRNAs to undergo immediate translation once they have entered the host cytoplasm enables fast, high-level transgene expression (evident as soon as 20 min post-administration) [17]. However, transgene expression is brief (approximately 2–6 days) [18]. Finally, modRNAs are hypoimmunogenic, as they purportedly evade activation of Toll-like receptors [19]; thus, repeat administration is feasible and could result in improved efficacy given the brief expression of the transgene. A modRNA-based approach (comprising intramyocardial injections of modRNA encoding vascular endothelial growth factor-A) has been tested preclinically in a mouse model of myocardial infarction with encouraging results [18]; however, modRNAs have not been tested yet in patients with cardiac disease.

Two types of *viral vectors* have been employed for gene transfer in gene therapy trials for heart failure: *adenoviruses* and *adeno-associated viruses* (AAVs). Adenoviruses are double-stranded DNA molecules that are capable of infecting cardiomyocytes (without however exhibiting specific tropism for cardiac cells). Adenoviruses result in high, albeit short-term (1–4 weeks), expression of the transgene. Nevertheless, a major drawback associated with the use of adenoviral vectors is their high immunogenicity [20], which may limit clinical applicability [21]. Adenoviral vectors have been used clinically in the AC6 gene transfer for CHF heart failure trial [22] and in the KAT [23], REVASC [24], and AGENT trials [25–27] for coronary artery disease (discussed later).

Adeno-associated viruses (AAVs) are the most widely used delivery systems for gene transfer in patients with heart failure. AAVs are small, single-stranded DNA molecules that can infect myocytes and produce long-term gene expression [10, 28]. AAVs have one significant advantage that renders them particularly attractive for cardiac applications: many AAV serotypes exhibit a specific tropism for myocytes [29], which presumably enables efficient cardiac infection even after systemic delivery of AAVs [30]. So far, AAVs have been tested clinically in the CUPID 1 and 2 trials [31, 32], in the SERCA-LVAD trial [33], and in the AGENT-HF trial [34] (discussed later). Regarding immunogenicity, AAVs do not seem to elicit a cellular immune response [10, 35]. However, the clinical efficacy of AAVs can be undermined by the presence of preformed neutralizing antibodies in the host (developed during a prior infection with wild-type AAVs), which block vector transduction. This is particularly relevant from a clinical standpoint as a) neutralizing antibodies against AAVs are present in ~60% of heart failure patients [36] and b) the presence of preformed neutralizing antibodies in the host appeared to severely compromise the efficacy of SERCA gene transfer in the CUPID 1 and 2 trials [31, 32, 35, 36]. In addition, the fact that recipients of AAV-based gene therapy typically develop neutralizing antibodies against AAVs post-therapy would presumably limit the effectiveness of repeat dosing [36]. Currently, research efforts have focused on circumventing this significant obstacle through generation of AAVs that are resistant to neutralizing antibodies, through concurrent use of immunosuppression during AAV delivery (which however does not seem to prevent formation of neutralizing antibodies [36]), through plasmapheresis (to deplete neutralizing antibodies prior to AAV administration), or through concurrent administration of empty capsids (that can serve as "decoys" and absorb the host's neutralizing antibodies [37]).

With regard to cardiac delivery of vectors, three methods have been used clinically so far: intracoronary delivery (employed in the CUPID 1 and 2 [31, 32], SERCA-LVAD [33, 38], AGENT-HF [34], and AC6 gene transfer for CHF [22] trials), retrograde delivery through the coronary sinus (employed in the RETRO-HF trial [12]), and intramyocardial delivery (employed in the STOP-HF trial [11]). Each delivery method is associated with a distinct set of advantages and disadvantages. Intracoronary delivery is technically straightforward (potentially allowing for broad clinical adoption) and results in homogeneous vector delivery throughout the heart (which can be important in the setting of diffuse myocardial diseases). However, it is limited by poor transgene expression, which may increase after concurrent administration of vasodilators that increase permeability of myocardial capillaries (adenosine, substance P, and nitroglycerin) [39]. Intramyocardial delivery (either via direct epicardial or catheter-guided transendocardial injections) produces increased transgene expression but is technically demanding and results in localized vector delivery (close to the injection sites [40]). Finally, retrograde infusion through the coronary sinus with simultaneous occlusion of antegrade coronary flow produces homogeneous vector delivery and results in increased transgene expression (presumably greater than intracoronary [41] or intramyocardial delivery [40]). However, it is technically challenging and may cause ischemic myocardial injury during the transient blockade of antegrade coronary flow.

18.3 Clinical Testing of Gene-Based Therapeutic Interventions in Heart Failure

Basic research has demonstrated that several signaling pathways are dysregulated at multiple levels in failing hearts. So far, clinical trials of gene therapy in heart failure have targeted genes involved in calcium handling, in key components of the beta-adrenergic signaling, and in paracrine signaling. With regard to coronary artery disease, gene therapy trials have focused on delivery of transgenes expression angiogenic growth factors. The aforementioned targets are considered individually below.

18.3.1 Gene Therapy Targeting Calcium Handling

Calcium handling is problematic in heart failure [42, 43], resulting in impaired contractility and arrhythmogenesis [44]. Several "molecular players" who play important roles in calcium cycling have been identified, including sarcoplasmic reticulum Ca^{2+}-ATPase activity *(SERCA2a)* [43, 45, 46], phospholamban [47, 48], small ubiquitin-like modifier type 1 (SUMO1) [49, 50], and S100A1 protein [51, 52]. The aforementioned proteins have been targeted by gene-based therapeutic interventions in several preclinical studies [30, 46, 49, 50, 53–57]. However, only SERCA2a has been used as a therapeutic target in clinical trials and will be discussed below.

Experimental studies in heart failure have highlighted the importance of SERCA2a in calcium homoeostasis and cardiomyocyte function [57]. The physiologic role of SERCA2a is to transfer calcium – released during contraction from the sarcoplasmic reticulum to the cytosol – back into the sarcoplasmic reticulum. Failing hearts (irrespective of heart failure etiology) have been found to have decreased levels of SERCA2a [42]. Restoring SERCA2a levels by gene transfer has been shown to improve cardiac inotropy and lusitropy [45], improve left ventricular mechanoenergetics [30, 46], decrease arrhythmogenesis [56], and augment coronary flow through activation of endothelial eNOS [58].

The Calcium Upregulation by Percutaneous Administration of Gene Therapy in Cardiac Disease 1 (CUPID 1) clinical trial was a first-in-human clinical trial that investigated the feasibility, safety, and potential efficacy of gene therapy aiming at restoring SERCA2a expression levels in patients with heart failure [31, 32]. CUPID 1 was a multicenter, Phase 1/2 study which enrolled patients with advanced heart failure (NYHA III/IV) and reduced ejection fraction (<35%). The deficient gene was administered using an AAV type-1 vector delivered via a single intracoronary infusion. CUPID consisted of an open-label Phase 1 portion (which enrolled nine patients [31]) and a subsequent, randomized, double-blinded, placebo-controlled Phase 2 portion (which enrolled 39 patients [32]). No significant safety concerns were raised during the Phase 1 portion of the study. Of note, while hints of efficacy were observed in the majority of Phase 1 patients, two patients who had preexisting anti-AAV1 neutralizing antibodies showed no signs of improvement [31]. Based on these results, the Phase 2 portion of CUPID 1 required eligible patients to have undetectable AAV1 neutralizing antibody titers.

In the Phase 2 portion of CUPID 1, 39 patients were randomized to receive either a low (6×10^{11} DNAse-resistant particles [DRP], $n = 8$), middle (3×10^{12} DRP, $n = 8$), and high dose (1×10^{13} DRP, $n = 9$) of AAV1/SERCA2a or placebo ($n = 14$) [32]. Patients were followed for 12 months, and the following efficacy parameters were evaluated: symptoms, functional status, cardiac biomarkers, left ventricular function/remodeling, and clinical outcomes. Administration of AAV1/SERCA2a was associated with a favorable safety profile. With regard to efficacy, patients receiving the high dose exhibited a significant increase in time to clinical events, a significantly decreased incidence of cardiovascular events, and a significantly decreased duration of cardiovascular hospitalizations compared to placebo-treated patients. PCR performed in myocardial tissue obtained from a subset of patients (procured during transplant, during LVAD placement, or at autopsy) revealed no persistence of the transgene in 1/1 low-dose patients and in 4/4 mid-dose patients. In contrast, long-term persistence (for up to 31 months postdelivery) of the transgene was observed in 3/4 patients that had received high-dose AAV1/SERCA2a therapy [28]. However, the detected levels of the transgene were very low (20–561 copies of vector per μg of DNA [28]), i.e., ~1000-fold lower compared to the levels measured in preclinical animal models [10]. The encouraging results of CUPID 1 provided the foundation for further investigation of AAV1/SERCA2a therapy in the larger follow-up CUPID 2 trial.

CUPID 2 was a pivotal, Phase 2b study that investigated the efficacy of a single intracoronary infusion of AAV1/SERCA2a administered at a dose of 1×10^{13} DRP (the high dose of CUPID 1) in patients with heart failure [35]. CUPID 2 was a multicenter, randomized, double-blind, placebo-controlled study which enrolled patients with moderate to advanced heart failure (NYHA II–IV), reduced ejection fraction (<35%), and undetectable AAV1 neutralizing antibody titers. A total of 250 patients were enrolled (making CUPID 2 the largest clinical trial of gene therapy in heart failure to date) and were randomized (1:1) to intracoronary AAV1/SERCA2a or placebo. No significant safety concerns related to AAV1/SERCA2a therapy were observed. The primary efficacy endpoint was time to recurrent events, defined as hospital admission or ambulatory treatment for worsening heart failure, and median follow-up was ~17 months. Despite the promising results of CUPID 1, CUPID 2 failed to reach its primary efficacy endpoint; time to recurrent heart failure events was comparable between groups (hazard ration 0.93, $p = 0.81$). In addition, none of the exploratory efficacy endpoints (changes in NYHA class, 6-min walk test, quality of life, or NT-proBNP) differed significantly between groups during follow-up. It is unclear how the discrepancy between the results of CUPID 1 and CUPID 2 can be explained. A simple explanation is that the small, pilot CUPID 1 trial may have been a "red herring," i.e., a trial that was positive by chance alone. Another explanation may be the difference in the proportion of empty viral capsids (i.e., viral capsids containing the protein capsid but not the AAV vector) between CUPID 1 (85%) and CUPID 2 (25%). While an association between an increased proportion of empty viral capsids and improved efficacy of gene therapy may appear paradoxical at first, it could be rationalized if one considers that empty capsids could act as "decoys" for host neutralizing antibodies [37].

AGENT-HF and SERCA-LVAD are two smaller studies, auxiliary to CUPID 2. The AGENT-HF trial aimed to investigate the effects of a single intracoronary infusion of AAV1/SERCA2a administered at a dose of 1×10^{13} DRP on ventricular remodeling, as assessed by computed tomography [34]. The investigators initially planned to enroll 40 patients, but enrollment was suspended following the negative results of CUPID 2. At the time of suspension, five patients had received AAV1/SERCA2a, and four patients had received placebo infusions. No differences in end-systolic volumes (the primary endpoint of the trial) were observed between groups, but the study was obviously underpowered to detect any differences. The SERCA-LVAD trial [33] aimed to investigate the effects of a single intracoronary infusion of AAV1/SERCA2a administered at a dose of 1×10^{13} DRP in patients receiving mechanical circulatory support with a left ventricular assist device [38]. Following the negative results of CUPID 2, enrollment in this trial was also suspended; at the time of suspension, five patients had received gene therapy with AAV1/SERCA2a. Despite the small cohort of patients, this trial provided important information as researchers were able to collect myocardial samples (procured by endomyocardial biopsy or at the time of cardiac transplantation) from the treated patients. No evidence of myocarditis was observed in the obtained samples, confirming the favorable safety profile observed in the other SERCA2a trials. Of note, PCR revealed the persistence of viral DNA in two patients; however, the DNA copy numbers were 25–250 times lower than those observed in animal studies. The detection of very low DNA copy numbers in the SERCA-LVAD trial is consistent with results from the CUPID 1 [28] trial and indicates that the inability of effective gene transfer into human cardiomyocytes remains a major limitation of cardiac gene therapy [59].

18.3.2 Gene Therapy Targeting Adenylyl Cyclase

Cyclic adenosine monophosphate (cAMP, a second messenger involved in beta-adrenergic signaling) is a key regulator of heart function [60]. *Adenylyl cyclase type 6* (AC6), the dominant AC type in cardiomyocytes, is a large (130 kD) membrane protein that served as an effector molecule in the beta-adrenergic signaling pathway and catalyzes the conversion of adenosine triphosphate (ATP) to cAMP. Additionally, AC6 has been found to also affect calcium handling, influencing cardiac function independently of intracellular cAMP levels [61]. This feature renders AC6 an attractive target for gene therapy, distinguishing it from conventional inotropic agents that increase intracellular cAMP and improve contractility (dobutamine, milrinone), at the cost of increased mortality in heart failure patients [62]. Failing hearts are deficient in AC6 [63, 64]. In addition, transgenic mice overexpressing AC6 exhibited improved cardiac function upon adrenergic stimulation [65], without having increased cardiac cAMP levels under basal conditions. Importantly from a therapeutic aspect, upregulation of AC6 via gene therapy has been shown to confer structural and functional benefits in a clinically relevant large animal model of heart failure [66].

AC6 gene transfer for heart failure was a first-in-man clinical trial that investigated the feasibility, safety, and potential efficacy of gene therapy aiming at restoring AC6 expression levels in patients with heart failure [22]. It was a randomized, multicenter, double-blind, placebo-controlled, dose-ranging Phase 1/2 study which enrolled patients with heart failure (NYHA II/III) and reduced ejection fraction

(<40%). AC6 was administered using an E1/E3-deleted human adenovirus type 5 encoding human AC6 (Ad5/AC6) via a single intracoronary infusion. A total of 56 patients were enrolled and were randomized (in a 3:1 ratio) to receive Ad5/AC6 ($n = 42$) or placebo ($n = 14$). Patients randomized to the gene therapy group received one of the following five intracoronary doses of Ad5/AC6: 3.2×10^9 virus particles ($n = 6$), 10^{10} virus particles ($n = 6$), 3.2×10^{10} virus particles ($n = 6$), 3.2×10^{11} virus particles ($n = 12$), or 10^{12} virus particles ($n = 12$). Patients were followed for 1 year. Ad5/AC6 administration did not raise significant safety concerns. With regard to efficacy, patients who received the two highest doses of Ad5/AC6 displayed a transient significant increase in ejection fraction (assessed by echocardiography) at 4 weeks postdelivery that did not remain significant at 12 weeks postdelivery. In contrast, no significant changes in ejection fraction were observed in the placebo group. In addition, patients who received the two highest doses of Ad5/AC6 displayed a significant improvement in dP/dT min (assessed by cardiac catheterization at 4 weeks postdelivery) compared to placebo-treated patients. Of note, a trend toward decreased rate of heart failure admissions was observed in Ad5/AC6-treated patients compared to controls (9.5% vs 28.9%, $p = 0.10$). The favorable safety profile combined with the encouraging efficacy signals observed in this study laid the foundation for the design of a Phase 3 follow-up trial, the FLOURISH trial [67]. The FLOURISH trial plans to enroll a total of 536 patients with heart failure and reduced ejection fraction (<35%), who will be randomized (1:1) to undergo a single intracoronary infusion of Ad5/AC6 (10^{12} virus particles, i.e., the highest dose administered in the dose-ranging study) or vehicle solution. The primary endpoint is the rate of heart failure hospitalizations over a 12-month follow-up period [67, 68].

18.3.3 Gene Therapy Targeting Paracrine Signaling

Gene-based therapeutic interventions targeting paracrine signaling have undergone extensive clinical testing in the setting of coronary artery disease. Specifically, gene therapy trials for coronary artery disease have focused on delivery of genes encoding *VEGF* and *fibroblast growth factor 4 (FGF4)*, which are known to promote angiogenesis [69]. Early-phase clinical testing of gene therapy aiming at amplifying expression of VEGF in the host tissue yielded encouraging preliminary results [70–72]. However, subsequent larger, pivotal, randomized trials were disappointing. Specifically, the majority of pivotal studies – including the VIVA trial [13], the Euroinject One trial [14], the NORTHERN trial [15], the GENASIS trial [73], and the REVASC trial [24] (but not the KAT trial [23]) – failed to demonstrate an objective increase in myocardial perfusion following gene therapy. Similarly to VEGF, intriguing hints of efficacy were observed during early-phase clinical testing of gene therapy aiming at increasing FGF4 expression in coronary artery disease (AGENT [25] and AGENT-2 [26] trials). However, these efficacy signals could not be reproduced in the subsequent, larger, pivotal AGENT-3 and AGENT-4 trials, which were prematurely terminated when an interim analysis of the AGENT-3 trial indicated that the trial would not reach its primary endpoint [27]. Despite the overall disappointing results, several clinical trials of angiogenic gene therapy in patients with coronary artery disease are currently ongoing or planned [69].

Gene therapy targeting paracrine signaling has also been tested clinically in patients with heart failure. *Stromal cell-derived factor 1 (SDF-1)* has been shown to promote cardiac tissue repair through activation of endogenous progenitor cells and stimulation of angiogenesis in animal models of ischemic cardiomyopathy and heart failure [74–79]. The Stromal Cell-Derived Factor-1 Plasmid Treatment for Patients with Heart Failure (STOP-HF) trial investigated the safety and potential efficacy of gene therapy aiming at increasing SDF-1 levels in patients with heart failure [11]. STOP-HF was a multicenter, randomized, double-blind, placebo-controlled Phase 2 study that enrolled patients with ischemic heart failure and reduced ejection fraction (<40%). Patients randomized to receive treatment underwent intramyocardial injection of JVS-100, a naked DNA plasmid encoding humans SDF-1 at a dose of 15 or 30 mg (based on the results of a Phase 1 dose-escalation study [80]). JSV-100 was administered in the infarct border zone (identified by echocardiography) by 15 transendocardial injections using a catheter that was advanced inside the left ventricle. A total of 93 patients were enrolled and were randomized (in a 1:1:1 ratio) to undergo intramyocardial injections of 15 mg JSV-100 (n = 32), 30 mg JSV-100 (n = 30), or vehicle (n = 31). The primary endpoint was a composite of change in 6-min walk distance and quality of life from baseline to 4 months from delivery. Transendocardial delivery of JSV-100 was safe, but the primary endpoint of the trial was not met. However, a prespecified subgroup analysis revealed that patients in the lowest tertile of baseline ejection fraction (<26%) treated with the high dose of JSV-100 demonstrated a significant increase in ejection fraction (~11%) compared to control patients at 1-year postdelivery. Currently, the feasibility, safety, and potential efficacy of retrograde infusion of JSV-100, administered into the coronary sinus, are being tested in the Phase 1/2 RETRO-HF trial [12]. RETRO-HF plans to enroll 72 patients with ischemic heart failure, and its primary endpoint is change in 6-min walk distance from baseline to 4 months postdelivery.

18.4 Gene Editing

Recently, *gene editing* technologies using programmable nucleases [81] have progressed rapidly toward clinical translation. Contrary to traditional gene-based therapeutic approaches (which use viral or nonviral vectors to achieve exogenous addition of deficient genes), gene editing technologies not only enable gene addition but also gene ablation or targeted gene correction [1]. In the heart, in vivo gene editing has been recently employed as a potential therapeutic approach for dystrophic cardiomyopathy in mice with Duchenne muscular dystrophy [82, 83]. While gene editing technologies are currently at their "translational infancy" [1], first-in-human clinical application in patients with Duchenne muscular dystrophy is expected to take place within the next 5 years [84].

In conclusion, to date, over 1000 patients have been enrolled in clinical trials of gene therapy for heart disease (either coronary artery disease or heart failure). Of note, gene transfer has been associated with an excellent safety profile so far, regardless of vector or delivery methods. However, therapeutic efficacy has been underwhelming; large pivotal, randomized, placebo-controlled trials have failed to reproduce the efficacy signals observed in earlier-phase clinical testing, and primary endpoints have not been met. Importantly, low efficiency of gene transfer into cardiomyocytes appears to remain a significant obstacle. Moving forward, research efforts should focus on development of better vectors, more efficient delivery systems, deeper understanding of disease pathophysiology, and improved clinical trial design (including selection of appropriate dosages, patients, and endpoints).

References

1. Dunbar CE, High KA, Joung JK, Kohn DB, Ozawa K, Sadelain M. Gene therapy comes of age. Science. 2018;359(6372 Epub 2018/01/13). https://doi.org/10.1126/science.aan4672. PubMed PMID: 29326244.
2. Friedmann T, Roblin R. Gene therapy for human genetic disease? Science. 1972;175(4025): 949–55. Epub 1972/03/03. PubMed PMID: 5061866.
3. Munyon W, Kraiselburd E, Davis D, Mann J. Transfer of thymidine kinase to thymidine kinaseless L cells by infection with ultraviolet-irradiated herpes simplex virus. J Virol. 1971;7(6):813–20. Epub 1971/06/01. PubMed PMID: 4327589; PubMed Central PMCID: PMCPMC356201.
4. Merril CR, Geier MR, Petricciani JC. Bacterial virus gene expression in human cells. Nature. 1971;233(5319):398–400. Epub 1971/10/08. PubMed PMID: 4940436.
5. Blaese RM, Culver KW, Miller AD, Carter CS, Fleisher T, Clerici M, et al. T lymphocyte-directed gene therapy for ADA- SCID: initial trial results after 4 years. Science. 1995;270(5235):475–80. Epub 1995/10/20. PubMed PMID: 7570001.
6. Jenks S. Gene therapy death—"everyone has to share in the guilt". J Natl Cancer Inst. 2000;92(2):98–100. Epub 2000/01/20. PubMed PMID: 10639505.
7. Orkin SH, Motulsky AG. Report and recommendations of the panel to assess the NIH investment in research on gene therapy; 1995.
8. Mathers CD, Loncar D. Projections of global mortality and burden of disease from 2002 to 2030. PLoS Med. 2006;3(11):e442. Epub 2006/11/30. https://doi.org/10.1371/journal.pmed.0030442. PubMed PMID: 17132052; PubMed Central PMCID: PMCPMC1664601.
9. Fargnoli AS, Katz MG, Bridges CR, Hajjar RJ. Gene therapy in heart failure. Handb Exp Pharmacol. 2017;243:395–421. Epub 2016/11/01. https://doi.org/10.1007/164_2016_81. PubMed PMID: 27796512.
10. Hulot JS, Ishikawa K, Hajjar RJ. Gene therapy for the treatment of heart failure: promise postponed. Eur Heart J. 2016;37(21):1651–8. Epub 2016/02/29. https://doi.org/10.1093/eurheartj/ehw019. PubMed PMID: 26922809; PubMed Central PMCID: PMCPMC4887702.
11. Chung ES, Miller L, Patel AN, Anderson RD, Mendelsohn FO, Traverse J, et al. Changes in ventricular remodelling and clinical status during the year following a single administration of stromal cell-derived factor-1 non-viral gene therapy in chronic ischaemic heart failure patients: the STOP-HF randomized Phase II trial. Eur Heart J. 2015;36(33):2228–38. Epub

2015/06/10. https://doi.org/10.1093/eurheartj/ehv254. PubMed PMID: 26056125; PubMed Central PMCID: PMCPMC4554960.

12. https://clinicaltrials.gov/ct2/show/NCT01961726.
13. Henry TD, Annex BH, McKendall GR, Azrin MA, Lopez JJ, Giordano FJ, et al. The VIVA trial: vascular endothelial growth factor in ischemia for vascular angiogenesis. Circulation. 2003;107(10):1359–65. Epub 2003/03/19. PubMed PMID: 12642354.
14. Kastrup J, Jorgensen E, Ruck A, Tagil K, Glogar D, Ruzyllo W, et al. Direct intramyocardial plasmid vascular endothelial growth factor-A165 gene therapy in patients with stable severe angina pectoris a randomized double-blind placebo-controlled study: the Euroinject one trial. J Am Coll Cardiol. 2005;45(7):982–8. Epub 2005/04/06. https://doi.org/10.1016/j.jacc.2004.12.068. PubMed PMID: 15808751.
15. Stewart DJ, Kutryk MJ, Fitchett D, Freeman M, Camack N, Su Y, et al. VEGF gene therapy fails to improve perfusion of ischemic myocardium in patients with advanced coronary disease: results of the NORTHERN trial. Molecular Ther. 2009;17(6):1109–15. Epub 2009/04/09. https://doi.org/10.1038/mt.2009.70. PubMed PMID: 19352324; PubMed Central PMCID: PMCPMC2835194.
16. Youn H, Chung JK. Modified mRNA as an alternative to plasmid DNA (pDNA) for transcript replacement and vaccination therapy. Expert Opin Biol Ther. 2015;15(9):1337–48. Epub 2015/07/01. https://doi.org/10.1517/14712598.2015.1057563. PubMed PMID: 26125492; PubMed Central PMCID: PMCPMC4696419.
17. Turnbull IC, Eltoukhy AA, Fish KM, Nonnenmacher M, Ishikawa K, Chen J, et al. Myocardial delivery of lipidoid nanoparticle carrying modRNA induces rapid and transient expression. Molecular Ther. 2016;24(1):66–75. Epub 2015/10/17. https://doi.org/10.1038/mt.2015.193. PubMed PMID: 26471463; PubMed Central PMCID: PMCPMC4754552.
18. Zangi L, Lui KO, von Gise A, Ma Q, Ebina W, Ptaszek LM, et al. Modified mRNA directs the fate of heart progenitor cells and induces vascular regeneration after myocardial infarction. Nature Biotechnol. 2013;31(10):898–907. Epub 2013/09/10. https://doi.org/10.1038/nbt.2682. PubMed PMID: 24013197; PubMed Central PMCID: PMCPMC4058317.
19. Kariko K, Buckstein M, Ni H, Weissman D. Suppression of RNA recognition by toll-like receptors: the impact of nucleoside modification and the evolutionary origin of RNA. Immunity. 2005;23(2):165–75. Epub 2005/08/23. https://doi.org/10.1016/j.immuni.2005.06.008. PubMed PMID: 16111635.
20. Alba R, Bosch A, Chillon M. Gutless adenovirus: last-generation adenovirus for gene therapy. Gene Ther. 2005;12(Suppl 1):S18–27. Epub 2005/10/19. https://doi.org/10.1038/sj.gt.3302612. PubMed PMID: 16231052.
21. Jooss K, Chirmule N. Immunity to adenovirus and adeno-associated viral vectors: implications for gene therapy. Gene Ther. 2003;10(11):955–63. Epub 2003/05/21. https://doi.org/10.1038/sj.gt.3302037. PubMed PMID: 12756416.
22. Hammond HK, Penny WF, Traverse JH, Henry TD, Watkins MW, Yancy CW, et al. Intracoronary gene transfer of adenylyl cyclase 6 in patients with heart failure: a randomized clinical trial. JAMA Cardiol. 2016;1(2):163–71. Epub 2016/07/22. https://doi.org/10.1001/jamacardio.2016.0008. PubMed PMID: 27437887; PubMed Central PMCID: PMCPMC5535743.
23. Hedman M, Hartikainen J, Syvanne M, Stjernvall J, Hedman A, Kivela A, et al. Safety and feasibility of catheter-based local intracoronary vascular endothelial growth factor gene transfer in the prevention of postangioplasty and in-stent restenosis and in the treatment of chronic myocardial ischemia: phase II results of the Kuopio angiogenesis trial (KAT). Circulation. 2003;107(21):2677–83. Epub 2003/05/14. https://doi.org/10.1161/01.cir.0000070540.80780.92. PubMed PMID: 12742981.
24. Stewart DJ, Hilton JD, Arnold JM, Gregoire J, Rivard A, Archer SL, et al. Angiogenic gene therapy in patients with nonrevascularizable ischemic heart disease: a phase 2 randomized, controlled trial of AdVEGF(121) (AdVEGF121) versus maximum medical treatment. Gene Ther. 2006;13(21):1503–11. Epub 2006/06/23. https://doi.org/10.1038/sj.gt.3302802. PubMed PMID: 16791287.

25. Grines CL, Watkins MW, Helmer G, Penny W, Brinker J, Marmur JD, et al. Angiogenic gene therapy (AGENT) trial in patients with stable angina pectoris. Circulation. 2002;105(11):1291–7. Epub 2002/03/20. PubMed PMID: 11901038.
26. Grines CL, Watkins MW, Mahmarian JJ, Iskandrian AE, Rade JJ, Marrott P, et al. A randomized, double-blind, placebo-controlled trial of Ad5FGF-4 gene therapy and its effect on myocardial perfusion in patients with stable angina. J Am Coll Cardiol. 2003;42(8):1339–47. Epub 2003/10/18. PubMed PMID: 14563572.
27. Henry TD, Grines CL, Watkins MW, Dib N, Barbeau G, Moreadith R, et al. Effects of Ad5FGF-4 in patients with angina: an analysis of pooled data from the AGENT-3 and AGENT-4 trials. J Am Coll Cardiol. 2007;50(11):1038–46. Epub 2007/09/11. https://doi.org/10.1016/j.jacc.2007.06.010. PubMed PMID: 17825712.
28. Zsebo K, Yaroshinsky A, Rudy JJ, Wagner K, Greenberg B, Jessup M, et al. Long-term effects of AAV1/SERCA2a gene transfer in patients with severe heart failure: analysis of recurrent cardiovascular events and mortality. Circ Res. 2014;114(1):101–8. Epub 2013/09/26. https://doi.org/10.1161/circresaha.113.302421. PubMed PMID: 24065463.
29. Zincarelli C, Soltys S, Rengo G, Rabinowitz JE. Analysis of AAV serotypes 1-9 mediated gene expression and tropism in mice after systemic injection. Molecular Ther. 2008;16(6):1073–80. Epub 2008/04/17. https://doi.org/10.1038/mt.2008.76. PubMed PMID: 18414476.
30. Sakata S, Lebeche D, Sakata N, Sakata Y, Chemaly ER, Liang LF, et al. Restoration of mechanical and energetic function in failing aortic-banded rat hearts by gene transfer of calcium cycling proteins. J Mol Cell Cardiol. 2007;42(4):852–61. Epub 2007/02/16. https://doi.org/10.1016/j.yjmcc.2007.01.003. PubMed PMID: 17300800; PubMed Central PMCID: PMCPMC1945057.
31. Jaski BE, Jessup ML, Mancini DM, Cappola TP, Pauly DF, Greenberg B, et al. Calcium upregulation by percutaneous administration of gene therapy in cardiac disease (CUPID Trial), a first-in-human phase 1/2 clinical trial. J Card Fail. 2009;15(3):171–81. Epub 2009/03/31. https://doi.org/10.1016/j.cardfail.2009.01.013. PubMed PMID: 19327618; PubMed Central PMCID: PMCPMC2752875.
32. Jessup M, Greenberg B, Mancini D, Cappola T, Pauly DF, Jaski B, et al. Calcium Upregulation by Percutaneous Administration of Gene Therapy in Cardiac Disease (CUPID): a phase 2 trial of intracoronary gene therapy of sarcoplasmic reticulum Ca2+-ATPase in patients with advanced heart failure. Circulation. 2011;124(3):304–13. Epub 2011/06/29. https://doi.org/10.1161/circulationaha.111.022889. PubMed PMID: 21709064; PubMed Central PMCID: PMCPMC5843948.
33. https://clinicaltrials.gov/ct2/show/NCT00534703.
34. Hulot JS, Salem JE, Redheuil A, Collet JP, Varnous S, Jourdain P, et al. Effect of intracoronary administration of AAV1/SERCA2a on ventricular remodelling in patients with advanced systolic heart failure: results from the AGENT-HF randomized phase 2 trial. Eur J Heart Fail. 2017;19(11):1534–41. Epub 2017/04/11. https://doi.org/10.1002/ejhf.826. PubMed PMID: 28393439.
35. Greenberg B, Butler J, Felker GM, Ponikowski P, Voors AA, Desai AS, et al. Calcium upregulation by percutaneous administration of gene therapy in patients with cardiac disease (CUPID 2): a randomised, multinational, double-blind, placebo-controlled, phase 2b trial. Lancet. 2016;387(10024):1178–86. Epub 2016/01/25. https://doi.org/10.1016/s0140-6736(16)00082-9. PubMed PMID: 26803443.
36. Greenberg B, Butler J, Felker GM, Ponikowski P, Voors AA, Pogoda JM, et al. Prevalence of AAV1 neutralizing antibodies and consequences for a clinical trial of gene transfer for advanced heart failure. Gene Ther. 2016;23(3):313–9. Epub 2015/12/25. https://doi.org/10.1038/gt.2015.109. PubMed PMID: 26699914.
37. Mingozzi F, Anguela XM, Pavani G, Chen Y, Davidson RJ, Hui DJ, et al. Overcoming preexisting humoral immunity to AAV using capsid decoys. Sci Transl Med. 2013;5(194):194ra92. Epub 2013/07/19. https://doi.org/10.1126/scitranslmed.3005795. PubMed PMID: 23863832; PubMed Central PMCID: PMCPMC4095828.

38. https://www.escardio.org/Congresses-&-Events/Heart-Failure/Congress-resources/serca-lvad-lessons-learned-for-gene-therapy-in-heart-failure, editor.
39. Woitek F, Zentilin L, Hoffman NE, Powers JC, Ottiger I, Parikh S, et al. Intracoronary cytoprotective gene therapy: a study of VEGF-B167 in a pre-clinical animal model of dilated cardiomyopathy. J Am Coll Cardiol. 2015;66(2):139–53. Epub 2015/07/15. https://doi.org/10.1016/j.jacc.2015.04.071. PubMed PMID: 26160630; PubMed Central PMCID: PMCPMC4499859.
40. Raake P, von Degenfeld G, Hinkel R, Vachenauer R, Sandner T, Beller S, et al. Myocardial gene transfer by selective pressure-regulated retroinfusion of coronary veins: comparison with surgical and percutaneous intramyocardial gene delivery. J Am Coll Cardiol. 2004;44(5):1124–9. Epub 2004/09/01. https://doi.org/10.1016/j.jacc.2004.05.074. PubMed PMID: 15337228.
41. Boekstegers P, von Degenfeld G, Giehrl W, Heinrich D, Hullin R, Kupatt C, et al. Myocardial gene transfer by selective pressure-regulated retroinfusion of coronary veins. Gene Ther. 2000;7(3):232–40. Epub 2000/03/01. https://doi.org/10.1038/sj.gt.3301079. PubMed PMID: 10694800.
42. Gwathmey JK, Copelas L, MacKinnon R, Schoen FJ, Feldman MD, Grossman W, et al. Abnormal intracellular calcium handling in myocardium from patients with end-stage heart failure. Circ Res. 1987;61(1):70–6. Epub 1987/07/01. PubMed PMID: 3608112.
43. Hasenfuss G, Pieske B. Calcium cycling in congestive heart failure. J Mol Cell Cardiol. 2002;34(8):951–69. Epub 2002/09/18. PubMed PMID: 12234765.
44. Lompre AM, Hajjar RJ, Harding SE, Kranias EG, Lohse MJ, Marks AR. Ca2+ cycling and new therapeutic approaches for heart failure. Circulation. 2010;121(6):822–30. Epub 2010/02/04. https://doi.org/10.1161/circulationaha.109.890954. PubMed PMID: 20124124; PubMed Central PMCID: PMCPMC2834781.
45. Kawase Y, Ly HQ, Prunier F, Lebeche D, Shi Y, Jin H, et al. Reversal of cardiac dysfunction after long-term expression of SERCA2a by gene transfer in a pre-clinical model of heart failure. J Am Coll Cardiol. 2008;51(11):1112–9. Epub 2008/03/18. https://doi.org/10.1016/j.jacc.2007.12.014. PubMed PMID: 18342232.
46. del Monte F, Williams E, Lebeche D, Schmidt U, Rosenzweig A, Gwathmey JK, et al. Improvement in survival and cardiac metabolism after gene transfer of sarcoplasmic reticulum Ca(2+)-ATPase in a rat model of heart failure. Circulation. 2001;104(12):1424–9. Epub 2001/09/19. PubMed PMID: 11560860; PubMed Central PMCID: PMCPMC1249503.
47. Chu G, Kranias EG. Phospholamban as a therapeutic modality in heart failure. Novartis Found Symp. 2006;274:156–71. discussion 72–5, 272–6. Epub 2006/10/06. PubMed PMID: 17019811.
48. Koss KL, Kranias EG. Phospholamban: a prominent regulator of myocardial contractility. Circ Res. 1996;79(6):1059–63. https://doi.org/10.1161/01.res.79.6.1059.
49. Kho C, Lee A, Jeong D, Oh JG, Chaanine AH, Kizana E, et al. SUMO1-dependent modulation of SERCA2a in heart failure. Nature. 2011;477(7366):601–5. Epub 2011/09/09. https://doi.org/10.1038/nature10407. PubMed PMID: 21900893; PubMed Central PMCID: PMCPMC3443490.
50. Tilemann L, Lee A, Ishikawa K, Aguero J, Rapti K, Santos-Gallego C, et al. <em>SUMO-1</em> Gene Transfer improves cardiac function in a large-animal model of heart failure. Sci Transl Med. 2013;5(211):211ra159–9. https://doi.org/10.1126/scitranslmed.3006487.
51. Ritterhoff J, Most P. Targeting S100A1 in heart failure. Gene Ther. 2012;19(6):613–21. Epub 2012/02/18. https://doi.org/10.1038/gt.2012.8. PubMed PMID: 22336719.
52. Most P, Seifert H, Gao E, Funakoshi H, Völkers M, Heierhorst J, et al. Cardiac S100A1 protein levels determine contractile performance and propensity toward heart failure after myocardial infarction. Circulation. 2006;114(12):1258–68. https://doi.org/10.1161/circulationaha.106.622415.
53. Ishikawa K, Fish KM, Tilemann L, Rapti K, Aguero J, Santos-Gallego CG, et al. Cardiac I-1c overexpression with reengineered AAV improves cardiac function in swine ischemic heart

failure. Molecular Ther. 2014;22(12):2038–45. Epub 2014/07/16. https://doi.org/10.1038/mt.2014.127. PubMed PMID: 25023328; PubMed Central PMCID: PMCPMC4429688.
54. Pathak A, del Monte F, Zhao W, Schultz JE, Lorenz JN, Bodi I, et al. Enhancement of cardiac function and suppression of heart failure progression by inhibition of protein phosphatase 1. Circ Res. 2005;96(7):756–66. Epub 2005/03/05. https://doi.org/10.1161/01.RES.0000161256.85833.fa. PubMed PMID: 15746443.
55. Watanabe S, Ishikawa K, Fish K, Oh JG, Motloch LJ, Kohlbrenner E, et al. Protein phosphatase inhibitor-1 gene therapy in a swine model of nonischemic heart failure. J Am Coll Cardiol. 2017;70(14):1744–56. Epub 2017/09/30. https://doi.org/10.1016/j.jacc.2017.08.013. PubMed PMID: 28958332; PubMed Central PMCID: PMCPMC5807083.
56. Prunier F, Kawase Y, Gianni D, Scapin C, Danik SB, Ellinor PT, et al. Prevention of ventricular arrhythmias with sarcoplasmic reticulum Ca2+ ATPase pump overexpression in a porcine model of ischemia reperfusion. Circulation. 2008;118(6):614–24. Epub 2008/07/23. https://doi.org/10.1161/circulationaha.108.770883. PubMed PMID: 18645052.
57. Hasenfuss G, Reinecke H, Studer R, Meyer M, Pieske B, Holtz J, et al. Relation between myocardial function and expression of sarcoplasmic reticulum ca(2+)-ATPase in failing and non-failing human myocardium. Circ Res. 1994;75(3):434–42. Epub 1994/09/01. PubMed PMID: 8062417.
58. Hadri L, Bobe R, Kawase Y, Ladage D, Ishikawa K, Atassi F, et al. SERCA2a gene transfer enhances eNOS expression and activity in endothelial cells. Molecular Ther. 2010;18(7):1284–92. Epub 2010/05/13. https://doi.org/10.1038/mt.2010.77. PubMed PMID: 20461063; PubMed Central PMCID: PMCPMC2911258.
59. Donahue JK. Cardiac gene therapy: a call for basic methods development. Lancet. 2016;387(10024):1137–9. Epub 2016/01/26. https://doi.org/10.1016/s0140-6736(16)00149-5. PubMed PMID: 26806516.
60. Sunahara RK, Dessauer CW, Gilman AG. Complexity and diversity of mammalian adenylyl cyclases. Annu Rev Pharmacol Toxicol. 1996;36:461–80. Epub 1996/01/01. https://doi.org/10.1146/annurev.pa.36.040196.002333. PubMed PMID: 8725398.
61. Gao MH, Tang T, Guo T, Sun SQ, Feramisco JR, Hammond HK. Adenylyl cyclase type VI gene transfer reduces phospholamban expression in cardiac myocytes via activating transcription factor 3. J Biol Chem. 2004;279(37):38797–802. Epub 2004/07/03. https://doi.org/10.1074/jbc.M405701200. PubMed PMID: 15231818.
62. DiBianco R, Shabetai R, Kostuk W, Moran J, Schlant RC, Wright R. A comparison of oral milrinone, digoxin, and their combination in the treatment of patients with chronic heart failure. N Engl J Med. 1989;320(11):677–83. Epub 1989/03/16. https://doi.org/10.1056/nejm198903163201101. PubMed PMID: 2646536.
63. Ping P, Anzai T, Gao M, Hammond HK. Adenylyl cyclase and G protein receptor kinase expression during development of heart failure. Am J Phys. 1997;273(2 Pt 2):H707–17. Epub 1997/08/01. https://doi.org/10.1152/ajpheart.1997.273.2.H707. PubMed PMID: 9277487.
64. Ishikawa Y, Sorota S, Kiuchi K, Shannon RP, Komamura K, Katsushika S, et al. Downregulation of adenylyl cyclase types V and VI mRNA levels in pacing-induced heart failure in dogs. J Clin Invest. 1994;93(5):2224–9. Epub 1994/05/01. https://doi.org/10.1172/jci117219. PubMed PMID: 8182154; PubMed Central PMCID: PMCPMC294370.
65. Gao MH, Lai NC, Roth DM, Zhou J, Zhu J, Anzai T, et al. Adenylyl cyclase increases responsiveness to catecholamine stimulation in transgenic mice. Circulation. 1999;99(12):1618–22. Epub 1999/03/30. PubMed PMID: 10096940.
66. Lai NC, Roth DM, Gao MH, Tang T, Dalton N, Lai YY, et al. Intracoronary adenovirus encoding adenylyl cyclase VI increases left ventricular function in heart failure. Circulation. 2004;110(3):330–6. Epub 2004/07/14. https://doi.org/10.1161/01.cir.0000136033.21777.4d. PubMed PMID: 15249510.
67. Penny WF, Henry TD, Watkins MW, Patel AN, Hammond HK. Design of a Phase 3 trial of intracoronary administration of human adenovirus 5 encoding human adenylyl cyclase type 6 (RT-100) gene transfer in patients with heart failure with reduced left ventricular ejection

fraction: the FLOURISH clinical trial. Am Heart J. 2018;201:111–6. Epub 2018/05/16. https://doi.org/10.1016/j.ahj.2018.04.005. PubMed PMID: 29763816.

68. https://clinicaltrials.gov/ct2/show/NCT03360448.
69. Yla-Herttuala S, Bridges C, Katz MG, Korpisalo P. Angiogenic gene therapy in cardiovascular diseases: dream or vision? Eur Heart J. 2017;38(18):1365–71. Epub 2017/01/12. https://doi.org/10.1093/eurheartj/ehw547. PubMed PMID: 28073865; PubMed Central PMCID: PMCPMC5837788.
70. Symes JF, Losordo DW, Vale PR, Lathi KG, Esakof DD, Mayskiy M, et al. Gene therapy with vascular endothelial growth factor for inoperable coronary artery disease. Ann Thorac Surg. 1999;68(3):830–6 discussion 6-7. Epub 1999/10/06 PubMed PMID: 10509970.
71. Rosengart TK, Lee LY, Patel SR, Sanborn TA, Parikh M, Bergman GW, et al. Angiogenesis gene therapy: phase I assessment of direct intramyocardial administration of an adenovirus vector expressing VEGF121 cDNA to individuals with clinically significant severe coronary artery disease. Circulation. 1999;100(5):468–74. Epub 1999/08/03. PubMed PMID: 10430759.
72. Losordo DW, Vale PR, Hendel RC, Milliken CE, Fortuin FD, Cummings N, et al. Phase 1/2 placebo-controlled, double-blind, dose-escalating trial of myocardial vascular endothelial growth factor 2 gene transfer by catheter delivery in patients with chronic myocardial ischemia. Circulation. 2002;105(17):2012–8. Epub 2002/05/01. PubMed PMID: 11980678.
73. Yla-Herttuala S, Baker AH. Cardiovascular gene therapy: past, present, and future. Molecular Ther. 2017;25(5):1095–106. Epub 2017/04/09. https://doi.org/10.1016/j.ymthe.2017.03.027. PubMed PMID: 28389321; PubMed Central PMCID: PMCPMC5417840.
74. Askari AT, Unzek S, Popovic ZB, Goldman CK, Forudi F, Kiedrowski M, et al. Effect of stromal-cell-derived factor 1 on stem-cell homing and tissue regeneration in ischaemic cardiomyopathy. Lancet. 2003;362(9385):697–703. Epub 2003/09/06. https://doi.org/10.1016/s0140-6736(03)14232-8. PubMed PMID: 12957092.
75. Penn MS, Pastore J, Miller T, Aras R. SDF-1 in myocardial repair. Gene Ther. 2012;19(6):583–7. Epub 2012/06/08. https://doi.org/10.1038/gt.2012.32. PubMed PMID: 22673496.
76. Ghadge SK, Muhlstedt S, Ozcelik C, Bader M. SDF-1alpha as a therapeutic stem cell homing factor in myocardial infarction. Pharmacol Ther. 2011;129(1):97–108. Epub 2010/10/23. https://doi.org/10.1016/j.pharmthera.2010.09.011. PubMed PMID: 20965212.
77. Sundararaman S, Miller TJ, Pastore JM, Kiedrowski M, Aras R, Penn MS. Plasmid-based transient human stromal cell-derived factor-1 gene transfer improves cardiac function in chronic heart failure. Gene Ther. 2011;18(9):867–73. Epub 2011/04/08. https://doi.org/10.1038/gt.2011.18. PubMed PMID: 21472007; PubMed Central PMCID: PMCPMC3169804.
78. Segers VF, Tokunou T, Higgins LJ, MacGillivray C, Gannon J, Lee RT. Local delivery of protease-resistant stromal cell derived factor-1 for stem cell recruitment after myocardial infarction. Circulation. 2007;116(15):1683–92. Epub 2007/09/19. https://doi.org/10.1161/circulationaha.107.718718. PubMed PMID: 17875967.
79. Malliaras K, Ibrahim A, Tseliou E, Liu W, Sun B, Middleton RC, et al. Stimulation of endogenous cardioblasts by exogenous cell therapy after myocardial infarction. EMBO Mol Med. 2014;6(6):760–77. Epub 2014/05/07. https://doi.org/10.1002/emmm.201303626. PubMed PMID: 24797668; PubMed Central PMCID: PMCPMC4203354.
80. Penn MS, Mendelsohn FO, Schaer GL, Sherman W, Farr M, Pastore J, et al. An open-label dose escalation study to evaluate the safety of administration of nonviral stromal cell-derived factor-1 plasmid to treat symptomatic ischemic heart failure. Circ Res. 2013;112(5):816–25. Epub 2013/02/23. https://doi.org/10.1161/circresaha.111.300440. PubMed PMID: 23429605.
81. Kim H, Kim JS. A guide to genome engineering with programmable nucleases. Nat Rev Genet. 2014;15(5):321–34. Epub 2014/04/03. https://doi.org/10.1038/nrg3686. PubMed PMID: 24690881.
82. El Refaey M, Xu L, Gao Y, Canan BD, Adesanya TMA, Warner SC, Akagi K, Symer DE, Mohler PJ, Ma J, Janssen PML, Han R. In vivo genome editing restores dystrophin expression and cardiac function in dystrophic mice. Circ Res. 2017;121:923–9. https://doi.org/10.1161/CIRCRESAHA.117.310996.

83. Amoasii L, Long C, Li H, Mireault AA, Shelton JM, Sanchez-Ortiz E, et al. Single-cut genome editing restores dystrophin expression in a new mouse model of muscular dystrophy. Sci Transl Med. 2017;9(418 pii: eaan8081). https://doi.org/10.1126/scitranslmed.aan8081.
84. King A. A CRISPR edit for heart disease. Nature. 2018;555(7695):S23–5. https://doi.org/10.1038/d41586-018-02482-4.
85. Naim C, Yerevanian A, Hajjar RJ. Gene therapy for heart failure: where do we stand? Curr Cardiol Rep. 2013;15(2):333. https://doi.org/10.1007/s11886-012-0333-3.

Index

A

Aborted myocardial infarction, 96
AC6 gene transfer, 379, 380, 383, 384
Accidental cell death (ACD), 106
ACE therapy, 66
Acidosis paradox, 89
Acute coronary syndromes (ACS), 227, 255
Acute MI Treated With or Without Reperfusion to Improve Outcome and Survival at Six Months Follow-Up (ALBATROSS) trial, 254
Acute myocardial infarction (AMI), 40, 114, 126, 130, 131, 173
Acute myocardial infarction contrast imaging (AMICI) trial, 250
Adenine nucleotide translocase (ANT), 111
Adeno-associated viruses (AAVs), 379, 380
Adenosine receptors, 93, 128
Adenoviruses, 379, 384
Adenylyl cyclase, 383, 384
Adiponectin, 259
Adipose derived-mesenchymal stromal cells, 360
AGENT-HF trial, 380, 382
Allogeneic CDCs, 362
Allopurinol, 258
α-adrenergic receptors, 68, 287
αβ-crystallin, 118, 178
American College of Cardiology/American Heart Association (ACC/AHA), 39, 40
American Society of Plastic Surgeons, 39
Anaerobic glycolysis, 89
Angina pectoris, 172, 173
Angiogenetic therapy, 259
Angiotensin receptor blockers (ARBs), 253, 254, 262
Angiotensin receptors, 68, 70, 71, 76
Angiotensin-converting-enzyme inhibitors, 254
Angiotensin-II, 127
Anomalous coronary artery, 2
Anti-apoptosis, 178
Antifibrotic action, 258
Aortic banding, 74
Aortic diseases, 329
Aortic regurgitation (AR), 73
Aortic stenosis, 75
Apoptosis (APO), 157, 221
Apoptosis-inducing factor (AIF), 111, 112, 132, 140
Apoptosome, 108–110, 112, 124
Arrhythmias, 290
Arrhythmic consequences, 75
Artificial intelligence (AI), 45
Association for Clinical Research Training (ACRT), 14
Atherosclerosis, 329, 330
Atherosclerotic cardiovascular disease, 2
Atrial fibrillation, 174, 189, 191
Atrial natriuretic factor, 65
Atrogin 5 (Atg) deletion, 72
ATTACH trials, 136
Autacoids, 284, 285, 291
Autophagic necrosis, 125
Autophagosome, 117, 118
Autophagy-related 5 homologue (Atg5), 116

D. V. Cokkinos (ed.), *Myocardial Preservation*,
https://doi.org/10.1007/978-3-319-98186-4

B

Basal, 119
Basic research, 11
Bcl-2 (B cell leukemia/lymphoma 2), 108
Bench to bedside, 12, 13
β-adrenergic receptor (BAR), 65, 66, 175, 223
β-arrestin, 68
β-myosin heavy chain, 65
β1 integrin, 127
Big data, 16
Biological networks, 54, 58
Biomedical Research Foundation of the Academy of Athens (BRFAA), 22
Biomimetic scaffolds, 367
BNIP3 activation, 119
Bone marrow cells (BMCs), 160
Bone marrow mononuclear cells (BMMNCs), 358
Bone marrow-derived mesenchymal stromal cells, 358, 359
Border zone (BOR), 220
Bottom-up analysis, 59
Bradykinin, 283–285, 291, 298
Broken heart syndrome, *see* Takotsubo cardiomyopathy
Bromocriptine, 76
Brugada syndrome, 2

C

Ca^{2+} overload, 115, 116, 121
Caenorhabditis elegans, 107, 111, 121, 122
Calcineurin/NFAT signaling, 67
Calcium cycling, 128
Calcium hypothesis, 177
Calcium responsiveness, 190
Calcium Upregulation by Percutaneous Administration of Gene Therapy in Patients with Cardiac Disease (CUPID) trial, 256, 381–383
Calpains, 108, 116, 119, 255
Calpastatin, 177
Canakinumab Anti-inflammatory Thrombosis Outcomes Study (CANTOS), 321
Capillary damage, 88
Cardiac arrhythmias, 88
Cardiac dysfunction, 77
Cardiac fibroblasts, 76
Cardiac homeobox transcription factor (Csx/NKX2–5), 207
Cardiac hypertrophy
- arrhythmic consequences, 75
- athlete's heart
  - ACE therapy, 66
  - cardiac plasticity, 65
  - pathological hypertrophy, 65
  - physiological hypertrophy, 65
  - thickness, 64
  - treadmill exercise, 65
- bioinformatics, 77
- calcineurin NFAT, 67
- cardiac fibroblasts, 76
- compensated/decompensated hypertrophy, 63
- definition, 63
- drugs, 76
- endothelial cells, 76
- exercise, 64
- gender differences, 75
- G-protein-coupled receptors, 67, 68
- inflammation, 69, 70
- insulin pathway, 69
- JNK class, 69
- MAPK pathways, 68, 69
- microRNAs
  - and HYP, 77
  - IGF-1 signaling, 77
  - miR-24, 77
  - miR-27b, 77
  - TGF-β signaling, 77
  - thyroid hormone, 77
- pregnancy, 64
- redox signaling
  - angiogenesis, 72, 73
  - autophagy, 72
  - caspase 3, 71
  - concentric hypertrophy, 73
  - eccentric hypertrophy, 73, 74
  - echocardiography, 74
  - energy metabolism, 71
  - oxidative stress, 71
  - VEGF, 73
- TLRs, 70, 71
- vascular smooth muscle cells, 76
- in ventricular pressure overload, 76

Cardiac magnetic resonance imaging (CMR), 193–195, 248, 249, 260, 261
Cardiac mass, 63
Cardiac plasticity, 65
Cardiac preservation, 4, 302
Cardiac remodeling (REM), 187, 189, 197
- adjunctive therapy in reperfusion, 252–253
- age, 220
- biomarkers, 266

cardiac contractility
  angiogenetic therapy, 259
  antifibrotic action, 258
  cardiac myosin activators, 256
  erythropoietin, 259
  histone deacetylase inhibitors, 257
  ischemia modifiers, 257
  ivabradine, 257
  levosimendan, 257
  metabolic modulators, 257
  monoamine oxidase inhibitors, 257, 258
  Nrf-2, 258
  sarcoplasmic/endoplasmic reticulum calcium ATPase-2α, 256
  tetracyclines, 258
  thyroid hormones, 259–260
cardiac magnetic resonance imaging, 248
cardiac myocyte death prevention
  angiotensin-converting-enzyme inhibitors, 254
  angiotensin receptor blockers, 254
  statins, 254, 255
  β2-blockers, 254
  β3-receptors, 254
  β-blockers, 254
cellular immune response, 229
chemokines, 228
chronic ischemia-hypoxia hypothesis, 232
CMC metabolism changes, 263–265
complement role, 228
continuous preconditioning, 261
cytokine induction, 228
definition, 215
device therapy
  electrical-mechanical, 261–263
  LVAD, 263
estradiol, 259
exercise rehabilitation, 260, 261
fibrosis, 223, 224
hypertension, 217
IL-10, 230, 231
inflammatory phase, 227
LV end-diastolic volume, 215
LV REM causes, 216, 217
mast cells, 229
metabolic remodeling, 231
metalloproteinases, 224, 225
miRNAs, 232, 234
MMP inhibitors, 225
molecular mechanisms
  apoptosis, 221
  border zone, 220, 222
  calcium cycling, 222
  cell death, 221
  culprit artery, 222
  HFrEF to HFpEF, 221
  hibernation, 221
  mechanotransduction, 220
  SERCA-2α, 222, 223
  stress-signaling kinases, 223
  systolic and diastolic tensions, 220
  thrombolysis, 222
  TIMI flow, 222
  tissue hypothyroidism, 221
monocytes-macrophages, 229
myosin heavy chains, 223
oxidative stress, 231
post-myocardial infarction, 218, 219
proliferative healing phase, 230
protein kinase C mechanisms, 232
proteotoxicity attenuation, 255, 256
RAAS, 223
radionuclide imaging
  AMICI trial, 250
  apoptosis, 250
  biomarkers, 250, 251
  inflammation, 249
  magnetic resonance imaging, 250
  molecular imaging, 249
  myocardial innervation, 249
  myocardial metabolism, 249
  myocardial perfusion, 249
  myocardial viability, 248
  PET, 249
remote region fibrosis, 226, 227
reverse REM, 216
ROS generation, 228
Starling's law, 215
valvular heart disease, 217, 218
Cardiac resynchronization therapy (CRT), 247, 248, 252, 262, 263
Cardioprotection, *see* Cardiac preservation
Cardiosphere-derived cells (CDCs), 160
Cardiovascular Cell Therapy Research Network, 19
Cardiovascular magnetic resonance, 193
Caspase 3, 71, 108, 109, 111, 112, 132, 133, 139, 289, 364
Caspases, 111, 112, 119, 124, 133
Catecholamines, 284
Cathepsins, 116, 129
CD4+ T-regulatory cells, 227
CD8+ T-cells, 227
Cell cycle arrest, 73

Cell death, 71, 88
  ACD, 106
  acute myocardial infarction, 130, 131
  aging heart, 133, 134
  apoptosis
    antiapoptotic members, 108
    CyPD, 111
    cytochrome c, 108
    entotic cell death, 112, 113
    extrinsic/death receptor pathway, 108
    intrinsic/canonical/mitochondrial pathway, 107, 108
    JNKs, 109
    MIM/IMM, 110, 111
    MITO, 107
    MOM/OMM, 109
    proapoptotic members, 108
    pyroptosis, 112
    tumor suppressor p53, 112
  autophagy
    autophagosome, 117
    basal, 119
    Bcl-2, 117
    BNIP3 activation, 119
    chaperone-mediated AUTO, 117
    definition, 116
    FoxO, 119
    microautophagy, 117
    MITO abnormalities, 118
    mitophagy, 118
    NIX, 119
    process, 118
    REDD1, 119
    UPS, 120
  calcium cycling, 128
  CD modality clarification, 120, 121
  chronic treatment, 136–138
  classification of, 107
  conditioning mechanism, 134, 135
  cross talk among processes, 121–124
  HSPs, 129, 130
  hypothermia, 135
  impact of inflammation, 131, 132
  induction of inflammation, 128–129
  mechanisms of conditioning, 135
  microRNAs, 138, 139
  modalities, 105, 106
  myocardial remodeling, 132, 133
  necrosis
    Ca^{2+} overload, 115
    causes, 114
    cyclophilin D, 116
    intracellular serpin-6, 115
    morphologic differences of apoptosis *vs.*, 113
    MPTP, 115, 116
    TMFR1, 115
  pharmaceutic interventions, 135
  PI3K/Akt pathway, 124–126
  RCD, 106, 107
  stress-activated protein kinases
    adrenergic receptors, 127, 128
    GPCRs, 127
    integrins/Fak, 127
    TNFα/NF-KB, 127
  therapeutic implications, 134
Cell death (CD), 221
Cell therapy, heart disease
  adipose derived-mesenchymal stromal cells, 360
  adult progenitor cells, 355, 356
  bone marrow-derived cells
    BMMNCs, 358
    mesenchymal stromal cells, 358, 359
  cell retention and survival, 366–368
  clinical trials, 361
  embryonic stem cells, 356, 357
  heart-derived progenitor cells, 359, 360
  LVEF, 361
  mechanical circulatory support, 363
  mechanism of action
    cardiac remodeling, 364, 365
    cardioprotective effect, 363
    endogenous regeneration, 363, 364
    immune modulation of inflammation, 364
    metabolism and contractility, 365
    neoangiogenesis, 365
    paracrine mechanisms, 363
  non-ischemic cardiomyopathy, 362
  preclinical and clinical studies, 365, 366
  refractory angina pectoris, 362
  skeletal myoblasts, 357
Cellular postconditioning, 363
Chaperone-mediated AUTO, 117
Chaperones, 129, 138, 255
Chemokines, 155, 156
Chronic obstructive pulmonary disease, 3
Chronic Oral Study of Myosin Activation to Increase Contractility (COSMIC) trial, 256–257
Clinical and Translational Science Awards (CTSA), 14, 18, 19
Clinical research, 11, 12
Collagen, 65, 68, 187
Computational simulation, 30

Conditioning of myocardium
 clinical applications
  acute myocardial infarction, 299–300
  cardiac surgery, 299
  cardiac transplantation, 301
  cardiopulmonary resuscitation, 301
 definition, 281
 postconditioning (*see* Postconditioning of myocardium)
 preconditioning, 282 (*see* Preconditioning of myocardium)
 therapeutic interventions
  effort angina, 297, 298
  prodromal angina, 298
 transfemoral transcatheter aortic valve, 301
Congestive heart failure (CHF), 105, 132, 133, 136, 379, 380
Contrast echocardiography, 248
Contrast ventriculography, 247
Cornification, 106, 121
Coronary artery disease (CAD), 216
Coronary stenosis, 187, 188, 197
Creatine phosphate, 188
Cromakalim, 282
Cyclic adenosine monophosphate (cAMP) pathway, 264, 383
Cyclooxygenase, 190
Cyclophilin D (CyPD), 111, 115, 288
Cyclosporine, 67, 93, 110, 111, 132, 134, 288, 301
Cyclosporine A in Reperfused Acute Myocardial Infarction (CYCLE) trial, 93, 253
Cyclosporine Improve Clinical Outcome in ST Elevation Myocardial Infarction Patients (CIRCUS) trial, 93, 253
Cytomegalovirus (CMV), 226
Cytoprotection, 178

D

Dahl salt-sensitive rats, 292
Damage-associated molecular patterns (DAMPs), 91, 129, 227
Data-as-a-Service Platform for Healthy Lifestyle and Preventive Medicine (DAPHNE) project, 47
Data sharing, 17
Death in USA, causes of, 3
Death valley, *see* Valley of death
Dementia, 3
Destination therapy, 5
Diabetes mellitus, 293, 294
Dilated cardiomyopathy, 2, 218
Dobutamine stress echocardiography, 191
Downward causation, 59
Doxorubicin, 189
Doxycycline, 258
Dry lab, 30, 31
Duchenne muscular dystrophy, 385, 386
Dyslipidaemia, 154

E

Edges/links, 55
8th Biennial Hatter Cardiovascular Institute Workshop, 291
Embryonic stem cells, 356, 357
Empagliflozin, 257
Endogenous cardiac regeneration
 adult cardiomyocytes, 347
 adverse outcomes, 347
 bitransgenic αMHC-MerCreMer/reporter mice, 348
 cardiosphere-derived cells, 348
 cell cycle activators, 346
 cell therapy, 348
 epicardial-derived endogenous progenitors, 348
 exercise, 348
 exogenous amplification, 345
 growth factor-based approach, 348
 Hippo signaling pathway, 347
 mechanical circulatory support, 348
 microRNA expression, 347
 mitogenic stimulation, 346
 myocyte proliferation, 346
 neuregulin signaling, 347
 oxidative DNA damage, 348
 therapeutic strategies, 345, 346
 YAP protein, 347
Endonuclease G (endoG), 109, 110, 140
Endothelial cells, 76, 92, 93
Endothelin receptor, 65, 68, 69, 71, 76
Endothelin-1, 127
Energy paradox, 89
Engineering bioartificial hearts, 368
Entotic cell death, 112, 113
Epinephrine (EPI), 249
Eritoran, 70
ERK 1/2 pathway, 68
Erythropoietin, 138, 259
Estradiol, 259
Euroinject One trial, 379, 384
European Society of Cardiology (ESC) guidelines, 40

Eutrophy, 63
Evaluation of Myocardial Effects of Bendavia for Reducing Reperfusion Injury in Patients With Acute Coronary Events (EMBRACE STEMI) study, 258
Evidence-based medicine (EBM)
  ACC/AHA guidelines, 39
  adverse effects, 43
  AHA/ACC guidelines, 40
  classes, 40
  Cochrane collaboration, 42
  comparative research *vs.* original science, 44
  cookbook medicine, 42
  definition, 37
  ESC guidelines, 40
  GRADE, 41, 42
  indication, 40
  levels of evidence, 38, 39
  long-term therapy, 43
  overdiagnosis, 43
  patient care, 42
  Pr Med (*see* Precision medicine (Pr Med))
  process, 39
  prognostic studies, 39
  systematic reviews, 41–42
Excitotoxicity, 130
Exercise rehabilitation, 260, 261
Exercise-induced ischemia, 173–174
Exercise in Left Ventricular Dysfunction and Chronic Heart Failure (ELVD-CHF) trial, 261
Exponential network, 56
Extracellular matrix (ECM)
  aortic diseases, 329
  cardiac remodeling, 223, 224
    atrial fibrillation, 329
    heart failure, 327
    hypertension, 328
    hypertrophic cardiomyopathy, 328
    myocardial fibrosis, 326
    myocardial infarction, 325–327
    myocarditis, 327
  cardiovascular risk factors, 325
  components, 322
  immune system, 321, 322
  MMP regulation, 323
  oxidative stress, 324
  peroxynitrite, 324
  proteolysis and degradation, 322, 323
  treatment, 331, 332
  wall stress, 325
Extracellular signal-regulated kinases 1 and 2 (ERK1/2), 126

F

Fas-associated death domain (FADD), 108, 122, 124
Ferroptosis, 112
Fetal phenotype
  α-actin, 205
  ANP expression
    diabetes, 206
    GATA- binding proteins, 207
    GATA4, 206
    hypothyroidism, 206
    Mef 2, 207
    NFAT, 207
    NKX2–5/CSX, 206
    SMAD family, 207
    stress, 206
  environmental changes, 204
  fetal gene program re-emergence, 203
  glycogen content, 203
  histone deacetylases, 208
  miR-1-133 cluster, 208
  PPAR-α, 204
  serum response factor, 207
  titin isoforms, 205
  βMHC, 204, 205
Fibroblast growth factor 4 (FGF4), 384
Fibroblasts, 223
Fibrosis, 65, 66, 68–73, 75–77
Fibrosis–inflammation
  atherosclerosis, 329, 330
  biomarkers, 321
  ECM (*see* Extracellular matrix (ECM))
  evaluation, 330, 331
  treatment, 331, 332
FLOURISH trial, 384
Focal adhesion kinase (FAK), 127
FoxO, 119

G

GATA- binding proteins, 207
GATA4, 73
GENASIS trial, 384
Gene editing, 385, 386
Gene therapy, 5
  adenylyl cyclase, 383, 384
  calcium handling
    AGENT-HF trial, 382
    CUPID 1 clinical trial, 381
    CUPID 2 clinical trial, 382
    SERCA2a, 381
    SERCA-LVAD trial, 383
  cardiac delivery of vectors, 380
  clinical translation, 377
  gene edting, 385–386

non-viral vectors, 378
modRNAs, 379
naked plasmid DNA, 379
paracrine signaling, 384, 385
viral vectors
adeno-associated viruses, 379, 380
adenoviruses, 379, 380
General Clinical Research Centers (GCRCs), 18
Genetic fate-mapping experiments, 341
Genome-wide association studies (GWAs), 24, 46
Genomics of protection, in STUN, 178
Ghrelin, 259
GPCR signaling, 68, 69
G-protein receptor kinase-2, 65
G-protein-coupled receptors (GPCRs), 67, 68, 127
Grading of Recommendations Assessment, Development, and Evaluation (GRADE) classification, 41, 42
GSK-3 (glycogen synthase kinase-3), 66, 126, 287, 289, 290

H

HAX-1, 128
Heart cell models, 59
Heart failure revascularization trial (HEART), 196
Heart failure with preserved ejection fraction (HFpEF), 217
Heart-derived progenitor cells, 359, 360
Hemodialysis, 174, 175
HF with a reduced EF (HFrEF), 261
Hibernating myocardium, 189
High-mobility group protein B1 (HMGB 1), 115
Histone aceryltransferases (HATs), 207
Histone deacetylases (HDACs), 208, 257
HIV/AIDS, 3
HORIZON research project, 30
HSP-70, 112, 116, 119
Hubs, 55, 56
Human-induced pluripotent stem cells (iPSCs), 160
Hydroxyephedrine (HED), 249
Hydrogen sulfide, 286
Hydroxy-methyl-glutaryl coenzyme (HMG-CoA), 331
Hypercholesterolemia, 294
Hypertension, 153, 154, 328
Hypertrophic cardiomyopathy (HCM), 2, 218, 328
Hypertrophy regression, 75
Hypothermia, 135
Hypoxia-inducible factor (HIF-1), 73

I

Immunoproteasome, 120
Incidental coronary artery disease, 176
Induced pluripotent stem cells (iPSCs), 160, 357
Inducible NO synthase (iNOS), 190
Informed consent, 12
Inhibitor of apoptosis proteins (IAPs), 109
Insulin/insulin receptor/Akt signaling, 69
Insulinomimetics, 257
Insulinotropics, 257
Intermaxillary bone/Goethe's bone, 1
Intramyocardial delivery, 380, 385
Ischemia modifiers, 257
Ischemia reperfusion injury (IRI), 5, 159, 160, 227
aborted myocardial infarction, 96, 97
acidosis paradox, 89
anaerobic glucosis, 89
calcium paradox, 90, 91
capillary damage, 88
cardiac arrhythmias, 88
cell death, 88
clinical perspectives, 97
diagnosis, 88
energy paradox, 89
expert groups, 95
inflammation, 91
innate immunity, 91
metabolic modulation, 89
microRNAs, 97
microvascular obstruction, 88
monocytes and macrophages
B-cells, 92
endothelial cells, 92, 93
mast cells, 92
microparticles, 92
neutrophils, 92
suppression/regulation T cells (Treg), 92
myocardial reperfusion injury, 87
no-reflow phenomenon, 87, 88
oxidative stress, 89
routine aspiration, 88
treatment
adenosine, 93
anticomplement therapy, 94
antileukocyte therapy, 94
antioxidant therapy, 94
cyclosporine, 93
nicorandil, 93

Ischemic contracture, 283, 294
Ischemic heart disease, 54
Ischemic preconditioning, 120, 124, 126
Isoproterenol, 124, 126
Isovolumic relaxation time adjusted for the heart rate (IVRT/HR), 247
Ivabradine, 257

J
JNK class, 69

K
Karyorrhexis, 107
KAT trial, 384
Keep it simple and stupid (KISS) principle, 24

L
Left bundle branch block (LBBB), 247, 262, 263
Left ventricular assist device (LVAD), 254, 261, 263–267
Left ventricular ejection fraction (LVEF), 361
Left ventricular hypertrophy, 292, 293
Levosimendan, 178, 257
Life expectancy, of Americans, 4
Links, 56
Long QT syndrome, 2
Lower respiratory infections, 3
LV end-diastolic volume (LVEDV), 216
LV end-systolic diameter (LVESD), 247
LV mass index (LVMI), 247
LV wall stress, 215
Lymphocytes, 92
Lysosomal rupture, 116
Lysosome, 117–120
Lysosome membrane permeabilization (LMP), 119

M
Macroautophagy, 117
Macrophage inflammatory proteins (MIP), 156
Mammalian heart
  endogenous cardiomyocyte replenishment, 339
    bitransgenic αMHC-MerCreMer/ZEG mice, 342
    cardiac c-kit+ cells, 343
    cardiac lineages, 343
    Cre recombinase activity, 342
    endogenous progenitors, 342
    fate-mapping studies, 343
    genetic fate-mapping experiments, 341
    green fluorescent protein (GFP), 342
    hypoxia-inducible factor 1a, 341
    during normal aging, 341
  myocyte turnover rates, 340, 341
  primary cardiac tumors, 339
  regenerative capacity, 339
  therapeutic strategies, 339
Mammalian target of rapamycin (mTOR), 70, 117
MAO inhibitors, 136
MAPK pathways, 68, 69
Marfan syndrome, 329
Mast cells, 92
Matrix metalloproteinase (MMP) activity, 156, 157, 162, 322
Matthew effect, 29, 56
Mechanical circulatory support (MCS), 266, 267
Mechanotransduction process, 220
Melusin, 138, 256
Metabolic flexibility, 204
Metabolic modulation, 89
Metabolic modulators, 257
Metabolic syndrome, 154
Metabolomic profiling, 57
Metaiodobenzylguanidine (MIBG), 249
Metalloproteinases (MMPs), 90
Metformin, 257
Metoprolol in Acute Myocardial Infarction (MIAMI) trial, 43
Microautophagy, 117
Microbubble imaging, 248
Microembolisation model, 190
MicroRNA-based therapy, 161
Microvascular obstruction, 88, 227
Minocycline, 135
MiR-1-133 cluster, 208
Mitochondrial calcium uniporter (MCU), 111
Mitochondrial outer membrane (MCMP), 123
Mitochondrial outer membrane (MOM), 108–110, 121, 122, 123
Mitochondrial outer membrane permeabilization (MOMP), 108
Mitochondrial permeability transition pore (MPTP), 109–111, 114–116, 121–123, 125, 130, 131, 134, 135, 140
Mitochondrial stampede, 118
Mitochondrial suicide, 123
Mitophagy, 118
Mitotic catastrophe, 121
Modified mRNAs (modRNAs), 379

Molecular autopsy, 2
Monoamine oxidase inhibitors, 257, 258
Monocyte chemoattractant protein (MCP)-1, 156
Multicenter Automatic Defibrillator Implantation Trial with Cardiac Resynchronization Therapy (MADIT-CRT) trial, 262
Myocardial fibrosis and necrosis
  dyslipidaemia, 154
  hypertension, 153, 154
  metabolic syndrome, 154
  smoking, 154, 155
  type 2 diabetes, 153
Myocardial flow, 187, 188
Myocardial healing
  apoptosis, 157
  cell therapy, 160
  clinical study, 161
  future perspectives, 162
  inflammatory process, 156
  ischaemia reperfusion, 159, 160
  microRNA-based therapy, 161
  MMPs, 156, 157
  osteopontin, 158, 159
  oxidative stress, 158
  protein-based therapy, 160, 161
  SLPI, 158
Myocardial hibernation
  cardiovascular magnetic resonance, 193
  cell death, 194
  definition, 185
  dobutamine stress echo cardiography, 191
  function, 194
  long-term HIB
    anaerobic metabolism, 187
    glycogen content, 188
    hibernating myocardium, 189, 190
    iNOS and cyclooxygenase 2, 190
    myocardial flow, 187, 188
    myocardial metabolism, 187
    myofibrils, 187
  metabolism, 194
  myocardial viability, 191
  PET, 192, 193
  renin-angiotensin system, 195–197
  short-term HIB, 186
  SPECT, 191–193
Myocardial infarction (MI)
  factors, 151
  healing (*see* Myocardial healing)
  pathophysiology of healing after, 152, 153
  risk factors (*see* Myocardial fibrosis and necrosis)
Myocardial innervation, 249
Myocardial ischemia, 88, 191
Myocardial Ischemia Reduction with Aggressive Cholesterol Lowering (MIRACL) study, 255
Myocardial metabolism, 249
Myocardial perfusion, 249
Myocardial preservation, 4
Myocardial remodeling, 132, 133
Myocardial reperfusion injury, 87
Myocardial stunning
  after cardiac surgery
    anti-apoptosis, 178
    cytoprotection, 178
    genomics of protection in, 178
    therapeutics, 178, 179
  hemodialysis, 174, 175
  percutaneous transcatheter coronary angioplasty
    acute myocardial infarction, 173
    angina pectoris, 172, 173
    atrial fibrillation, 174
    exercise-induced ischemia, 173, 174
    at PTCA, 172
  sepsis, 175
  takotsubo syndrome (*see* Takotsubo cardiomyopathy)
Myocardial viability (VIA), 191, 248
Myocarditis, 327
Myocyte enhancer factor 2 (Mef 2), 207
Myofibrils, 187–189
Myosin heavy chain (MHC) isoform switching, 260–261

N

Na+/H+ exchanger (NHE) activity, 71
National Center for Advancing Translational Services (NCATS), 19
National Heart, Lung, and Blood Institute (NHLBI) working group, 266
Necroptosis, 122–125, 129, 138, 255
Necrosome, 122
Necrostatin (Nec)-1, 122, 132, 134
Neoangiogenesis, 152, 160
Neonatal cardiac regeneration, 344, 345
Neuregulin, 255
Neutrophil extracellular traps (NETs), 113
Neutrophils, 88, 91, 92, 95, 229
NFkB, 127
NF-kB activity, 69, 70
Nicorandil, 93, 257
Nitrosative stress, 90
Nodes, 55–57

Non-functional polypeptides (XTENylation), 161
Non-ischemic cardiomyopathy, 362
No-reflow phenomenon, 87, 88, 93
NORTHERN trial, 379, 384
Nuclear factor erythroid 2–related factor 2 (Nrf-2), 258
Nuclear factor of activated T-cells (NFAT), 207

O
Obesidome, 58
Omecamtiv mecarbil, 256
Omics technology, 53
Oncosis, 113, 114, 121
Osteopontin, 158
Oxidative stress, 71, 89, 90, 158, 324
Oxygen paradox, *see* Oxidative stress
Oxyradical hypothesis, 177

P
p38–MAPK signaling, 69
p62, 123
Pan-caspase inhibitors, 255
Paracrine signaling, 160, 384, 385
Parathyroid hormone, 259
Parthanatos, 112
Pathogen-associated molecular patterns (PAMPs), 123
Pathological or maladaptive hypertrophy, 63–69, 74, 77
Pediatric Cardiovascular Translational Bench to Bassinet program, 19
Pentose phosphate pathway (PPP), 117
Pentoxifylline, 136
Percutaneous transcatheter coronary angioplasty (PTCA)
  acute myocardial infarction, 173
  angina pectoris, 172, 173
  at PTCA, 172
  atrial fibrillation, 174
  exercise-induced ischemia, 173–174
Peripartum cardiomyopathy, 64, 76
Peroxisome proliferator-activated receptor (PPAR), 71, 204
Perturbation score, 250
PH domain leucine-rich repeat protein phosphatase (PHLPP), 126
Phenylephrine, 68, 69, 71
Pheochromocytoma, 176
Phosphatidylinositol-3 kinase (PI3K), 117, 156
Phosphodiesterase-5 Inhibition to Improve Clinical Status and Exercise Capacity in Heart Failure with Preserved Ejection Fraction (RELAX) trial, 256
Phospholipase A2 (PLA2), 120
Physicians/ clinicians challenges, 5
Physiological/adaptive hypertrophy, 63–66, 68, 69, 71, 72, 74, 75, 77
PI3K (p110γ) signaling, 69
PI3K/Akt pathway, 66, 124–126
Placental growth factor (PLGF), 259
Plasmid DNA, 379
Platelet deposition, 95
Platelet-rich plasma (PRP), 160
Poly-ADP ribose polymerase (PARP), 111, 116, 124
Polyethylene glycol polymer chains (PEGylation), 161
Positron emission tomography (PET), 192, 193, 249
Postconditioning of myocardium
  apoptosis, 289
  arrhythmias, 290
  brain, 296
  cyclophilin D, 288
  cyclosporine, 288
  diabetes mellitus, 296
  effectiveness of, 287
  kidney, 296
  liver, 297
  no-reflow phenomenon, 289
  PKG/c GMP pathway, 288
  remote ischemic post C, 291, 292
  time and dosage, 289
Precision medicine (Pr Med)
  acceptance, 45
  artificial intelligence, 45
  big data sources, 48
  data management, 47
  definition, 44
  FDA, 48
  genetic and environmental factors, 45
  GWAS, 46
  medical practice, 47
  next-generation sequencing, 47
  vs. personalized medicine, 46
  physical branch, 48
  systems biology, 47
  virtual branch, 48
Preconditioning of myocardium
  age, 293
  chronic kidney disease, 295
  classical preconditioning

effectors, 284
intracellular mediator cascade, 284
ischemic contracture, 283
K^+ATP channels, 282
PI3K/Akt pathway, 283
SAFE pathway, 283
triggers, 284
tyrosine kinase, 283
delayed/second window
bradykinin, 285
definition, 284
hydrogen sulfide, 286
opiods, 285
proteins, 285
ROS, 286, 287
diabetes mellitus, 293, 294
heart failure, 295
hypercholesterolemia, 294
left ventricular hypertrophy, 292, 293
RIPC (*see* Remote pre C (RIPC))
thyroid abnormalities, 294, 295
Presbycardia, 4
Prinzmetal's angina, 173
Prodromal angina, 4
Pro-inflammatory cytokines, 156
Propofol, 300
Protein-based therapy, 160, 161
Protein kinase C (PKC), 128
Protein kinase Cε, 65
Protein/lipid phosphatase and tensin homologue (PTEN), 124, 126
Pyroptosis, 112, 130

R

Random network, 56
Ranolazine, 138, 257
Rasagiline, 258
Reactive Oxygen Species (ROS) generation, 228
REDD1, 119
Refractory angina pectoris, 362
Regulated cell death (RCD), 106, 107, 119
Remodelling, 151, 154 (also *see* Cardiac Remodelling)
Remote ischemic post C, 291, 292
Remote pre C (RIPC)
application, 290
cardiac remodeling prevention, 301, 302
humoral pathway, 290, 291
neural pathway, 291
repeated, 292
Remote preconditioning, 5
RENEWAL trials, 136
Renin-angiotensin system, 195–197
Renin–angiotensin–aldosterone (RAAS) system, 223, 260
Repeated RIPC, 292
Reperfusion arrhythmias, 87, 290
Reperfusion injury salvage kinase (RISK) pathway, 135, 283, 284, 288
Research
definition, 9, 10
practical considerations, 10
steps in, 10
Resveratrol, 258
RETRO-HF clinical trials, 379, 380, 385
REVASC trial, 384
Revascularization, 186, 188, 190, 191, 194–197
Reverse remodeling, 197
Rheumatic fever, 1
RPI-RIP3 signaling, 132

S

SAFE pathway activation, 95
Sarcoplasmic reticulum Ca^{2+}-ATPase activity (SERCA2a), 222, 223, 256, 380–383
Scale-free networks, 56, 57
Second window of cardioprotection (SWOP), 284
Secreted protein acidic and rich in cysteine (SPARC), 158
Secretory leukocyte protease inhibitor (SLPI), 158
Sepsis, 175
SERCA-LVAD trial, 380, 383
Serotonin receptor, 68
Serpin-6, 115
Serum response factor (SRF), 207
Sestamibi, 192
Sevoflurane, 300
Sildenafil, 256
Silico biology, 60
Single-photon emission tomography (SPECT), 191, 192
Sirtuins, 66
Skeletal myoblasts, 357
Small mother against decapentoplegic (SMAD) family, 207
Smoking, 154, 155, 220
Social justice, 17
Speckle tracking, 248
Sphingomyelin/sphingosine, 120
Spironolactone, 254

Spontaneous hypertensive rats (SHR), 292, 296
Starling's law, 215
STAT- 5 isoform, 95
Statins, 136, 254–255
Sterile inflammation, 91, 132
STOP-HF clinical trials, 379, 380
STREAM trial, 97
Stress-signaling kinases, 223
Stromal cell-derived factor 1 (SDF-1), 385
Stromal Cell-Derived Factor-1 Plasmid Treatment for Patients with Heart Failure (STOP-HF) trial, 385
Sudden non traumatic death, 2
Sudden unexplained death (SUD), 2
Sulforaphane, 258
Survival activating factor enhancement (SAFE), 135, 283, 284
Systems biology
  bottom-up analysis, 59
  definition, 53, 54
  exponential network, 56
  framework of, 55
  genetics, 57
  human disease, 57, 58
  linear pathways, 55
  nodes, 57
  obesidome, 58
  "omics" technology, 53
  random network, 56
  scale-free network, 56
  silico biology, 60
  system-based definition, 54
  US highway system, 56
Systolic Heart Failure Treatment with the I_f Inhibitor Ivabradine trial (SHIFT), 257

T

Tachycardia, 176
Tachycardia-induced cardiomyopathy, 326
Takotsubo cardiomyopathy
  coronary artery disease, 176
  pathophysiology of stunning, 177–178
  tachycardia, 176
  thyroid disorders, 176
TASTE trial, 26
T-cell migration, 226
Testosterone, 259
Tetracyclines, 258
Tetrofosmin, 192
Theranostics, 95, 96
Thioredoxin, 258
3D organ printer, 30
Thyroid disorders, 176
Thyroid hormone, 66, 77, 259–260
Thyroid Hormone Replacement Therapy in ST Elevation Myocardial Infarction (THiRST) study, 260
Thyroid-stimulating hormone (TSH) levels, 260
Tissue engineering methods, 367
Tissue hypothyroidism, 221
Tissue inhibitors of metalloproteinases (TIMPs), 156, 225, 260
TNF-α induced hypertrophy, 71
TNFα neutralization, 136
Tollip (Toll- interacting protein), 70
Toll-like receptors (TLRs), 70, 71
Torasemide (Prolonged Release) on Myocardial Fibrosis in Patients With Heart Failure (TORAFIC) trial, 258
Transcriptomic profiles, 250
Transfemoral transcatheter aortic valve (TAVR), 301
Translational epidemiology, 16
Translational research (TR)
  basic science to the clinical area, 10
  big data, 16
  blocks, 17, 18
    clinical trials, 24, 25
    managing, 27
    meta-analyses, 27
    RCTS, 25, 26
  bottom-up approach, 15
  collaborations value, 19
  data sharing, 17
  definition, 13
  dry lab, 30, 31
  ethical principles, 17
  evaluation, 17
  experimental translational therapeutic pathway, 15
  four-legged stool, 13
  importance, 9
  Institute of Medicine Clinical Research Roundtable, 13
  ischemic preconditioning, 15
  leadership, 23
  NIH roadmap for clinical research, 14
  organizational aspects, 18, 19
  six steps, 14
  social justice, 17

strategy, 15
TR continuum, 16
training scientists, 20–22
valley of death, 28, 29
wet lab, 30
Transthoracic echo (TTE), 247
Transverse aortic constriction (TAC), 72, 73, 256, 358
Treadmill exercise, 65, 66, 174, 297
Tree of research, 21
Tuberculosis, 3
Tumor necrosis factor-α receptor 1 (TMFR1), 115
Twenty-first-century human translational investigator's laboratory, 21
Type 2 diabetes, 153
Tyrosine kinase, 283, 285, 286

U
Ubiquitin (Ub), 120
Ubiquitin proteasome system (UPS), 120
US Preventive Services Task Force, 38

V
Valley of death, 28, 29
Valproic acid, 136
Valvular heart disease, 217, 218
Vascular endothelial growth factor (VEGF), 384
Vascular smooth muscle cells, 76
Ventricular arrhythmias, 191
Ventricular mass, 64
Ventricular tachycardia, 190
Vesicular translocation, 68
Vitamin D supplementation, 259
VIVA trial, 384
Voltage-dependent anion channel (VDAC), 110

W
Wet lab, 30

Y
Yes-associated protein (YAP), 126, 347

MIX
Papier aus verantwortungsvollen Quellen
Paper from responsible sources
FSC® C105338

If you have any concerns about our products,
you can contact us on
ProductSafety@springernature.com

In case Publisher is established outside the EU,
the EU authorized representative is:
Springer Nature Customer Service Center GmbH
Europaplatz 3, 69115 Heidelberg, Germany

Printed by Libri Plureos GmbH
in Hamburg, Germany